Handbook of Perception and Action

Volume 2: Motor skills

Handbook of Perception and Action

Volume 2: Motor skills

Edited by

Herbert Heuer[1] and Steven W. Keele[2]

[1]*Institut für Arbeitsphysiologie an der Universität Dortmund, Germany*

[2]*Department of Psychology, University of Oregon, Eugene, USA*

ACADEMIC PRESS
Harcourt Brace & Company, Publishers

London, San Diego, New York, Boston, Sydney, Tokyo, Toronto

ACADEMIC PRESS LIMITED
24–28 Oval Road
LONDON NW1 7DX

U.S. Edition Published by
ACADEMIC PRESS INC.
San Diego, CA 92101

This book is printed on acid-free paper

The German original is published under the title, "Psychomotorik"
as volume 3 of the "Enzyklopädie für Psychologie".
Copyright © 1994 by Hogrefe-Verlag
Rohnsweg 25, 37085 Göttingen, Germany

A catalogue record for this book is available from the British Library

ISBN 0 12 516162 X

Typeset by Doyle Graphics, Tullamore, Co. Offaly, Republic of Ireland
Printed and bound in Great Britain by Hartnolls Ltd, Bodmin, Cornwall

Contents

I General Concepts

II Particular Skills

Marjorie Hines Woollacott and Jody L. Jensen

List of Contributors

Carol A. Fowler
Haskins Laboratories
270 Crown Street
New Haven
CT 06511
USA

Herbert Heuer
Institut für Arbeitsphysiologie
an der Universität Dortmund
Ardeystraße 67
D-44139 Dortmund 1
Germany

Richard Ivry
Department of Psychology
University of California
Berkeley
CA 94720
USA

Marc Jeannerod
INSERM-Unite 94
Laboratoire de
  Neuropsychologie Experimentale
16 Avenue du Doyen Lepine
F 69500 Bron
France

Jody L. Jensen
Department of Exercise and
  Movement Science
University of Oregon
Eugene
OR 97403-1240
USA

Michael I. Jordan
Department of Brain and
  Cognitive Sciences
MIT
Cambridge
MA 02139
USA

Steven W. Keele
Department of Psychology
University of Oregon
Eugene
Oregon 97403-1273
USA

Horst Krist
Institut für Psychologie der
  J.-W. Goethe Universität
Georg-Voigt-Straße 8
D-60054 Frankfurt 11
Germany

David A. Rosenbaum
Department of Psychology
621 Moore Building
Pennsylvania State University
University Park
PA 16802
USA

Geert J. P. Savelsbergh
Faculty of Human Movement Sciences
Free University
Van der Boechorststraat 9
NL 1081 BT Amsterdam
The Netherlands

Hans-Leo Teulings
Exercise Science and
   Physical Education
PE East
Arizona State University
Tempe
AZ 85287-0404
USA

Dirk Vorberg
Institut für Psychologie
   der Tu Braunschweig
Spielmannstraße 19
D-38023 Braunschweig
Germany

Harold T. A. Whiting
Department of Psychology
University of York
Heslington
York Y01 5DD
UK

Alan M. Wing
MRC Applied Psychology Unit
15 Chaucer Road
Cambridge CB2 2EF
UK

Majorie H. Woollacott
Department of Exercise and Movement
   Science and Institute of Neuroscience
Gerlinger Annex
University of Oregon
Eugene
OR 97403-1240
USA

Preface

This book is part of a three-volume set on perception and action. The other two volumes deal with perception (edited by W. Prinz and B. Bridgeman) and attention (edited by O. Neumann and A. F. Sanders).

There are moments in the process of editing a book that are rather pleasant. These come from the pleasures of reading excellent chapters and from the dialogs on substantive issues between editor, author and reviewers. For these moments we wish to thank first and foremost the contributors to this volume. Second we wish to thank those who have commented on drafts of the chapters. We solicited help from some individuals in editing chapters, and we would like to acknowledge the assistance of H. Forssberg, D. Lee, D. G. MacKay, D. A. Rosenbaum and R. A. Schmidt.

In a project of this size, many people work to improve the quality. Others provide technical services. Without them, the project would not succeed. We extend our gratitude to Margit Groll, Margot Ahrens and Marietta Widynski who have handled a variety of technical aspects associated with the project. This handbook series is published simultaneously in German and in English. All the chapters were originally submitted and edited in English. For the translation to German we wish to thank Michael Basten, Rose Shaw and Jörg Sangals. Karin Brandt adapted the figures for the German version and redrew all the figures that were in need of being redrawn for the English edition.

Herbert Heuer and Steven W. Keele
Dortmund, Germany and Eugene, USA

Introduction

Steven W. Keele* and Herbert Heuer†

*University of Oregon, Eugene and †Universität Dortmund

Humans are spectacular, compared with other animals, in matters of mental capability. They memorize new materials, employing systematic processes of rehearsal and organization to do so. Once stored in declarative memory, the contents can be expressed in arbitrary ways – by speech, by writing, by demonstration. Humans have an enormous capacity to reason. They solve problems. They create. Humans have capacities of language nowhere approached by other animals. No wonder psychology has expended so much effort in understanding cognition in all its manifestations.

Still, it has often been remarked that cognitive psychology, the study of these various capacities, leaves an organism stranded in thought, unable to engage in action (Guthrie, 1935). This criticism makes clear that the study of action – the study of movement and skill and the internal processes that lead to them – is a legitimate area of psychological investigation. Indeed, in modern psychology the study of action, or what is commonly called the study of motor control, is a vigorous field of investigation.

At first glance one might suppose the study of motor control is the study of only peripheral processes, such as how neurons control muscles, and how muscles are activated. Were this so, motor control would be in the domain of physiology and biomechanics with little to be gained from psychology. It is unlikely, however, that an organism so highly developed in cognition would have evolved a system in which action is independent of cognition itself. Indeed, human intelligence manifests itself not only in cognition but in the action products of cognition. Not only do humans express language, but they also have amazing flexibility in the motor systems for such expression – speech, typing, handwriting, even the singing telegram and sign language. Only humans knit sweaters, build cabinets, play the trombone. Only humans dance, play soccer, and engage in gymnastics. The variety of human skills is practically endless, and new skills are invented every day.

Such competence in skill led a pioneer in the study of motor control, Karl Lashley (1951), to comment that human ability to produce sequential action is as much a mark of their intelligence as any other human endeavor. Human motoric capabilities are no less impressive than those of memory, of reasoning, of language. Indeed, some have suggested and even argued (e.g. Bruner, 1968) that human cognition has grown out of some of the same evolutionary developments in the human brain that led to extraordinary motor skill.

Handbook of Perception and Action, Volume 2
ISBN 0-12-516162-X

Rozin (1976) argued that what has made humans intelligent in so many domains is a kind of brain organization in which computations that may have evolved for particular purposes have become accessible for a variety of tasks. Thus, brain systems that code phonetics and are useful for speech, according to Rozin, also are accessible to visual inputs in the course of reading. Such shareability of computational systems among different task domains also extends to computations involved in motor control. Greenfield (1991) has argued that brain systems that support hierarchical organization in language, one of the key features of human language, also support the hierarchical control of action. Ivry (1993) has argued that cerebellar systems involved in motor timing also are employed in a wide variety of perceptual timing. Such modular organization, in which computations supplied by a brain system are accessible both for motor control and for other acts of cognition, may help to explain why it is that human intelligence manifests itself in the motor domain as well as in cognition.

The great diversity of human skills poses a problem regarding how to research them. It would make little sense in a handbook to describe each skill separately: how to play cricket, how to bowl, how to dance the tango. Such an endeavor would be of interest only to practitioners of each activity. On the other hand, sometimes lessons can be extracted only from particular and highly practiced skills. This may be because some aspects of skill only emerge once the performer becomes unusually proficient. Moreover, some principles of skill may be particular to certain activities. Beyond this, some skills are considered to be particularly important or characteristic for humans, and on that basis deserve full investigation. Such considerations argue that the study of skill is best approached in two ways.

One approach is to search for general principles that apply to a large class of skills. Approximately half of this handbook analyzes skill from this perspective. The second approach examines particular skills, and the other half of this handbook analyzes skill from that perspective.

There are five chapters that deal with general processes. Although these often make reference to particular skills, their focus is on principles that should be manifest in many domains. One chapter, by Rosenbaum and Krist, is concerned with the planning of action. Clearly, one feature that distinguishes human motor control and makes it such an integral part of cognition is that human action involves planning. However, planning is not sufficient for being able to actually produce what has been planned. The human body is a biomechanical system that operates in a physical environment and, for example, to move a finger in a certain way requires deriving the input signals that are needed to achieve the desired output. This is the problem of control as discussed by Jordan. Moreover, the human body consists of several limbs. For several skills the limbs have to cooperate, and such cooperation faces constraints. Heuer's chapter on coordination deals with such constraints on multilimb movements.

Movements evolve in time. This is a trivial statement. However, there are many skills for which timing is not a secondary aspect but is specified by task requirements instead. Musical skills belong most obviously to this class, and precise timing in such tasks is not at all trivial. Vorberg and Wing develop a variety of theoretical issues with respect to explicitly controlled timing of motor action. It is trivial also to say that motor skills can be improved through practice. Again, understanding how this happens is another and less easy matter. Much effort has been invested in determining how practice can be optimized. Ivry in his chapter takes a different approach, one less focused on training procedures *per se,* but rather on what is learned during the course of learning. Understanding the latter perhaps will have deeper implications for training procedures than a direct attack on procedures themselves. Moreover, emphasis on the structure of what is learned should lead to a better understanding of why some procedures are better than others.

The second half of this handbook is composed of five chapters dealing with individual skills. Given the extensive variety of skills of which people are capable, how should one choose which ones are most worthy of discussion? One possibility is to consider skills that are universal, or nearly so, such as speaking or writing. A second possibility is to study subskills that are components of several other more complex skills. Both possibilities are exercised in the five chapters of the second half of the handbook.

The most basic as well as probably most important subskill that plays a large role in many other skills is posture and locomotion. Woollacott and Jensen examine these activities from different theoretical perspectives. Almost of the same generality is reaching and grasping – that is, transporting the hand to a spatial location and adjusting the fingers to the shape of the object in that location so that it can be grasped. Jeannerod's chapter discusses both of these components as well as their relationships. Although catching does not have the same generality as posture and locomotion or reaching and grasping, it is a critical component of a large number of other skills. Moreover, it is a sufficiently general subskill that it may have an innate basis, being found in rudimentary form in the youngest of infants. A variety of issues, including how catching is adjusted to precise spatiotemporal parameters of the environment, are discussed in the chapter by Savelsbergh and Whiting.

The final two chapters deal with rather universal skills of language production. Fowler reviews what is known about speaking, while Teulings deals with handwriting and includes some discussion of typing. While speech may in some sense be special in that parts of the brain may have evolved in large part to support it, it is quite unlikely that the brain has evolved specifically for handwriting. There is enough difference between these two language production skills to justify separate treatments, although similarities may be discovered at the higher levels of control.

The organization of the material covered by this volume into two sections – one on general concepts and the other on particular skills – represents two different perspectives on related issues. Thus the reader should expect to see some overlap between the main sections. Such repetition is beneficial. Repetition in different contexts, as we have learned from the concept of 'elaboration' in memory research, helps to build the web of ideas that represents knowledge. It is the hope of the editors of this volume that the knowledge assembled herein will find its way from one material substrate – paper – to another one: 'mind stuff'.

REFERENCES

Bruner, J. S. (1968). *Processes of Cognitive Growth: Infancy.* Worcester, MA: Clark University Press.

Greenfield, P. M. (1991). Language, tools and brain: The ontogeny and phylogeny of hierarchically organized sequential behavior. *Behavioral and Brain Sciences,* **14,** 531–595.

Guthrie, E. R. (1935). *The Psychology of Learning.* New York: Harper.

Ivry, R. (1993). Cerebellar involvement in the explicit representation of temporal information. In P. Tallal, A. Galaburda, R. R. Llinas and C. von Euler (Eds), *Temporal Information Processing in the Nervous System: Special Reference to Dyslexia and Dysphasia*. Annals of the New York Academy of Sciences, vol. 682, 214–230.

Lashley, K. S. (1951). The problem of serial order in behavior. In L. A. Jeffress (Ed.), *Cerebral Mechanisms in Behavior* (pp. 112–136). New York: John Wiley.

Rozin, P. (1976). The evolution of intelligence and access to the cognitive unconscious. In J. M. Sprague and A. N. Epstein (Eds), *Progress in Psychobiology and Physiological Psychology*, vol. 6. New York: Academic Press.

Part I

General Concepts

Chapter 1

Antecedents of Action

David A. Rosenbaum* and Horst Krist[†]

*Pennsylvania State University, USA and
†University of Frankfurt, Germany

1 INTRODUCTION

In seeking to understand the control of motor behavior, it is natural to inquire into the antecedents of action – the events that precede and allow for the execution of voluntary movements. In this chapter, we consider the *representations* formed before movements are carried out and which are vital for the successful realization of the actor's intentions. Such representations have been called *plans* or *motor programs*. The term 'motor program' connotes a representation of forthcoming activity that codes details about movements. The term 'plan' connotes a higher-level representation. Regardless of which term is used – here we will generally use 'motor program' or simply 'program' – two main questions have generally occupied the attention of those concerned with the representations presaging movement: (1) What aspects of movements are represented in advance? (2) What is the time course of the programming process?

A third question is logically related to the two questions raised above: (3) When is it possible to *avoid* postulation of representations for forthcoming motor acts? We introduce the latter question not out of antipathy for mentalistic accounts of behavior, nor because we believe that the nervous system should be viewed as a 'black box'. On the contrary, progress in cognitive and neural science indicates that such aversions have little place in modern research. The reason for avoiding the assumption of representations when possible is that we respect a major new focus in the study of motor control, namely, a focus on *physical constraints*. This focus originated with Bernstein (1967), who argued that what the body can do is largely shaped by its physical characteristics and by its physical interactions with the external environment. Bernstein's ideas about action are similar to Gibson's (1979) ideas about perception. Gibson argued that one may be mistaken in assuming that the perceiver engages in problem-solving or unconscious inference (Helmholtz, 1866/1962) to pick up useful perceptual information. He argued that the structure of optic arrays directly reveals properties of the environment. Hence, in the same way that structured properties of optic

Handbook of Perception and Action, Volume 2
ISBN 0-12-516162-X

arrays may obviate perceptual representations, physical properties of the actor–environment system may obviate motoric representations. If the physical characteristics of the actor–environment system can 'take care' of details of forthcoming movements, it may be unnecessary to specify them in motor programs.

Accepting this perspective implies that a careful analysis of the physical properties of the actor–environment system can suggest opportunities for relieving the burden on the motor programming system. On the other hand – and this is how our approach differs from those who endorse the Gibsonian perspective (Turvey, 1990) – when a careful analysis of the actor – environment system provides little indication of how physical parameters alone can give rise to behavior, one may be ill-advised to eschew representations altogether.

Bernstein (1967) made another point that influences our thinking: although physical constraints often limit what can be done, many physically acceptable options are usually available for carrying out a task. Bernstein called this the *degrees of freedom* problem. He used this term when referring to the fact that the degrees of freedom of the motor system, expressed in mechanical, muscular, or neural terms, usually exceed the degrees of freedom inherent in the description of a task to be performed. A well-known example is the task of touching a point in three-dimensional space. Such a point, by definition, has just three degrees of freedom. Yet the body has many more degrees of freedom. Hence, to select a reaching movement, a decision must be made about which of the infinite number of movements that *can* be used to reach the point should be performed. The problem is mathematically ill-posed. Nevertheless, under normal circumstances it is solved instantly, effortlessly and without conscious awareness. Understanding how it is solved constitutes the degrees of freedom problem. The relevance of the problem for the study of the antecedents of action is that, as long as one assumes that a movement pattern has been selected, the solution to the degrees of freedom problem can be assumed to have been represented before the pattern was carried out.

Considering the degrees of freedom problem naturally suggests a metric of complexity. In general, the more complex an action, the larger the number of degrees of freedom it has. Because it is convenient to consider actions of varying complexity, this chapter is organized with respect to a complexity metric, from actions that are ostensibly simplest to those that are ostensibly most complex. It is sensible to organize the discussion this way because, as has been argued by many authors, behavior can be broken into constituents. A trip to the supermarket, for example, can be broken into a set of behavioral episodes: going to the store, selecting and purchasing the items that are needed, bringing them home, putting them away, and so forth. Each of these episodes can be broken into smaller episodes, each of these can be subdivided still further, and so forth. The smallest behavioral acts that might be considered while remaining within the realm of behavioral science are discrete movements involving one mechanical degree of freedom. We begin our review with such acts. Next we turn to discrete movements involving more than one mechanical degree of freedom. In the final section we consider entire series of motor acts involving many degrees of freedom.

Before turning to these topics, we turn to matters of evidence. We consider those factors that can be taken to suggest antecedent representations and which, just as strongly, seem not to admit of purely physical determinations of action selection or control.

2 FACTORS SUGGESTING ANTECEDENT REPRESENTATIONS

How can one tell that a motor program has been established for an observed action? We have already suggested one answer: when an action is carried out, although other actions are possible, some decision must have been made to favor the action that occurred. Logically, all the factors distinguishing the action that occurred from those that did not are candidates for the factors contained in the motor program. The number of such factors is potentially limitless; they correspond to all possible ways in which an action can be characterized. What is more likely is that the only factors that are represented are those that are necessary and sufficient to specify the action that will be performed at a given time. A major aim of research on motor programming is to determine just what those factors are. A number of measures, criteria and inferential methods have been devised for this purpose.

2.1 Anticipation

A major source of information about programs for forthcoming movements are changes in the way movements are performed depending on what movements will follow. Many examples of anticipation have been described in the literature on motor control. Domains in which anticipation has been studied include speaking, jumping, and reaching and grasping. Examples of anticipatory behavior from these domains are, respectively, anticipatory lip rounding (Bengueral and Cowan, 1974), bending down to facilitate forthcoming upward jumps (Alexander, 1984), and preshaping the hand in anticipation of forthcoming grasps (Jeannerod, 1981, and this volume).

These examples are interesting from different perspectives. Jeannerod's (1981, and this volume) observations concerning hand preshaping might be attributed to the perception of affordances (Gibson, 1979): the actor might be assumed to pick up information about the properties of objects to be grasped, and the action system might be assumed to be tuned to that information. Provided there is tight coupling between the perception of the object to be grasped and the corresponding grasping behavior, one might conclude that complex transformations do not exist between the percept and the act. This argument has been put forward by those favoring an ecological view of behavior.

While we do not deny the importance of the ecological view – indeed, we think it is an important methodological advance because it discourages postulation of cognitive events when physical or low-level sensory events might suffice to explain phenomena of interest – we wonder how informative the ecological account is in this context. We ask whether the ecological description begs more questions than it answers. What is the nature of the coupling that ensures proper hand grasps and the proper unfolding in time of the hand shape that is used? As anyone familiar with robotics knows, getting a robot to reach for and grasp a seen object is a nontrivial problem. The presence of perceptual information may indeed guide action, as Lee and Thomson (1982) and others have suggested, but this cannot be the whole story. Preshaping the hand is just one example of an anticipatory behavior that seems to demand postulation of *knowledge* of objects, *knowledge* of the hand's capabilities, and skillful mapping between the two.

Bending down to prepare upward jumps is another interesting example of anticipation. As in the case of manual preshaping, one might argue that the jump is tuned to the perceptual information of the object for which the actor is aiming. Still, the fact that downward motion is incompatible with the ultimate upward motion seems problematic for a simple ecological account. The reason for moving down before moving up is easy to understand in mechanical terms, and therefore in terms congenial to the ecological perspective: bending down stretches the tendons, which allows for the storage of elastic energy; when this stored elastic energy is released, it adds upward momentum (Alexander, 1984). The *decision* to move down is harder to explain, however. Limb tendons may store elastic energy, but deliberately moving down to store elastic energy cannot be explained without recourse to learning and memory. The point is that postulating motor programs need not imply willful ignorance of physics, as some critics of motor program theory have charged (Kelso, 1981). What is programmed is in most cases programmed with respect to the physical properties of the motor system as well as the perceptual environment in which performance occurs. It would be foolish to think otherwise, and no one pursuing a motor programming perspective has, as far as we know, ever suggested that cognition should replace rather than complement physics.

The last example of anticipation that we wish to mention at this point is anticipatory lip rounding, as in pursing the lips before saying the /t/ in 'tulip'. Anticipatory lip rounding demonstrates that information about the /u/ is available before production of /t/. This example of anticipatory behavior differs from the two examples discussed above in that it does not involve visual perception. Anticipatory lip rounding presumably does not depend on having seen others purse their lips in advance of /u/. There is, in fact, no obvious way to explain anticipatory lip rounding in terms of picking up perceptual information. A more straightforward explanation is that the speaker simply has a plan or program for the entire utterance, and that as the /t/ is being prepared, so too is the imminent /u/. Every detailed account of anticipation effects in speech production makes just such an assumption (Jordan, 1986). That anticipation effects in speech span only certain numbers and types of linguistic elements (Fromkin, 1980) provides support for the view that the effects are mainly governed by cognitive factors.

2.2 Errors

Not all overt anticipatory behaviors are adaptive. Some appear by accident and reveal underlying mechanisms for planning and control. One example is the exchange error in speech. Reversing initial phonemes, as in 'The queer old dean' instead of the 'The dear old queen', suggests that the initial phoneme of the later word ('queen') was available before the initial phoneme of the earlier word ('dear'). Exchange and other types of speech errors allow one to develop detailed models of the representations underlying forthcoming utterances (see, for example, Dell, 1986; Fowler, this volume; Fromkin, 1980). In general, errors in any performance domain, speech or otherwise, reveal hidden properties of the mechanisms underlying those domains, whether the mechanisms are motivational (Freud, 1901/1971) or computational (Norman, 1981). Analyses of errors have, in fact, permitted detailed accounts of programs for speech (Dell, 1986; MacKay, 1987), typewriting (Grudin, 1983; see Rosenbaum, 1991, for review), keyboard performance (Rosenbaum, Kenny and Derr, 1983) and handwriting (Ellis and Young, 1988). What these models share is the major assumption that there are distinct levels of representation, with levels activated earlier providing information about wide spans of behavior (e.g. the entire word, in typewriting), and levels activated later providing information about smaller constituents (e.g. individual keystrokes). That the errors being modeled correspond to errors made by patients with localized brain damage (Ellis and Young, 1988) suggests that the representations are rooted in physical (neurological) reality.

2.3 Reaction Time

Another indication of motor programs is the time taken for an action to begin. The time can be measured in different contexts: (1) when the actor is informed in advance about which action will be required but has to wait for an imperative signal (*simple* reaction time); (2) when the actor is informed in advance that one of a number of possible actions will be required but has to wait for a signal indicating which action should be performed (*choice* reaction time); and (3) when the actor is informed in advance that a given action will either be required or not and must wait for a signal indicating whether or not to perform the response (*go/no-go* reaction time). In all these conditions, one component of the reaction time corresponds to the time to process the signal (i.e. to detect or recognize it), another corresponds to the time to select the response (i.e. deciding *which* response to perform, *whether* to perform the response, and/or *when* to perform the response), and a third corresponds to the time physically to initiate the response.

Based on these assumptions, it is possible to draw inferences about motor programs from observed reaction times. For example, one can rely on the simple reaction time to begin a sequence of movements, where across conditions the sequence begins with the same movement but is completed with different movements. If the first movement is the same across the conditions but the simple reaction time depends on the number or identity of subsequent movements, the change in the initial reaction time can be taken to suggest that information about the entire sequence was represented in advance.

This logic has been pursued by a number of investigators (Henry and Rogers, 1960; Sternberg *et al.*, 1978). Henry and Rogers (1960) studied the performance of *n* successive manual responses, where the value of *n* varied. When *n* equalled 1, the task was to lift the hand as quickly as possible from a start button. When *n* equalled 2, the task was first to lift the hand from the start button (as in the $n = 1$ case) and then to grab a tennis ball. When *n* equalled 3, the first two tasks were the same as for $n = 2$, but a third task (striking an obstacle) was added. Henry and Rogers found that the time to lift the hand from the start button increased with *n*. Hence the same response took longer to initiate depending on the additional tasks to be performed. Because subjects were aware of what task was supposed to be performed and were highly motivated to perform rapidly and accurately, it is hard to interpret the result in terms unrelated to motor preparation (e.g. identifying a choice signal). Henry and Rogers argued, in fact, that instructions for the forthcoming movement sequence were loaded into a buffer after the imperative signal appeared. The loading time, by hypothesis, increased with the number of instructions, which in turn was assumed to increase with the number of movements to be performed.

Analogous sequence length effects were obtained by Sternberg *et al.* (1978) using other kinds of response sequences (speaking and typewriting). They explained their results in similar terms, although they favored a buffer *search* model rather than a buffer *loading* model. The important point for the present discussion is that the changes in simple reaction time observed by Sternberg *et al.* were not artifacts of the tasks they employed, such as changes in the musculature with task context, or variation in the amount of air held in the lungs prior to uttering long as opposed to short phrases (Sternberg *et al.*, 1980; but see Fowler, this volume). Instead, their simple reaction time effects reflected the internal state of the actor, which, judging from the data, varied systematically with properties of the sequence to be performed.

In considering the implications of reaction time effects for inferences about motor programs, it is important not to insist that, for programs to be implicated, reaction times must increase with response complexity. This requirement has been propounded by some. Consider the following quotation:

'Bernstein . . . showed that the sprinter reacts to the starter's gun with the same latency as it takes to lift a finger off a button. Yet, the sprinter has to perform a highly coordinated activity involving a larger number of muscles and body segments (plenty of "elements"!). One answer to the dilemma is that the skilled athlete has discovered ways to reduce the degrees of freedom of the motor system, so that the action is performed as a single, functional unit.' (Kelso, 1982, pp. 237–238)

As the above quotation indicates, a metric of response complexity may not always be apparent. Nonetheless, the *absence* of a complexity effect need not be attributed to the absence of motor programming, nor to bankruptcy of the motor program concept. The true measure of complexity might differ from the one the investigator assumes or surmises; in this connection it is a *virtue* of the reaction time method that it allows one to determine what factors do in fact define complexity. (Note that Kelso implicitly used this logic in the above argument.) For example, Sternberg *et al.* (1978, 1980) showed that the number of stressed syllables was the key determinant of the simple reaction time to begin saying a phrase. On the basis of this result, they concluded that the stress group is a fundamental unit of speech production. This conclusion differed from earlier hypotheses, such as the view that syllables (stressed *and* unstressed) comprise the basic units of speech (Klapp, 1974).

A second reaction to Kelso's (1982) complaint is that we are too ignorant of the inner workings of the motor programming system to insist that any one measure – particularly one as indirect as reaction time – should always be expected to vary with sequence complexity. After all, the biological system may have evolved to promote rapid initiation of complex but adaptive action patterns (e.g. sprinting toward prey). The fact that the time to initiate those patterns is no longer than the time to initiate simpler patterns for which rapid initiation has not been selected need not cast doubt on the role of preparation.

A third reaction to Kelso's (1982) challenge is that other sorts of reaction time measure can be used to great advantage to shed light on motor programs.

Consider choice reaction times. When a given response is paired with other possible responses, the choice reaction time for the common response changes depending on what other response is possible (Heuer, 1984; Kornblum, 1965). Such choice context effects provide fuel for the argument that actors' preparatory states shape their performance. Choice context effects are not merely due to peripheral interactions related, say, to muscle tension extending across effectors poised for action. They also appear when choices are made between alternative *sequences* of responses. When a given finger-tapping sequence is paired with various alternative sequences, for example, the choice reaction time for the common sequence decreases with the serial position of the first difference between the sequences (Figure 1.1). Thus, if the two sequences share all but the first response, the choice reaction time is longer than if the two sequences share all but a later response (Rosenbaum, Inhoff and Gordon, 1984). Because these choice context effects appear when the same response sequence is produced following the same stimulus and where the alternative stimulus is the same in all conditions, it is difficult to accept the idea that the effects result from factors other than the actor's internal state. Detailed modeling of choice reaction times in sequence-choice experiments has led to the idea that programs for forthcoming response

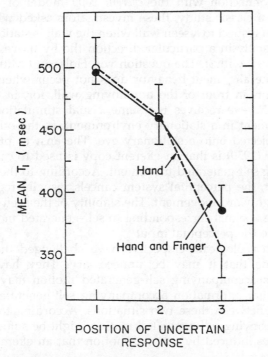

Figure 1.1. *Choice reaction time to initiate a finger-tapping sequence when the position of the uncertain response was at the first, second or third serial position (i.e. when the alternative sequences shared only the same second and third responses, only the first and third responses, or only the first and second responses). The uncertain response either differed with respect to hand or to finger and hand. The two possible sequences in each trial were revealed ahead of time and were highly practiced. [From Rosenbaum, Inhoff and Gordon, 1984.]*

sequences are organized hierarchically, and that information needed to differentiate the sequence to be performed from the sequence that was possible but not required is added to the program after the choice signal is identified, but before the early portions of the sequence are physically produced (Rosenbaum, 1987).

2.4   Perceptual–Motor Interactions

Another source of evidence for motor programming is the fact that registration of perceptual information, or response to it, depends on the preparatory state of the actor. Consider the fact that the subjective amplitude of the sounds of one's own speech or chewing is considerably lower than would be expected from the actual amplitudes of those sounds. Afferent signals generated during these oral activities are suppressed, in part via inhibitory efferent signals to the peripheral receptors and initial relay nuclei (Granit, 1955). Through these centrifugal effects, appreciation of one's self-generated speaking and chewing sounds is attenuated by central neural activity.

Central gating of sensory input related to one's own behavior has been studied most intensively in connection with the *efferent copy* model of von Holst and Mittelstaedt (1950). In a classic study, these investigators asked why the housefly can move laterally with respect to a seen wall when the wall is stationary, but when the wall is moved laterally in a particular direction the fly moves with the wall, maintaining its alignment with it. The question von Holst and Mittelstaedt sought to answer was why the alignment behavior does not occur when the fly makes spontaneous movements in front of the nonmoving wall, for, in either case, the receptive surface of the eye receives the same visual stimulation – in one case induced by eye movement in a stationary environment, in the other by environmental movement projected onto a stationary eye. The answer put forth by von Holst and Mittelstaedt (1950) is that an efferent copy is used to cancel perceptual changes accompanying self-generated movement. According to their model, if the fly turns $x°$ to the left, the perceptual system cancels visually registered motion corresponding to $x°$ rightward movement. The stability of the seen environment is ensured by subtracting a signal corresponding to self-generated movement from a signal corresponding to the perceptual input.

Some who favor an ecological perspective have challenged the efferent copy model on the grounds that it may be unnecessary. They have argued that perceptual information accompanying self-generated motion may be sufficiently different from perceptual information accompanying self-generated stability that there is no ambiguity between these two situations. According to this view, the visual changes accompanying self-generated motion might be sufficiently different from the visual changes induced by external motion that an efferent copy system would be superfluous.

This argument may be valid in some circumstances. For example, given that proprioceptive feedback from the extraocular muscles is richer than was previously thought (Skavenski and Hansen, 1978), it may be unnecessary to invoke an efferent copy mechanism to explain the stability of the visual world accompanying eye movements. Thus, inflow from the eye muscles might help distinguish self-generated retinal motion from externally generated retinal motion. Another possibility is that retinally registered visual change may indicate whether the actor, environment, or both are moving. On the other hand, perceptual processing is affected by motor activity in such a wide range of contexts that it is difficult to dismiss the efferent copy idea entirely. In fact, several results seem to *demand* acceptance of the efferent copy model. Two are mentioned below.

One result is that responses of the cat's limb to mechanical disturbances depend on when during the step cycle the disturbance is applied (Forssberg, Grillner and Rossignol, 1975). If pressure is applied to the dorsum of the cat's paw during the *stance* phase (when the leg is extended and the paw is planted on the ground), the response is greater downward pressure, as if the cat were trying to get a firmer foothold. However, if pressure is applied to the dorsum of the cat's paw during the *swing* phase (when the leg is moving forward toward the next footfall), the response is greater upward motion, as if the cat were trying to avoid an obstacle. The change in the response to sensory input depending on the phase of the walking cycle demonstates that information about motor activity shapes perceptual or perceptual-motor processing, as assumed in the efferent copy model.

The second source of information for efferent copy is a recent report concerning the discharge properties of neurons in the monkey parietal lobe related to visual stimuli presented at varying times relative to saccadic eye movements (Duhamel, Colby and Goldberg, 1992). As shown in Figure 1.2, at first, when the monkey fixated a stimulus in one part of the visual field (the mountain), the receptive field

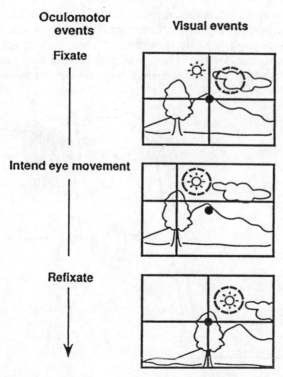

Figure 1.2. *Changes in the receptive field properties of a parietal cortex neuron in relation to current and forthcoming eye positions. See text for details. [From Duhamel, Colby and Goldberg, 1992.]*

of a given cell in the parietal cortex was to the right and above that location (the cloud). As the animal prepared to make a saccade to a new location (the tree), the receptive field of that cell changed to a location to the right and above where the eye *would* land (the sun). When the eye finally reached the new location (the tree), the receptive field of the cell remained on the spot to the right and above the now-fixated location (the sun). This outcome shows that there is anticipation of the retinal consequences of intended eye movements, registered in (or possibly emanating from) the parietal cortex. Similar psychophysical results (not necessarily implicating the parietal cortex) have been obtained with human subjects (Matin, 1972). Matin's subjects mislocalized briefly seen stimuli in anticipation of forthcoming saccades. This result, like the parietal cortex results of Duhamel, Colby and Goldberg (1992), indicates that the circuitry of the brain permits programming of forthcoming movements along with expectancies about their perceptual consequences.

2.5   Corrections

The way actors respond to externally imposed disturbances provides another source of information about motor programs. Those aspects of motion or stability that are reinstituted after a disturbance provide information about aspects of performance that comprise reference or target conditions for the performance system.

Consider the observation of Abbs, Gracco and Cole (1984) that downward perturbation of the jaw results in greater than normal downward movement of the upper lip. The apparatus used for this experiment is shown in Figure 1.3. One of the most important outcomes of the Abbs *et al.* study was that the exaggerated downward motion of the upper lip occurred only when the speaker produced

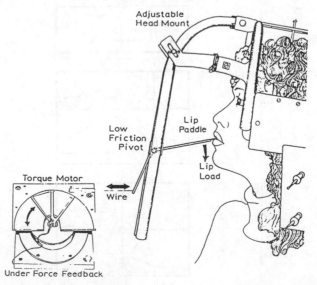

Figure 1.3. *Apparatus used to impose loads on the lower lip during speech. [From Abbs, Gracco and Cole, 1984. Reproduced by kind permission.]*

utterances for which bilabial closure was important. When bilabial closure was unimportant, the compensatory descent of the upper lip did not occur (Kelso *et al.*, 1984).

The latter observation implies that the compensatory motion of the upper lip was functionally related to the actor's internal state. Understanding how the state is represented and how it brings about the observed compensation is an important research problem. A possible solution to the problem (Rosenbaum, 1991, pp. 315–317) is described below.

As seen in Figure 1.4, the model consists of a controller for upper lip movement, a controller for lower lip movement, intermediate units (interneurons) for communication between the two controllers, and a 'bilabial closure unit' that potentiates the intermediate units. When the bilabial closure unit turns on (as is assumed to occur when bilabial closure is desired), it permits the lower lip to inhibit the upper lip controller in proportion to the lower lip's distance from its resting position (assumed to be the open-mouth position). Likewise, when the bilabial closure unit turns on, it permits the upper lip to inhibit the lower lip controller in proportion to the upper lip's distance from the upper lip's resting position (assumed also to be the open-mouth position). Thus, each lip controller becomes less and less active as the opposite lip gets farther and farther from its resting position (i.e. closer and closer to the bilabial closure position). The important feature of this circuit is that if one of the lips happens not to approach the closure position, or to approach it less than usual, the opposite lip becomes more active

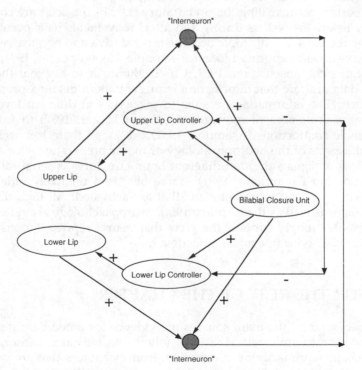

Figure 1.4. *Model of two-lip coordination during production of bilabial consonants. [Adapted from Rosenbaum, 1991.]*

than usual. Furthermore, the compensatory action by the opposite lip occurs only when the bilabial closure unit permits cross-talk between the lips.

This proposed circuit can be generalized to other kinds of response systems. For example, it may apply to the task of pinching together the index finger and thumb; when one of these fingers is held back, the other finger immediately approaches more vigorously than usual (Cole, Gracco and Abbs, 1984). As in the case of bilabial closure, the free finger closes more rapidly than normal only when the task is to pinch the two fingers together. In terms of the model, this goal would be represented by a 'pinch unit' that encourages mutual inhibition between the fingers. For the appropriate compensation to occur, the pinch unit would have to be activated before pinching begins.

2.6   Physiological Changes

Changes in the activity of the muscles or nervous system prior to action provide another source of information about the antecedents of action. The electrical activity of muscles, for example, can reveal subtle aspects of preparation for forthcoming motor acts. Changes in the electrical activity of the postural muscles prior to reaching, for example, indicate that, before a person extends the arm, muscles of the legs and back contract to counteract the forthcoming change in the body's center of gravity (Belen'kii, Gurfinkel and Pal'tsev, 1967). Which postural muscles become activated depends on which arm will be raised (El'ner, 1973).

No less important for revealing the preparatory state of the actor are changes in neural activity before (as well as during and after) movements have occurred. We will not review the work on this topic because it is massive and because reviews of the material have already appeared (see, for example, Georgopoulos, 1991; Kalaska and Crammond, 1992; Rosenbaum, 1991, Ch. 2). Suffice it to say that the neuro-physiological data indicate that information is present about detailed properties of forthcoming acts. The information pertains to properties at different levels, from features of entire sequences of movements (Wiesendanger, 1987) to features of individual muscle contractions (Asanuma, 1981). Although there has been debate about detailed aspects of the neurophysiology of motor preparation – for example, whether the flow of signals through different brain structures is serial rather than parallel (Kalaska and Crammond, 1992) – there has been relatively little dispute about the specificity of the representations that are activated. All told, the neuro-physiological data, as well as the accompanying neuropsychological evidence (Ellis and Young, 1988), strongly support the view that neural representations presage skilled voluntary behavior in considerable detail.

3   PLAN FOR THE REST OF THE CHAPTER

Having outlined some of the main sources of evidence for antecedent representations, we now wish to anticipate what will follow. As indicated earlier, we will organize the chapter primarily by complexity, from behaviors that are ostensibly simplest to those that are ostensibly most complex. Given the above survey, we could present the main sources of evidence for each level of complexity, in effect filling a matrix whose rows and columns correspond to level-of-complexity and type-of-evidence. However, some of the cells would be empty, for questions about motor performance and methods used to answer them have often been conflated in the literature; many questions have been addressed only with particular methods. Given this state of affairs, the organization of the rest of the chapter will be more flexible so we may satisfy the major aims of this review – to identify antecedent representations for action, describe the representations in as much detail as possible, and trace the time course of their development and implementation. As we consider different kinds of behavior, we will often go into considerable detail about the behavior itself without specific reference to what happens before the behavior is produced. Typically this will occur for cases in which little is known about the relevant preprogramming. Our rationale for examining regularities in behaviors as produced is that they can suggest how the behaviors are planned.

4 ONE DEGREE-OF-FREEDOM MOVEMENTS

The spatiotemporal course of a movement (or muscular activity) is commonly called its *trajectory*. Researchers have focused on different aspects of trajectory formation using different methodologies and theoretical concepts. In this section we provide a selective review of this area of study, concentrating on the issue of predictive control in voluntary movements with one mechanical degree of freedom. The question is: which parameters or aspects of a trajectory are specified in advance and how do the specifications depend on task demands?

4.1 Equilibrium-Point Control

The well-known fact that muscles contract if they are stimulated was established in the seventeenth century (Needham, 1971). How muscle contraction is accomplished and how it yields force was only recently clarified (Partridge, 1983).

A major insight stemming from this field of research is that muscles, in conjunction with their attachments (connective tissues and tendons), behave roughly like tunable springs. The idea that the motor system exploits this spring-like property in order to control posture and movement was first elaborated by Feldman and his collaborators (Asatryan and Feldman, 1965; Feldman, 1966a, b), although it appears to have been conceived earlier and independently by Crossman and Goodeve (1963/1983). Related approaches have been pursued by other investigators (Bizzi, 1980; Cooke, 1980; Hogan, 1984; Kelso and Holt, 1980). Collectively, the conception of muscles as tunable springs has been called the *mass-spring model* (Schmidt, 1988).

The essential assumption of the mass-spring model is the *equilibrium-point hypothesis*, which states that postures and movements are controlled by shifts of equilibrium positions. The term 'equilibrium position' has been defined in various ways. Feldman (1986) defined the equilibrium point in the physical sense as that

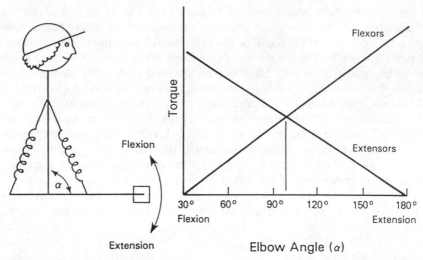

Figure 1.5. *The mass-spring model. Left: forearm represented as a lever rotating about a hinge axis; flexor and extensor muscles represented as springs. Right: length–tension diagrams for flexor and extensor muscles seen as ideal springs; the intersection yields the elbow angle at which flexor and extensor torques are equal and opposite. (Note: the fact that the torque exerted by each spring is also a function of the angle of force application, and hence α, is not considered in the diagram.) [From Schmidt, 1988.]*

muscle length or angular position of a joint at which internal and external forces balance out. According to this definition, the equilibrium point is load dependent. Bizzi and his colleagues (Bizzi, Polit and Morasso, 1976; Bizzi *et al.*, 1984) defined the equilibrium point as the position at which the internal forces of agonist and antagonist muscles cancel each other out. According to this definition, the actual position of the limb corresponds to the equilibrium position only if no net external force is present. In the following we will use the term 'equilibrium point' in Feldman's sense and designate Bizzi's notion as 'virtual position' (Hogan, 1984; Bizzi *et al.*, 1992).[1]

Equilibrium-point control can be easily understood by considering a simplified mechanical model. A lever rotates about a hinge axis by means of an 'agonist' and an 'antagonist' spring (Figure 1.5). The lever represents a limb segment that moves about a single joint (with one mechanical degree of freedom), and the springs represent agonist and antagonist muscle groups.

Hooke's law says that a spring, if stretched by an amount *x*, exerts a force proportional to *x*. The constant of proportionality is called the *stiffness* of the spring. Increasing the stiffnesses of opposing springs by equal amounts increases the stiffness of the entire system without shifting its equilibrium position. The consequence of increased stiffness is that a higher external force is needed to move the lever.

---

[1]Both the concept of an equilibrium point and that of a virtual position refer to statics; they are also defined for dynamics, however, as the simple example of a swinging pendulum illustrates (Feldman, 1986; see also Hogan, 1984 and Bizzi *et al.*, 1992).

Shifting the equilibrium position can be achieved through two methods. One is to adjust the relative stiffnesses of the springs, that is, to make one spring stiffer than the other. The other method is to alter the springs' resting lengths. Muscles, unlike conventional springs, are indeed tunable with respect to their resting lengths and stiffnesses (Houk and Rymer, 1981). Thus, at least in principle, the motor system can program postures and movements by adjusting resting lengths and/or relative stiffnesses.

Feldman (1986) termed his version of the equilibrium-point hypothesis the *lambda* model. A basic assumption of this model is that movements are generated by central commands that alter the thresholds of the stretch reflexes of agonist and antagonist muscles. Thus, the lambda model treats the feedback system underlying the stretch reflex as the entire controlled mass-spring system, rather than the muscle–tendon unit only. Consistent with this view, a muscle with intact reflexes behaves more like a spring (of constant stiffness) than does a muscle deprived of the afferent connections that allow it to behave reflexively (see Stein, 1982).

Feldman (1986) distinguished between voluntary and involuntary movements. Involuntary movements result from shifts in the equilibrium position caused by external load perturbations. Several experiments (Feldman, 1980; Vincken, Gielen and Denier van der Gon, 1983) have shown that involuntary responses to load perturbations exhibit a so-called *invariant characteristic* (IC). The defining feature of the IC is that the relationship between length and tension of the intact muscle remains the same over wide variation in the external forces applied to or removed from it. For human subjects ICs are only observed if the subject 'lets go' (i.e. does not compensate for perturbations).

Voluntary movements, according to Feldman's lambda model, are programmed by choosing appropriate ICs, mainly by shifting the minimum muscle length required to trigger a reflex response; this minimum length is denoted by lambda. According to the model, if the muscle length exceeds lambda a reflex response ensues, but if the muscle length is less than lambda the muscle becomes inactive and exerts no force. The lambda model offers at least a qualitative account of electromyographic (EMG) recordings (Abdusamatov, Adamovitch and Feldman, 1987; Feldman, 1986).[2]

Because, in the lambda model, central commands do not affect muscle contractions or electromyograms (EMGs) directly but only via modulations of peripheral reflexes, the proposed style of control is indirect. In this sense, the model resembles Merton's (1953) servocontrol model, which draws on the fact that the central motor system sends messages to the periphery via two routes. One route, called *alpha*, involves neurons that terminate on muscles that directly cause movement. The other route, called *gamma*, terminates on specialized muscles that are incapable of causing movement themselves. Instead, they change the length of a sensor, so that the sensor is itself stimulated when the primary muscles activated by the alpha

---

[2]Feldman (Abdusamatov, Adamovitch and Feldman, 1987; Adamovitch and Feldman, 1989; Feldman, 1974a, b, 1986) has also worked on the problem of speed control. We will not dwell on this extension of the lambda model here, because it appears to us that the cited articles do not yet present a clear picture. The relationship between the different proposals (1) to control the speed of equilibrium-point shifts by corresponding lambda shifts (Abdusamatov *et al.*, 1987; Adamovitch and Feldman, 1989), and (2) to control a damping coefficient which in turn affects the dynamic reflex threshold (Feldman, 1974a, b, 1986) requires further clarification.

system differ from the sensor's own length setting. When the sensor becomes active, it feeds back through the spinal cord to increase the level of activity in the alpha route, causing activity in the main, movement producing, muscles. According to Merton's model, then, which is the one just described, movement is produced indirectly via gamma activity followed by alpha activity.

Although Feldman's model is similar to Merton's, it differs from Merton's model in two respects. First, only Merton's model postulates that the stretch reflex functions like a length servo: the gamma system specifies a desired muscle length, and the difference between actual and desired length induces subsequent large-scale compensation in the alpha system. By contrast, in the lambda model, descending commands specify reflex thresholds, not muscle lengths, causing the resulting muscle length to be load dependent. Second, in contrast to Merton's servocontrol hypothesis, the lambda model does not include the assumption that activation of gamma motor neurons always drives, and hence precedes, alpha activity. This assumption is not necessary in the lambda model because reflex thresholds can also be modulated by the alpha system. In fact, alpha and gamma motor neurons are often activated at the same time (Vallbo, 1981).

One problem both models share, however, is that the gain of the stretch reflex is insufficient to produce movements. As can be appreciated from the above discussion, although stimulation of muscles through the alpha system causes movement, activation of a stretch receptor can only augment the power already coming through the alpha system; in the absence of any pre-existing alpha activity, gamma activity cannot produce movement by itself. Feldman (1986) argued that a meaningful gain is not necessary to assure postural stability. Nonetheless, it remains to be shown whether reflex activity is sufficient for movement production. This problem is one that has motivated other researchers to seek an alternative to the lambda model (Bizzi, 1980; Cooke, 1980; Hogan, 1984; Kelso and Holt, 1980).

Another problem that led others to develop an alternative model is that reflexes are not always necessary for adaptive movement. Not only is the gamma system unable to cause movement, but movement can also occur when reflex systems, including the gamma system, are eliminated altogether. Several investigators (see, for example, Taub and Berman, 1968) have shown that monkeys can engage in locomotor and grasping behavior when all kinesthetic feedback is eliminated. Moreover, in some neurological disturbances, humans without kinesthetic sensibility can produce at least moderately accurate limb movements. Given such findings, the question that remained was whether the capacity for adaptive movement in the absence of reflexes could be attributed to a mass-spring controller. Work by Bizzi and his collaborators (Bizzi, Polit and Morasso, 1976; Polit and Bizzi, 1978, 1979) suggested that it could be.

In a classic experiment, Polit and Bizzi (1978, 1979) trained monkeys to perform a positioning task. The monkeys rotated the forearm about the elbow joint so the forearm and hand pointed to a designated target, which was indicated by a light. If the hand remained for at least one second within the designated target area (target width = 12 to 15 degrees) the monkey received a reward. Polit and Bizzi showed that unexpectedly displacing the forearm just prior to movement onset did not significantly diminish pointing accuracy. Because the movements were performed without sight of the arm or hand, the animals could not use visual information to update their postures. Most remarkably, the monkeys could still point accurately to the target after dorsal rhizotomy, which eliminated proprioceptive feedback from the limb. This result provided the main impetus for the formulation of Bizzi's equilibrium-point hypothesis.[3]

Several studies lent further credibility to the equilibrium-point hypothesis (Kelso and Holt, 1980; Schmidt and McGown, 1980). A noteworthy study, by Bizzi *et al.* (1984), modified the paradigm used by Polit and Bizzi (1978, 1979) in the following respect. Instead of displacing the monkey's limb prior to movement onset, perturbations were applied only after voluntary muscle contraction began. The beginning of contraction was indexed by EMG activity. In some test trials, the monkey's arm was held in its initial position for a variable amount of time and was then released. The initial acceleration after release of the arm was found to increase with the duration of the holding period. For deafferented monkeys, the time to peak (isometric) torque was reached between 350 and 500 ms after EMG onset. Forcing the arm of the deafferented animal to the target position and holding it there for a variable amount of time had the effect that the arm first traveled back toward the initial position before returning to the target position (Figure 1.6). The amplitude of the return movement also depended on the duration of the holding action. Only if at least one second elapsed between activation of the target light and termination of the holding action did the arm stay at the target position. Return movements were also observed in intact animals in trials where the arm was rapidly driven toward the target and then released.

These findings support the mass-spring view, at least for movements of large amplitude, moderate speed and low accuracy. The findings suggest, according to Bizzi *et al.* (1984), that the central nervous system specifies a gradual shift of the virtual position, or what Bizzi and his colleagues called a *virtual trajectory* (Hogan, 1984). Insofar as the virtual trajectory idea is correct, series of equilibrium positions would have to be specified in advance.

4.2 Control of Isometric Contractions

In a sense, amount of muscular force or tension is the basic unit of motor control. Activation of motor units, via central pathways or reflex circuits, activates the contractile portions of muscle fibers to produce force. Hence, the idea that motor programs specify patterns of muscular force appears straightforward. There are reasons, however, to doubt that muscle tension is the sole or even the most important variable in motor control (Stein, 1982). The major reason is that many factors affect muscle force in an interactive and nonlinear way (e.g. the length–tension relationship, mentioned earlier), and it seems unlikely that these influences can be accounted for completely by feedback or feedforward mechanisms (but see Bawa and Dickinson, 1982).

The equilibrium-point hypothesis circumvents these problems by assuming that entire length–tension curves are selected so that muscle force is only indirectly controlled. This feature appears to be a major strength of the equilibrium-point hypothesis, but it may also be a weakness. Because muscular contractions *need not* be specified directly, equilibrium-point control is computationally simple. On the

---

[3]It may be that the deafferented animals switched to a different control strategy than the one they would normally use (Feldman, 1986), but this seems unlikely given that the deafferented animals had great difficulty compensating for bias loads (Polit and Bizzi, 1978, 1979).

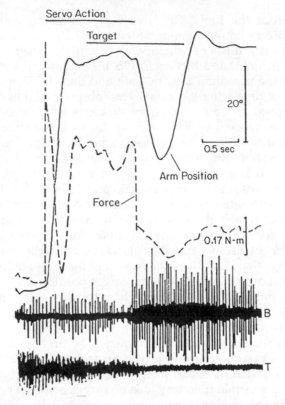

Figure 1.6. *Reversal movement of the forearm of a deafferented monkey. A servomechanism moved the arm to the target position and was later turned off. A target light appeared during application of the servo action. The upper bar (Servo Action) indicates duration of the servo action; the lower bar (Target) indicates onset of the target light. Arm position is shown by the solid curve, and torque exerted by the arm (Force) is shown by the dashed curve. Electromyograms of the biceps flexor (B) and triceps extensor (T) are shown at the bottom. [From Bizzi et al., 1984.]*

other hand, if muscular contractions *cannot* be specified directly, but the control of muscle contraction is key, additional control structures are needed.

Consider the task of producing targeted force impulses. This task has been studied most systematically by Ghez and his colleagues (Ghez and Gordon, 1987; Ghez, Hening and Favilla, 1990; Ghez and Martin, 1982; Ghez and Vicario, 1978a, b; Gordon and Ghez, 1987a, b). They focused on simple isometric flexion – extension responses. Unlike isotonic contractions, isometric contractions are relatively unaffected by reflex effects and the complex relationship between changes in muscle force and length (Ghez and Gordon, 1987; Ghez, Hening and Favilla, 1990). To the extent, then, that muscle tension is directly related to efferent signals, the measurement of isometric forces and concomitant EMG activity can reveal underlying control principles.

In a first series of experiments, Ghez and colleagues (Ghez and Martin, 1982; Ghez and Vicario, 1978a, b) trained cats in a discrete step-tracking task (Poulton, 1974). The cats had to exert variable amounts of elbow flexion or extension force on a manipulandum to compensate for displacements of a lever rotating in the

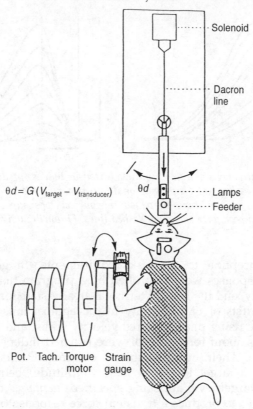

$$\theta d = G (V_{\text{target}} - V_{\text{transducer}})$$

Figure 1.7. *Schematic drawing of the experimental arrangement used by Ghez and Vicario. When the cat pushed or pulled on the manipulandum, the display device moved from side to side. The angular position of the device (Θd) was a function (G) of the voltage difference between the target level (V_{target}) and the output from the force transducer ($V_{\text{transducer}}$). Reinforcement was provided when the solenoid was released and the feeder came close to the cat's mouth. [From Ghez and Vicario, 1978a.]*

horizontal plane (Figure 1.7). A feeder was attached to the tip of the lever, and a reward was delivered if the cat managed to bring the feeder back to its mouth after the lever was suddenly displaced.

Ghez and Vicario (1978a, b) found that the animals achieved a high level of skill in this task. They responded to the perturbations with short latencies (70–120 ms), mostly while the lever was still in motion. Response latencies were the same for random and blocked presentations of different perturbation amplitudes (in a constant direction). Nevertheless, there was a high correlation between perturbation amplitude and both the initial force adjustment and peak force velocity (i.e. peak rate of change of force), even when amplitude was randomly varied from trial to trial. Peak force was linearly related to peak force velocity, which in turn was linearly related to peak force acceleration. When peak force was achieved by a single impulse, time to peak force velocity was independent of peak force velocity, and time to peak force was independent of peak force. Ghez and Vicario (1978b) concluded that the responses were

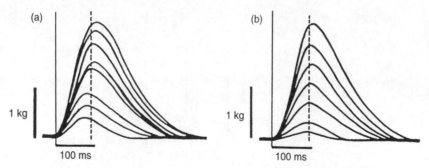

Figure 1.8. *Isometric contractions of a finger muscle (extensor indicis) producing different levels of peak force as quickly as possible. (a) Nontarget condition, in which the subject could produce any desired amplitude; (b) target condition, in which the subject was supposed to produce target amplitudes. Mean times to peak force shown by dashed lines. [From Freund and Büdingen, 1978.]*

scaled from their inception to the task requirements. In general, the results suggested that the responses were controlled by a program that specified the rate of rise of force velocity, and the level of terminal steady-state force. Consistent with this interpretation, bursts of EMG activity in the agonist muscle showed a close correspondence to the rising phase of force velocity (Ghez and Martin, 1982).

Similar conclusions about force control were reached independently by Freund and Büdingen (1978). Their human subjects contracted muscles as quickly as possible, with either a target level (i.e. peak amplitude) being specified (*target* condition) or with a target level not being specified (*nontarget* condition). Subjects were instructed always to produce a transient force response (i.e. a fast voluntary contraction followed by a passive return of force to baseline). Force rise time increased only slightly with increasing peak force in the nontarget condition, whereas rise time was approximately constant in the target condition (Figure 1.8). There was a strong linear relationship between average force velocity and peak force in the target condition. Unlike in cats' tracking responses (Ghez and Vicario, 1978a, b), EMG bursts were observed in both agonist and antagonist muscles.[4] These bursts largely overlapped in time and had approximately constant durations. Freund and Büdingen (1978) summarized their results in terms of 'speed-control'. They argued that the velocity of contraction was adjusted to its amplitude such that contraction time remained approximately constant. They assumed that these adjustments were achieved by neural mechanisms whose activity is reflected in EMG bursts of constant duration but varying spike density. In other words, the chief means of controlling muscle contractions, according to Freund and Büdingen (1978), is pulse-height modulation.

At first glance, the cocontraction of agonist and antagonist muscles observed by Freund and Büdingen (1978) may appear wasteful, because there was no need to counter external perturbations by stiffening the joint in these tasks (but see Hasan, 1986). To shed light on the functional role of opposing muscles, Ghez and Gordon (1987) recorded EMGs from the biceps and triceps muscles while human subjects

---

[4]Antagonist activity was virtually absent in cats performing isometric force steps in the tracking task described above (Ghez and Martin, 1982). Ghez and Gordon (1987, p. 238) ascribed this result to the fact that the forces and rates of force change produced by the cats were relatively modest.

produced isometric force trajectories. Subjects exerted flexor forces of different amplitudes and in different rise times. Target rise times were specified by visual and auditory templates which subjects were supposed to match. A complex pattern of results was obtained. For short force rise times (<120 ms), a pattern of alternating EMG activity in agonist and antagonist muscles (biceps and triceps) was found, with the antagonist burst beginning when agonist activity just reached its peak. The antagonist burst had a relatively constant duration, but the duration of the agonist burst tended to increase with force amplitude. Nevertheless, the peaks and troughs of force velocity and acceleration were stereotypically related to the timing of the EMG bursts in the opposing muscles. For intermediate rise times (120–200 ms), a discrete agonist burst was observed, which terminated at peak force velocity and was followed by a silent period before onset of the antagonist muscle. Force trajectories with long rise times (>200 ms) closely followed the EMG activity in the agonist muscle. In general, the integrated magnitude of the agonist activity was closely related to peak force, while the magnitude of the antagonist activity was most closely related to force rise time (with rise times greater than about 140 ms). Similar bursts of antagonist activity were found in both rapid force impulses and steps. Moreover, it was shown that these bursts were not obligatory, but could be voluntarily suppressed. Apparently, the antagonist burst served to truncate the rising force when brief rise times were required, thereby compensating for the low-pass filter properties of the agonist muscle.

From these findings, it may be suggested that variation of force rise time cannot be achieved without changing the pattern of neuromuscular activity. Hence, by keeping force rise time constant, subjects can produce different peak forces using the same sequence of commands. That subjects actually select a particular force rise time if they are asked to perform as accurately as possible without temporal constraints has been demonstrated by Gordon and Ghez (1987a). Their subjects performed transient elbow flexor forces either as quickly as possible or as accurately as possible. Average force rise time was longer in the *accurate* condition than in the *fast* condition (100 versus 80 ms). While there was a slight dependence of rise time on amplitude in the fast condition, in the accurate condition rise time was constant (cf. Freund and Büdingen, 1978). In both conditions, peak of force acceleration strongly predicted peak force achieved, indicating that responses were largely preprogrammed (Figure 1.9).

A curious result from Gordon and Ghez's (1987a) study was that, although rise times were longer in the accurate than in the fast condition, they were still very brief (100 ms). This seems to be at odds with the speed–accuracy tradeoff usually found with other paradigms (see Section 5.1). Given that there were no time constraints for subjects in the accurate condition, why did subjects choose to produce very rapid responses? Gordon and Ghez (1987a) speculated that for each range of required response amplitudes there may be an optimal force rise time that minimizes overall response variability. While this still remains to be shown, it should be noted that subjects in Gordon and Ghez's experiment were trained not to make overt corrections. It may be that for certain types of ballistic contractions – possibly those that do not include an active braking component – there is no speed–accuracy tradeoff. This idea would be consistent with simple impulse variability considerations and the fact that no speed–accuracy tradeoff has been found with so-called ballistic timing tasks (Schmidt *et al.*, 1979; and see Section 5.1.4). On the other hand, although the subjects in Gordon and Ghez's (1987a)

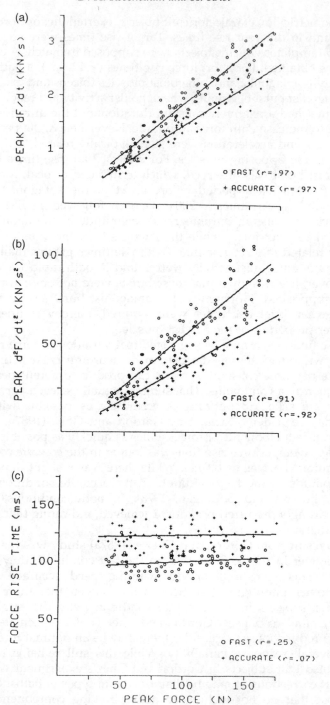

Figure 1.9. *Relationship of peak force to: (a) peak force velocity (dF/dt); (b) peak force acceleration (d^2F/dt^2); and (c) force rise time. Data are from a single subject. Linear regression lines are shown for trials within both a fast condition (speed more important than accuracy) and an accurate condition (accuracy more important than speed). [From Gordon and Ghez, 1987a.]*

experiment were quite successful in performing ballistic contractions, a small but significant proportion of their response adjustments (1–14%) was compensatory, in the sense that errors in initial response programming were corrected online, presumably by feedforward processes (see Gordon and Ghez, 1987b). Further research is needed to explore the exact nature of the balance between preprogrammed, ballistic performance and error correction in tasks like those studied by Gordon and Ghez (cf. Corcos *et al.*, 1990, p. 1042).

From the research reviewed in this section, the ultimate question is whether muscle tension is directly controlled. A definite affirmative answer would, in our opinion, be premature. Indeed, none of the authors cited in this section has made such a strong claim. What we wish to conclude, however, is that the motor system may not control only equilibrium points or virtual positions. The evidence reviewed above suggests that direct control of muscular activity, or parameters related directly to muscle activity, may also be possible. The manner in which direct control is accomplished is by regulating amplitudes of both agonist and antagonist impulses and their temporal relationships. The temporal effects, in particular, argue for active programming of particular force and force–duration combinations.

4.3 Control of Isotonic Contractions

As stated earlier, the work of Bizzi, Taub and others indicates that the major features of limb movements can be produced without feedback. What role, then, does feedback play? Answering this question is important for understanding the antecedents of action, because if a limb is brought to a position by relying extensively on feedback, the program guiding the movement can be judged simple. On the other hand, if the limb is brought to the target with little or no reliance on feedback, the program guiding the movement is probably more complex. From these observations it follows that determining the importance of feedback can help shed light on the complexity of motor programs. In addition, finding out which aspects of feedback are most important for shaping movements can help to show what aspects of movements are controlled.

Consider the hypothesis that positioning a single joint is achieved with a closed-loop mechanism (Adams, 1971): the position of the limb is continually adjusted until its seen and/or felt position matches that of a seen, felt or remembered target. Evidence for such a servomechanism has been presented by Sittig, Denier van der Gon and Gielen (1985). By applying vibration to the tendon of the biceps or triceps, they induced systematic misperceptions of forearm position in their subjects. Because subjects were not allowed to see their limbs, position was merely perceived proprioceptively (probably based on afferent information from the muscle spindles). Misperceptions were indexed by subjects' mispositionings of the unaffected forearm in trying to match the felt position of the affected forearm. Sittig *et al.* replicated two findings from previous vibration experiments (Goodwin, McCloskey and Matthews, 1972; McCloskey, 1973): (1) vibrating the biceps or triceps, respectively, led to the illusion of the forearm being more extended or flexed than it really was; and (2) in trying to match a certain target position, subjects flexed the affected forearm excessively if vibration was applied to the biceps, or extended the affected forearm excessively if vibration was applied to the triceps.

Additionally, Sittig, Denier van der Gon and Gielen (1985) found that both kinds of error – misperception and mispositioning – closely corresponded to each other.

Muscle vibration not only gives rise to misperceptions of position but also to misperceptions of velocity. Particularly striking is the fact that vibrating a restrained arm can lead to a misperception of position while the arm can simultaneously be perceived as moving continuously. This phenomenon, and the fact that loading the vibrated muscle has different effects on position and velocity perception (McCloskey, 1973), suggests that position and velocity are controlled by separate feedback mechanisms (Sittig, Denier van der Gon and Gielen, 1985). Further evidence for this view was obtained by Sittig *et al.* in the experiment just described: if subjects were instructed to match a slow target velocity instead of (and independent of) position, the vibration-induced errors corresponded to those expected from misperception of limb velocity. This was true, even though perception and matching of velocity were found to be disturbed by vibration in different ways than perception and matching of position.

In a follow-up experiment, Sittig, Denier van der Gon and Gielen (1987) investigated which mode of control subjects spontaneously adopted when performing elbow flexions and extensions at different speeds. They did so by assessing the effects of vibration rate on tracking performance in different task conditions and by comparing those effects with the vibration rate dependence of position and velocity perception, respectively. Sittig *et al.* concluded that subjects relied on position feedback in slow movements and on velocity feedback in moderately fast movements. The fact that the latter movements were not affected by vibration (even if the vibration started well before the target displacement) until at least 300 ms after movement onset (Figure 1.10) suggests that velocity feedback may play a crucial role in the timing of the braking of moderately fast movements (Sittig, Denier van

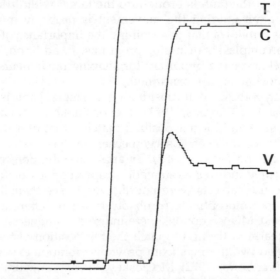

Figure 1.10. *Effect of biceps tendon vibration on elbow extension performed at moderate speed. T, target trajectory; C, trajectory produced in the control condition (no vibration applied); V, trajectory produced in the experimental condition (vibration applied). Horizontal calibration: 1 s; vertical calibration: 10 degrees. [From Sittig, Denier van der Gon and Gielen, 1987.]*

der Gon and Gielen, 1987). This interpretation is also supported by the finding that vibration applied to the antagonist during acceleration of the limb led to an undershoot error, whereas the same vibration applied during deceleration did not affect the final limb position (Capaday and Cooke, 1983; see also MacKay, 1989). Thus, there is reason to believe that, at least in moderately fast movements, speed may play a role similar to position in slow positioning movements. It may therefore be misleading to reduce the behavioral problem of speed control, as it arises, for example, in shooting a basket (cf. Krist, Fieberg and Wilkening, 1993), to a problem of equilibrium-point control *or* impulse timing. The dissociation between position and velocity control observed in vibration experiments suggests that separate 'move' and 'hold' programs (Brooks, 1986) may control different kinds of motor responses and that the same movement task may be accomplished by different control mechanisms. 'Phasic' and 'tonic' control mechanisms are by no means mutually exclusive, and both mechanisms may even operate simultaneously within the same discrete response (Abrams, Meyer and Kornblum, 1990; Ghez and Vicario, 1978b).

At present it remains unclear whether force and velocity, or more generally the dynamics and kinematics of a movement, are controlled separately. Often it is assumed that response specification proceeds from more abstract codes to more concrete, muscle-related codes. There is indeed neurophysiological and behavioral evidence indicating that motor responses are coded on different levels of representation within the nervous system (Kalaska and Crammond, 1992; Rosenbaum, 1991; Saltzman, 1979). However, there is no simple one-to-one mapping from different brain structures to different levels of representation, even with respect to narrowly defined motor tasks. It is as if the structures and substructures involved in motor control are only partially specialized for monitoring or specifying certain aspects of forthcoming or ongoing motor responses and the architecture of the motor system is not strictly hierarchical (Kalaska and Crammond, 1992).

Given this complexity, it has proven useful, especially in studies of the control of dynamics, to focus on patterns of EMG activity. This approach has been taken by several researchers studying rapid single-joint movements – most notably elbow flexions and extensions (Hallett, Shahani and Young, 1975; Lestienne, 1979; Wadman *et al.*, 1979). A well-known finding from this line of research is the so-called triphasic EMG: an initial burst of agonist activity is followed by a burst in the antagonist and a second agonist burst. It is generally accepted that the initial agonist burst is responsible for the initial acceleration of the limb, whereas the antagonist burst yields most of the force needed to brake the movement. The second agonist burst is less well defined and is sometimes absent, particularly if the movement is slow. Brown and Cooke (1990; Cooke and Brown, 1990) suggested that the triphasic pattern should be conceived as a blending of an acceleration and a deceleration phase, where both phases result from paired agonist–antagonist activation. The acceleration phase is assumed to be determined by an agonist–antagonist burst pair, whereas the deceleration phase is assumed to be determined by an antagonist–agonist burst pair. Interestingly, this account agrees with Ghez and Gordon's (1987) conjecture that, in rapid isometric contractions, the antagonist burst serves to truncate the rising force (see Section 4.2).

Recently, Gottlieb, Corcos and Agarwal (1989b) attempted to organize the disparate findings of EMG research related to rapid, discrete single-joint movements. They focused on the initial agonist burst, but suggested that similar

considerations apply to the antagonist burst. They proposed that at least two
control strategies should be distinguished: a speed-insensitive (SI) strategy and a
speed-sensitive (SS) strategy. Gottlieb, Corcos and Agarwal (1989b) defined a
strategy as 'a set of rules between a movement task and measured variables,
sufficient to perform the task' (p. 192). Gottlieb *et al.* (1990) proposed that the SI
strategy is the default, but that the SS strategy comes into play whenever speed
and/or movement time is constrained to meet task requirements. According to the
model, the SI strategy is implemented by varying the 'width' of the excitation pulse
delivered to the motoneuron pool, keeping its 'height' constant as task parameters
vary. By contrast, the SS strategy is equivalent to a pulse-height control policy.
According to Gottlieb *et al.* (1990), the (rectified and filtered) EMG signal is
proportional to the sum of all the action potentials within the relevant motoneuron
pool, and the activation of the motoneuron pool itself, and hence the EMG as well,
is taken to be a low-pass filtered version of the excitation pulse. Assuming that the
activation of the motoneuron pool is amplitude limited and, for the sake of
simplicity, that the excitation pulse is rectangular, pulse-height and pulse-width
modulation yield distinct patterns of EMG activity (Figure 1.11).

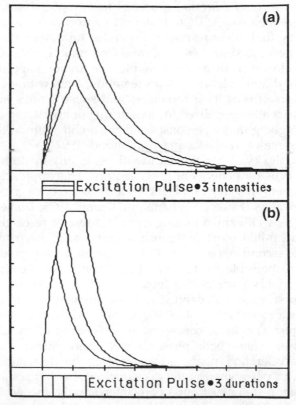

Figure 1.11. *Theoretical effect of rectangular excitation pulses of different (a) intensities and (b)
durations on rectified and filtered electromyograms. EMG amplitude is shown on the vertical axis
(arbitrary units). Time is shown on the horizontal axis (arbitrary units). The model assumes that the
pulses are low-pass filtered according to a linear first-order differential equation followed by an
amplitude-limiting nonlinearity. [From Gottlieb, Corcos and Agarwal, 1989b.]*

The main feature distinguishing the SI and SS EMG patterns is the initial slope of the curves. The EMG slope should ideally be the same if only the duration of the pulse (i.e. its width) is modulated (SI strategy). Consequently, the torque produced by the agonist should initially be the same, too. If the limb's inertial load is varied, the initial joint acceleration should scale inversely according to the inertia. On the other hand, if the intensity of the pulse (its height) is modulated (SS strategy), EMG slopes, joint torques and accelerations should differ from the outset.

Gottlieb, Corcos and Agarwal (1989b) showed that existing data on rapid single-joint movements can be partitioned into the SI and SS categories. The usefulness of the classification scheme was further demonstrated by Gottlieb, Corcos and Agarwal (1989a), who varied movement distance (joint angular displacement) and inertial load. Subjects were required to move rapidly and accurately to targets of fixed size (9 degrees of elbow rotation). The rising phase of the agonist EMG as well as the initially developed torque were found to be independent of the distance or load moved, indicating use of the SI strategy in both cases (Figure 1.12). This was true even though peak inertial torque, peak acceleration, peak velocity and movement time were all highly correlated with distance and load.

Gottlieb, Corcos and Agarwal (1989b) did not strictly equate the SS strategy with an excitation pulse of constant duration. While experiments in which either speed or accuracy (i.e. target width) were manipulated yielded results suggesting pure pulse-height control (Corcos, Gottlieb and Agarwal, 1989), experiments in which movement time was varied (Shapiro and Walter, 1986) did not. Experiments in which movement time was held constant while distance or load was varied (Sherwood, Schmidt and Walter, 1988) produced equivocal results. Because the correspondence between pulse width and EMG burst duration is theoretically imperfect (especially if the pulse is not rectangular), and because the observed correspondence also depends on the method of EMG measurement, the issue of whether there are different types of SS strategies remains unresolved (Gottlieb, Corcos and Agarwal, 1989b).

These problems notwithstanding, the central point made by Gottlieb *et al.* is that subjects rely on the SI strategy as a default. Gottlieb *et al.* (1990) showed that uniform EMG slopes can be observed over a wide range of movement speeds. Thus, if a task is unconstrained with respect to movement time or speed, it seems to be up to the subject to use the default. If target width is varied experimentally, an implicit temporal constraint is induced that renders the SI strategy suboptimal. Corcos, Gottlieb and Agarwal (1989) showed that when target width is varied subjects do indeed control their movements as if speed were explicitly constrained.

As appealing as the framework of Gottlieb, Corcos and Agarwal (1989b) may be, it appears unable to account for the pulse-height policy observed in experiments on isometric contractions (see Section 4.1). The reason is that subjects seem to follow this policy only in experiments where control of speed or movement time is not required.[5] If one adopts the perspective suggested by Gottlieb *et al.*, it remains unclear why subjects do not rely on the default (SI) strategy to produce forces of different amplitudes. We have already noted, however, that the control policy adopted by subjects in isometric tasks is not always of the SS type and that subtle

---

[5]The *target* condition in the Freund and Büdingen (1978) study may be viewed as an exception, because here target width was kept at a constant proportion (10%) of response amplitude. This manipulation may have had the effect of implicitly constraining response duration (see Section 5.1).

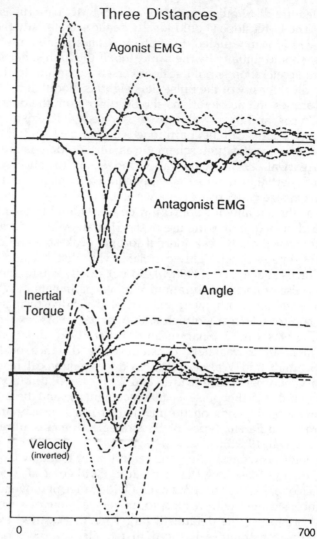

Figure 1.12. *Averaged electromyograms (EMGs), inertial torques, joint angles and velocities from one subject making elbow flexion movements over three target distances as quickly and as accurately as possible. The uniformity of the initial portions of the agonist EMGs and inertial torques suggests that the subject used a speed-insensitive strategy. [From Gottlieb, Corcos and Agarwal, 1989b.]*

aspects of the experimental procedure may influence the way subjects meet the task demands (Corcos *et al.*, 1990). It should also be mentioned that width control frequently occurs when subjects attempt to achieve a new steady-state force rather than a transient force impulse (Cordo, 1987; Hening, Vicario and Ghez, 1983). The latter finding is of particular interest because width control has also been diagnosed with respect to (larger) saccadic eye movements (Bahill, Clark and Stark, 1975; Harris, Wallman and Scudder, 1990). These similarities between the control of force steps and saccades on the one hand, and arm movements against different loads and over various distances on the other, are intriguing and may be more than superficial (Bridgeman, 1989). In all these cases, possible influences of external and/or internal feedback loops on the duration of the agonist burst and the latency and intensity of the antagonist burst must be considered (cf. Gielen and Denier van der Gon, 1989; MacKay, 1989). Thus, one may speculate that width control (the SI strategy) relies on a closed-loop mode of response modulation, whereas height control (the SS strategy) is a purely open-loop or predictive mode of control. The two modes of control could then be viewed as extreme cases of a continuum, rather than two distinct categories.

We started this section on one degree-of-freedom movements by describing the implementation of movement as simply planning the trajectory of a moving equilibrium point. What we have seen is that the planning process is actually more complex. Humans are capable of more than one movement strategy. The availability of such strategies suggests that subjects must build an internal model of the motor apparatus and shape inputs to the skeletal–muscular system that produce movements in a desired manner. The situation is not one of simply moving equilibrium points along a desired path.

5 DISCRETE MULTI-DEGREE-OF-FREEDOM MOVEMENTS

In the previous sections we discussed movements involving one mechanical degree of freedom – typically movements involving flexion or extension of the elbow. Relatively few real-world tasks are this simple, however. To develop a theory that relates to the full range of behaviors that skilled agents carry out, it is necessary to broaden the perspective. We do so in this section by considering discrete multi-degree-of-freedom movements. The behavior we consider in most detail is discrete positioning of the limb (usually the arm) to bring the end-effector (usually the hand) to a target. First, we consider the kinematics of the hand, with special reference to speed–accuracy tradeoffs observed in aiming performance. Then we turn to issues pertaining to the *selection* of reaching movements. Regarding the latter topic, we first consider the selection of global features of reaching movements, such as the direction and amplitude of the reach. Then we turn to selection of the specific limb segment patterns that permit particular positioning movements to be performed.

5.1 Speed–Accuracy Tradeoffs

It appears intuitively plausible that the speed of an aiming movement should be lower the higher its accuracy demands. To thread the eye of a needle, for example, it would be more efficient to proceed slowly rather than quickly. The problem of trading speed for accuracy becomes especially important if time is costly, as, for example, in swatting at a mosquito about to bite one's skin. In this case, the spatial-accuracy demand is given while the actor tries to minimize the duration of the movement. Tasks of this kind have been used widely in research on speed–accuracy tradeoffs. In another major research paradigm, the subject is not asked to minimize time while spatial-accuracy demands are fixed. Instead, the subject tries to minimize spatial error while movement time is fixed. The former type of problem is a *time-minimization* task; the latter is a *time-matching* task (Meyer *et al.*, 1990).

Before beginning this section, we wish to comment on its placement in this part of the chapter. We include the treatment of speed–accuracy tradeoff here because most studies in which such tradeoffs have been analyzed have used discrete multi-degree-of-freedom movements (e.g. moving a stylus from one place to another). The concepts and methods that have been developed to study speed–accuracy tradeoffs apply as well to other kinds of movements and movement sequences. Nonetheless, the style of analysis represents a convenient bridge to the study of more complex tasks.

5.1.1   Woodworth's Pioneering Work

Woodworth (1899) was among the earliest pioneers in the study of aiming performance. Indeed, he may be considered the founder of research on speed–accuracy tradeoffs (Meyer *et al.*, 1990). In his experiments Woodworth used the time-matching paradigm. Subjects tried to draw lines of specified lengths on a moving roll of paper by moving a pencil back and forth through a slit. The back-and-forth movements were paced by a metronome set at different rates. Woodworth analyzed the spatial error of the movements as a function of movement rate. He found that the absolute error in movement distance increased monotonically with movement rate. This was not true, however, if subjects had to draw the lines with their eyes closed; then, accuracy was low even for slow movements.

Woodworth assumed that a regular aiming movement consists of an initial adjustment phase and a current control phase. Whereas the former reflected preprogramming, the latter served the function of homing in on the target. Because only the current control phase could be based on visual feedback, Woodworth interpreted his results by attributing the speed–accuracy tradeoff solely to error corrections during the current control phase.

5.1.2   Fitts' Law

More than half a century later, Fitts (1954) developed another paradigm to examine speed–accuracy relationships. In contrast to Woodworth, who used a time-matching task, Fitts adopted a time-minimization task. His subjects used a hand-held stylus to alternately tap two target plates. The subjects were instructed to move as rapidly as possible, but were cautioned not to miss the target in more than 5% of their taps. Fitts manipulated the width (W) of the target areas and the distance (D) between the target centers. He found that the average movement time (MT) was a logarithmic function of the ratio of the target distance to the target width:

$$MT = a + b \log_2(2D/W) \qquad (1)$$

where a and b denote empirical constants. Because this quantitative relationship has been shown to hold in many task contexts and for many subject populations, it has come to be known as *Fitts' law.*

Fitts framed his interpretation of this relationship in terms of information theory. He assumed: (1) that the term $\log_2(2D/W)$, which he called the *index of difficulty*, corresponded to the amount of information needed to specify the motor output sufficiently in the presence of (adjustable) background noise; and (2) that movement time increases linearly with the index of difficulty because the channel capacity of the motor system is fixed (Fitts, 1954; Fitts and Peterson, 1964).

5.1.3 Iterative Corrections Model

Although Fitts' quantitative description of the dependence of movement time on distance and required accuracy stood the test of time with only minor alterations, his explanation of the function met with criticism. In the 1960s, an alternative theory, the *iterative corrections* model, was presented by Crossman and Goodeve (1963/1983); it remained the best-known explanation of Fitts' law for many years. Crossman and Goodeve revived Woodworth's assumption that the locus of the speed–accuracy tradeoff is in the current control phase. They postulated that an aiming movement consists of a series of submovements, each of which is programmed to travel a constant proportion of the remaining target distance. They conceptualized the control process as a discrete servomechanism that uses feedback about the remaining target distance as error information.

The logic of the iterative corrections model may be explained by considering a numerical example. Assume the limb always moves 70% of the (remaining) distance to the target.[6] Thus, it would successively cover the following proportions of the initial target distance (D) in sequence: 70, 91, 97.3, 99.19, 99.76, 99.93%, and so forth. Formally, each submovement would cover a distance of $p(1 - p)^{n-1}D$, where p is a constant proportion and n is the ordinal position of the submovement in the sequence. Theoretically, this scheme guarantees that the aiming error eventually approaches a lower limit solely determined by the measurement error of the system, given that the number of possible submovements is unlimited. The theory does not predict that this limit will always be reached, but it assumes that the movement sequence stops once the target area has been captured. As can be shown formally (Crossman and Goodeve, 1963/1983; Keele, 1968), it follows that the number of submovements is approximately proportional to the index of difficulty, $\log_2(2D/W)$. The model's additional assumption, that each submovement takes an equal amount of time, yields Fitts' law.

In support of the iterative corrections model, discrete submovements have been documented in several studies (Jagacinski *et al.*, 1980; Langolf, Chaffin and Foulke, 1976; Vince, 1948; Woodworth, 1899). On the other hand, submovements are not always observed, even though Fitts' law still applies in these situations (Langolf, Chaffin and Foulke, 1976). Furthermore, submovements, when they are discernible, do not travel a constant portion of the distance between the starting position and the target (Jagacinski *et al.*, 1980), nor do they take an equal amount of time (Jagacinski *et al.*, 1980; Langolf, Chaffin and Foulke, 1976). Finally, in violation of the iterative corrections model, the duration of the initial part of the movement trajectory is sensitive to the index of difficulty rather than being constant in duration (Jagacinski *et al.*, 1980; Langolf, Chaffin and Foulke, 1976). These and other failures

---

[6]This example is meant to illustrate the quantitative formulation of the model. It would be unrealistic, of course, to assume that the limb would always travel *exactly* a certain proportion of the target distance (cf. Keele, 1968). If this were the case, a mechanism for error correction would be superfluous because the movement could be programmed to cover the entire distance in a single movement.

of the iterative corrections model (see Meyer *et al.*, 1988, 1990) do not argue against the importance of feedback mechanisms in general but do indicate that the attempt to attribute the speed–accuracy tradeoff solely to the current control phase may be inappropriate.

5.1.4 Impulse Variability Models

A different approach to the speed–accuracy tradeoff was developed by Schmidt and his collaborators (Schmidt, Zelaznik and Frank, 1978; Schmidt *et al.*, 1979). Open-loop control, according to Schmidt (1975), is achieved by specifying certain parameters of a generalized motor program. The generalized motor program is conceived as an abstract representation that specifies the general characteristics of a class of movements (e.g. throwing, or writing the letter 'a'). Schmidt (1988; Schmidt *et al.*, 1979) suggested that the relative forces in the contractions involved in a movement as well as the relative timing of their application (their 'phasing') are invariant features of movements governed by the same motor program. The actual forces and time intervals, by contrast, are modulated by specifying a scaling parameter for each aspect. This view of motor control is called the *impulse timing* hypothesis (Schmidt, 1988; Wallace, 1981). It rests on the assumption that patterns of muscle contraction are modulated by scaling two global parameters: a force parameter and a time parameter.

In conjunction with certain, more specific assumptions, the impulse timing hypothesis can be used to derive formal predictions about the variability of motor output. Schmidt *et al.* (1979) first introduced such a stochastic elaboration of the impulse timing hypothesis; their model came to be known as the *impulse variability* model. In it, movements are viewed as caused by a series of impulses – that is, a series of forces (or torques) that act on one or more joints over a period of time. Recall from elementary physics that an impulse is defined as the integral of force over time. Thus, it seems straightforward to account for the speed–accuracy tradeoff in terms of impulse variability (i.e. in terms of fluctuations in force and/or time parameters).

Schmidt *et al.* (1979) started out with a version of the impulse timing hypothesis according to which: (1) the relative timing of forces remains constant when movements are programmed to travel different distances in different times; and (2) the individual impulses are (linearly) scaled by two independent parameters – a force parameter and a duration parameter, the former determining the 'height' of the impulse and the latter its 'width'. Based on experiments concerning the variability of isometric force production and of impulse duration (Schmidt, Zelaznik and Frank, 1978; Schmidt *et al.*, 1979), as well as studies of the variability of interresponse intervals in tapping (Michon, 1967; Wing, 1980; Wing and Kristofferson, 1973), Schmidt *et al.* treated the force and time parameters of each impulse as stochastic variables, the standard deviation of which was proportional to the respective mean.[7] From the aforementioned premises, it can be shown how the variability of a given impulse affects the spatial and temporal variability of the trajectory. It is also possible to predict how variable errors in space and time should

---

[7]Recent studies suggest that the relationship between force and force variability may be more complicated, at least for high force values (see Schmidt *et al.*, 1985, for a discussion). Exceptions to the rule that time and time variability are proportional have also been reported (Rosenbaum and Patashnik, 1980).

relate to the mean amplitude and duration of movements (performed under constant conditions).

Formally, the impulse variability model predicts that spatial variability (i.e. the variable error about the mean distance) should be proportional to movement distance, and that temporal variability should be proportional to movement time (cf. Meyer, Smith and Wright, 1982 (Appendix A); Schmidt *et al.*, 1979 (Appendix), 1985). Therefore, the (original) impulse variability model predicts a *distance*–accuracy tradeoff, not a *speed*–accuracy tradeoff. This is true with respect to spatial accuracy only. With respect to temporal accuracy, the model predicts a *time*–accuracy tradeoff, which, for a fixed distance, actually amounts to an *inverse* speed–accuracy tradeoff.

Counterintuitive as these predictions may seem, they have nevertheless received considerable empirical support, at least in the original experiments in which the model was tested, using so-called ballistic timing and reciprocal movement tasks. In the ballistic timing paradigm, the subject typically moved a lever in the horizontal plane and was supposed to cover a given distance in a prescribed time. After a series of practice trials, in which knowledge of results about temporal accuracy was given, the variable error in timing was assessed. This procedure was repeated for different combinations of movement time and amplitude. Schmidt *et al.* (1979) found that the variable error in timing was virtually independent of movement distance and nearly proportional to movement time. Schmidt *et al.* also analyzed the spatial variability of the trajectories at the instant when the prescribed duration elapsed. The predictions were confirmed for this dependent variable, too. There was no effect of movement time, and spatial variability was nearly proportional to movement amplitude. The latter result was essentially replicated for the reciprocal movement task studied by Schmidt *et al.* (1979), in which subjects made rapid oscillating movements of a lever in time to a metronome.

Subsequent studies of similar tasks (for a review, see Schmidt *et al.*, 1985) provided only partial support for the impulse variability model. While spatial and temporal variability generally were linearly related to movement distance and movement time, respectively, repeated demonstrations of so-called *velocity effects* (Newell, 1980) failed to confirm the predictions of the model. Here it was shown that spatial accuracy tends to *decrease* with increased speed (shorter movement time), whereas temporal accuracy tends to *increase* with higher speed (greater movement distance).

Ironically, the greatest failure of the impulse variability model concerns the single aiming paradigm, the type of movement task that originally motivated the model (Schmidt *et al.*, 1985, p. 115). The single aiming paradigm is similar to the ballistic timing task except that subjects move a hand-held stylus swiftly through space (to hit a target line), instead of performing a uniplanar follow-through movement (to achieve a certain movement time). Unlike in the Fitts task, subjects are supposed to match movement times, with spatial error, rather than absolute movement time, being the main dependent variable. Schmidt *et al.* (1979) discovered that for this paradigm a strong linear relation holds between the average movement speed and the variable error in movement distance (Figure 1.13). The relationship can be expressed as:

$$W_e = a + b(D/MT) \qquad (2)$$

where W_e is the standard deviation of movement end-points, the so-called *effective target width, D,* is the mean movement distance, *MT* is the mean movement time,

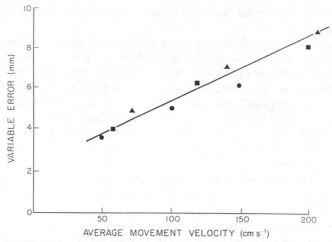

Figure 1.13. *Linear speed–accuracy tradeoff obtained in a task in which subjects tried to move the arm over three distances (10, 20 or 30 cm) for durations matching three target durations:* ▲, *140 ms;* ■, *170 ms; or* ●, *200 ms. [From Schmidt et al., 1979.]*

and *a* and *b* are empirical constants. This 'law of rapid actions' (Keele, 1986) resembles Fitts' law, although it posits a linear speed–accuracy tradeoff rather than the logarithmic relationship assumed by Fitts. The linear tradeoff has been replicated (Zelaznik, Shapiro and McColsky, 1981; Zelaznik *et al.*, 1988) and has been shown to apply not only to tapping movements but also to wrist rotations (Wright and Meyer, 1983) and saccadic eye movements (Abrams, Meyer and Kornblum, 1989; Patla *et al.*, 1985).

Hence, the most reliable finding that grew out of the early work on the impulse variability model seems to be the one with which the model conflicts the most. Initially, Schmidt *et al.* (1979) thought they could account for the linear speed–accuracy tradeoff in a straightforward manner, but they were in error in this, as pointed out by Meyer, Smith and Wright (1982).[8] There seems to be no simple way, if any, to account for the speed–accuracy tradeoff in terms of the original model. Meyer, Smith and Wright (1982) showed, however, that a linear (or, more precisely, a proportional) speed–accuracy tradeoff is compatible with a modified impulse variability model, which they called the *symmetric impulse variability* model. This model rests on similar assumptions to those made in the original model but makes the additional claim that the force–time curve has certain symmetrical properties. Under the symmetric impulse variability model, the proportionality between speed and spatial variability holds if and only if the force–time curve has a particular shape. Meyer, Smith and Wright (1982) did not try to fit the predicted kinematics to data, but the predictions of their model were qualitatively supported.

Why can the symmetric impulse variability model account for a speed–accuracy tradeoff, whereas the original model cannot? The way Meyer, Smith and Wright (1982) presented their model may lead one to think that this outcome was obtained because their model, unlike the original model, allows for force–time curves other than the special square-wave case. Yet this is not the case. Leikind (1985) (cited in

---

[8]It is worth noting, however, that Meyer, Smith and Wright (1982) misrepresented the original impulse variability model in certain respects (for clarifications, see Schmidt *et al.*, 1985).

Schmidt *et al.*, 1985) showed that the displacement of a particle subject to any acceleration is always proportional to the amplitude of the acceleration and to the square of the time of acceleration. For this to be true, the mathematical form of the acceleration function, or force–time curve, has to be preserved as time is varied. This so-called *shape constancy* assumption is part of both impulse variability models. Therefore, it is not the case that Schmidt *et al.* (1979) oversimplified movement dynamics in this respect, as Meyer, Smith and Wright (1982) claimed. Nor is it true that the original model did not consider both acceleration and deceleration (Schmidt *et al.*, 1985). As for the particular shape of the force–time curve, the issue of whether there is a deceleration phase, or whether it is a mirror image of the acceleration phase, is simply inconsequential in the original model. The reason that Meyer, Smith and Wright (1982) could account for a proportional speed–accuracy tradeoff is subtle and, as far as we can tell, not sufficiently elaborated in their article.

Meyer, Smith and Wright (1982) introduced a weighting function to calibrate the amplitude of the prototypical time curve. Particular force–time curves are assumed to be arrived at by first rescaling the prototypical time curve (to provide shape constancy) and then by multiplying the rescaled time function by the weighting function as well as a force parameter. The weighting function is constrained such that rescaling the prototype does not change the distance moved in half the movement time, all other factors being equal. This constraint is crucial in the derivations of Meyer *et al.* because it makes the weighting function a function of movement time. Hence, the amplitude of the force–time curve not only reflects the force but also the time parameter. Recall that in the original model the 'height' of the impulse is solely determined by the force parameter. If there were no weighting function, a proportional speed–accuracy tradeoff would not be possible under the symmetric impulse variability model (Meyer, Smith and Wright, 1982, p. 465). There is no direct way to prove the existence of the weighting function. Meyer *et al.* argued, however, that they were justified in postulating it, together with the above-mentioned constraint, based on considerations of efficiency of movement programming and the fact that the assumptions are necessary to account for the speed–accuracy tradeoff under their model (Meyer, Smith and Wright, 1982, pp. 465–466).

Regardless of whether one is willing to accept their arguments, there is reason to suspect that the impulse timing hypothesis underlying both variability models may be wrong, at least for rapid aiming movements. Zelaznik, Schmidt and Gielen (1986) found that the shape constancy assumption is seriously violated in stylus-tapping movements. Time to peak acceleration as well as time from peak deceleration through movement termination remained virtually constant in their study (i.e. these peaks occurred at the same moment in absolute, not relative, time). Whether the shape constancy assumption is seriously violated in uniplanar aiming movements or in other movement paradigms still has to be assessed systematically. Nonetheless, it seems clear that future impulse variability models will have to acknowledge biomechanical principles, such as the force–velocity relationship in muscular contractions (Hill, 1938), as well as neurophysiological data.

5.1.5 Optimized Submovement Model

Although a fully satisfying explanation of the linear speed–accuracy tradeoff (equation 2) is still missing, the fact that this tradeoff exists for a well-defined class of rapid aiming movements suggests two things: (1) a vital part of the speed–

accuracy tradeoff in aiming movements stems from what Woodworth called the initial adjustment phase; and (2) the difference between the linear tradeoff found in time-matching tasks (equation 2) and the logarithmic tradeoff found in time-minimization tasks (equation 1) may be accounted for by the fact that only the time-minimization task allows for secondary submovements, or, in Woodworth's terms, for current control. Thus, it seems straightforward to seek an integrative theoretical framework that includes both the acknowledgement of variability in the execution of rapid, preprogrammed movements and the potential influence of submovements on motor performance in the Fitts paradigm.

Meyer et al. (1988) developed such a model: the *stochastic optimized submovement* model. This model is eclectic in the sense that it incorporates assumptions about impulse variability (Meyer, Smith and Wright, 1982; Schmidt et al., 1979), ideas contained in the iterative corrections model (Crossman and Goodeve, 1963/1983; Keele, 1968), and the optimization concept of normative motor control theory (Hogan, 1984; Hollerbach, 1982; Nelson, 1983). Meyer et al. (1988) postulated that an aiming movement, in the typical time-minimization task, starts with a primary submovement programmed to hit the center of the target area. Due to neuromotor noise, the end-points of the primary submovements vary from trial to trial, with their standard deviation being proportional to the average movement velocity (as expected if the linear speed–accuracy tradeoff held for this submovement). If the primary submovement is successful, action terminates, but if it misses the target, a secondary, corrective, submovement follows without delay (Figure 1.14). The end-point variability of the secondary submovement is also assumed to be proportional to its average velocity. Therefore, the secondary submovement may occasionally miss the target. No further corrective movements are assumed in the simplest, dual submovement, version of the model.

According to the model, one faces the problem of finding an ideal compromise between the mean duration of primary submovements and the mean duration of secondary submovements. The problem derives from the fact that, in trying to reach the target as quickly as possible while attaining a high proportion of final target hits, one should not increase the speed of the primary submovements too much, because this would increase the relative frequency of secondary submovements. On the other hand, the primary submovement should not take too long.

Through elementary differential calculus, the optimal values for the average durations of the primary and secondary submovements can be determined, given a desired proportion of target hits and given the target width and target distance (Meyer et al., 1988). The optimal average duration of primary submovements, secondary submovements and total movements can each be approximated by square-root functions of the form:

$$MT = a + b(D/W)^{1/2} \tag{3}$$

where MT is the average (sub)movement duration, a and b are nonnegative constants, D is the target distance, and W is the target width. Because Meyer et al. (1988) assumed that humans perform optimally, they predicted that these relationships would predict real motor behavior.

To test their model, Meyer et al. (1988) performed two experiments on wrist rotations. Subjects rotated a handle as quickly and accurately as possible to move

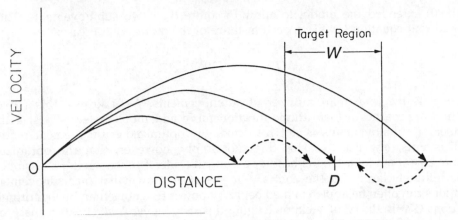

Figure 1.14. *Sequences of submovements toward a target region of width* W *whose center is* D *distance units from the starting point, as assumed in the optimized dual-submovement model. [From Meyer et al., 1988.]*

a cursor on a computer screen to a target area. The cursor was either visible throughout (experiment 1) or, on every other trial, only at the beginning and end of the movement (experiment 2). Meyer *et al.* (1988) obtained strong support for their model: (1) as predicted, the end-point variability of primary submovements increased, approximately in proportion to average speed; (2) the average durations of the total movements as well as the durations of the primary and secondary submovements could be fitted by equation (3); and (3) the relative frequencies of secondary submovements and of errors increased monotonically with D/W, as they were expected to according to the model.

Interestingly, the same qualitative effects as in experiment 1 were also observed in experiment 2, regardless of whether the cursor was visible or not. The only quantitative effects of removing visual feedback were an increase in error rates and an attenuated effect of target difficulty on the average duration of secondary submovements. These results indicated that subjects did not switch to a one-submovement strategy in trials where they could not use visual feedback to guide their corrective submovements. The results also indicated that the primary sub-movements were unaffected by visual feedback. The increased error rates in the reduced-feedback condition, on the other hand, showed that visual feedback is used for error correction in aiming performance (cf. Keele and Posner, 1968).[9]

The optimized submovement model as described above has great explanatory power. Nevertheless, it does not predict Fitts' law exactly. More recently, Meyer *et*

---

[9]Keele and Posner (1968) estimated that it takes about 200 ms to use vision to correct aiming movements. Even though subsequent research has yielded somewhat lower estimates (Carlton, 1981; Zelaznik, Hawkins and Kisselburgh, 1983), the fact that there is a lower bound for visual error correction (at least 100 ms) should be taken into account in further refinements of the optimized submovement model. In order to optimize performance it would be useless to push the duration of the primary submovement below this level, unless the target were wide enough to allow for single-shot movements. The experimental results obtained by Meyer *et al.* (1988) suggest that subjects were more reluctant to program very brief durations (below about 200 ms) for primary submovements than expected under the optimized (dual) submovement model (Meyer *et al.*, 1988, p. 367).

al. (1990) extended the model to allow for more than two submovements. They showed that equation (3) is a special instance of the more general case:

$$MT = a + b(D/W)^{1/n} \qquad (4)$$

where n is the (maximal) number of submovements. As n grows, this power function approaches a logarithmic function more and more closely. Thus, if the number of submovements is not restricted, the optimized submovement model predicts Fitts' law exactly. This does not imply, however, that the optimized submovement model accounts best for empirical tradeoff functions if n is assumed to be infinitely large. On the contrary, it has been shown that mean movement durations can often be approximated better by power functions than by logarithmic functions (Kvalseth, 1980). Acknowledging this fact, Meyer *et al.* (1990) reanalyzed some of Fitts' (1954) data and found that the optimized submovement model yielded the best fit if the maximal number of submovements equaled three. A power function with an exponent of about $1/3$ also best describes the results of Crossman and Goodeve (1963/1983). With respect to their own wrist rotation data (Meyer *et al.*, 1988, experiment 1), Meyer *et al.* (1990) found that assuming four or more submovements yielded the best fit. Therefore, Meyer *et al.* (1990) also reanalyzed the individual trajectories from this experiment (using a refined parsing algorithm), and in this way diagnosed up to four submovements; this number of submovements is consistent with their prediction.

Although the optimized submovement model, in its present form, may not be the final word on rapid aiming movements (Meyer *et al.*, 1988, p. 366), it has performed so well that it seems unlikely that an entirely different theory could do significantly better. Probably, Fitts' law cannot be accounted for without recognizing the 'law of rapid actions' (equation 2) as well as people's capacity to employ sophisticated strategies to optimize performance, even while engaging in activities as seemingly mundane as bringing the hand to a target (Rosenbaum, 1991).

5.2   Selection of Major Kinematic Features of Aiming Movements

In the foregoing discussion, we focused on relatively fine-grained aspects of aiming performance. It is important, however, not to lose sight of the more macroscopic decisions that must be made in programming positioning movements. Such issues as which hand to use and which direction to pursue must be resolved. How they are is a basic question for research on the antecedents of action.

In 1980, one of us introduced a general hypothesis about motor programming, along with a technique for testing it (Rosenbaum, 1980). The hypothesis is stated at the beginning of Section 2. It holds that any factors that distinguish actions that occur from those that do not may be represented in motor programs. If one wishes to investigate this hypothesis, two main questions come to mind: (1) Which features are represented in motor programs? and (2) How are the features specified in time? An experimental method – the *movement precuing* technique (Rosenbaum, 1980, 1983) – was designed to answer these questions.

The procedure used in the movement precuing technique is as follows. First, one establishes a set of response alternatives which vary with respect to one or more dimensions. The subject's task is to wait for the appearance of a signal indicating the response that must be performed and then to carry out the designated response as quickly as possible after the signal appears. Before the appearance of the choice signal, advance information (the precue) is given about some, none, or all of the features of the response that will be required. In most cases, the precue is always valid; it gives reliable information about properties of the response to be tested. However, this need not always be the case.

The rationale behind the movement precuing technique is that advance information about features of forthcoming movements should help subjects preprogram movements if the motor programming system is configured to take advantage of the precue information. The preprogramming should be reflected in a saving in the choice reaction time. Thus, if the program for an aimed hand movement normally contains information about: (1) the hand used to carry out the movement; (2) the direction of the movement; and (3) the amplitude or extent of the movement, then precues concerning those features should aid programming. In terms of observables, the precue should effect a reduction in reaction time. Moreover, the amount of reduction in the reaction time relative to the control condition (where no features are precued) should provide an index of the time savings associated with each feature or combination of features. If some features cannot be preprogrammed, then precues about them should not be helpful, and no reaction time benefit should accrue. Similarly, if a given feature cannot be preprogrammed until some other feature has been preprogrammed, then a precue about the former feature should not be helpful if a precue about the latter feature is withheld.

The movement precuing experiment reported by Rosenbaum (1980) used the apparatus shown schematically in the top panel of Figure 1.15. Subjects placed their left and right index fingers on two square buttons in the center of the response panel. The circular targets on the right could be reached with the right hand, and the circular targets on the left could be reached with the left hand; thus, hand (or 'arm') was one choice dimension. The circular targets also called for movements that brought the hand *toward* or *away* from the frontal plane of the body; thus direction of movement was another choice dimension. Finally, the targets called for movements that brought the hand over a *long* or *short* distance from the home positions; thus, amplitude or 'extent' of movement was another choice dimension. Prior to the signal indicating which of the eight targets would have to be reached on a trial, a precue was given about: (a) arm; (b) direction; (c) extent; (d) arm and direction; (e) arm and extent; (f) direction and extent; (g) arm, direction and extent; or (h) none of these features.

The choice reaction time data appear in the bottom panel of Figure 1.15. Choice reaction times increased as fewer dimensions were precued. Such an outcome is expected from the principle, established in information processing research (Hick, 1952; Hyman, 1953), that the larger the number of stimulus–response alternatives, the longer the choice reaction time. Nevertheless, this interpretation would apply to the precuing situation only if the precues could reduce uncertainty about the defining features of the forthcoming response. That the choice reaction times followed the usual uncertainty effect indicates that subjects could take advantage of the precues. Furthermore, assuming that the precues were used to choose features of the forthcoming motor response, the results rule out a model in which arm, direction, or extent must be chosen in a fixed order – say, with extent only chosen after arm or direction.

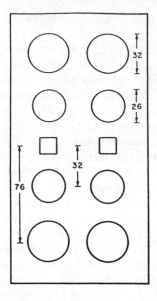

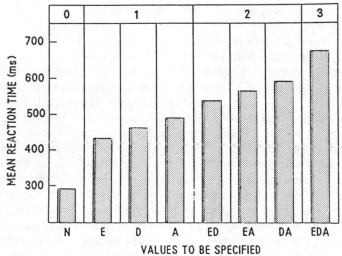

Figure 1.15. *Apparatus (top panel) and mean reaction times (bottom panel) from a movement precuing experiment on the programming of aimed hand movements. [From Rosenbaum, 1983.]*

How does one know that precues were used to choose features of the forthcoming motor response? Another possibility is that precues helped subjects to identify spatial locations of the targets, but did not help subjects prepare motorically. To test the nonmotor preparation interpretation, Rosenbaum (1980) conducted another experiment in which subjects made True–False judgements about stimuli presented after precues were shown. On a given trial, a precue gave information about one or more feature(s), such as the direction and extent of a target, and then the target was divulged. The subject's task was to indicate as quickly as possible, by saying 'True' or 'False', whether the target had the indicated properties (e.g. the previously specified direction and extent). The result differed from the results of the manual positioning experiment. In the True–False task, there was an overall uncertainty effect (i.e. reaction times depended on the number of precued features), but there was no effect of the *type* of precued feature. This result led to the conclusion that precues about arm, direction and extent aided stimulus identification as well as motor preparation. The differential effects of the *types* of features were attributed to motor programming.

Not all investigators were convinced that precues facilitated programming of specific response features, however. Goodman and Kelso (1980) used a modified form of the precuing paradigm in which, on any trial, a set of lights corresponding to possible targets was presented before just one of the lights was illuminated. (In Rosenbaum's (1980) experiment, the precues took the form of letters, and the targets were colored dots presented in a tachistoscope; the movements were made without sight of the hand.) Goodman and Kelso varied the dimensional coherence of the targets presented in the precued set. Thus, when two lights were presented, the corresponding targets could differ with respect to just one dimension (e.g. direction only), with respect to two dimensions (e.g. direction and extent), or with respect to three dimensions (e.g. lateral side of the response panel, direction and extent). Goodman and Kelso argued that, if motor programs are organized dimensionally, subjects should be better able to take advantage of precued target sets whose elements differ with respect to few dimensions rather than many. This prediction was not supported, leading Goodman and Kelso to conclude that motor programs are not dimensionalized.

Other results, from neurophysiology and motor psychophysics, have failed to support the holistic view of Goodman and Kelso (1980), however. Studies of motor cortex neurons, for example, have shown that directional precues give rise to more sustained activity in the motor cortex than do amplitude (distance) precues (Requin, Riehle and Seal, 1993; Riehle and Requin, 1989). Similarly, many brain studies, including studies of the motor cortex, basal ganglia, cerebellum and colliculus, have shown that in a wide variety of tasks cells are tuned to specific aspects of forthcoming movements. For example, as emphasized by Georgopoulos (1991), cells in the monkey motor cortex discharge preferentially to forthcoming *directions* of movement but show little or no selectivity to forthcoming *amplitudes* of movement. A similar dissociation was reported by Soechting and Flanders (1989) in a study of movement recall: their subjects consistently made distance errors but not direction errors (for further discussion, see Flanders, Helms Tillery and Soechting, 1992). Finally, as shown by Favilla, Hening and Ghez (1989) using a variant of the movement precuing technique, force direction and force magnitude appear to be distinct programming parameters. Collectively, the results appear to support the view that the nervous system dimensionalizes forthcoming movements.

5.3 Selecting Limb Segment Combinations

Once decisions have been made about where a limb should be positioned, decisions must be made about how the limb should move there. In general, understanding how the decision is made is difficult because for any end-effector position (e.g. for any given spatial location of the index finger) an infinite number of postures allows the position to be achieved. If one considers entire trajectories that could bring the end-effector to the terminal position, the indeterminacy problem is compounded because a trajectory can be viewed as a series of postures.

In computational analyses of motor control, the indeterminacy associated with the assignment of postures to locations is called the *inverse kinematics* problem. The term 'inverse' refers to the fact that one must map back from a desired end-effector location to joint angles capable of achieving that location. The term 'kinematics' refers to the fact that one is dealing with motions without regard to the forces that cause them; when one considers underlying forces, one is dealing with 'kinetics'. The inverse kinematics problem is fundamental to the study of motor control because much of everyday activity seems to be driven by the desire to move to spatial locations (e.g. pressing the 'third floor' button in the elevator, touching one's nose, reaching for an apple, etc.). Only in specialized contexts (e.g. exercise or dance) do we move for the sake of movement.

A number of solutions to the inverse kinematics problem have been proposed (for reviews, see Atkeson, 1989; Jordan, this volume; Jordan and Rosenbaum, 1989). However, none of the proposed solutions appears to be as simple or as compatible with known facts of behavior and physiology as one might like (Rosenbaum *et al.*, 1993a). This sentiment led Rosenbaum *et al.* to develop an alternative solution. Their central idea was that there are motor control modules which continually evaluate their respective capabilities for achieving physical tasks. The modules contribute to overt behavior in proportion to their evaluations. The advantage of modules is that they can function largely autonomously. In addition, allowing the modules to act in concert but in proportion to their capabilities accords with current views of the neural control of movement, most notably the *population coding* strategy (for reviews, see Erickson, 1984; Georgopoulos, 1990, 1991; Wise and Desimone, 1988).

5.3.1   Optimal Selection Model

The first modular model developed by Rosenbaum and his colleagues was the *optimal selection* model (Rosenbaum *et al.*, 1991). It was assumed here that modules make 'bids' to a higher-level mechanism which integrates the bids and allocates work to the effectors according to the bids' relative strengths.

The experimental context in which the model was developed was a task in which subjects moved the tip of the extended index finger back and forth between two locations in the horizontal plane. Performance was done with the right hand, and the hand was held such that the base of the thumb was up and the index finger pointed out. The target locations were on a line parallel to the frontal plane of the body, at a forearm's length away from the subject, and at stomach level. The distance between the locations was varied, as was the rate of back-and-forth movement (prescribed by a metronome). Because the fingertip had to get from one location to another in time with the metronome but did not have to travel in a straight line or path of fixed curvature, the task could be completed in several ways: (1) by moving only the index finger (rotating the finger about the metacarpophalangeal joint); (2) by moving only the hand (rotating the hand about the wrist); (3) by moving only the forearm (rotating the forearm about the elbow); or (4) combinations of the above. The question was which combination of limb segments would be used depending on the required amplitude and frequency of fingertip oscillation.

In the model, it was assumed that each limb segment has an optimal amplitude and frequency of movement, traceable to its properties as a damped oscillator (cf. French, 1971; Holt, Hamill and Andres, 1990). From physical mechanics, it was assumed that the forearm (i.e. the forearm plus rigid hand and finger) would be optimally suited for low-frequency oscillations covering small angular amplitudes about the elbow, that the hand (i.e. the hand plus rigid finger) would be optimally suited for medium-frequency oscillations covering medium angular amplitudes about the wrist, and that the finger would be optimally suited for high-frequency oscillations covering large angular amplitudes about the metacarpophalangeal joint. These assumptions were tested in the first phase of the study reported by Rosenbaum *et al.* (1991). The method was to have subjects move only the finger, hand or forearm at preferred amplitudes given required frequencies, or at preferred frequencies given required amplitudes. The results confirmed the expectations (Figure 1.16).

In the second phase of the study, the same subjects covered different distances at different frequencies with whatever three-segment combination they preferred. The main prediction was that the relative contributions of the limb segments would be related to their fits to task demands (i.e. to how close their optimal amplitudes and frequencies came to the required amplitude and frequency of fingertip motion). In the model, it was assumed that movement modules for the finger, hand and forearm made 'bids' to a higher-level task-controller based on their respective capacities to achieve the task on their own. Thus, the finger module determined how costly it would be for the finger alone to do the task, the hand module determined how costly it would be for the hand alone to do the task, and the forearm module determined how costly it would be for the forearm alone to do the task. The individual limb segments were made to work in proportion to the relative strengths of their bids.

The model accounted successfully for the data (Figure 1.17). As predicted, the forearm had a larger relative contribution the larger the amplitude and the lower the frequency of fingertip oscillation; the finger had a larger relative contribution the smaller the amplitude and the higher the frequency of fingertip oscillation; and the hand had a larger relative contribution the more the amplitudes and frequencies of fingertip oscillation approximated intermediate values.[10]

The optimal selection model was also applied to other, related, tasks. Whereas subjects in the experiment of Rosenbaum *et al.* (1991) waved the fingertip back and forth in an unobstructed fashion, subjects in experiments reported by Vaughan *et al.* (in press) tapped the fingertip against one stop or two. Subjects were responsible for controlling two variables: the *frequency* of finger-tapping and the *impact of collision* against the stop(s). Vaughan *et al.* were interested in finger-tapping because this behavior has been used widely in studies of motor timing (Wing, 1980), and because many movements are deliberately made to have an impact on a surface (e.g. hammering or boxing).

---

[10]The finger was predicted to be used most for small fingertip displacements even though the finger was found to have the largest preferred angular excursion because large angular displacements at the metacarpophalangeal joint give rise to *small* fingertip displacements. Likewise, the forearm was predicted to be used most for large fingertip displacements even though the forearm was found to have the smallest preferred angular excursion because small angular displacements at the elbow give rise to *large* fingertip displacements.

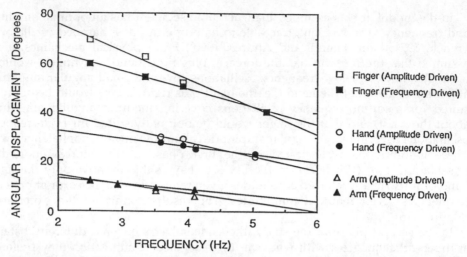

Figure 1.16. *Angular displacement of the finger, hand and arm in frequency-driven conditions (in which the fingertip was supposed to move at different prescribed frequencies over subjects' preferred amplitudes) or in amplitude-driven conditions (in which the fingertip was supposed to cover different prescribed amplitudes at subjects' preferred frequencies). [From Rosenbaum et al., 1991.]*

Because Vaughan *et al.* wished to understand the control of impact forces, but the optimal selection model was designed with respect to optimal amplitudes and frequencies of motion, they suggested that the impact control problem might be treated as a problem of spatial control. They reasoned that, if the limb were moved to an impact surface as if the target was *beyond* the surface, the impulse of collision, for any movement frequency, would increase with the distance beyond the surface to which the movement was aimed. Vaughan *et al.* called this point beyond the impact surface the *virtual* target. By estimating the locations of the virtual targets from the kinematics of subjects' movements, they estimated the amplitudes of the movements that subjects, by hypothesis, tried to generate. Vaughan *et al.* then tested the prediction of the optimal selection model that relative contributions of the finger, hand and forearm would depend on the functional proximity of those limb segments' optima to the frequency and (estimated) amplitude that had to be produced. The model did well: the finger was used most for tasks demanding high frequencies and low impulses of collision; the hand was used most for tasks demanding intermediate frequencies and intermediate impulses of collision; and the arm was used most for tasks demanding low frequencies and high impulses of collision.

Another task for which the optimal selection proved successful was drawing. Meulenbroek *et al.* (1992) analyzed the relative contribution of the fingers, hand and forearm to displacement of a pen in back-and-forth drawing tasks. In each trial, subjects produced back-and-forth drawing motions of a pen so the lines that were drawn became steadily longer or shorter, and the performance was completed in a short, medium or long time. Meulenbroek *et al.* (1992) made SELSPOT recordings of the effectors during this task and found that the fingers were used most for small-amplitude, high-frequency drawing; the hand was used most for medium-amplitude, medium-frequency drawing; and the forearm was used most for

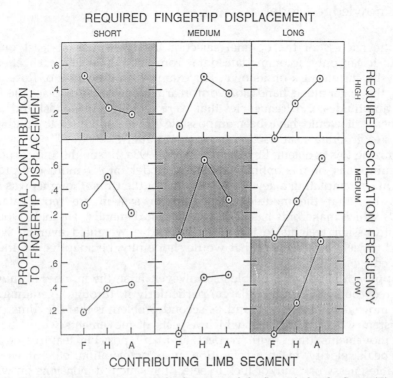

REQUIRED FINGERTIP DISPLACEMENT

Figure 1.17. *Proportional contribution to displacement of the fingertip by the finger (F), hand (H) and forearm (A) when the required fingertip displacement was best for the finger (short), best for the hand (medium), or best for the forearm (long), and when the required oscillation frequency was best for the finger (high), best for the hand (medium), or best for the forearm (low), as well as all other combinations of these displacement and frequency values. [From Rosenbaum et al., 1991.]*

large-amplitude, low-frequency drawing. Thus, the results agreed with the predictions of the optimal selection model. An additional finding was that there were hysteresis effects: when subjects steadily increased the amplitudes of the lines, the amplitude at which the forearm began to be used was higher than it was when the amplitude steadily decreased. A similar result was obtained for the fingers.

These asymmetries – the defining feature of hysteresis – were accounted for in terms of 'computational inertia': given that selection of limb segments may be computationally demanding, it may be adaptive to persist for as long as possible with a given limb segment combination. The trigger for switching to a different limb segment combination may in turn depend on feedback. The feedback strategy would relieve the burden on the central control mechanisms responsible for determining how much work should be done by the effectors. The latter proposal was offered in an earlier study concerning choices of hand grips in sequential reaching tasks (Rosenbaum and Jorgensen, 1992).[11]

---

[11]Another possible advantage of hysteresis is that it can serve to prevent oscillation when the system occupies a region near a threshold.

5.3.2   Knowledge Model

Despite the success of the optimal selection model, it has at least one major limitation: it can only accommodate data from tasks in which each effector can complete the current task on its own. For example, in the study of Rosenbaum *et al.* (1991), the finger alone, hand alone or forearm alone could displace the fingertip over the amplitudes and frequencies that were required. If the task did not have this property, it would have been impossible for the modules to combine their influences to generate a satisfactory movement pattern.

Recognizing this problem, Rosenbaum *et al.* (1993a, b) sought to incorporate the basic assumptions of the optimal selection model into a more comprehensive account. In contemplating a new approach, one of their first thoughts was that one could assume that the modules of the motor system are representations of *movements* which make bids based on fits to task demands. The bids would then be used to assign weights to the modules, and a weighted average would be generated to yield a movement that would, hopefully, be adaptive for the task to be achieved.

This approach has several problems, however. First, the number of movements to be stored could be extremely large, particularly if, through averaging, a truly adaptive movement had to be found. A second problem is that the dimensionality of the system would be unclear: which aspects of movements would be stored? Because movements differ with respect to many possible features (e.g. mean velocity, peak velocity, mean acceleration, peak acceleration, etc.), it would take considerable guesswork and/or luck to select the salient dimensions on which the stored movements differ. A third problem is that research on memory for movements indicates that people do not remember movements accurately. When asked to reproduce movement amplitudes, for example, subjects do poorly (Smyth, 1984). Insofar as movement amplitudes might be viewed as primary features of movement representations, people's inability to remember amplitudes suggests that movements *per se* are not remembered and hence are not stored.

What people do seem to remember in 'memory-for-movement' tasks are *positions* to which they previously moved (Smyth, 1984). For example, in one particularly dramatic study (Kelso and Holt, 1980), subjects who were temporarily deprived of sensation from the thumb were able to reproduce the position to which they just brought the thumb, even if the thumb was passively displaced from its original starting position. Kelso and Holt accounted for this result with the mass-spring model. According to the model as applied to this task, subjects recalled the equilibrium position to which they brought the thumb. Rosenbaum *et al.* (1993a, b) reasoned that if equilibrium positions are primary from the point of view of motor *generation*, they may also be primary from the point of view of *storage*.

Based on this line of reasoning, Rosenbaum *et al.* (1993a, b) proposed that the motor system selects movements by relying on stored *postures*. A posture – or at least an adopted posture – can be viewed as an equilibrium position, in the mass-spring sense. Rosenbaum *et al.* hypothesized that postures are the basic stored elements of motor control. The set of stored postures is part of the knowledge used for motor performance. Emphasizing knowledge in this way, Rosenbaum *et al.* dubbed their system the *knowledge* model.[12]

If postures are the stored elements of the motor system, how does the motor system select *movements*? The solution proposed in the knowledge model is as follows. When a spatial location is chosen, stored postures are evaluated for their potential for bringing the hand to that location. (One can also conceptualize the process as one in which posture modules become activated according to their own self-determined evaluations.) Each posture is evaluated with respect to two costs: a *spatial error cost* and a *travel cost*. A posture's spatial error cost is the Euclidean distance between the location the hand would occupy if the candidate posture were adopted and the spatial location of the target. (Note that there is no guarantee a posture will be available with a negligible spatial error cost for a given spatial target, because the number of spatial targets is infinite, whereas the number of stored postures is limited.) A posture's travel cost is related to the difficulty of moving from the starting posture, which is assumed to be known, to the candidate posture. The travel cost for a given posture is the sum of the angular displacements of all the joints, where each joint's angular displacement is multiplied by a cost-of-movement factor specific to each joint, and where the sum is divided by the required movement time. The cost-of-movement factor for a joint depends on the joint's stiffness, friction and the average moments of inertia of the limb segments attached to it; the exact form of the dependency has not yet been specified in the model, although in the modeling done so far (which has concentrated on the movement patterns of a seated stick figure capable of generating movements in the sagittal plane by rotating the hip, shoulder and elbow), the hip has generally been assigned a higher cost-of-movement value than the shoulder, and the shoulder has generally been assigned a higher cost-of-movement value than the elbow. The knowledge model allows the cost-of-movement factors of the joints to change as a function of experience. For example, if the elbow is injured, making it difficult to bend, its cost-of-movement factor increases. One advantage of this capacity for change is that other joints can compensate for the relative immobility of the injured joint. How this occurs can be understood by considering other basic aspects of the knowledge model, which are discussed below.

Consider again the instant when a spatial target has been designated and the knowledge system polls its stored postures. All the postures are assigned (or provide their own) spatial error costs and travel costs, and the two costs for each posture are combined into a *total cost*. Based on the total costs for all the stored postures, they are assigned weights so that, ultimately, a weighted average of the postures is derived. This weighted average constitutes the single *target posture* to which a movement will be made.[13]

The final step is to move physically from the starting posture to the target posture. The movement is governed by joint interpolation. At each moment, the

---

[12]The model was also given this name to highlight the fact that skillful movement requires knowledge – a point that has not been adequately appreciated by most cognitive psychologists today. Witness the fact that few if any cognitive psychology textbooks include a discussion of action control.

angular velocity of each joint is given by the following equation:

$$\omega_j(t) = \eta_j \omega_j(t-1) + (1 - \eta_j)\omega_j^*(t) \tag{5}$$

where $\omega_j(t)$ denotes the angular velocity of the j-th joint at time t, η_j $(0 \leqslant \eta_j \leqslant 1)$ is an index of inertia, and $\omega_j^*(t)$ is proportional to the angular distance still to be covered by the j-th joint at time t.[14] Equation (5) can be rewritten:

$$\omega_j(t) = \eta_j \omega_j(t-1) + (1 - \eta_j)\beta(|x_j(t) - x_j(T)|) \tag{6}$$

where β is a positive constant, x_j denotes the j-th joint angle, and T denotes the required movement time. Implementing this equation successively over time allows the joints to reduce their angular distances from their respective target positions.

Figure 1.18 shows a typical set of angular velocity profiles produced by the model. The curves are asymmetrically bell-shaped, as observed in many studies (for review, see Bullock and Grossberg, 1988). The reason for the curves' shape is that inertia causes speed to increase when the limb starts from rest, whereas the drive to reach the target, which coresponds to $\omega_j^*(t)$ in equation (5), simultaneously causes speed to *decrease* as the limb approaches the target. The concept of letting drive decrease as a target is approached is common in servosystems and has been used in other simulation models of limb kinematics, notably the model of Bullock and Grossberg (1988).

In Figure 1.18, the elbow has the highest peak angular velocity and the hip has the lowest peak angular velocity. This is because, in this particular example, the hip has the highest index of inertia and the elbow has the lowest index of inertia. The inertial index is not the only determinant of peak velocity, however. Peak velocity also depends on the total angular displacement to be covered. This feature of the

---

[13]The way that weights are assigned to postures is as follows. The total costs of the postures serve as inputs to a Gaussian function. Because all the total costs have nonnegative values and the peak of the Gaussian is set to a total cost of zero, postures with small total costs receive large Gaussian values, whereas postures with large total costs receive small Gaussian values. After Gaussian values have been assigned to all postures, a weight is assigned to each posture, where the weight for each posture equals the posture's Gaussian value divided by the sum of the Gaussian values assigned to all the postures. Finally, the weights are applied to their respective postures and a weighted sum of the postures is obtained. It is possible to obtain a weighted posture sum because postures can be viewed as vectors in joint space; the dimensionality of the space corresponds to the number of mechanical degrees of freedom of the body (i.e. the number of ways the joints can move). Note that the process of taking a weighted sum is analogous to population coding, which is used widely in the nervous system (Erickson, 1984; Georgopoulos, 1990, 1991; Wise and Desimone, 1988). The reason for taking a weighted sum of the postures rather than using the posture with the smallest total cost is to allow new postures to be generated deliberately.

[14]η_j is an index of inertia but not equal to inertia itself, because η_j is dimensionless, whereas (rotational) inertia is expressed in kg m^2.

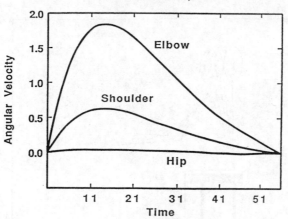

Figure 1.18. *Theoretical angular velocity profiles of the hip, shoulder and elbow produced by the knowledge model. [From Rosenbaum et al., 1993a.]*

model is consistent with the finding that peak velocity increases with the distance to be traversed (Soechting and Lacquaniti, 1981).

The most important achievement of the knowledge model is the way it selects limb segment patterns. Figure 1.19 shows that the model allows intact joints to compensate for joints whose normal mobility has been impaired. In this example, the stick figure brings its hand from one location to another, where in one case the elbow has the lowest cost of movement and in the other case the elbow has the highest cost of movement (as might occur if the elbow were injured). In the disabled elbow case, the other joints contribute more than usual. The compensation occurs because the stored postures that require large elbow displacements are assigned high total costs and are therefore given low weights. The ultimately chosen target

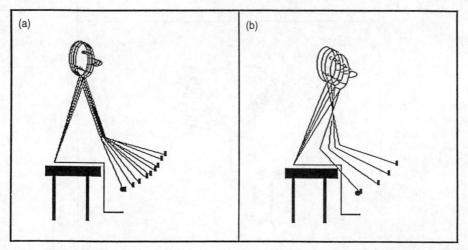

Figure 1.19. *(a) Reaches from one point to another when the cost of movement is highest for the hip, lower for the shoulder and lowest for the elbow; or (b) when the cost of movement is highest for the elbow, lower for the shoulder and lowest for the hip. [From Rosenbaum et al., 1993a.]*

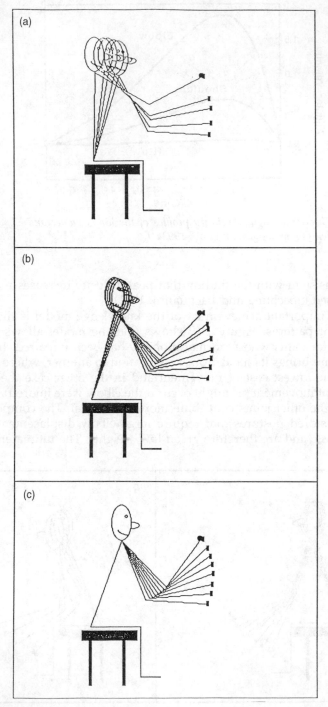

Figure 1.20. *Reaches from one point to another when the speed is: (a) low, (b) medium, or (c) high.* *[From Rosenbaum et al., 1993a.]*

posture is one that demands more hip movement and more shoulder movement than would normally occur.

Besides allowing for variation in limb segment patterns depending on the relative costs of movement of the joints, the knowledge model also predicts that limb segment patterns should depend on the required speed of motion. (Recall that this was the main result of the study reported by Rosenbaum *et al.*, 1991.) Specifically, the prediction is that as the required speed of motion increases, the contribution of high cost-of-movement joints should decrease. For example, if the hip has a high cost of movement and the shoulder and elbow have lower costs of movement, increased speed should result in reduced hip rotation. This prediction has been confirmed through computer simulation (Figure 1.20) and in a recent experiment with human subjects (Fischer *et al.*, in press).

5.3.3 Extensions of the Knowledge Model

Although the knowledge model has so far been developed using a simple stick figure with only three degrees of freedom, it can be applied to more complex motion systems. Indeed, the computations assumed in the model are extendable to systems with arbitrary numbers of degrees of freedom. Several extensions of the model have been implemented. It is worth mentioning them here to indicate how the model is expected to change at the time of writing.

One change is to allow for feedforward correction. In the original model, the hand sometimes missed the spatial target because the weighted average did not bring the hand close enough to the target to count as an accurate reach. (Such inaccuracies are common in averaging schemes; see Jordan and Rosenbaum, 1989.) A solution to this problem is to aim for spatial targets that are equal and opposite in sign to the spatial positions the hand would occupy if proposed target postures were adopted. The latter positions are estimable by relying on forward kinematics (i.e. using the limb lengths and joint angles of the proposed target posture to compute the hand's spatial location). The idea is to acknowledge biases in the system and compensate for them by exploiting them. The way the procedure works can be understood by considering the following example.

When one of us (DAR) goes bowling, he often inadvertently rolls the ball too far to the left. To compensate for this error, he deliberately aims to the right of the original target, and his performance often improves. The method used in the extended knowledge model is analogous (Figure 1.21). If the hand position associated with a proposed target posture is too far to the right, say by x_1 distance units, and too high, say by y_1 units, the system aims for a new target that is x_1 units to the *left* and y_1 units *below* the original spatial target (i.e. at $-x_1, -y_1$); this new target can be called a *virtual* target. If aiming for the virtual target leads to the hand still being too far removed from the target, this time by x_2 and y_2, then another virtual target can be aimed for, located at $-x_2$ and $-y_2$ with respect to the original spatial target. If the next hand position is still too far from the original spatial target, the process can be repeated. The entire *virtual targeting* procedure can be used over and over again until the hand's final position is acceptably close to the target. The method appears to work well, judging from simulation work done so far.

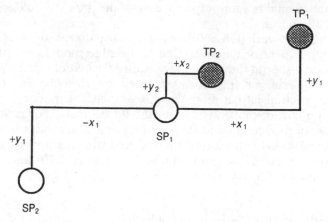

Figure 1.21. *Virtual targeting procedure. The spatial position of the hand associated with the first target posture* (TP$_1$) *deviates from the first spatial target* (SP$_1$) *by a horizontal distance* $+x_1$ *and a vertical distance* $+y_1$. *To compensate for the bias, a second spatial target* (SP$_2$) *is aimed for, located at* $-x_1$ *and* $-y_1$ *with respect to* SP$_1$. *Aiming for* SP$_2$ *gives rise to a second target posture* (TP$_2$) *for which the spatial position of the hand deviates from* SP$_1$ *by a horizontal distance* $+x_2$ *and a vertical distance* $+y_2$.

Notice that, for the above system to work, it is necessary to assume that forward kinematics can be computed. It is an empirical question whether it can be. If it can, then one not only can achieve feedforward correction, as assumed in the virtual targeting scheme outlined above, but one can also wield tools effectively. That is, by knowing the length of the hand-held tool, the spatial location of its end-point (or any point of interest along its length) can be determined. The result is that the tool can be used to reach objects without extensive reliance on feedback. From the fact that people can use tools effectively for this purpose (Solomon and Turvey, 1988), it is reasonable to assume that forward kinematics can be computed, although other explanations need to be considered as well.

Another reason to believe that forward kinematics is naturally computable is that people can swat instantly at mosquitoes biting them on unpredictable skin locations, even when the skin covers a part of the body that may occupy different positions with respect to the swatting hand (e.g. on the left hand, which can occupy different positions with respect to the right hand). What is impressive about this feat is that people can reach instantly for the appropriate location defined not just in body (skin) space, but also in extracorporeal space, which accords with the idea that forward kinematics is easily computed.

A second extension of the model is related to learning. In the original knowledge model, learning occurred through the accumulation of new postures, each of which was a newly generated target posture. As more postures became available for creating weighted averages, the weighted averages improved. In particular, the spatial errors and travel costs of the target postures decreased with the number of postures in the knowledge base.

As appealing as this outcome may be, it is difficult to accept a simple accumulation model of learning, because as more postures have to be considered, processing time should increase (unless the system operates in a perfectly parallel fashion). The learning strategy used in the extended knowledge model avoids this problem by assuming a fixed number of stored postures, where the identities of the postures are random 'at birth', but where the strengths of the postures reflect a cumulative history of their weights. If the strength of a posture gets too low, it is dumped (or 'dies'), and when this happens a new random posture takes its place. Learning carried out in this manner mimics a Darwinian process. More postures become available for regions of joint space that have proven useful over time. As a result, more precise averaging should become possible for regions that have more available postures, and the number of virtual target cycles needed to arrive at an acceptably accurate posture – and hence the time needed to find such target postures – should diminish with the number of postures close to the posture ultimately chosen as the target.

The final extension of the knowledge model concerns the production of *sequences* of movements. The task of interest is motion to one target followed immediately by motion to another target. The extended model can generate two-movement sequences by relying on the following principles. First, target postures can be selected for both spatial targets before movement to either target begins. This makes it possible to avoid long delays between completion of the reach to the first target and initiation of the reach to the second target. Second, movements to the two targets can be orchestrated such that movement begins to the first target posture only, and then, when the achieved posture has become acceptably close to the first target posture, movement begins to the second target posture. By initiating the second movement before the first target posture has been reached, and by allowing inertia from the first movement to carry into the second movement, it should be possible to generate smooth, curved movements. It is expected (but has not yet been proved) that this procedure will cause the tangential velocity of the hand to increase as the hand path becomes less and less curved, as has been reported by Lacquaniti, Terzuolo and Viviani (1984).

Of course, the latter ideas are still speculative. Nonetheless, the knowledge model holds considerable promise, even as already formulated. Regardless of how the model ultimately fares, we believe it is likely that computational models will play an increasingly important role in studies of the antecedents (and ongoing control) of action. Such models allow for more detailed, exact accounts of complex processes, like those involved in action planning, than have been possible in the past (see also Jordan, this volume).

6 SERIES OF MULTI-DEGREE-OF-FREEDOM MOVEMENTS

The final section of this chapter is concerned with sequences of multi-degree-of-freedom movements. Because the control of movement sequencing is considered in depth in Ivry's chapter (this volume) and has been the subject of other reviews (Keele, Cohen and Ivry, 1990; Rosenbaum, 1991, Ch. 2 and 8; Sternberg, Knoll and Turock, 1990), our discussion is limited to aspects of sequencing that point to the combined importance of biomechanics and cognition.

6.1 End-State Comfort

As indicated earlier, the analysis of sequential behavior demands the postulation of detailed, internal programs. This point was made nearly 50 years ago by Lashley (1951) who argued, as we have, that the structure of successively performed behaviors, and especially the presence of anticipatory effects in such behaviors, indicates that the motor act performed at a given time is usually not triggered by feedback from the act performed just before it. Instead, a plan or program is needed to explain the timing and sequencing that is observed.

It is ironic, given this state of affairs, that some researchers have not accepted the program construct. Those who have not, have tended to avoid discussion of complex, nonrepetitive motor sequences, such as those that occur in spontaneous speech or keyboard performance. Instead, they have focused either on repetitive movements (Haken, Kelso and Bunz, 1985; Kugler and Turvey, 1987) or on discrete movements assumed to be closely tied to continuously available perceptual input (e.g. Bootsma and van Wieringen, 1990). In focusing on the latter kind of behavior there has been an assumption that the perceptual input is a trigger for the immediately succeeding action event. Although this may be true in some cases, the problem with this notion is that it denies anticipation and, more generally, independence between perception and action. A hallmark of voluntary behavior is that it can (though need not) be independent of the information available to the perceiver. As the children's book author, Dr Seuss, once wrote (Geisel and Geisel, 1990):

> You have brains in your head.
> You have feet in your shoes.
> You can steer yourself any direction you choose.
> You're on your own.
> And you know what you know.
> And YOU are the guy who'll decide where to go!

If poetry is not convincing, consider the following experiment. Subjects in a study reported by Rosenbaum *et al.* (1990) were asked to use the right hand to pick up a stick lying horizontally on a cradle. The stick could be picked up with an overhand grip or with an underhand grip. In one set of conditions, subjects were asked to grab the stick and point the left end down on a target located to the left of the cradle or on a target to the right of the cradle. In another pair of conditions, subjects were asked to grab the stick and point the *right* end down on either of the targets. *A priori*, subjects could have grabbed the stick in whatever way was most comfortable when it was first grabbed. From the fact that an overhand grip was more comfortable than an underhand grip, as confirmed in a rating study (Rosenbaum *et al.*, 1990), it would have been plausible for subjects always to use the overhand grip. However, as shown in Figure 1.22, subjects grabbed the stick differently depending on which end would be brought to the target. When the right end would be brought to the target, subjects grabbed the stick with the overhand grip, but when the left end would be brought to the target, subjects grabbed the stick with the underhand grip.

Through a further series of experiments, it was shown that the source of this effect was a preference for completing the task with the arm in a comfortable

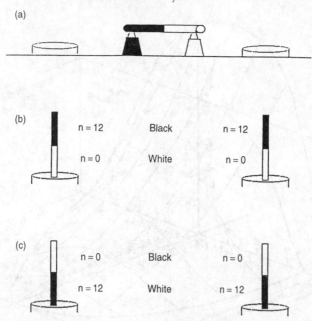

Figure 1.22. *Object manipulation task. (a) The experimental arrangement, consisting of a stick lying in a cradle and the two targets on which the black or white end could be placed. (b) When the white end was placed on the left or right target, 12 of 12 subjects grabbed the stick with the thumb toward the black end. (c) When the black end was placed on the left or right target, 12 of 12 subjects grabbed the stick with the thumb toward the white end. [From Rosenbaum* et al., *1992b.]*

position (i.e. at or near the middle of its range of motion). The preference was also manifested in tasks in which either end of the stick was carried to targets occupying different heights (Rosenbaum and Jorgensen, 1992), tasks in which the stick was moved from one vertical position to another under reaction-time pressure (Rosenbaum *et al.*, 1992a), and tasks in which a handle was turned so one end or the other pointed to a designated clock position (Rosenbaum *et al.*, 1992b). The most important feature of this widespread *end-state comfort* effect is that it cannot be attributed to the optic array or to simple coupling between the perceiver and the actor. Because subjects saw the same physical arrangement in virtually all the conditions of the experiments, all that was varied was what the subjects knew they were supposed to do (based on the experimenter's verbal instructions). This knowledge, coupled with what subjects had learned earlier about the capabilities of their bodies, led them to exhibit the end-state comfort effect.

Attributing subjects' choices to what they know leaves open the question of why they preferred what they did. Why were subjects willing to sacrifice initial comfort for final comfort? Many possible answers were considered (Rosenbaum *et al.*, 1992b). The answer that appeared most compelling was that the middle of the range of motion of the arm is the part of the range that affords the quickest back-and-forth motion, which is the sort of movement that is needed for rapid positioning of an object on a target. Consistent with this explanation, it was recently shown that the arm can make more rapid back-and-forth motions near the middle

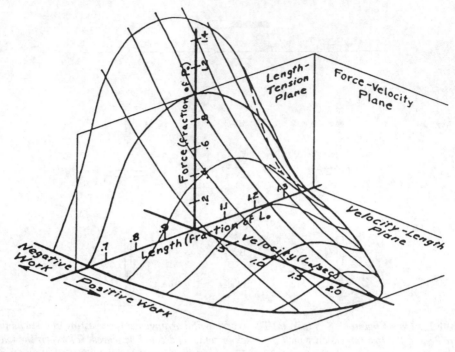

Figure 1.23. *Force–length–velocity surface. [From Winter, 1990.]*

of its range of motion than at the extremes (Rosenbaum, Heugten and Caldwell, in press).

The latter effect may have grounds in biomechanics, as shown in Figure 1.23, which presents the functional relationship between muscle force, length and velocity. As indicated in the figure, both the highest velocities and the highest forces can be achieved in the middle of the muscle's length range (and so, in the middle of its range of motion). Note that these curves represent contributions of *active* muscle forces only; contributions of *passive* forces are not depicted. Nonetheless, to the extent that the curves provide a simple explanation of greater speed at intermediate muscle lengths (the midrange of supination–pronation) than at extreme muscle lengths (full supination or full pronation), it is reasonable to hypothesize that active muscle forces are the main determinant of movement speed for these sorts of movements. Apparently, subjects had implicit knowledge of this fact when they selected their reaching and grasping motions in the object manipulation studies reviewed above.

6.2   Throwing and Related Tasks

A final activity that illustrates the joint importance of biomechanics and cognition is throwing and related acts involving propulsion of an object with the body. A variety of skills require an object to be projected at high speeds, such as throwing, striking or kicking for maximum distance. Perfection of these skills requires optimization of multilink movements with respect to the timing and sequencing of segmental submovements. Professional baseball pitchers, for example, achieve release speeds of more than $30\,\mathrm{m\,s}^{-1}$ (Hay, 1985). They achieve peak angular velocities in the rotation of the pelvis about the hip joint first, and in rotation of the hand about the wrist last (Atwater, 1979). Similar sequences are observed for the javelin throw (Menzel, 1986), the tennis serve (van Gheluwe and Hebbelinck, 1985), the badminton smash (Gowitzke and Waddell, 1979), the shot-put (Zatsiorsky, Lanka and Shalmanov, 1981), the golf swing (Milburn, 1982) and soccer kicking (Robertson and Mosher, 1985).

Although it is possible to ascribe the timing of these body segment motions to cognitive planning alone, it would be a mistake to do so. All the skills involve a system of segmental links that constitute an open kinetic chain. A defining feature of an open kinetic chain is that the system of links is free to move at its most distal segment (hand, foot or implement). The motion of a whip provides an example: the external torque applied at the handle of the whip accelerates the system as a whole and gives it angular momentum. Because of the elastic properties of the whip, it does not rotate all at once; rather, the more distal the segment the later it is affected by the motion of the handle. The angular momentum of the system travels from the handle to the tip, expressing itself in ever smaller parts of the system. Therefore, the rotational inertia of the system decreases as well. According to the law of conservation of momentum, the angular velocity increases at the same rate as the rotational inertia decreases. This effect outstrips the concurrent reduction of the radius of rotation, so the tip of the whip eventually acquires a speed that can be supersonic; in fact, the 'crack' of the whip is literally a sonic boom. What occurs in throwing, kicking and whipping, then, is the transfer of kinetic energy and momentum from proximal to distal body segments and finally to the ball or whip itself. That a whip, by virtue of its physical structure, can allow for the transfer of kinetic energy and momentum from the source of the energy to its tip indicates that the transfer need not be deliberately planned or programmed. Throwing and related skills may similarly exploit the whip-like characteristics of the extremities. The fact that the elbow can be extended much more quickly in a normal throwing movement than in the isolated act of extending the elbow as quickly as possible (Toyoshima *et al.*, 1974) accords with the view that the arm is passively swung like a whip during throwing. The whip metaphor implies that all the details of the throwing motion need not be programmed in advance.

Nevertheless, active muscular torque production, especially in the base segments, plays an important role in generating maximum velocities in the end-effector. Alexander (1991) showed that the proper sequencing of muscular contractions is indeed essential for the perfection of skills like shot-putting or throwing. Using simple mathematical models that included two muscles, one of which moved a more distal part of the body than the other, he investigated the consequences of varying the delay between activation of the more proximal muscle and activation of the more distal one. He found that it is usually best to activate the proximal muscle before the distal muscle and that there is an optimal delay that maximizes the kinetic energy given to the projectile. Alexander (1991) also found that under special circumstances the order of activation has to be reversed: in his model of shot-putting, the distal muscle must be activated first if the shot is very heavy (30% of the body mass). As this modeling work shows, and as related experiments have confirmed (Robertson and Mosher, 1985), successful throwing relies on skillful sequencing and timing adaptively tuned to the mechanics of the system being controlled. It is just this blend of exploiting or coping with mechanics on the one hand and governing the many degrees of freedom of the body in single and extended series of movements on the other that typifies the problems to be solved by the systems involved in selecting, preparing and executing the actions we carry out every day.

ACKNOWLEDGEMENTS

Preparation of this chapter was aided by grants BNS-8710933, BNS-9008665 and SBR 9308671 from the National Science Foundation, NIMH Research Scientist Development Award (KO2 MH00977-01A1), and a University of Massachusetts BRSG Faculty Research Grant (all to the first author), and grant Kr1213/1-1 from the Deutsche Forschungsgemeinschaft (to the second author). We thank Herbert Heuer and Steven Keele for helpful comments. Correspondence should be sent to the first author at the Department of Psychology, Moore Building, Pennsylvania State University, University Park, Pennsylvania 16802, USA (electronic mail: DAR12@CAC.PSU.EDU) or to the second author at Fachbereich Psychologie, Johann Wolfgang Goethe-Universität, Frankfurt am Main, Georg-Voigt Strasse 8, Postfach 11 19 32, D-6000 Frankfurt am Main 11, Germany (electronic mail: Horst.Krist@psych.uni-frankfurt.d400.de).

REFERENCES

Abbs, J. H., Gracco, V. L. and Cole, K. J. (1984). Control of multimovement coordination: Sensorimotor mechanisms in speech motor programming. *Journal of Motor Behavior*, **16**, 195–231.

Abdusamatov, R. M., Adamovitch, S. V. and Feldman, A. G. (1987). A model for one-joint motor control in man. In G. N. Gantchev, B. Dimitrov and P. Gatev (Eds), *Motor Control* (pp. 183–187). New York: Plenum Press.

Abrams, R. A., Meyer, D. E. and Kornblum, S. (1989). Speed and accuracy of saccadic eye movements: Characteristics of impulse variability in the oculomotor system. *Journal of Experimental Psychology: Human Perception and Performance*, **15**, 529–543.

Abrams, R. A., Meyer, D. E. and Kornblum, S. (1990). Eye–hand coordination: Oculomotor control in rapid aimed limb movements. *Journal of Experimental Psychology: Human Perception and Performance*, **16**, 248–267.

Adamovitch, S. V. and Feldman, A. G. (1989). The prerequisites for one-joint motor control theories. *Behavioral and Brain Sciences*, **12**, 210–211.

Adams, J. A. (1971). A closed-loop theory of motor learning. *Journal of Motor Behavior*, **3**, 111–149.

Alexander, R. M. (1984). Walking and running. *American Scientist*, **72**, 348–354.

Alexander, R. M. (1991). Optimum timing of muscle activation for simple models of throwing. *Journal of Theoretical Biology*, **150**, 349–372.

Asanuma, H. (1981). The pyramidal tract. In V. B. Brooks (Ed.), *Handbook of Physiology*, Vol. 2: *Motor Control* (pp. 703–733). Bethesda, MD: American Physiological Society.

Asatryan, D. G. and Feldman, A. G. (1965). Functional tuning of the nervous system with control of movement or maintenance of a steady posture. I. Mechanographic analysis of the work of the joint on execution of a postural task. *Biophysics*, **10**, 925–935.

Atkeson, C. G. (1989). Learning arm kinematic and dynamics. *Annual Review of Neuroscience,* **12,** 157–183.

Atwater, A. E. (1979). Biomechanics of overarm throwing movements and of throwing injuries. *Exercise and Sport Science Reviews,* **7,** 43–85.

Bahill, A. T., Clark, M. and Stark, L. (1975). The main sequence, a tool for studying human eye movements. *Mathematical Biosciences,* **24,** 191–204.

Bawa, P. N. S. and Dickinson, J. (1982). Force as the controlling muscle variable in limb movement. *Behavioral and Brain Sciences,* **5,** 543.

Belen'kii, V. E., Gurfinkel, V. S. and Pal'tsev, E. I. (1967). Control elements of voluntary movements. *Biofizika,* **12,** 135–141.

Bengueral, A. P. and Cowan, H. A. (1974). Coarticulation of upper lip protrusion in French. *Phonetica,* **30,** 41–55.

Bernstein, N. (1967). *The Coordination and Regulation of Movements.* London: Pergamon.

Bizzi, E. (1980). Central and peripheral mechanisms in motor control. In G. E. Stelmach and J. Requin (Eds), *Tutorials in Motor Behavior* (pp. 131–144). Amsterdam: North-Holland.

Bizzi, E., Accornero, N., Chapple, W. and Hogan, W. (1984). Posture control and trajectory formation during arm movement. *Journal of Neuroscience,* **4,** 2738–2744.

Bizzi, E., Hogan, N., Mussa-Ivaldi, F. A. and Giszter, S. (1992). Does the nervous system use equilibrium-point control to guide single and multiple joint movements? *Behavioral and Brain Sciences,* **15,** 603–613.

Bizzi, E., Polit, A. and Morasso, P. (1976). Mechanisms underlying achievement of final head position. *Journal of Neurophysiology,* **39,** 435–444.

Bootsma, R. J. and van Wieringen, P. C. (1990). Timing an attacking forehand drive in table tennis. *Journal of Experimental Psychology: Human Perception and Performance,* **16,** 21–29.

Bouma, H. and Bouwhuis, D. G. (Eds). (1983). *Attention and Performance X: Control of Language Processes.* Hillsdale, NJ: Erlbaum.

Bridgeman, B. (1989). Skeletal and oculomotor control systems compared. *Behavioral and Brain Sciences,* **12,** 212.

Brooks, V. B. (1986). *The Neural Basis of Motor Control.* New York: Oxford University Press.

Brown, S. H. and Cooke, J. D. (1990). Movement-related phasic muscle activation. I. Relations with temporal profile of movement. *Journal of Neurophysiology,* **63,** 455–464.

Bullock, D. (1989). Saturation is not an evolutionarily stable strategy. *Behavioral and Brain Sciences,* **12,** 212–214.

Bullock, D. and Grossberg, S. (1988). Neural dynamics of planned arm movements: Emergent invariants and speed–accuracy properties during trajectory formation. *Psychological Review,* **95,** 49–90.

Capaday, C. and Cooke, J. D. (1983). Vibration-induced changes in movement-related EMG activity in humans. *Experimental Brain Research,* **52,** 139–146.

Carlton, L. G. (1981). Visual information: The control of aiming movements. *Quarterly Journal of Experimental Psychology,* **33A,** 87–93.

Cole, K. J., Gracco, V. L. and Abbs, J. H. (1984). Autogenic and nonautogenic sensorimotor actions in the control of multiarticulate hand movements. *Experimental Brain Research,* **56,** 582–585.

Cooke, J. D. (1980). The organization of simple, skilled movements. In G. E. Stelmach and J. Requin (Eds), *Tutorials in Motor Behavior* (pp. 199–212). Amsterdam: North-Holland.

Cooke, J. D. and Brown, S. H. (1990). Movement–related phasic muscle activation. II. Generation and functional role of the triphasic pattern. *Journal of Neurophysiology,* **63,** 465–472.

Corcos, D. M., Agarwal, G. C., Flaherty, B. P. and Gottlieb, G. L. (1990). Organizing principles for single joint movements. IV. Implications for isometric contractions. *Journal of Neurophysiology,* **64,** 1033–1042.

Corcos, D. M., Gottlieb, G. L. and Agarwal, G. C. (1989). Organizing principles for single joint movements. II. A speed-sensitive strategy. *Journal of Neurophysiology,* **62,** 358–368.

Cordo, P. J. (1987). Mechanisms controlling accurate changes in elbow torque. *Journal of Neuroscience,* **7,** 432–442.

Crossman, E. R. F. W. and Goodeve, P. J. (1963/1983). Feedback control of hand-movement and Fitts' law. *Quarterly Journal of Experimental Psychology*, **35A**, 251–278.

Dell, G. S. (1986). A spreading activation theory of retrieval in sentence production. *Psychological Review*, **93**, 283–321.

Duhamel, J. R., Colby, C. L. and Goldberg, M. E. (1992). The updating of the representation of visual space in parietal cortex by intended eye movements. *Science*, **255**, 90–92.

Ellis, A. W. and Young, A. W. (1988). *Human Cognitive Neuropsychology*. Hove and London: Erlbaum.

El'ner, A. N. (1973). Possibilities of correcting the urgent voluntary movements and associated postural activity of human muscles. *Biophysics*, **18**, 966–971.

Erickson, R. P. (1984). On the neural bases of behavior. *American Scientist*, **72**, 233–241.

Favilla, M., Hening, W. and Ghez, C. (1989). Trjaectory control in targeted force impulses. VII. Independent setting of amplitude and direction in response preparation. *Experimental Brain Research*, **79**, 530–538.

Feldman, A. G. (1966a). Functional tuning of the nervous system with control of movement or maintenance of a steady posture: II. Controllable parameters of the muscles. *Biophysics*, **11**, 565–578.

Feldman, A. G. (1966b). Functional tuning of the nervous system with control of movement or maintenance of a steady posture: III. Mechanographic analysis of execution by man of the simplest motor tasks. *Biophysics*, **11**, 766–775.

Feldman, A. G. (1974a). Change of muscle length as a consequence of a shift in equilibrium in the muscle-load system. *Biophysics*, **19**, 544–548.

Feldman, A. G. (1974b). Control of the length of a muscle. *Biophysics*, **19**, 776–771.

Feldman, A. G. (1980). Superposition of motor programs. I. Rhythmic forearm movements in man. *Neuroscience*, **5**, 81–90.

Feldman, A. G. (1986). Once more on the equilibrium-point hypothesis (model) for motor control. *Journal of Motor Behavior*, **18**, 17–54.

Fischer, M. H., Rosenbaum, D. A., and Vaughan, J. (in press). Speed and sequential effects in posture and movement selection. *Journal of Experimental Psychology: Human Perception and Performance*.

Fitts, P. M. (1954). The information capacity of the human motor system in controlling the amplitude of movement. *Journal of Experimental Psychology*, **47**, 381–391.

Fitts, P. M. and Peterson, J. R. (1964). Information capacity of discrete motor responses. *Journal of Experimental Psychology*, **67**, 103–112.

Flanders, M., Helms Tillery, S. I. and Soechting, J. F. (1992). Early stages in a sensorimotor transformation. *Behavioral and Brain Sciences*, **15**, 309–362.

Forssberg, H., Grillner, S. and Rossignol, S. (1975). Phase dependent reflex reversal during walking in chronic spinal cats. *Brain Research*, **55**, 247–304.

French, A. P. (1971). *Vibrations and Waves*. New York: Norton.

Freud, S. (1901/1971). *The Psychopathology of Everyday Life*. [Translated by A. Tyson.] New York: Norton.

Freund, H.-J. and Büdingen, H. J. (1978). The relationship between speed and amplitude of the fastest voluntary contractions of human arm muscles. *Experimental Brain Research*, **31**, 1–12.

Fromkin, V. A. (Ed.). (1980). *Errors in Linguistic Performance*. New York: Academic Press.

Geisel, T. S. and Geisel, A. S. (1990). *Oh, The Places You'll Go!* New York: Random House.

Georgopoulos, A. (1990). Neurophysiology of reaching. In M. Jeannerod (Ed.), *Attention and Performance*, vol. XIII (pp. 227–263). Hillsdale, NJ: Erlbaum.

Georgopoulos, A. P. (1991). Higher order motor control. *Annual Review of Neuroscience*, **14**, 361–377.

Ghez, C. and Gordon, J. (1987). Trajectory control in targeted force impulses. I. Role of opposing muscles. *Experimental Brain Research*, **67**, 225–240.

Ghez, C., Hening, W. and Favilla, M. (1990). Parallel interacting channels in the initiation and specification of motor response features. In M. Jeannerod (Ed.), *Attention and Performance*, vol. XIII (pp. 265–293), Hillsdale, NJ: Erlbaum.

Ghez, C. and Martin, J. H. (1982). The control of rapid limb movement in the cat. III. Agonist–antagonist coupling. *Experimental Brain Research*, **45**, 115–125.

Ghez, C. and Vicario, D. (1978a). The control of rapid limb movement in the cat. I. Response latency. *Experimental Brain Research*, **33**, 173–189.

Ghez, C. and Vicario, D. (1978b). The control of rapid limb movement in the cat. II. Scaling of isometric force adjustments. *Experimental Brain Research*, **33**, 191–202.

Gibson, J. J. (1979). *The Ecological Approach to Visual Perception*. Boston, MA: Houghton-Mifflin.

Gielen, C. C. A. M. and Denier van der Gon, J. J. (1989). If a particular strategy is used, what aspects of the movement are controlled? *Behavioral and Brain Sciences*, **12**, 218–219.

Goodman, D. and Kelso, J. A. S. (1980). Are movements prepared in parts? Not under compatible (naturalized) conditions. *Journal of Experimental Psychology: General*, **109**, 475–495.

Goodwin, G. M., McCloskey, D. I. and Matthews, P. B. C. (1972). The contribution of muscle afferents to kinaesthesia shown by vibration-induced illusions of movement and by the effect of paralysing joint afferents. *Brain*, **95**, 705–748.

Gordon, J. and Ghez, C. (1987a). Trajectory control in targeted force impulses. II. Pulse height control. *Experimental Brain Research*, **67**, 241–252.

Gordon, J. and Ghez, C. (1987b). Trajectory control in targeted force impulses. III. Compensatory adjustments for initial errors. *Experimental Brain Research*, **67**, 253–269.

Gottlieb, G. L., Corcos, D. M. and Agarwal, G. C. (1989a). Organizing principles for single joint movements. I. A speed-insensitive strategy. *Journal of Neurophysiology*, **62**, 342–357.

Gottlieb, G. L., Corcos, D. M. and Agarwal, G. C. (1989b). Strategies for the control of single mechanical degrees of freedom voluntary movements. *Journal of Neurophysiology* **12**, 189–210.

Gottlieb, G. L., Corcos, D. M., Agarwal, G. C. and Latash, M. L. (1990). Organizing principles for single joint movements. III. The speed-insensitive strategy as default. *Journal of Neurophysiology*, **63**, 625–636.

Gowitzke, B. and Waddell, D. B. (1979). Techniques of badminton stroke production. In J. Terauds (Ed.), *Science in Racket Sports* (pp. 17–42). Del Mar, CA: Academic Publishers.

Granit, R. (1955). *Receptors and Sensory Perception*. New Haven, CT: Yale University Press.

Grudin, J. G. (1983). Error patterns in novice and skilled typists. In W. E. Cooper (Ed.), *Cognitive Aspects of Skilled Typewriting* (pp. 121–143). New York: Springer.

Haggard, P. and Wing, A. M. (1991). Remote responses to perturbation in human prehension. *Neuroscience Letters*, **122**, 103–108.

Haken, H., Kelso, J. A. S. and Bunz, H. (1985). A theoretical model of phase transitions in human hand movements. *Biological Cybernetics*, **51**, 347–356.

Hallett, M., Shahani, B. T. and Young, R. R. (1975). EMG analysis of stereotyped voluntary movements in man. *Journal of Neurology, Neurosurgery, and Psychiatry*, **38**, 1154–1161.

Harris, C. M., Wallman, J. and Scudder, C. A. (1990). Fourier analysis of saccades in monkeys and humans. *Journal of Neurophysiology*, **63**, 877–886.

Hasan, Z. (1986). Optimized movement trajectories and joint stiffness in unperturbed, inertially loaded movements. *Biological Cybernetics*, **53**, 373–382.

Hay, J. G. (1985). *The Biomechanics of Sports Techniques*, 3rd edn. Englewood Cliffs, NJ: Prentice-Hall.

Helmholtz, H. von (1866/1962). *Handbook of Physiological Optics*. New York: Dover. [Translation of *Handbuch der physiologischen Optik*. Hamburg: Voss.]

Hening, W., Vicario, D. and Ghez, C. (1983). Choice reaction time conditions after response dynamics in an isometric tracking task in humans. *Society for Neuroscience Abstracts*, **9**, 1031.

Henry, F. M. and Rogers, D. E. (1960). Increased response latency for complicated movements and a 'memory drum' theory of neuromotor reaction. *Research Quarterly*, **31**, 448–458.

Heuer, H. (1984). Binary choice reaction time as a function of the relationship between durations and forms of responses. *Journal of Motor Behavior*, **16**, 392–404.

Hick, W. E. (1952). On the rate of gain of information. *Quarterly Journal of Experimental Psychology*, **4**, 11–26.

Hill, A. V. (1938). The heat of shortening and dynamic constants of muscle. *Proceedings of the Royal Society, B*, **126**, 136–195.

Hogan, N. (1984). An organizing principle for a class of voluntary movements. *Journal of Neuroscience*, **4**, 2745–2754.

Hollerbach, J. M. (1982). Computers, brains and the control of movement. *Trends in Neurosciences*, **5**, 189–192.

Holt, K. G., Hamill, J. and Andres, R. O. (1990). The force-driven harmonic oscillator as a model for human locomotion. *Human Movement Science*, **9**, 55–68.

Houk, J. C. and Rymer, J. C. (1981). Neural control of muscle length and tension. In V. B. Brooks (Ed.), *Handbook of Physiology*, vol. 2: *Motor Control*. Bethesda, MD: American Physiological Society.

Hyman, R. (1953). Stimulus information as a determinant of reaction time. *Journal of Experimental Psychology*, **45**, 188–196.

Jagacinski, R. J., Repperger, D. W., Moran, M. S., Ward, S. L. and Glass, B. (1980). Fitts' law and the microstructure of rapid discrete movements. *Journal of Experimental Psychology: Human Perception and Performance*, **6**, 309–320.

Jeannerod, M. (1981). Intersegmental coordination during reaching at natural objects. In J. Long and A. Baddeley (Eds), *Attention and Performance*, vol. IX (pp. 153–169). Hillsdale, NJ: Erlbaum.

Jeannerod, M. (1988). *The Neural and Behavioral Organization of Goal-directed Movements*. Oxford: Oxford University Press.

Jeannerod, M. (Ed.) (1990). *Attention and Performance*, vol. XIII: *Motor Control and Representation*. Hillsdale, NJ: Erlbaum.

Jordan, M. I. (1986). *Serial Order: A Parallel, Distributed Processing Approach*. Technical Report No. 8604. La Jolla, CA: University of California, San Diego, Institute for Cognitive Science.

Jordan, M. I. and Rosenbaum, D. A. (1989). Action. In M. I. Posner (Ed.), *Foundations of Cognitive Science* (pp. 727–767). Cambridge, MA: MIT Press.

Kalaska, J. F. and Crammond, D. J. (1992). Cerebral cortical mechanisms of reaching movements. *Science*, **255**, 1517–1523.

Keele, S. W. (1968). Movement control in skilled motor performance. *Psychological Bulletin*, **70**, 387–403.

Keele, S. W. (1986). Motor control. In J. K. Boff, L. Kaufman and J. P. Thomas (Eds), *Handbook of Human Perception and Performance*, vol. II (pp. 1–60). New York: John Wiley.

Keele, S. W., Cohen, A. and Ivry, R. (1990). Motor programs: Concepts and issues. In M. Jeannerod (Ed.), *Attention and Performance*, vol. XIII: *Motor Representation and Control* (pp. 77–110). Hillsdale, NJ: Erlbaum.

Keele, S. W. and Posner, M. I. (1968). Processing of visual feedback in rapid movements. *Journal of Experimental Psychology*, **77**, 155–158.

Kelso, J. A. S. (1981). Contrasting perspectives on order and regulation in movement. In J. Long and A. Baddeley (Eds), *Attention and Performance*, vol. IX (pp. 437–457). Hillsdale, NJ: Erlbaum.

Kelso, J. A. S. (1982). Editor's remarks. In J. A. S. Kelso (Ed.) *Human Motor Behavior: An Introduction* (pp. 237–238). Hillsdale, NJ: Erlbaum.

Kelso, J. A. S. and Holt, K. G. (1980). Exploring a vibratory systems analysis of human movement production. *Journal of Neurophysiology*, **43**, 1183–1196.

Kelso, J. A. S., Tuller, B., Vatikiotis-Bateson, E. and Fowler, C. A. (1984). Functionally specific articulatory cooperation following jaw perturbations during speech: Evidence for coordinative structures. *Journal of Experimental Psychology: Human Perception and Performance*, **10**, 812–832.

Klapp, S. T. (1974). Syllable-dependent pronunciation latencies in number naming: A replication. *Journal of Experimental Psychology*, **102**, 1138–1140.

Kornblum, S. (1965). Response competition and/or inhibition in two choice reaction time. *Psychonomic Science*, **2**, 55–56.

Krist, H., Fieberg, E. L. and Wilkening, F. (1993). Intuitive physics in action and judgment: The development of knowledge about projectile motion. *Journal of Experimental Psychology: Learning, Memory and Cognition*, **19**, 952–966.

Kugler, P. N. and Turvey, M. T. (1987). *Information, Natural Law and Self-Assembly of Rhythmic Movements: A Study in the Similitude of Natural Law*. Hillsdale, NJ: Erlbaum.

Kvalseth, T. O. (1980). An alternative to Fitts' law. *Bulletin of the Psychonomic Society*, **16**, 371–373.

Lacquaniti, F., Terzuolo, C. and Viviani, P. (1984). Global metric properties and preparatory processes in drawing movements. In S. Kornblum and J. Requin (Eds), *Preparatory States and Processes* (pp. 357–370). Hillsdale, NJ: Erlbaum.

Langolf, G. D., Chaffin, D. B. and Foulke, J. A. (1976). An investigation of Fitts' law using a wide range of movement amplitudes. *Journal of Motor Behavior*, **8**, 113–128.

Lashley, K. S. (1951). The problem of serial order in behavior. In L. A. Jeffress (Ed.), *Cerebral Mechanisms in Behavior* (pp. 112–131). New York: John Wiley.

Lee, D. N. and Thomson, J. A. (1982). Vision in action: The control of locomotion. In D. J. Ingle, M. A. Goodale and R. J. W. Mansfield (Eds), *Analysis of Visual Behavior* (pp. 411–433). Cambridge, MA: MIT Press.

Leikind, B. J. (1985). A generalization of constant acceleration formulas of Newtonian kinematics. Unpublished manuscript, UCLA.

Lestienne, F. (1979). Effects of inertial load and velocity on the braking process of voluntary limb movements. *Experimental Brain Research*, **35**, 407–418.

McCloskey, D. I. (1973). Differences between the senses of movement and position shown by the effects of loading and vibration of muscles in man. *Brain Research*, **61**, 119–131.

MacKay, D. G. (1987). *The Organization of Perception and Action: A Theory for Language and Other Cognitive Skills*. New York: Springer.

MacKay, W. A. (1989). Braking may be more critical than acceleration. *Behavioral and Brain Sciences*, **12**, 227–228.

Marteniuk, R. G., MacKenzie, C. L., Jeannerod, M., Athenes, S. and Dugas, C. (1987). Constraints on human arm movement trajectories. *Canadian Journal of Psychology*, **4**, 365–378.

Matin, L. (1972). Eye movements and perceived visual direction. In D. Jameson and L. Hurvich (Eds), *Handbook of Sensory Physiology*, Vol. 7 (pp. 331–380). Berlin: Springer.

Menzel, H. J. (1986). Biomechanik des Speerwurfs. In R. Ballreich and A. Kuhlow (Eds), *Biomechanik der Sportarten* (pp. 110–120). Stuttgart: Enke.

Merton, P. A. (1953). Speculations on the servo-control of movement. In G. E. W. Wolstenholme (Ed.), *CIBA Foundation Symposium, The Spinal Cord* (pp. 247–255). London: Churchill.

Meulenbroek, R. G. J., Rosenbaum, D. A., Thomassen, A. J. W. M. and Schomaker, L. R. B. (1992). Limb-segment selection in drawing behavior. *Quarterly Journal of Experimental Psychology*, **46A**, 273–299.

Meyer, D. E., Abrams, R. A., Kornblum, S., Wright, C. E. and Smith, J. E. K. (1988). Optimality in human motor performance: Ideal control of rapid aimed movements. *Psychological Review*, **95**, 340–370.

Meyer, D. E., Smith, J. E. K., Kornblum, S., Abrams, R. A. and Wright, C. E. (1990). Speed–accuracy tradeoffs in aimed movements: Toward a theory of rapid voluntary action. In M. Jeannerod (Ed.), *Attention and Performance*, vol. XIII (pp. 173–226). Hillsdale, NJ: Erlbaum.

Meyer, D. E., Smith, J. E. K. and Wright, C. E. (1982). Models for the speed and accuracy of aimed movements. *Psychological Review*, **89**, 449–482.

Michon, J. A. (1967). *Timing in Temporal Tracking*. Soesterberg, The Netherlands: Institute for Perception.

Milburn, P. D. (1982). Summation of segmental velocities in the golf swing. *Medicine and Science in Sports and Exercise*, **14**, 60–64.

Miller, J. (1982). Discrete versus continuous stage models of human information processing. *Journal of Experimental Psychology: Human Perception and Performance*, **8**, 273–296.

Needham, D. M. (1971). *Machina Carnia: The Biochemistry of Muscular Contraction in its Historical Development*. Cambridge: Cambridge University Press.

Nelson, W. L. (1983). Physical principles for economies of skilled movements. *Biological Cybernetics*, **46**, 135–147.

Newell, K. M. (1980). The speed–accuracy paradox in movement control: Error of time and space. In G. E. Stelman and J. Requin (Eds), *Tutorials in Motor Behavior* (pp. 501–510). Amsterdam: North-Holland.

Norman, D. A. (1981). Categorization of action slips. *Psychological Review*, **88**, 1–15.

Partridge, L. D. (1983). Neural control drives a muscle spring: A persisting yet limited motor theory. *Experimental Brain Research Supplementum*, **7**, 280–290.

Patla, A. E., Frank, J. S., Allard, R. and Thomas, E. (1985). Speed–accuracy characteristics of saccadic eye movements. *Journal of Motor Behavior*, **17**, 411–419.

Polit, A. and Bizzi, E. (1978). Processes controlling arm movements in monkeys. *Science*, **201**, 1235–1237.

Polit, A. and Bizzi, E. (1979). Characteristics of motor programs underlying arm movements in monkeys. *Journal of Neurophysiology*, **42**, 183–194.

Poulton, E. C. (1974). *Tracking Skill and Manual Control*. New York: Academic Press.

Reeve, T. G. and Proctor, R. W. (1984). On the advance preparation of discrete finger responses. *Journal of Experimental Psychology: Human Perception and Performance*, **10**, 541–553.

Reeve, T. G. and Proctor, R. W. (1985). Nonmotoric translation processes in the preparation of discrete finger responses: A rebuttal of Miller's (1985) analysis. *Journal of Experimental Psychology: Human Perception and Performance*, **11**, 234–241.

Requin, J., Riehle, A. and Seal, J. (1993). Neuronal networks for motor preparation. In D. E. Meyer and S. Kornblum (Eds), *Attention and Performance*, vol. XIV: *Synergies in Experimental Psychology, Artificial Intelligence and Cognitive Neuroscience* (pp. 745–769). Cambridge, MA: MIT Press, Bradford Books.

Requin, J. and Stelmach, G. E. (Eds). (1991). *Tutorials in Motor Neuroscience*. Netherlands: Kluwer.

Riehle, A. and Requin, J. (1989). Monkey primary motor and premotor cortex: Single-cell activity related to prior information about direction and extent of an intended movement. *Journal of Neurophysiology*, **61**, 534–549.

Robertson, S. and Mosher, R. E. (1985). Work and power of the leg muscles in soccer kicking. In D. A. Winter, R. W. Norman and R. P. Wells (Eds), *Biomechanics*, vol. IX–B (pp. 533–538). Champaign, IL: Human Kinetics.

Rosenbaum, D. A. (1980). Human movement initiation: Specification of arm, direction, and extent. *Journal of Experimental Psychology: General*, **109**, 444–474.

Rosenbaum, D. A. (1983). The movement precuing technique: Assumptions, applications, and extensions. In R. A. Magill (Ed.), *Memory and Control of Action* (pp. 231–274). Amsterdam: North-Holland.

Rosenbaum, D. A. (1987). Successive approximations to a model of human motor programming. In G. H. Bower (Ed.), *Psychology of Learning and Motivation*, vol. 21 (pp. 153–182). Orlando, FL: Academic Press.

Rosenbaum, D. A. (1991). *Human Motor Control*. San Diego, CA: Academic Press.

Rosenbaum, D. A., Engelbrecht, S. E., Bushe, M. M. and Loukopoulos, L. D. (1993a). Knowledge model for selecting and producing reaching movements. *Journal of Motor Behavior* **25**, 217–227. [Special issue edited by T. Flash and A. Wing: *Modeling the control of upper limb movement*.]

Rosenbaum, D. A., Engelbrecht, S. E., Bushe, M. M. and Loukopoulos, L. D. (1993b). A model for reaching control. *Acta Psychologica, 82*, 237–250.

Rosenbaum, D. A., Heugten, C. and Caldwell, G. C. (in press). From cognition to biomechanics and back: The end-state comfort effect and the middle-is-faster effect. *Acta Psychologica*.

Rosenbaum, D. A., Inhoff, A. W. and Gordon, A. M. (1984). Choosing between movement sequences: A hierarchical editor model. *Journal of Experimental Psychology: General, 113*, 372–393.

Rosenbaum, D. A. and Jorgensen, M. J. (1992). Planning macroscopic aspects of manual control. *Human Movement Science, 11*, 61–69.

Rosenbaum, D. A., Kenny, S. and Derr, M. A. (1983). Hierarchical control of rapid movement sequences. *Journal of Experimental Psychology: Human Perception and Performance, 9*, 86–102.

Rosenbaum, D. A., Marchak, F., Barnes, H. J., Vaughan, J., Slotta, J. and Jorgensen, M. (1990). Constraints for action selection: Overhand versus underhand grips. In M. Jeannerod (Ed.), *Attention and Performance*, vol. XIII (pp. 321–342). Hillsdale, NJ: Erlbaum.

Rosenbaum, D. A. and Patashnik, O. (1980). A mental clock-setting process revealed by reaction times. In G. E. Stelman and J. Requin (Eds), *Tutorials in Motor Behavior* (pp. 487–499). Amsterdam: North-Holland.

Rosenbaum, D. A., Slotta, J. D., Vaughan, J. and Plamondon, R. J. (1991). Optimal movement selection. *Psychological Science, 2*, 86–91.

Rosenbaum, D. A., Vaughan, J., Barnes, H. J. and Jorgensen, M. J. (1992a). Time course of movement planning: Selection of hand grips for object manipulation. *Journal of Experimental Psychology: Learning, Memory, and Cognition, 18*, 1058–1073.

Rosenbaum, D. A., Vaughan, J., Jorgensen, M. J., Barnes, H. J. and Stewart, E. (1992b). Plans for object manipulation. In D. E. Meyer and S. Kornblum (Eds), *Attention and Performance*, vol. XIV: *A Silver Jubilee: Synergies in Experimental Psychology, Artificial Intelligence and Cognitive Neuroscience* (pp. 803–820). Cambridge, MA: MIT Press, Bradford Books.

Saltzman, E. (1979). Levels of sensorimotor representation. *Journal of Mathematical Psychology, 20*, 91–163.

Schmidt, R. A. (1975). A schema theory of discrete motor skill learning. *Psychological Review, 82*, 225–260.

Schmidt, R. A. (1988). *Motor Control and Learning*, 2nd edn. Champaign, IL: Human Kinetics.

Schmidt, R. A. and McGown, C. (1980). Terminal accuracy of unexpectedly loaded rapid movements: Evidence for a mass-spring mechanism in programming. *Journal of Motor Behavior, 12*, 149–161.

Schmidt, R. A., Sherwood, D., Zelaznik, H. N. and Leikind, B. (1985). Speed–accuracy trade-offs in motor behavior: Theories of impulse variability. In H. Heuer, U. Kleinbeck and K.-H. Schmidt (Eds), *Motor Behavior: Programming, Control, and Acquisition* (pp. 79–123). Berlin: Springer.

Schmidt, R. A., Zelaznik, H. N. and Frank, J. S. (1978). Sources of inaccuracy in rapid movement. In G. E. Stelmach (Ed.), *Information Processing in Motor Control and Learning* (pp. 183–203). New York: Academic Press.

Schmidt, R. A., Zelaznik, H. N., Hawkins, B., Frank, J. S. and Quinn, J. T., Jr (1979). Motor output variability: A theory for the accuracy of rapid motor acts. *Psychological Review, 86*, 415–451.

Shaffer, L. H. (1984). Timing in musical performance. In J. Gibbon and L. Allan (Eds), *Timing and Time Perception* (pp. 420–428). New York: New York Academy of Sciences.

Shapiro, D. C. and Walter, C. B. (1986). An examination of rapid positioning movements with spatiotemporal constraints. *Journal of Motor Behavior, 18*, 372–395.

Sherwood, D. E., Schmidt, R. A. and Walter, C. B. (1988). Rapid movements with reversals in direction. II. Control of movement amplitude and inertial load. *Experimental Brain Research, 69*, 355–367.

Sittig, A. C., Denier van der Gon, J. J. and Gielen, C. C. A. M. (1985). Separate control of arm position and velocity demonstrated by vibration of muscle tendon in man. *Experimental Brain Research, 60*, 445–453.

Sittig, A. C., Denier van der Gon, J. J. and Gielen, C. C. A. M. (1987). The contribution of afferent information on position and velocity to the control of slow and fast human forearm movements. *Experimental Brain Research*, **67**, 33–40.

Skavenski, A. A. and Hansen, R. M. (1978). Role of eye position information in visual space perception. In J. Senders, D. Fisher and R. Monty (Eds), *Eye Movements and the Higher Psychological Functions* (pp. 15–34). Hillsdale, NJ: Erlbaum.

Smyth, M. M. (1984). Memory for movements. In M. M. Smyth and A. M. Wing (Eds), *The Psychology of Human Movement* (pp. 83–117). London: Academic Press.

Soechting, J. F. and Flanders, M. (1989). Sensorimotor representations for pointing to targets in three-dimensional space. *Journal of Neurophysiology*, **62**, 582–594.

Soechting, J. F. and Lacquaniti, F. (1981). Invariant characteristics of a pointing movement in man. *Journal of Neuroscience*, **1**, 710–720.

Solomon, H. Y. and Turvey, M. T. (1988). Haptically perceiving the distances reachable with hand-held objects. *Journal of Experimental Psychology: Human Perception and Performance*, **14**, 404–427.

Stein, R. B. (1982). What muscle variable(s) does the nervous system control in limb movements? *Brain and Behavioral Sciences*, **5**, 535–577.

Sternberg, S., Knoll, R. L. and Turock, D. L. (1990). Hierarchical control in the execution of action sequences: Tests of two invariance properties. In M. Jeannerod (Ed.), *Attention and Performance*, vol. XIII (pp. 1–55). Hillsdale, NJ: Erlbaum.

Sternberg, S., Monsell, S., Knoll, R. L. and Wright, C. E. (1978). The latency and duration of rapid movement sequences: Comparisons of speech and typewriting. In G. E. Stelmach (Ed.), *Information Processing in Motor Control and Learning* (pp. 117–152). New York: Academic Press.

Sternberg, S., Wright, C. E., Knoll, R. L. and Monsell, S. (1980). Motor programs in rapid speech. In R. Cole (Ed.), *Perception and Production of Fluent Speech*. Hillsdale, NJ: Erlbaum.

Taub, E. and Berman, A. J. (1968). Movement and learning in the absence of sensory feedback. In S. J. Freeman (Ed.), *The Neuropsychology of Spatially Oriented Behavior* (pp. 173–192). Homewood, IL: Dorsey.

Toyoshima, S., Hoshikawa, T., Miyashita, M. and Oguri, T. (1974). Contribution of the body parts to throwing performance. In R. C. Nelson and C. A. Morehouse (Eds), *Biomechanics*, vol. IV (pp. 169–174). Baltimore, MD: University Park Press.

Turvey, M. T. (1990). The challenge of a physical account of action: A personal view. In H. T. A. Whiting, O. G. Meijer and P. C. van Wieringen (Eds), *The Natural–Physical Approach to Movement Control* (pp. 57–93). Amsterdam: VU University Press.

Van Gheluwe, B. and Hebbelinck, M. (1985). The kinematics of the service movement in tennis: A three-dimensional cinematographical approach. In D. A. Winter, R. W. Norman and R. P. Wells (Eds), *Biomechanics*, vol. IX-B (pp. 521–526). Champaign, IL: Human Kinetics.

van Heugten, C. (1992). The end-state comfort effect revisited: Biomechanical considerations. Unpublished doctoral dissertation. Leiden University, Leiden, The Netherlands.

Vallbo, A. (1981). Basic patterns of muscle spindle discharge in man. In A. Taylor and A. Prochazka (Eds), *Muscle Receptors and Movement* (pp. 263–275). London: Macmillan Press.

Vaughan, J., Rosenbaum, D. A., Moore, C. and Diedrich, F. (in press). Cooperative selection of movements: The optimal selection model. *Psychological Research*.

Vince, M. A. (1948). Corrective movements in a pursuit task. *Quarterly Journal of Experimental Psychology*, **1**, 85–103.

Vincken, M. H., Gielen, C. C. A. M. and Denier van der Gon, I. J. (1983). Intrinsic and afferent components in apparent muscle stiffness in man. *Neuroscience*, **9**, 529–534.

von Holst, E. and Mittelstaedt, H. (1950). Das Reafferenzprinzip. Wechselwirkungen zwischen Zentralnervensystem und Peripherie. *Naturwissenschaften*, **37**, 464–476. [English translation in von Holst, E. (1973). The reafference principle. *The Behavioral Physiology of Animals and Man: The Collected Papers of Erich von Holst*, vol. 1, Translator R. Martin. London: Methuen.]

Wadman, W. J., Denier van der Gon, J. J., Genze, R. H. and Mol, C. R. (1979). Control of fast goal-directed arm movements. *Journal of Human Movement Studies*, **5**, 3–17.

Wallace, S. A. (1981). An impulse-timing theory for reciprocal control of muscular activity in rapid, discrete movements. *Journal of Motor Behavior*, **13**, 144–160.

Wiesendanger, M. (1987). Initiation of voluntary movements and the supplementary motor area. In H. Heuer and C. Fromm (Eds), *Generation and Modulation of Action Patterns* (pp. 3–13). Berlin: Springer.

Wing, A. M. (1980). The long and short of timing in response sequences. In G. E. Stelmach and J. Requin (Eds), *Tutorials in Motor Behavior* (pp. 469–486). Amsterdam: North-Holland.

Wing, A. M. and Kristofferson, A. B. (1973). Response delays and the timing of discrete motor responses. *Perception and Psychophysics*, **14**, 5–12.

Winter, D. A. (1990). *Biomechanics and Motor Control of Human Movement*, 2nd edn. New York: John Wiley.

Wise, S. P. and Desimone, R. (1988). Behavioral neurophysiology: Insights into seeing and grasping. *Science*, **242**, 736–741.

Woodworth, R. S. (1899). The accuracy of voluntary movement. *Psychological Review Monograph Supplements*, **3**, No. 3.

Wright, C. E. and Meyer, D. E. (1983). Conditions for a linear speed–accuracy trade-off in aimed movements. *Quarterly Journal of Experimental Psychology*, **35A**, 279–296.

Zatsiorsky, V. M., Lanka, G. E. and Shalmanov, A. A. (1981). Biomechanical analysis of shot putting technique. *Exercise and Sport Science Reviews*, **9**, 353–389.

Zelaznik, H. N., Hawkins, B. and Kisselburgh, L. (1983). Rapid visual feedback processing in single-aiming movements. *Journal of Motor Behavior*, **15**, 217–236.

Zelaznik, H. N., Mone, S., McCabe, G. P. and Thaman, C. (1988). Role of temporal and spatial precision in determining the nature of the speed–accuracy trade-off in aimed-hand movements. *Journal of Experimental Psychology: Human Perception and Performance*, **14**, 221–230.

Zelaznik, H. N., Schmidt, R. A. and Gielen, C. C. A. M. (1986). Kinematic properties of aimed hand movements. *Journal of Motor Behavior*, **18**, 353–372.

Zelaznik, H. N., Shapiro, D. C. and McColsky, D. (1981). Effects of a secondary task on the accuracy of single aiming movements. *Journal of Experimental Psychology: Human Perception and Performance*, **7**, 1007–1018.

Chapter 2

Computational Aspects of Motor Control and Motor Learning

Michael I. Jordan

Massachusetts Institute of Technology, USA

1 Introduction

This chapter provides a basic introduction to various of the computational issues that arise in the study of motor control and motor learning. A broad set of topics is discussed, including feedback control, feedforward control, the problem of delay, observers, learning algorithms, motor learning and reference models. The goal of the chapter is to provide a unified discussion of these topics, emphasizing the complementary roles that they play in complex control systems. The choice of topics is motivated by their relevance to problems in motor control and motor learning. However, the chapter is not intended to be a review of specific models; rather, we emphasize basic theoretical issues with broad applicability.

Many of the ideas described here are developed more fully in standard textbooks in modern systems theory, particularly textbooks on discrete-time systems (Åström and Wittenmark, 1984), adaptive signal processing (Widrow and Stearns, 1985) and adaptive control systems (Åström and Wittenmark, 1989; Goodwin and Sin, 1984). These texts assume a substantial background in control theory and signal processing, however, and many of the basic ideas that they describe can be developed in special cases with a minimum of mathematical formalism. There are also issues of substantial relevance to motor control that are not covered in these standard sources, particularly problems related to nonlinear systems and time delays. As we shall see, consideration of these problems leads naturally to a focus on the notion of an 'internal model' of a controlled system. Much of the discussion in the chapter will be devoted to characterizing the various types of internal models and describing their role in complex control systems.

In the next several sections, we develop some of the basic ideas in the control of dynamical systems, distinguishing between *feedback* control and *feedforward* control. In general, controlling a system involves finding an input to the system that will cause a desired behavior at its output. Intuitively, finding an *input* that will produce a desired *output* would seem to require a notion of 'inverting' the process that leads from inputs to outputs; that is, controlling a dynamical system would seem to involve the notion of 'inverting' the dynamical system. As we will see, this notion

Handbook of Perception and Action, Volume 2
ISBN 0-12-516162-X

can be made precise and made to serve as a useful unifying principle for understanding control systems. Indeed, feedback control and feedforward control can both be understood as techniques for inverting a dynamical system. Before developing these ideas we first discuss some mathematical representations for dynamical systems.

2 DYNAMICAL SYSTEMS

A fundamental fact about many systems is that knowledge of only the input to the system at a given time is not sufficient to predict its output. For example, to predict the flight of a ping-pong ball, it is not enough to know how it was struck by the paddle but it is also necessary to know its velocity and spin prior to being struck. Similarly, to predict the effects of applying a torque around the knee joint one must know the configuration and motion of the body. In general, to predict the effect of the input to a dynamical system, one must know the values of an additional set of variables known as *state variables*. Knowing the state of a system and its input at a given moment in time is sufficient to predict its state at the next moment in time.

In physical systems, the states of a system often have a natural physical interpretation. For example, knowing the position and velocity of a mass together with the force acting on the mass is sufficient to predict the position and velocity of the mass at the next instant of time. Thus position and velocity are the state variables and force is the input variable.

It is also common to specify an *output* of a dynamical system. Mathematically the output is simply a specified function of the state of the system. In many cases, the output has a physical interpretation as the set of measurements made by an external measuring device. In other cases, the choice of the output variables is dictated more by the goals of the modeler than by the existence of a measuring device. For example, the modeler of the ping-pong ball may be interested in tracking the kinetic and potential energy of the ball, perhaps as part of a theoretical effort to understand the ball's motion. In such a case the kinetic and potential energy of the ball, both of which are functions of the state, would be the output variables.

In general, a dynamical system can be characterized by a pair of equations: a *next-state equation* that expresses how the state changes as a function of the current state $\mathbf{x}[n]$ and the input $\mathbf{u}[n]$:

$$\mathbf{x}[n + 1] = f(\mathbf{x}[n], \mathbf{u}[n]) \tag{1}$$

where n is the time step, and an *output equation* that specifies how the output $\mathbf{y}[n]$ is obtained from the current state:[1]

$$\mathbf{y}[n] = g(\mathbf{x}[n]) \tag{2}$$

The functions f and g are referred to as the next-state function and the output function, respectively. It is often useful to combine these equations and write a

---

[1]We use discrete time throughout the chapter, mainly for pedagogical reasons. In the following section an example is given of converting a continuous-time dynamical system to a corresponding discrete-time dynamical system.

composite equation that describes how states and inputs map into outputs:

$$\mathbf{y}[n + 1] = h(\mathbf{x}[n], \mathbf{u}[n]) \tag{3}$$

where h is the composition of f and g.

Many sensorimotor transformations are naturally expressed in terms of state space models. To model speech production, for example, one might choose the positions and velocities of the speech articulators as state variables and the muscular forces acting on the articulators as input variables. The next-state equation would characterize the motion of the articulators. A natural choice of output variables for speech would be a spectral representation of the speech signal, thus the output equation would model the acoustics of the vocal tract.

There is another representation for dynamical systems that does away with the notion of state in favor of a representation in terms of sequences of input vectors. Consider again the ping-pong example: the velocity and spin of the ping-pong ball at a given moment in time can be analyzed in terms of the way the ball was struck at the preceding time step, the time step before that, and so on. In general, a dynamical system can be treated as a transformation from an infinite sequence of input vectors to an output vector:

$$\mathbf{y}[n + 1] = F(\mathbf{u}[n], \mathbf{u}[n - 1], \mathbf{u}[n - 2], \ldots) \tag{4}$$

This representation emphasizes the fact that a dynamical system can be treated as a mapping from an input sequence to an output sequence. The disadvantage of this representation is that the function F is generally much more complex than its counterparts f and g. In the remainder of this chapter we assume that a dynamical system can be expressed in terms of a set of state variables and a pair of functions f and g.[2]

---

[2]It is worth noting that in many dynamical systems the influence of the input dies away over time, so that an input–output relationship involving an infinite sequence of previous inputs (as in equation 4) can often be *approximated* by a truncated relationship involving only the last K inputs:

$$\mathbf{y}[n + 1] \approx \hat{F}(\mathbf{u}[n], \mathbf{u}[n - 1), \ldots, \mathbf{u}[n - K + 1]) \tag{5}$$

If we define the state variable $\mathbf{x}[n]$ as the sequence $\mathbf{u}[n - 1], \mathbf{u}[n - 2], \ldots, \mathbf{u}[n - K]$, then equation (5) can be represented in terms of the state equations:

$$\mathbf{x}[n + 1] = f(\mathbf{x}[n], \mathbf{u}[n])$$

and

$$\mathbf{y}[n] = g(\mathbf{x}[n])$$

where g is equal to $\hat{F}$ and f simply shifts the current input $\mathbf{u}[n]$ into the state vector while shifting $\mathbf{u}[n - K]$ out. Thus truncated input–output representations can be easily converted to state variable representations.

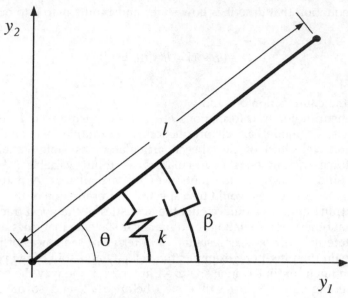

Figure 2.1. *A one-link mechanical system. A link of length* l *is subject to torques from a linear spring with spring constant* k *and a linear damper with damping constant* β.

2.1 Dynamics and Kinematics

The term 'dynamics' is used in a variety of ways in the literature on motor control. Two of the most common uses of the term derive from robotics (Hollerbach, 1982; Saltzman, 1979) and from dynamical systems theory (Haken, Kelso and Bunz, 1985; Turvey, Shaw and Mace, 1978). Let us review some of the relevant distinctions by way of an example.

Consider the one-link mechanical system shown in Figure 2.1. Newton's laws tell us that the angular acceleration of the link is proportional to the total torque acting on the link:

$$I\ddot{\theta} = -\beta\dot{\theta} - k(\theta - \theta_0) \tag{6}$$

where θ, $\dot{\theta}$, and $\ddot{\theta}$ are the angular position, velocity and acceleration, respectively, I is the moment of inertia, β is the damping coefficient, k is the spring constant, and θ_0 is the equilibrium position of the spring. This equation can be approximated by a discrete-time equation of the form:[3]

$$\theta[t + 2] = a_1\theta[t + 1] + a_2\theta[t] + b\theta_0[t] \tag{7}$$

where $a_1 = 2 - h\beta/I$, $a_2 = h\beta/I - h^2k/I - 1$, $b = h^2k/I$, and h is the time step of the discrete-time approximation.

---

[3]There are many ways to convert differential equations to difference equations. We have utilized a simple Euler approximation in which $\ddot{\theta}$ is replaced by $(\theta[t+2h]-2\theta[t + h] + \theta[t])/h^2$, and $\dot{\theta}$ is replaced by $(\theta[t+h]-\theta[t])/h$. For further discussion of discrete-time approximation of continuous-time dynamical systems, see Åström and Wittenmark (1984).

Let us suppose that movement of the link is achieved by controlled changes in the equilibrium position of the spring. Thus we define the control signal $\mathbf{u}[t]$ to be the time-varying equilibrium position $\theta_0[t]$ (cf. Hogan, 1984). Let us also define two state variables:

$$x_1[t] = \theta[t + 1]$$
$$x_2[t] = \theta[t]$$

Note that $x_2[t + 1] = x_1[t]$. We combine this equation with equation (7) to yield a single vector equation of the form:

$$\begin{pmatrix} x_1[t + 1] \\ x_2[t + 1] \end{pmatrix} = \begin{pmatrix} a_1 & a_2 \\ 1 & 0 \end{pmatrix} \begin{pmatrix} x_1[t] \\ x_2[t] \end{pmatrix} + \begin{pmatrix} b \\ 0 \end{pmatrix} u[t] \tag{8}$$

which is of the general form of a next-state equation (cf. equation 1).

Let us also suppose that we want to describe the position of the tip of the link at each moment in time by a pair of Cartesian coordinates y_1 and y_2. Elementary trigonometry gives us:

$$\begin{pmatrix} y_1[t] \\ y_2[t] \end{pmatrix} = \begin{pmatrix} l \, \cos(x_2[t]) \\ l \, \sin(x_2[t]) \end{pmatrix} \tag{9}$$

where l is the length of the link. This equation is an output equation of the form of equation (2).

Let us now return to the terminological issues that we raised earlier. We have described a dynamical system in terms of a next-state equation (equation 8) and an output equation (equation 9). For a roboticist, the next-state equation in this example is the *dynamics* of the link and the output equation is the *kinematics* of the link. In general, a roboticist uses the term 'dynamics' to refer to an equation that relates forces or torques to movement (e.g. accelerations). Such an equation generally corresponds to the next-state equation of a dynamical system. The term 'kinematics' is used to refer to a transformation between coordinate systems (e.g. angular coordinates to Cartesian coordinates). This generally corresponds to the output equation of a dynamical system. To a dynamical systems theorist, on the other hand, the next-state equation and the output equation together constitute a 'dynamical system'. In this tradition, the term 'dynamics' is used more broadly than in the mechanics tradition: any mathematical model that specifies how the state of a system evolves specifies the 'dynamics' of the system. No special reference need be made to forces or torques, nor, in many cases, to any notion of causality. Many useful dynamical systems models are simply descriptive models of the temporal evolution of an interrelated set of variables.

3 FORWARD AND INVERSE MODELS

The term 'model' is also used with a variety of meanings in the motor control literature. Most commonly, a model is a formal system that a scientist uses to describe or explain a natural phenomenon. There are models of muscle dynamics, models of reaching behavior, or models of the cerebellum. Another usage of the term model is in the sense of 'internal model'. An internal model is a structure or process in the central nervous system that mimics the behavior of some other natural process. The organism may have an internal model of some aspect of the external world, an internal model of its own musculoskeletal dynamics, or an internal model of some other mental transformation. Note that it is not necessary for the internal structure of a model to correspond in any way to the internal structure of the process being modeled. For example, an internal model might predict the distance that a propelled object will travel, without integrating the equations of motion, either explicitly or implicitly. (The prediction could be based, for example, on extrapolation from previous observations of propelled objects.) These two senses of 'model' are also often merged, in particular when a scientist's model of a phenomenon (e.g. reaching) posits an internal model of a sensorimotor transformation (e.g. an internal kinematic model). This dual or composite sense of 'model' captures the way in which we will often use the term in the remainder of the chapter. Thus a model of reaching may include a piece of formal machinery (generally a state space representation) that models the posited internal model.

Earlier sections introduced state space representations of dynamical systems. This mathematical framework requires a choice of variables to serve as inputs and a choice of variables to serve as outputs. For any particular dynamical system, the choice of variables is generally nonarbitrary and is conditioned by our understanding of the causal relationships involved. For example, in a dynamical model of angular motion it is natural to treat torque as an input variable and angular acceleration as an output variable. Models of motor control also tend to treat the relationships between variables in terms of a causal, directional flow. Certain variables are distinguished as motor variables and other variables are distinguished as (reafferent) sensory variables. In a dynamical model the motor variables are generally treated as inputs and the sensory variables are generally treated as outputs.

There are other transformations in motor control that are not generally conceived of in terms of causality, but which nonetheless are usefully thought of in terms of a directional flow. For example, the relationship between the joint coordinates of an arm and the spatial coordinates of the hand is not a causal relationship; however, it is still useful to treat spatial coordinates as being derived from joint coordinates. This is due to the *functional* relationship between joint coordinates and spatial coordinates. As is well known (Bernstein, 1967), the relationship between joint angles and spatial positions is many-to-one; that is, to any given spatial position of the hand there generally corresponds an infinite set of possible configurations of the joints. Thus the joint coordinates and the spatial coordinates have asymmetric roles in describing the geometry of the limb. This functional asymmetry parallels the asymmetry that arises from causal considerations and allows us to impose a directionality on sensorimotor transformations. We refer to the many-to-one, or causal, direction as a *forward* transformation, and to the one-to-many, or anticausal, direction as an *inverse* transformation.

The preceding considerations lead us to distinguish between forward models and inverse models of dynamical systems. Whereas a forward model of a dynamical system is a model of the transformation from inputs to outputs, an inverse model is a model of the transformation from outputs to inputs. Because the latter transformation need not be unique, there may be an infinite number of possible

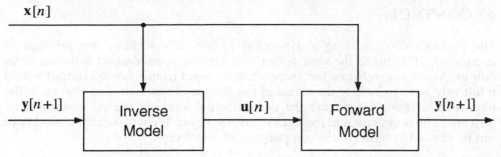

Figure 2.2. *The mathematical relationship between forward models and inverse models.*

inverse models corresponding to any given dynamical system.[4] The forward model
is generally unique.

Consider a dynamical system in the form of equation (3):

$$\mathbf{y}[n + 1] = h(\mathbf{x}[n], \mathbf{u}[n]) \tag{10}$$

Assuming that the transformation from $\mathbf{u}$ to $\mathbf{y}$ is a causal or many-to-one transformation, any system that produces $\mathbf{y}$ as a function h of $\mathbf{x}$ and $\mathbf{u}$ constitutes a forward
model of the dynamical system. Thus a forward model is a mapping from inputs
to outputs, in the context of a given state vector. Similarly, an inverse model is a
mapping from outputs to inputs, again in the context of a given state vector.
Mathematically, this relationship is expressed as follows:

$$\mathbf{u}[n] = h^{-1}(\mathbf{x}[n], \mathbf{y}[n + 1]) \tag{11}$$

Note that we use the symbol h^{-1} even though this equation is not strictly speaking
a mathematical inverse (it is not simply a swapping of the left and right sides of
equation 10). Nonetheless, equation (11) is to be thought of as inverting the
relationship between inputs and outputs in equation (10), with the state thought of
as a context. These relationships are summarized in Figure 2.2.

The terms 'forward model' and 'inverse model' are generally used to refer to
internal models of dynamical systems and it is in this sense that we use the terms
in the remainder of the chapter. Note that an internal model is a model of some
particular dynamical system; thus, it is sensible to speak of an 'approximate
forward model' or an 'approximate inverse model'. It is also important to distinguish between actual values of variables and internal estimates of variables, and to
distinguish between actual values of variables and desired values of variables. For
example, a ball flying through the air has an actual position and velocity, but an
internal model of the ball dynamics must work with internal estimates of position
and velocity. Similarly, we must distinguish between the desired position of the ball
and its actual or estimated position. We postpone a further discussion of these
issues until later sections in which we see how forward models and inverse models
can be used as components of control systems.

---

[4]The issue of *existence* of an inverse model will not play a significant role in this chapter; we will
generally assume that an inverse exists. We also ignore the issue of how noise affects questions of
existence and uniqueness.

4   CONTROL

The problem of controlling a dynamical system is essentially the problem of computing an input to the system that will achieve some desired behavior at its output. As we suggested earlier, computing an input from a desired output would intuitively seem to involve the notion of the inverse of the controlled system. In the next three sections we discuss the two principal kinds of control systems: feed forward control systems and feedback control systems. We will see that indeed both can be viewed in terms of the computation of an inverse.

4.1   Predictive Control

Suppose that the system to be controlled – the *plant* – is currently believed to be in state $\hat{x}[n]$. Suppose further that the desired output at the next time step is a particular vector $\mathbf{y}^*[n + 1]$.[5] We wish to compute the control signal $\mathbf{u}[n]$ that will cause the plant to output a vector $\mathbf{y}[n + 1]$ that is as close as possible to the desired vector $\mathbf{y}^*[n + 1]$.[6] Clearly the appropriate computation to perform is that given by equation (11); that is, we require an inverse model of the plant. An inverse model of the plant allows the control system to compute a control signal that is predicted to yield the desired future output. The use of an explicit inverse model of the plant as a controller is referred to as 'predictive control'. Predictive control comes in different varieties depending on the way the states are estimated.

A First-Order Example
Let us consider the simple first-order plant given by the following next-state equation:

$$x[n + 1] = 0.5x[n] + 0.4u[n] \tag{12}$$

and the following output equation:

$$y[n] = x[n] \tag{13}$$

Substituting the next-state equation into the output equation yields the forward dynamic equation:

$$y[n + 1] = 0.5x[n] + 0.4u[n] \tag{14}$$

If the input sequence $u[n]$ is held at zero, then this dynamical system decays exponentially to zero, as shown in Figure 2.3a.

A predictive controller for this system can be obtained by solving for $u[n]$ in equation (14):

$$u[n] = -1.25\hat{x}[n] + 2.5y^*[n + 1] \tag{15}$$

---

[5]We will use the 'hat' notation ($\hat{x}$) throughout the paper to refer to *estimated* values of signals and the 'asterisk' notation ($\mathbf{y}^*$) to refer to *desired* values of signals.
[6]This idea will be generalized in the section on model-reference control.

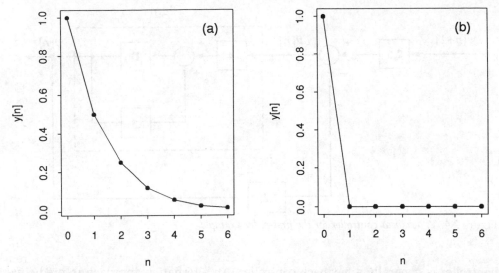

Figure 2.3. *(a) The output of the uncontrolled dynamical system in equation (14) with initial condition x[0]= 1. (b) The output of the dynamical system using the feedforward controller in equation (15). The desired output y*[n] is fixed at zero. The controller brings the actual output y[n] to zero in a single time step.*

Because this is an equation for a controller we treat y as the desired plant output rather than the actual plant output. Thus, the signal $y^*[n + 1]$ is the input to the controller and denotes the desired future plant output. The controller output is $u[n]$. Note that we also assume that the state $x[n]$ must be estimated.

Suppose that the controller has a good estimate of the state and suppose that it is desired to drive the output of the dynamical system to a value d as quickly as possible. Setting $y^*[n + 1]$ to d, letting $\hat{x}[n]$ equal $x[n]$, and substituting equation (15) into equation (14), we see that indeed the output y at time $n + 1$ is equal to d (Figure 2.3b). A predictive controller that can drive the output of a dynamical system to an arbitrary desired value in k time steps, where k is the order of the dynamical system (i.e. the number of state variables), is referred to as a *deadbeat* controller. In the following section, we provide a further example of a deadbeat controller for a second-order system.

How should the state be estimated in the deadbeat controller? Because the output equation (equation 13) shows that the state and the output are the same, a natural choice for the state estimate is the current output of the plant. Thus, the controller can be written in the more explicit form:

$$u[n] = -1.25y[n] + 2.5y^*[n + 1] \tag{16}$$

This choice of state estimator is not necessarily the best choice in the more realistic case in which there are disturbances acting on the system, however. In the section on observers, we shall discuss a more sophisticated approach to state estimation. Even in this more general framework, however, the state estimate is generally computed based on feedback from the output of the plant. Thus a deadbeat

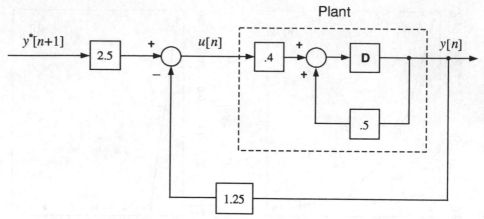

Figure 2.4. *A deadbeat controller for the first-order example.*

controller is generally a feedback controller. An alternative approach to predictive control design – open-loop feedforward control – is discussed below.

Figure 2.4 shows the deadbeat controller for the first-order example. The symbol 'D' in the figure refers to a one-time-step delay: a signal entering the delay is buffered for one time step. That is, if the signal on the right-hand side of the delay is $y[n]$, then the signal on the left-hand side of the delay is $y[n + 1]$. It can be verified from the figure that $y[n + 1]$ is equal to the sum of $0.5y[n]$ and $0.4u[n]$, as required by the dynamical equations for this system (equations 14 and 13).

A Second-Order Example
Higher-order dynamical systems are characterized by the property that the control signal does not normally have an immediate influence on the output of the system, but rather exerts its influence after a certain number of time steps, the number depending on the order of the system. In this section we design a deadbeat controller for a second-order plant to indicate how this issue can be addressed.

Consider a second-order dynamical system with the following next-state equation:

$$\begin{pmatrix} x_1[n + 1] \\ x_2[n + 1] \end{pmatrix} = \begin{pmatrix} a_1 & a_2 \\ 1 & 0 \end{pmatrix} \begin{pmatrix} x_1[n] \\ x_2[n] \end{pmatrix} + \begin{pmatrix} 1 \\ 0 \end{pmatrix} u[n] \tag{17}$$

and output equation:

$$y[n] = (0 \quad 1) \begin{pmatrix} x_1[n] \\ x_2[n] \end{pmatrix} \tag{18}$$

From the second row of equation (17) it is clear that the control signal cannot affect the second state variable in one time step. This implies, from equation (18), that the control signal cannot affect the output in a single time step. The control signal can affect the output in *two* time steps, however. Therefore we attempt to obtain a predictive controller in which the control signal is a function of the desired output two time steps in the future. Extracting the first component of the next-state equation and solving for $u[n]$ in terms of $x_2[n + 1]$, we obtain the following:

$$u[n] = -a_1\hat{x}_1[n] - a_2\hat{x}_2[n] + y^*[n + 2] \qquad (19)$$

where we have used the fact that $x_1[n + 1]$ is equal to $x_2[n + 1]$ (from the second next-state equation) and $x_2[n + 2]$ is equal to $y[n + 2]$ (from the output equation). Although this equation relates the control signal at time n to the desired output at time $n + 2$, there is a difficulty in estimating the states. In particular, $x_1[n]$ is equal to $y[n + 1]$, thus we would need access to a future value of the plant output in order to implement this controller. As it stands, the controller is unrealizable.

To remove the dependence on the future value of the output in equation (19), let us substitute the next-state equation into itself, thereby replacing $x_1[n]$ and $x_2[n]$ with $x_1[n - 1]$, $x_2[n - 1]$ and $u[n - 1]$. This substitution yields:

$$\begin{pmatrix} x_1[n + 1] \\ x_2[n + 1] \end{pmatrix} = \begin{pmatrix} a_1^2 + a_2 & a_1 a_2 \\ a_1 & a_2 \end{pmatrix} \begin{pmatrix} x_1[n - 1] \\ x_2[n - 1] \end{pmatrix} + \begin{pmatrix} a_1 \\ 1 \end{pmatrix} u[n - 1] + \begin{pmatrix} 1 \\ 0 \end{pmatrix} u[n]$$

Extracting the first component from this equation and solving for $\mathbf{u}[n]$ yields:

$$u[n] = -(a_1^2 + a_2)\hat{x}_1[n - 1] - a_1 a_2\hat{x}_2[n - 1] - a_1 u[n - 1] + y^*[n + 2]$$

This equation depends only on quantities defined at time n or earlier. In particular, $\hat{x}_1[n - 1]$ can be estimated by $y[n]$ and $\hat{x}_2[n - 1]$ can be estimated by $y[n - 1]$. This yields the following deadbeat controller:

$$u[n] = -(a_1^2 + a_2)y[n] - a_1 a_2 y[n - 1] - a_1 u[n - 1] + y^*[n + 2] \qquad (20)$$

The technique that we have described in this section is applicable to dynamical systems of any order. Because a state variable can always be expressed in terms of inputs and states at earlier moments in time, an unrealizable controller can always be converted into a realizable controller by expanding the next-state equation. It is worth pointing out that the technique is also applicable to nonlinear systems, assuming that we are able to invert the equation relating the control signal to the future desired output signal. In cases in which this equation cannot be inverted analytically it may be possible to use numerical techniques.[7] These issues will arise again in the section on motor learning.

4.1.1 Open-Loop Feedforward Control

The second class of predictive control systems is the class of open-loop feedforward control systems. Like the deadbeat controller, the open-loop feedforward controller is based on an explicit inverse model of the plant. The logic behind the open-loop

---

[7]It is also worth raising a cautionary flag: there is an important class of systems, including some linear systems, for which the techniques that we are discussing do not suffice and must be extended. Some systems are *uncontrollable*, which means that there are state variables that cannot be affected through a particular control variable. A proper treatment of this topic requires the notion of a *controllability gramian*. For further discussion, see Åström and Wittenmark (1984).

feedforward controller is the same as that behind the deadbeat controller: the controller computes a control signal which is predicted to yield a desired future output. The difference between the two approaches is the manner in which the state is estimated.

Example

In the previous section, we saw that a deadbeat controller for the first-order plant has the form:

$$u[n] = -1.25y[n] + 2.5y^*[n + 1]$$

where the signal $y[n]$ is considered to be an estimate of the state of the plant. We might also consider a controller of the following form:

$$u[n] = -1.25y^*[n] + 2.5y^*[n + 1] \tag{21}$$

in which the state is estimated by the desired plant output $y^*[n]$ rather than the actual plant output $y[n]$. Figure 2.5 shows a diagrammatic representation of this controller. Note that there is no feedback from the plant to the controller; the loop from plant to controller has been 'opened'. Because of the lack of a feedback term in the control equation, the open-loop approach allows the entire control signal to be 'preprogrammed' if the desired output trajectory is known in advance. The justification for the open-loop approach is that a good controller will keep the actual output and the desired output close together, so that replacing $y[n]$ by $y^*[n]$ in estimating the state may not incur much error. This is a strong assumption, however, because there are many sources of inaccuracy that can degrade the performance of a feedforward controller. In particular, if there are disturbances acting on the plant, then the state of the plant will diverge from the internal estimate of the state. Of course, no controller can control a system perfectly in the presence of disturbances. A system that utilizes feedback, however, has its state estimate continually reset and is therefore less likely to diverge significantly from reality than an open-loop controller. Another source of error is that the controller itself may be an inaccurate inverse model of the plant. Feedback renders the control system less sensitive to such inaccuracies.

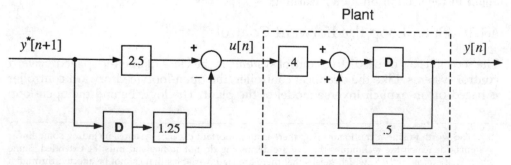

Figure 2.5. *An open-loop feedforward controller for the first-order example.*

One disadvantage of controllers based on feedback is that feedback can introduce stability problems. For this reason, open-loop feedforward controllers have important roles to play in certain kinds of control problems. As we discuss in a later section, stability is particularly of concern in systems with delay in the feedback pathway; thus an open-loop controller may be a reasonable option in such cases. Open-loop controllers also have an important role to play in composite control systems, when they are combined with an error-correcting feedback controller (see below). The division of labor into open-loop control and error-correcting control can be a useful way of organizing complex control tasks.

4.1.2   Biological Examples of Feedforward Control

There are many examples of open-loop feedforward control systems in the motor control literature. A particularly clear example is the vestibulo-ocular reflex (VOR). The VOR couples the movement of the eyes to the motion of the head, thereby allowing an organism to keep its gaze fixed in space. This is achieved by causing the motion of the eyes to be equal and opposite to the motion of the head. The VOR control system is typically modeled as a transformation from head velocity to eye velocity (Robinson, 1981). The head velocity signal, provided by the vestibular system, is fed to a control system that provides neural input to the eye muscles. In our notation, the head velocity signal is the controller input $-\mathbf{y}^*[n]$, the neural command to the muscles is the control signal $\mathbf{u}[n]$, and the eye velocity signal is the plant output $\mathbf{y}[n]$. Note that the plant output (the eye velocity) has no effect on the control input (the head motion), thus the VOR is an open-loop feedforward control system. This implies that the neural machinery must implement an open-loop inverse model of the oculomotor plant. It is generally agreed in the literature on the VOR that such an inverse model exists in the neural circuitry and there have been two principal proposals for the neural implementation of the inverse model. Robinson (1981) has proposed a model based on an open-loop feedforward controller of the form shown in Figure 2.5. In this model, as in the figure, the inverse model is implemented by adding the signals on a pair of parallel channels: a feed-through pathway and a pathway incorporating a delay (which corresponds to an integrator in Robinson's continuous-time model). An alternative model, proposed by Galliana and Outerbridge (1984), implements the inverse model by placing a forward model of the plant in an internal feedback pathway. (A closely related technique is described later; see Figure 2.8).

Another interesting example of feedforward control arises in the literature on speech production. Lindblom, Lubker and Gay (1979) studied an experimental task in which subjects produced vowel sounds while their jaw was held open by a bite block. They observed that the vowels produced by the subjects had formant frequencies in the normal range, despite the fact that unusual articulatory postures were required to produce these sounds. Moreover, the formant frequencies were in the normal range during the first pitch period, before any possible influence of acoustic feedback. This implies feedforward control of articulatory posture (with respect to the acoustic goal). Lindblom *et al.* proposed a qualitative model of this feedforward control system that again involved placing a forward model of the plant in an internal feedback pathway (see Figure 2.8).

4.2   Error-Correcting Feedback Control

In this section we provide a brief overview of error-correcting feedback control systems. Error-correcting feedback control differs from predictive control in that it does not rely on an explicit inverse model of the plant. As we shall see, however, an error-correcting feedback control system can be thought of as implicitly computing an approximate plant inverse; thus, these two forms of control are not as distinct as they may seem.

An error-correcting feedback controller works directly to correct the error at the current time step between the desired output and the actual output. Consider the first-order system presented earlier. A natural choice for an error-correcting feedback signal would be the weighted error:

$$u[n] = K(y^*[n] - y[n]) \qquad (22)$$

where the scalar K is referred to as a *gain*. Note that the reference signal for this controller is the current desired output ($y^*[n]$) rather than the future desired output ($y^*[n + 1]$) as in the predictive control approach. The performance of this feedback controller is shown in Figure 2.6 for several values of K. As K increases, the feedback controller brings the output of the plant to the desired value more rapidly.

A block diagram of the error-correcting feedback control system is shown in Figure 2.7, to be compared with the predictive controllers in Figures 2.4 and 2.5.

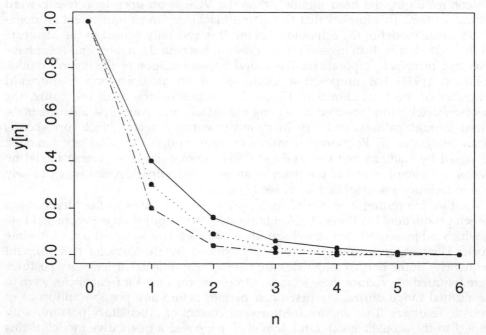

Figure 2.6. *Performance of the error-correcting feedback controller as a function of the gain. The desired output $y^*[n]$ is fixed at zero.* —, $K = 0.25; \dots, K = 0.50; -\cdot-, K = 0.75$.

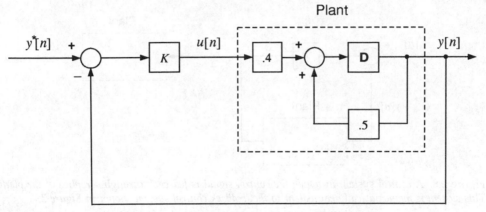

Figure 2.7. *An error-correcting feedback controller for the first-order example.*

Several general distinctions can be drawn from comparing these control systems. One important distinction between predictive and error-correcting control is based on the temporal relationships that are involved. In predictive control, the control signal is a function of the future desired output. If the predictive controller is a perfect inverse model of the plant, and if there are no unmodeled disturbances acting on the plant, then the future desired output will indeed by achieved by using the computed control signal. That is, an ideal predictive controller operates without error. An error-correcting feedback controller, on the other hand, corrects the error after the error has occurred, thus even under ideal conditions such a controller exhibits a certain amount of error. The assumption underlying error-correcting control is that the desired output changes relatively slowly; thus, correcting the error at the current time step is likely to diminish the error at the following time step as well. Another distinction between predictive control and error-correcting control has to do with the role of explicit knowledge about the plant. Predictive control requires explicit knowledge of the dynamics of the plant (a predictive controller is an inverse model of the plant). For example, the coefficients 1.25 and 2.5 in the predictive controllers in the previous section are obtained explicitly from knowledge of the coefficients of the plant dynamic equation. Error-correcting control does not require the implementation of an explicit plant model. The design of an error-correcting controller (i.e. the choice of the feedback gain) generally depends on knowledge of the plant. However the knowledge that is required for such control design is often rather qualitative. Moreover, the performance of an error-correcting controller is generally rather insensitive to the exact value of the gain that is chosen. The predictive controllers based on feedback (i.e. the deadbeat controllers) are also somewhat insensitive to the exact values of their coefficients. This is in contrast to open-loop controllers, for which the performance is generally highly sensitive to the values of the coefficients. For example, choosing a value other than 2.5 in the forward path of the open-loop controller in the previous section yields a steady-state error at the output of the plant. Finally, as we have stated earlier, feedback controllers tend to be more robust to unanticipated disturbances than open-loop controllers.

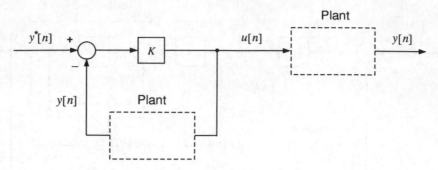

Figure 2.8. *A control system in which the control signal is fed back through a replica of the plant. This system is mathematically equivalent to the feedback control system shown in Figure 2.7.*

4.2.1   Feedback Control and Plant Inversion

Let us now establish a relationship between error-correcting feedback control and the notion of inverting a dynamical system. To simplify the argument we restrict ourselves to the first-order plant considered previously (Figure 2.7). Consider now the system shown in Figure 2.8, in which a replica of the plant is placed in a feedback path from the control signal to the error signal. This system is entirely equivalent to the preceding system, if we assume that there are no disturbances acting at the output of the plant. That is, the control signal in both diagrams is exactly the same:

$$u[n] = K(y^*[n] - y[n])$$

This error equation can be expanded using the next-state equation (12) and the output equation (13):

$$u[n] = Ky^*[n] - 0.5Ky[n-1] - 0.4Ku[n-1]$$

Dividing by K and moving $\mathbf{u}[n-1]$ to the left-hand side yields:

$$\frac{1}{K}u[n] + 0.4u[n-1] = y^*[n] - 0.5y[n-1]$$

If we now let the gain K go to infinity, the first term drops away and we are left with an expression for $u[n-1]$:

$$0.4u[n-1] = y^*[n] - 0.5y[n-1]$$

Shifting the time index and rearranging yields:

$$u[n] = -1.25y[n] + 2.5y^*[n+1]$$

This expression is an inverse dynamic model of the plant (cf. equation 16).

What we have shown is that, for large values of the gain, the internal loop in Figure 2.8 computes approximately the same control signal as an explicit inverse model of the plant.[8] Thus an error-correcting feedback control system with high gain is equivalent to an open-loop feedforward system that utilizes an explicit inverse model. This is true even though the feedback control system is clearly not computing an explicit plant inverse. We can think of the feedback loop as *implicitly* inverting the plant.

In many real feedback systems, it is impractical to allow the gain to grow large. One important factor that limits the magnitude of the gain is the presence of delays in the feedback loop, as we will see in the following section. Other factors have to do with robustness to noise and disturbances. It is also the case that some plants – so-called 'nonminimum phase' plants – are unstable if the feedback gain is too large (Åström and Wittenmark, 1984). Nonetheless, it is still useful to treat a feedback control system with a finite gain K as computing an *approximation* to an inverse model of the plant. This approximation is ideally as close as possible to a true inverse of the plant, subject to constraints related to stability and robustness.

The notion that a high-gain feedback control system computes an approximate inverse of the plant makes intuitive sense as well. Intuitively, a high-gain controller corrects errors as rapidly as possible. Indeed, as we saw in Figure 2.6, as the gain of the feedback controller grows, its performance approaches that of a deadbeat controller (Figure 2.3b).

It is also worth noting that the system shown in Figure 2.8 can be considered in its own right as an implementation of a *feedforward* control system. Suppose that the replica of the plant in the feedback loop in Figure 2.8 is implemented literally as an internal forward model of the plant. If the forward model is an accurate model of the plant, then in the limit of high gain this internal loop is equivalent to an explicit inverse model of the plant. Thus the internal loop is an alternative implementation of a feedforward controller. The controller is an open-loop feedforward controller because there is no feedback from the actual plant to the controller. Note that this alternative implementation of an open-loop feedforward controller is consistent with our earlier characterization of feedforward control: (1) the control system shown in Figure 2.8 requires explicit knowledge of the plant dynamics (the internal forward model); (2) the performance of the controller is sensitive to inaccuracies in the plant model (the loop inverts the forward model, not the plant); and (3) the controller does not correct for unanticipated disturbances (there is no feedback from the actual plant output).

4.3 Composite Control Systems

Because feedforward control and error-correcting feedback control have complementary strengths and weaknesses, it is sensible to consider composite control systems that combine these two kinds of control. There are many ways that

---

[8]In fact, the mathematical argument just presented is not entirely correct. The limiting process in our argument is well defined only if the discrete-time dynamical system is obtained by approximating an underlying continuous-time system, and the time step of the approximation is taken to zero as the gain is taken to infinity. Readers familiar with the Laplace transform will be able to justify the argument in the continuous-time domain.

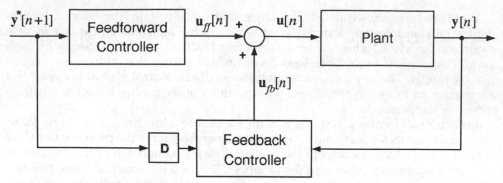

Figure 2.9. *A composite control system composed of a feedback controller and a feedforward controller.*

feedforward and feedback can be combined, but the simplest scheme – that of adding the two control signals – is generally a reasonable approach. Justification for adding the control signals comes from noting that because both kinds of control can be thought of as techniques for computing a plant inverse, the sum of the control signals is a sensible quantity.

Figure 2.9 shows a control system that is composed of a feedforward controller and an error-correcting feedback controller in parallel. The control signal in this composite system is simply the sum of the feedforward control signal and the feedback control signal:

$$\mathbf{u}[n] = \mathbf{u}_{ff}[n] + \mathbf{u}_{fb}[n]$$

If the feedforward controller is an accurate inverse model of the plant, and if there are no disturbances, then there is no error between the plant output and the desired output. In this case the feedback controller is automatically silent. Errors at the plant output, whether due to unanticipated disturbances or to inaccuracies in the feedforward controller, are corrected by the feedback controller.

5 DELAY

The delays in the motor control system are significant. Estimates of the delay in the visuomotor feedback loop have ranged from 100 to 200 ms (Carlton, 1981; Keele and Posner, 1968). Such a large value of delay is clearly significant in reaching movements, which generally last from 250 ms to a second or two.

Many artificial control systems are implemented with electrical circuits and fast-acting sensors, such that the delays in the transmission of signals within the system are insignificant when compared with the time constants of the dynamical elements of the plant. In such cases the delays are often ignored in the design and analysis of the controller. There are cases, however, including the control of processes in a chemical plant and the control of the flight of a spaceship, in which the delays are significant. In this section we make use of some of the ideas developed in the study of such problems to describe the effects of delays and to present tools for dealing with them.

What is the effect of delay on a control system? The essential effect of delay is that it generally requires a system to be operated with a small gain in the feedback loop. In a system with delay, the sensory reading that is obtained by the controller reflects the state of the system at some previous time. The control signal corresponding to that sensory reading may no longer be appropriate for the current state of the plant. If the closed-loop system is oscillatory, for example, then the delayed control signal can be out of phase with the true error signal and may contribute to the error rather than correct it. Such an out-of-phase control signal can destabilize the plant.

To illustrate the effect of delay in the closed loop, consider the first-order plant looked at previously (see equation 12):

$$y[n + 1] = 0.5y[n] + 0.4u[n]$$

which decays geometrically to zero when the control signal u is zero, as shown earlier in Figure 2.3a. Let us consider four closed-loop control laws with delays of zero, one, two and three time steps, respectively. With no delay, we set $u[n] = -Ky[n]$, and the closed loop becomes:

$$y[n + 1] = 0.5y[n] - 0.4Ky[n]$$

where K is the feedback gain. Letting K equal 1 yields the curve labeled $T = 0$ in Figure 2.10, where we see that the regulatory properties of the system are improved when compared with the open loop. If the plant output is delayed by one time step,

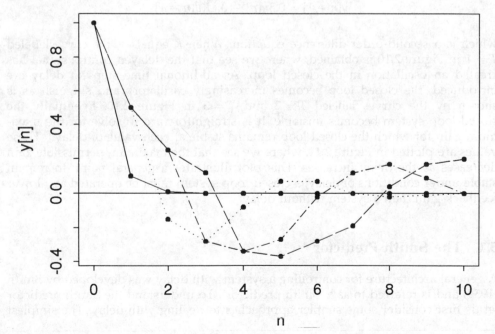

Figure 2.10. *Performance of the feedback controller with delays in the feedback path.* —, $T = 0$; ·····, $T = 1$; ———, $T = 2$; --, $T = 3$.

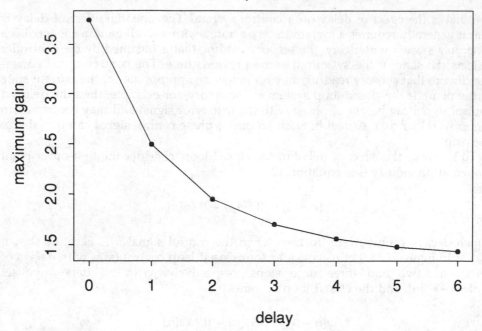

Figure 2.11. *Maximum possible gain for closed-loop stability as a function of feedback delay.*

we obtain $u[n] = -Ky[n-1]$, and the closed-loop dynamics are given by:

$$y[n+1] = 0.5y[n] - 0.4Ky[n-1]$$

which is a second-order difference equation. When K equals 1, the curve labeled $T = 1$ in Figure 2.10 is obtained, where we see that the delayed control signal has created an oscillation in the closed loop. As additional time steps of delay are introduced, the closed loop becomes increasingly oscillatory and sluggish as is shown by the curves labeled $T = 2$ and $T = 3$ in Figure 2.10. Eventually the closed-loop system becomes unstable. It is straightforward to solve for the maximum gain for which the closed loop remains stable at each value of delay.[9] These values are plotted in Figure 2.11, where we see that the maximum permissible gain decreases as the delay increases. This plot illustrates a general point: to remain stable under conditions of delay, a closed-loop system must be operated at a lower feedback gain than a system without delay.

5.1 The Smith Predictor

A general architecture for controlling a system with delay was developed by Smith (1959) and is referred to as a 'Smith predictor'. To understand the Smith predictor let us first consider some simpler approaches to dealing with delay. The simplest

---

[9]These are the values of gain for which one of the roots of the characteristic equation of the closed-loop dynamics crosses the unit circle in the complex plane (see, for example, Åstrom and Wittenmark, 1984).

scheme is simply to utilize an open-loop feedforward controller. If the feedforward controller is a reasonable approximation to an inverse of the plant then this scheme will control the plant successfully over short intervals of time. The inevitable disturbances and modeling errors will make performance degrade over longer time intervals; nonetheless, the advantages of feedforward control are not to be neglected in this case. By ignoring the output from the plant, the feedforward system is stable despite the delay. It might be hoped that a feedforward controller could provide coarse control of the plant without compromising stability, thereby bringing the magnitude of the performance errors down to a level that could be handled by a low-gain feedback controller.

Composite feedforward and feedback control is indeed the idea behind the Smith predictor, but another issue arises due to the presence of delay. Let us suppose that the feedforward controller is a perfect inverse model of the plant and that there are no disturbances. In this case there should be no performance errors to correct. Note, however, that the performance error cannot be based on the difference between the current reference signal and the current plant output, because the output of the plant is delayed by T time steps with respect to the reference signal. One approach to dealing with this problem would be simply to delay the reference signal by the appropriate amount before comparing it with the plant output. This approach has the disadvantage that the system is unable to anticipate potential future errors. Another approach – that used in the Smith predictor – is to utilize a forward model of the plant to predict the influence of the feedforward control signal on the plant, delay this prediction by the appropriate amount, and add it to the control signal to cancel the anticipated contribution of the feedback controller.

The control system now has both an inverse model for control and a forward model for prediction. Recall that one way to implement a feedforward controller is to utilize a forward model in an internal feedback loop (cf. Figure 2.8). Thus a forward model can be used both for implementing the feedforward controller and for predicting the plant output. Placing the forward model in the forward path of the control system yields the Smith predictor, as shown in Figure 2.12. Note that if the forward model and the delay model in the Smith predictor are perfect, then the outer loop in the diagram is canceled by the positive feedback loop that passes through the forward model and the delay model. The remaining loop (the negative

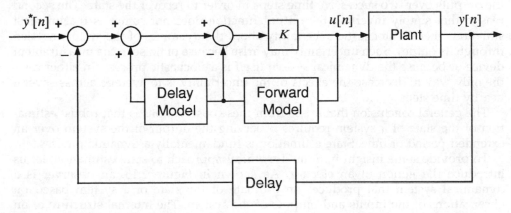

Figure 2.12. *The Smith predictor.*

feedback loop that passes through the forward model) is exactly the feedforward control scheme described previously in connection with Figure 2.8. Because this internal loop is not subject to delay from the periphery, the feedback gain, K, can be relatively large and the inner loop can therefore provide a reasonable approximation to an inverse plant model.

Although the intuitions behind the Smith predictor have been present in the motor control literature for many years, only recently has explicit use been made of this technique in motor control modeling. Miall *et al.* (1993) have studied visuomotor tracking under conditions of varying delay and have proposed a physiologically based model of tracking in which the cerebellum acts as an adaptive Smith predictor.

6 OBSERVERS

In this section we briefly discuss the topic of state estimation. State estimation is a deep topic with rich connections to dynamical systems theory and statistical theory (Anderson and Moore, 1979). Our goal here is simply to provide some basic intuition for the problem, focusing on the important role of internal forward models in state estimation.

In the first-order example that we have discussed, the problem of state estimation is trivial because the output of the system is the same as the state (equation 13). In most situations the output is a more complex function of the state. In such situations it might be thought that the state could be recovered by simply inverting the output function. There are two fundamental reasons, however, why this is not a general solution to the problem of state estimation. First, there are usually more state variables than output variables in dynamical models, thus the function g is generally not uniquely invertible. An example is the one-joint robot arm considered earlier. The dynamical model of the arm has two state variables: the joint angle at the current time step and the joint angle at the previous time step. There is a single output variable: the current joint angle. Thus the output function preserves information about only one of the state variables, and it is impossible to recover the state by simply inverting the output function. Minimally, the system must combine the outputs over two successive time steps in order to recover the state. The second reason that simply inverting the output function does not suffice is that in most situations there is stochastic uncertainty about the dynamics of the system as seen through its output. Such uncertainty may arise because of noise in the measurement device or because the dynamical system itself is a stochastic process. In either case, the only way to decrease the effects of the uncertainty is to average across several nearby time steps.

The general conclusion that arises from these observations is that robust estimation of the state of a system requires observing the output of the system over an extended period of time. State estimation is fundamentally a dynamic process.

To provide some insight into the dynamical approach to state estimation, let us introduce the notion of an *observer*. As shown in Figure 2.13, an observer is a dynamical system that produces an estimate of the state of a system based on observations of the inputs and outputs of the system. The internal structure of an observer is intuitively very simple. The state of the observer is the variable $\hat{x}[n]$, the

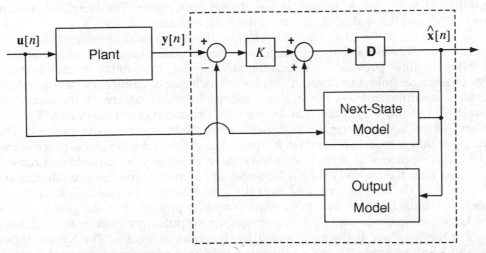

Figure 2.13. *An observer. The inputs to the observer are the plant input and output, and the output from the observer is the estimated state of the plant.*

estimate of the state of the plant. The observer has access to the input to the plant, so it is in a position to predict the next state of the plant from the current input and its estimate of the current state. To make such a prediction the observer must have an internal model of the next-state function of the plant (the function f in equation 1). If the internal model is accurate and if there is no noise in the measurement process or the state transition process, then the observer will accurately predict the next state of the plant. The observer is essentially an internal simulation of the plant dynamics that runs in parallel with the actual plant. Of course, errors will eventually accumulate in the internal simulation, thus there must be a way to couple the observer to the actual plant. This is achieved by using the plant output. Because the observer has access to the plant output, it is able to compare the plant output to its internal prediction of what the output should be, given its internal estimate of the state. To make such a prediction requires the observer to have an internal model of the output function of the plant (the function g in equation 2). Errors in the observer's estimate of the state will be reflected in errors between the predicted plant output and the observed plant output. These errors can be used to correct the state estimate and thereby couple the observer dynamics to the plant dynamics.

The internal state of the observer evolves according to the following dynamical equation:

$$\hat{x}[n + 1] = \hat{f}(\hat{x}[n], u[n]) + K(y[n] - \hat{g}(\hat{x}[n])) \tag{23}$$

where $\hat{f}$ and $\hat{g}$ are internal forward models of the next-state function and the output function, respectively. The first term in the equation is the internal prediction of the next state of the plant, based on the current state estimate and the known input to the plant. The second term is the coupling term. It involves an error between the actual plant output and the internal prediction of the plant output. This error is multiplied by a gain K, known as the *observer gain matrix*. The weighted error is then added to the first term to correct the state estimate.

In the case of linear dynamical systems, there is a well-developed theory to provide guidelines for setting the observer gain. In deterministic dynamical models, these guidelines provide conditions for maintaining the stability of the observer. Much stronger guidelines exist in the case of stochastic dynamical models, in which explicit assumptions are made about the probabilistic nature of the next-state function and the output function. In this case the observer is known as a 'Kalman filter', and the observer gain is known as the 'Kalman gain'. The choice of the Kalman gain is based on the relative amount of noise in the next-state process and the output process. If there is relatively more noise in the output measurement process, then the observer should be conservative in changing its internal state on the basis of the output error and thus the gain K should be small. Conversely, if there is relatively more noise in the state transition process, then the gain K should be large. An observer with large K averages the outputs over a longer span of time, which makes sense if the state transition dynamics are noisy. The Kalman filter quantifies these tradeoffs and chooses the gain that provides an optimal tradeoff between the two different kinds of noise. For further information on Kalman filters, see Anderson and Moore (1979).

In the case of nonlinear dynamical systems, the theory of state estimation is much less well developed. Progress has been made, however, and the topic of the nonlinear observer is an active area of research (Misawa and Hedrick, 1989).

7 LEARNING ALGORITHMS

In earlier sections we have seen several ways in which internal models can be used in a control system. Inverse models are the basic building block of feedforward control. Forward models can also be used in feedforward control, and have additional roles in state estimation and motor learning. It is important to emphasize that an internal model is a form of knowledge about the plant. Many motor control problems involve interacting with objects in the external world, and these objects generally have unknown mechanical properties. There are also changes in the musculoskeletal system due to growth or injury. These considerations suggest an important role for adaptive processes. Through adaptation the motor control system is able to maintain and update its internal models of external dynamics.

The next several sections develop some of the machinery that can be used to understand adaptive systems. Before entering into the details, let us first establish some terminology and introduce a distinction. The adaptive algorithms that we will discuss are all instances of a general approach to learning known as *error-correcting learning* or *supervised learning*. A supervised learner is a system that learns a transformation from a set of inputs to a set of outputs. Examples of pairs of inputs and outputs are presented repeatedly to the learning system, and the system is required to abstract an underlying law or relationship from these data so that it can generalize appropriately to new data. Within the general class of supervised learning algorithms, there are two basic classes of algorithms that it is useful to distinguish: *regression* algorithms and *classification* algorithms. A regression problem involves finding a functional relationship between the inputs and outputs. The form of the relationship depends on the particular learning architecture, but generally it is real-valued and smooth. By way of contrast, a classification problem involves associating a category membership label with each of the input patterns. In a classification problem the outputs are generally members of a discrete set and the functional relationship from inputs to outputs is characterized by sharp decision boundaries.

The literature on supervised learning algorithms is closely related to the classical literature in statistics on regression and classification. Let us point out one salient difference between these traditions. Whereas statistical algorithms are generally based on processing a batch of data, learning algorithms are generally based on *online* processing – that is, a learning system generally cannot afford to wait for a batch of data to arrive, but must update its internal parameters immediately after each new learning trial.

The next two sections present two simple learning algorithms that are representative of classification algorithms and regression algorithms, respectively.

7.1 The Perceptron

In this section we describe a simple classification learner known as the *perceptron* (Rosenblatt, 1962). The perceptron learns to assign a binary category label to each of a set of input patterns. For example, the input pattern might represent the output of a motion detection stage in the visual system and the binary label might specify whether or not an object can be caught before it falls to the ground. The perceptron is provided with examples of input patterns paired with their corresponding labels. The goal of the learning procedure is to extract information from the examples so that the system can generalize appropriately to novel data. That is, the perceptron must acquire a decision rule that allows it to make accurate classifications for those input patterns whose label is not known.

The perceptron is based on a thresholding procedure applied to a weighted sum. Let us represent the features of the input pattern by a set of real numbers x_1, $x_2, \ldots, x_n$. For each input value x_i there is a corresponding *weight* w_i. The perceptron sums up the weighted feature values and compares the weighted sum to a threshold θ. If the sum is greater than the threshold, the output is one; otherwise the output is zero. That is, the binary output y is computed as follows:

$$y = \begin{cases} 1 & \text{if } w_1x_1 + w_2x_2 + \cdots + w_nx_n > \theta \\ 0 & \text{otherwise} \end{cases} \tag{24}$$

The perceptron can be represented diagrammatically as shown in Figure 2.14a.

The perceptron learning algorithm is a procedure that changes the weights w_i as a function of the perceptron's performance on the training examples. To describe the algorithm, let us assume for simplicity that the input values x_i are either zero or one. We represent the binary category label as y^*, which also is either zero or one. There are four cases to consider. Consider first the case in which the desired output y^* is one, but the actual output y is zero. There are two ways in which the system can correct this error: either the threshold can be lowered or the weighted

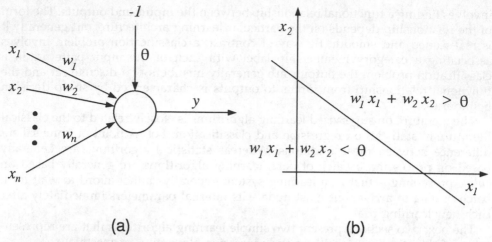

(a)   (b)

Figure 2.14. (a) A perceptron. The output y is obtained by thresholding the weighted sum of the inputs. The threshold θ can be treated as a weight emanating from an input line whose value is fixed at −1 (see below). (b) A geometric representation of the perceptron in the case of two input values x_1 and x_2. The line $w_1x_1 + w_2x_2 = \theta$ is the decision surface of the perceptron. For points lying above the decision surface the output of the perceptron is one. For points lying below the decision surface the output of the perceptron is zero. The parameters w_1 and w_2 determine the slope of the line and the parameter θ determines the offset of the decision surface from the origin.

sum can be increased. To increase the weighted sum it suffices to increase the weights. Note, however, that it is of no use to increase the weights on the input lines that have a zero input value, because those lines do not contribute to the weighted sum. Indeed, it is sensible to leave the weights unchanged on those lines so as to avoid disturbing the settings that have been made for other patterns. Consider now the case in which the desired output y^* is zero, but the actual output y is one. In this case the weighted sum is too large and needs to be decreased. This can be accomplished by increasing the threshold and/or decreasing the weights. Again the weights are changed only on the active input lines. The remaining two cases are those in which the desired output and the actual output are equal. In these cases, the perceptron quite reasonably makes no changes to the weights or the threshold.

The algorithm that we have described can be summarized in a single equation. The change to a weight w_i is given by:

$$\Delta w_i = \mu(y^* - y)x_i \tag{25}$$

where μ is a small positive number referred to as the *learning rate*. Note that, in accordance with the description given above, changes are made only to those weights that have a nonzero input value x_i. The change is of the appropriate sign due to the $(y^* - y)$ term. A similar rule can be written for the threshold θ:

$$\Delta\theta = -\mu(y^* - y) \tag{26}$$

which can be treated as a special case of the preceding rule if we treat the threshold as a weight emanating from an input line whose value is always −1.

Geometrically, the perceptron describes a hyperplane in the n-dimensional space of the input features, as shown in Figure 2.14b. The perceptron learning algorithm adjusts the position and orientation of the hyperplane to attempt to place all of the input patterns with a label of zero on one side of the hyperplane and all of the input patterns with a label of one on the other side of the hyperplane. It can be proven that the perceptron is guaranteed to find a solution that splits the data in this way, if such a solution exists (Duda and Hart, 1973).

7.2 The LMS Algorithm

The perceptron is a simple, online scheme for solving classification problems. What the perceptron is to classification, the least mean squares (LMS) algorithm is to regression (Widrow and Hoff, 1960). In this section we derive the LMS algorithm from the point of view of optimization theory. We shall see that it is closely related to the perceptron algorithm.

The LMS algorithm is essentially an online scheme for performing multivariate linear regression. Recall that the supervised learning paradigm involves the repeated presentation of pairs of inputs and desired outputs. In classification the desired outputs are binary, whereas in regression the desired outputs are real-valued. For simplicity let us consider the case in which a multivariate input vector is paired with a single real-valued output (we consider the generalization to multiple real-valued outputs below). In this case, the regression surface is an $n + 1$-dimensional hyperplane, where n is the number of input variables. The equation describing the hyperplane is as follows:

$$y = w_1 x_1 + w_2 x_2 + \cdots + w_n x_n + b \qquad (27)$$

where the *bias* b allows the hyperplane to have a nonzero intercept along the y-axis. The bias is the analog of the negative of the threshold in the perceptron.

The regression equation (27) can be computed by the simple processing unit shown in Figure 2.15a. As in the case of the perceptron, the problem is to develop an algorithm for adjusting the weights and the bias of this processing unit based on the repeated presentation of input–output pairs. As we will see, the appropriate algorithm for doing this is exactly the same as the algorithm developed for the perceptron (equations 25 and 26). Rather than motivate the algorithm heuristically as we did in the previous section, let us derive the algorithm from a different perspective, introducing the powerful tools of optimization theory. We consider a *cost function* that measures the discrepancy between the actual output of the processing unit and the desired output. In the case of the LMS algorithm this cost function is one-half the squared difference between the actual output y and the desired output y^*:

$$J = \frac{1}{2} (y^* - y)^2 \qquad (28)$$

Note that J is a function of the parameters w_i and b (because y is a function of these parameters). J can therefore be optimized (minimized) by proper choice of the

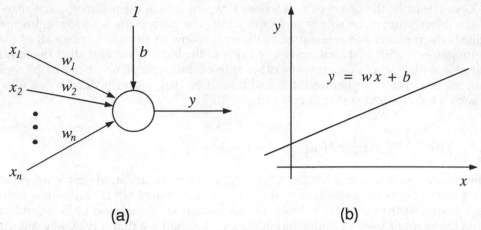

(a)   (b)

Figure 2.15. *(a) A least mean squares (LMS) processing unit. The output y is obtained as a weighted sum of the inputs. The bias can be treated as a weight emanating from an input line whose value is fixed at 1. (b) A geometric representation of the LMS unit in the case of a single input value x. The output function is $y = wx + b$, where the parameter w is the slope of the regression line and the parameter b is the y-intercept.*

parameters. We first compute the derivatives of J with respect to the parameters; that is, we compute the *gradient* of J with respect to w_i and b:

$$\frac{\partial J}{\partial w_i} = -(y^* - y)\frac{\partial y}{\partial w_i} \tag{29}$$

$$= -(y^* - y)x_i \tag{30}$$

and

$$\frac{\partial J}{\partial b} = -(y^* - y)\frac{\partial y}{\partial b} \tag{31}$$

$$= -(y^* - y) \tag{32}$$

The gradient points in the direction in which J increases most steeply (Figure 2.16); therefore, to decrease J we take a step in the direction of the negative of the gradient:

$$\Delta w_i = \mu(y^* - y)x_i \tag{33}$$

and

$$\Delta b = \mu(y^* - y) \tag{34}$$

where μ is the size of the step. Note that we have recovered exactly the equations that were presented in the previous section (equations 25 and 26). The difference between these sets of equations is the manner in which y is computed. In equations

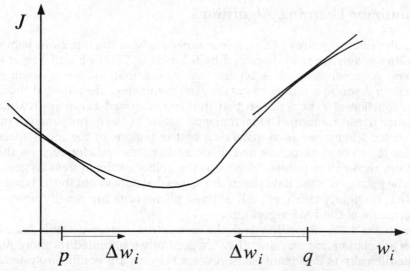

Figure 2.16. *The logic of gradient descent: if the derivative of J with respect to w_i is positive (as it is at q), then to decrease J we decrease w_i. If the derivative of J with respect to w_i is negative (as it is at p), we increase w_i. The step Δw_i also depends on the magnitude of the derivative.*

(33) and (34), y is a *linear* function of the input variables (equation 27), whereas in equations (25) and (26), y is a *binary* function of the input variables (equation 24). This seemingly minor difference has major implications – the LMS algorithm (equations 27, 33 and 34) and the perceptron algorithm (equations 24, 25 and 26) have significantly different statistical properties and convergence properties, reflecting their differing roles as a regression algorithm and a classification algorithm, respectively. For an extensive discussion of these issues see Duda and Hart (1973).

Although we have presented the LMS algorithm and the perceptron learning algorithm in the case of a single output unit, both algorithms are readily extended to the case of multiple output units. Indeed, no new machinery is required – we simply observe that each output unit in an array of output units has its own set of weights and bias (or threshold), so that each output unit learns independently and in parallel. In the LMS case, this can be seen formally as follows. Let us define a multi-output cost function:

$$J = \frac{1}{2} \|\mathbf{y}^* - \mathbf{y}\|^2 = \frac{1}{2} \sum_i (y_i^* - y_i)^2 \tag{35}$$

where y_i^* and y_i are the i-th components of the desired output vector and the actual output vector, respectively. Letting w_{ij} denote the weight from input unit j to output unit i, we have:

$$\frac{\partial J}{\partial w_{ij}} = \sum_k \frac{\partial J}{\partial y_k} \frac{\partial y_k}{\partial w_{ij}} \tag{36}$$

$$= -(y_i^* - y_i)x_j \tag{37}$$

which shows that the derivative for weight w_{ij} depends only on the error at output unit i.

7.3 Nonlinear Learning Algorithms

The LMS algorithm captures in a simple manner many of the intuitions behind the notion of the *motor schema* as discussed by Schmidt (1975), Koh and Meyer (1991) and others. A motor schema is an internal model that utilizes a small set of parameters to describe a family of curves. The parameters are adjusted incrementally as a function of experience so that the parameterized curve approximates a sensorimotor transformation. The incremental nature of the approximation implies that the motor schema tends to generalize best in regions of the input space that are nearby to recent data points and to generalize less well for regions that are further from recent data points. Moreover, the ability of the system to generalize can often be enhanced if the data points are somewhat spread out in the input space than if they are tightly clustered. All of these phenomena are readily observed in the performance of the LMS algorithm.

Although the LMS algorithm and the perceptron are serviceable for simple models of adaptation and learning, they are generally too limited for more realistic cases. The difficulty is that many sensorimotor systems are nonlinear systems and the LMS algorithm and the perceptron are limited to learning linear mappings. There are many ways to generalize the linear approach, however, to treat the problem of the incremental learning of nonlinear mappings. This is an active area of research in a large number of disciplines and the details are beyond the scope of this paper (see, for example, Geman, Bienenstock and Doursat, 1992). Nonetheless it is worth distinguishing a few of the trends. One general approach is to consider systems that are nonlinear in the inputs but linear in the parameters. An example of such a system would be a polynomial:

$$y = ax^3 + bx^2 + cx + d \tag{38}$$

where the coefficients a, b, c and d are the unknown parameters. By defining a new set of variables $z_1 = x^3$, $z_2 = x^2$ and $z_3 = x$, we observe that this system is linear in the parameters and also linear in the transformed set of variables. Thus an LMS processing unit can be used after a preprocessing level in which a fixed set of nonlinear transformations is applied to the input x. There are two difficulties with this approach – first, in cases with more than a single input variable, the number of cross-products (e.g. $x_1 x_5 x_8$) increases exponentially; and second, high-order polynomials tend to oscillate wildly between the data points, leading to poor generalization (Duda and Hart, 1973).

A second approach which also does not stray far from the linear framework is to use *piecewise* linear approximations to nonlinear functions. This approach generally requires all of the data to be stored so that the piecewise fits can be constructed on the fly (Atkeson, 1990). It is also possible to treat the problem of splitting the space as part of the learning problem (Jordan and Jacobs, 1992).

Another large class of algorithms are both nonlinear in the inputs and nonlinear in the parameters. These algorithms include the generalized splines (Poggio and Girosi, 1990; Wahba, 1990), the feedforward neural network (Hinton, 1989) and regression trees (Breiman *et al.*, 1984; Friedman, 1990; Jordan and Jacobs, 1992). For example, the standard two-layer feedforward neural network can be written in the form:

$$y_i = f\left(\sum_j w_{ij} f\left(\sum_k v_{jk} x_k \right) \right) \tag{39}$$

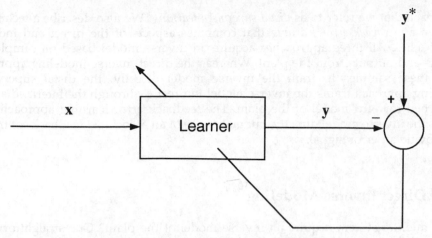

Figure 2.17. *A generic supervised learning system.*

where the parameters w_{ij} and v_{jk} are the weights of the network and the function f is a fixed nonlinearity. Because the weights v_{jk} appear 'inside' the nonlinearity, the system is nonlinear in the parameters and a generalization of the LMS algorithm, known as 'backpropagation', is needed to adjust the parameters (Rumelhart, Hinton and Williams, 1986; Werbos, 1974). The generalized splines and the regression trees do not utilize backpropagation, but rather make use of other forms of generalization of the LMS algorithm.

A final class of algorithms are the nonparametric approximators (Specht, 1991). These algorithms are essentially smoothed lookup tables. Although they do not utilize a parameterized family of curves, they nonetheless exhibit generalization and interference due to the smoothing.

In the remainder of this chapter, we lump all of these various nonlinear learning algorithms into the general class of supervised learning algorithms. That is, we simply assume the existence of a learning algorithm that can acquire a nonlinear mapping based on samples of pairs of inputs and corresponding outputs. The diagram that we use to indicate a generic supervised learning algorithm is shown in Figure 2.17. As can be seen, the generic supervised learning system has an input **x**, an output **y**, and a desired output **y***. The error between the desired output and the actual output is used by the learning algorithm to adjust the internal parameters of the learner. This adjustment process is indicated by the diagonal arrow in the figure.

8   MOTOR LEARNING

In this section we put together several of the ideas that have been introduced in earlier sections and discuss the problem of motor learning. To fix ideas, we consider feedforward control; in particular, we discuss the problem of learning an inverse model of the plant (we discuss a more general learning problem in the following section). We distinguish between two broad approaches to learning an inverse model: a direct approach that we refer to as *direct inverse modeling*, and an indirect approach that we refer to as *distal supervised learning*. We also describe a technique known as *feedback error learning* that combines aspects of the direct and indirect approaches. All three approaches acquire an inverse model based on samples of inputs and outputs from the plant. Whereas the direct inverse modeling approach uses these samples to train the inverse model directly, the distal supervised learning approach trains the inverse model indirectly, through the intermediary of a learned forward model of the plant. The feedback error learning approach also trains the inverse model directly, but makes use of an associated feedback controller to provide an error signal.

8.1   Direct Inverse Modeling

How might a system acquire an inverse model of the plant? One straightforward approach is to present various test inputs to the plant, observe the outputs, and provide these input–output pairs as training data to a supervised learning algorithm by reversing the role of the inputs and the outputs. That is, the plant output is provided as an input to the learning controller, and the controller is required to produce as output the corresponding plant input. This approach, shown diagrammatically in Figure 2.18, is known as *direct inverse modeling* (Atkeson and Reinkensmeyer, 1988; Kuperstein, 1988; Miller, 1987; Widrow and Stearns, 1985). Note that we treat the plant output as being observed at time n. Because an inverse model is a relationship between the state and the plant input at one moment in time with the plant output at the following moment in time (cf. equation 11), the plant input ($\mathbf{u}[n]$) and the state estimate ($\hat{\mathbf{x}}[n]$) must be delayed by one time step to yield the proper temporal relationships. The input to the learning controller is therefore the current plant output $\mathbf{y}[n]$ and the delayed state estimate $\hat{\mathbf{x}}[n-1]$. The controller is required to produce the plant input that gave rise to the current output, in the context of the delayed estimated state. This is generally achieved by the optimiz-

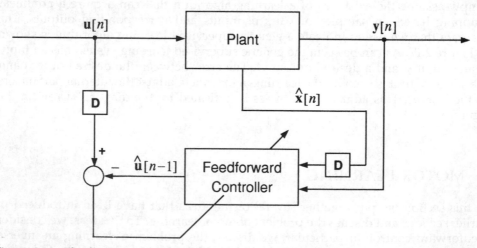

Figure 2.18. *The direct inverse modeling approach to learning a feedforward controller. The state estimate* $\hat{\mathbf{x}}[n]$ *is assumed to be provided by an observer (not shown).*

ation of the following sum-of-squared-error cost function:

$$J = \frac{1}{2} \|\mathbf{u}[n-1] - \hat{\mathbf{u}}[n-1]\|^2 \tag{40}$$

where $\hat{\mathbf{u}}[n-1]$ denotes the controller output.

Example
Consider the first-order plant:

$$y[n+1] = 0.5x[n] + 0.4u[n] \tag{41}$$

As we have seen previously, the inverse model for this plant is linear in the estimated state and the desired output (cf. equation 15). Let us assume that we do not know the appropriate values for the coefficients in the inverse model; thus we replace them with unknown values v_1 and v_2:

$$\hat{u}[n] = v_1 \hat{x}[n] + v_2 y[n+1] \tag{42}$$

This equation is linear in the unknown parameters, thus we can use the LMS algorithm to learn the values of v_1 and v_2. We first shift the time index in equation 42 to write the inverse model in terms of the current plant output ($y[n]$). This

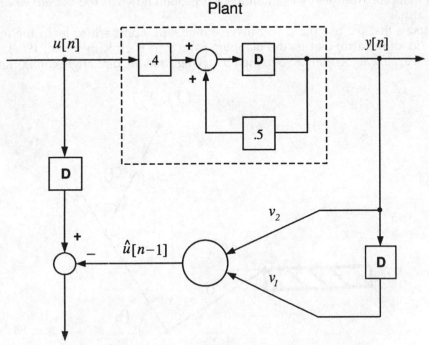

Figure 2.19. *An example of the direct inverse modeling approach. An LMS processing unit is connected to the first-order plant. The bias has been omitted for simplicity.*

requires delaying the control input and the state estimate by one time step. Connecting the LMS unit to the plant with the appropriate delays in place yields the wiring diagram in Figure 2.19. Note that we assume that the state is estimated by feedback from the plant, thus the delayed state $x[n-1]$ is estimated by the delayed plant output $y[n-1]$ (cf. equation 16). The inputs to the LMS processing unit are the plant output $y[n]$ and the delayed plant output $y[n-1]$. The target for the LMS unit is the delayed plant input $u[n-1]$. Note that if the unit is equipped with a bias, the bias value will converge to zero because it is not needed to represent the inverse model for this plant.

8.1.1   The Nonconvexity Problem

The direct inverse modeling approach is well behaved for linear systems and indeed can be shown to converge to correct parameter estimates for such systems under certain conditions (Goodwin and Sin, 1984). For nonlinear systems, however, a difficulty arises that is related to the general 'degrees-of-freedom problem' in motor control (Bernstein, 1967). The problem is due to a particular form of redundancy in nonlinear systems (Jordan, 1992). In such systems, the 'optimal' parameter estimates (i.e. those that minimize the cost function in equation 40) in fact yield an incorrect controller.

To illustrate, let us consider the planar kinematic arm shown in Fgure 2.20. The arm has three joint angles, which we denote by θ_1, θ_2 and θ_3. The tip of the arm can be described by a pair of Cartesian coordinates, which we denote by y_1 and y_2. For every vector of joint angles $\boldsymbol{\theta}$ there is a corresponding Cartesian position vector **y**. The mapping from $\boldsymbol{\theta}$ to **y** is a nonlinear function known as the *forward kinematics* of the arm.

Suppose that we use the direct inverse modeling approach to learn the *inverse kinematics* of the arm; that is, the mapping from **y** to $\boldsymbol{\theta}$ (cf. Kuperstein, 1988). Data for the learning algorithm are obtained by trying random joint angle configurations

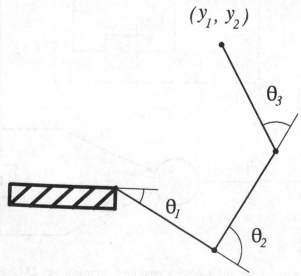

Figure 2.20. *A three-joint planar arm.*

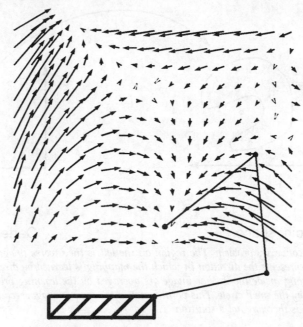

Figure 2.21. *Near-asymptotic performance of direct inverse modeling. Each vector represents the error at a particular position in the workspace.*

and observing the corresponding position of the tip of the arm. A nonlinear supervised learning algorithm is used to learn the mapping from tip positions to joint angles. Figure 2.21 shows the results of a simulation of this approach for the planar arm. The figure is an error vector field; that is, the tail of each arrow is a desired position, and the head of each arrow is the position produced by utilizing the inverse model to produce a set of joint angles. As can be observed, there are substantial errors throughout the workspace.

It is possible to rule out a number of possible explanations for the errors. The errors are not explained by possible local minima, by insufficient training time, or by poor approximation capability of the inverse model (Jordan and Rumelhart, 1992). The particular inverse model used in the simulation was a feedforward neural network trained with backpropagation, but it can be shown that any least-squares based nonlinear approximator would give a similar result. To understand the difficulty, let us consider the direct inverse modeling approach geometrically, as shown in Figure 2.22. The figure shows the joint space on the left and the Cartesian space on the right. The arm is a redundant kinematic system; that is, to every tip position inside the workspace, there are an infinite set of joint angle configurations that achieve that position. Thus, to every point on the right side of the figure, there is a corresponding region (the *inverse image*) on the left. The direct inverse modeling approach samples randomly in joint space, observes the corresponding points in Cartesian space and learns the mapping in the reverse direction. Let us suppose that three sample points happen to fall in a particular inverse image (Figure 2.22). All three of these points correspond to a single point in Cartesian space, thus the direct inverse learner is presented with data that are one-to-many: a single input maps to three different target outputs. The optimal least-squares

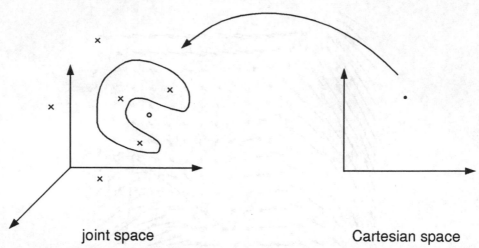

joint space   **Cartesian space**

Figure 2.22. *The convexity problem. The region on the left is the inverse image of the point on the right. The arrow represents the direction in which the mapping is learned by direct inverse modeling. The three points lying inside the inverse image are averaged by the learning procedure, yielding the vector represented by the small circle. This point is not in the inverse image, because the inverse image is not convex, and is therefore not a solution.*

solution is to produce an output that is an average of the three targets. If the inverse image has a nonconvex shape, as shown in the figure, then the average of the three targets lies outside of the inverse image and is therefore not a solution.

It is easy to demonstrate that linear systems always have convex inverse images, thus the nonconvexity problem does not arise for such systems.[10] The problem does arise for nonlinear systems, however. In particular, Figure 2.23 demonstrates that the problem arises for the planar kinematic arm. The figure shows two particular joint angle configurations that lie in the same inverse image (i.e. map into the same Cartesian position). The figure also shows the joint-space average of these two configurations (the dashed configuration in the figure). An average of two points lies on the straight line joining the points, thus the fact that the average configuration does not itself lie in the inverse image (i.e. does not map into the same Cartesian position) demonstrates that the inverse image is nonconvex. Interestingly, the Cartesian error observed in Figure 2.23 is essentially the same error as that observed in the corresponding position of the error vector field in Figure 2.21. This provides support for the assertion that the error vector field is due to the nonconvexities of the inverse kinematics.

---

[10]Let $\mathbf{y} = f(\mathbf{x})$ be a linear function, and consider a particular point $\mathbf{y}^*$ in the range of f. The convex combination of any two points $\mathbf{x}_1$ and $\mathbf{x}_2$ that lie in the inverse image of $\mathbf{y}^*$ also lies in the inverse image of $\mathbf{y}^*$:

$$f(\alpha\mathbf{x}_1 + (1 - \alpha)\mathbf{x}_2) = \alpha f(\mathbf{x}_1) + (1 - \alpha)f(\mathbf{x}_2)$$
$$= \alpha\mathbf{y}^* + (1 - \alpha)\mathbf{y}^*$$
$$= \mathbf{y}^*$$

where $0 < \alpha < 1$. Thus the inverse image is a convex set.

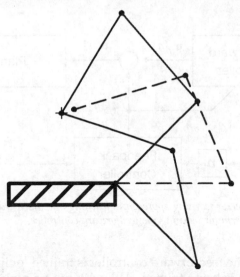

Figure 2.23. *The nonconvexity of inverse kinematics. The dotted configuration is an average in joint space of the two solid configurations.*

8.2 Feedback Error Learning

Kawato, Furukawa and Suzuki (1987) have developed a direct approach to motor learning that avoids some of the difficulties associated with direct inverse modeling. Their approach, known as *feedback error learning*, makes use of a feedback controller to guide the learning of the feedforward controller. Consider the composite feedback–feedforward control system discussed earlier (cf. Figure 2.9), in which the total control signal is the sum of the feedforward component and the feedback component:

$$\mathbf{u}[n] = \mathbf{u}_{ff}[n] + \mathbf{u}_{fb}[n]$$

In the context of a direct approach to motor learning, the signal $\mathbf{u}[n]$ is the target for learning the feedforward controller (cf. Figure 2.18). The error between the target and the feedforward control signal is $(\mathbf{u}[n] - \mathbf{u}_{ff}[n])$, which in the current case is simply $\mathbf{u}_{fb}[n]$. Thus an error for learning the feedforward controller can be provided by the feedback control signal (Figure 2.24).

An important difference between feedback error learning and direct inverse modeling regards the signal used as the controller input. In direct inverse modeling the controller is trained 'offline'; that is, the input to the controller for the purposes of training is the actual plant output, not the desired plant output. For the controller actually to participate in the control process, it must receive the desired plant output as its input. The direct inverse modeling approach therefore requires a switching process – the desired plant output must be switched in for the purposes of control and the actual plant output must be switched in for the purposes of training. The feedback error learning approach provides a more elegant solution to this problem. In feedback error learning, the desired plant output is used for both

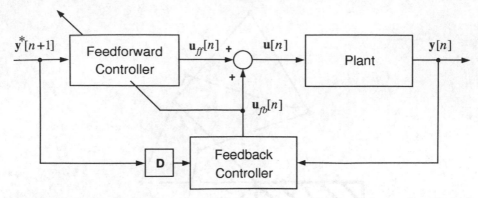

Figure 2.24. *The feedback error learning approach to learning a feedforward controller. The feedback control signal is the error term for learning the feedforward controller.*

control and training. The feedforward controller is trained 'online'; that is, it is used as a controller while it is being trained. Although the training data that it receives – pairs of actual plant inputs and desired plant outputs – are not samples of the inverse dynamics of the plant, the system nonetheless converges to an inverse model of the plant because of the error-correcting properties of the feedback controller.

By utilizing a feedback controller, the feedback error learning approach also solves another problem associated with direct inverse modeling. Direct inverse modeling is not *goal directed*; that is, it is not sensitive to particular output goals (Jordan and Rosenbaum, 1989). This is seen by simply observing that the goal signal ($y^*[n + 1]$) does not appear in Figure 2.18. The learning process samples randomly in the control space, which may or may not yield a plant output near any particular goal. Even if a particular goal is specified before the learning begins, the direct inverse modeling procedure must search throughout the control space until an acceptable solution is found. In the feedback error learning approach, however, the feedback controller serves to guide the system to the correct region of the control space. By using a feedback controller, the system makes essential use of the error between the desired plant output and the actual plant output to guide the learning. This fact links the feedback error learning approach to the indirect approach to motor learning that we discuss in the following section. In the indirect approach, the learning algorithm is based directly on the output error.

8.3 Distal Supervised Learning

In this section we describe an indirect approach to motor learning known as *distal supervised learning*. Distal supervised learning avoids the nonconvexity problem and also avoids certain other problems associated with direct approaches to motor learning (Jordan, 1990; Jordan and Rumelhart, 1992). In distal supervised learning, the controller is learned indirectly, through the intermediary of a forward model of the plant. The forward model must itself be learned from observations of the inputs and outputs of the plant. The distal supervised learning approach is therefore composed of two interacting processes: one process in which the forward model is learned and another process in which the forward model is used in the learning of the controller.

In the case of a linear plant, the distal supervised learning approach is a cross between two techniques from adaptive control theory: indirect self-tuning control and indirect model reference adaptive control (Åström and Wittenmark, 1989). Let us begin by describing the basic idea of indirect self-tuning control, to provide some insight into how a forward model can be used as an intermediary in the learning of an inverse model. Consider once again the first-order example (equation 41). Suppose that instead of learning an inverse model of the plant directly, the system first learns a forward model of the plant. We assume a parameterized forward plant model of the following form:

$$\hat{y}[n + 1] = w_1\hat{x}[n] + w_2u[n] \tag{43}$$

where the weights w_1 and w_2 are unknown parameters. This equation is linear in the unknown parameters, thus the LMS algorithm is applicable. As in the previous section, we shift the time index backward by one time step to express the model in terms of the current plant output $y[n]$. This yields the wiring diagram shown in Figure 2.25. The forward model is an LMS processing unit with inputs $u[n - 1]$ and $y[n - 1]$, where $y[n - 1]$ is the estimate $\hat{x}[n - 1]$. The output of the LMS unit is the

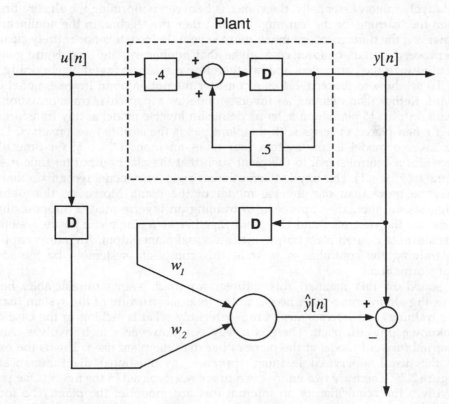

Figure 2.25. *An example of the learning of the forward model in the distal supervised learning approach. An LMS processing unit is connected to the first-order plant. The bias has been omitted for simplicity.*

predicted plant output $\hat{y}[n]$ and the target for the learning algorithm is the actual plant output $y[n]$. By minimizing the *prediction error* ($y[n] - \hat{y}[n]$), the system adjusts the weights in the forward model.

Let us suppose that the learner has acquired a perfect forward model; that is, the predicted plant output is equal to the actual plant output for all states and all inputs. Equation 43 can now be inverted algebraically to provide an inverse model of the following form:

$$u[n] = -\frac{w_1}{w_2}\hat{x}[n] + \frac{1}{w_2}y^*[n+1] \tag{44}$$

Note that, in this equation, the weights of the forward model are being used to construct the inverse model. If the forward model is perfect, that is, if w_1 is equal to 0.5 and w_2 is equal to 0.4, then the inverse model is also perfect – the coefficients in equation 44 are 1.25 and 2.5 (cf. equation 15).

8.3.1   The Nonlinear Case

In the case of a linear plant, the differences between the direct approach to learning an inverse model and the indirect approach to learning an inverse model are relatively minor. Essentially, the choice is between performing the algebra first and then the learning, or the learning first and then the algebra. In the nonlinear case, however, the differences are much more salient. Indeed, it is not entirely clear how to proceed in the nonlinear case, given that nonlinear plant models are generally nonlinear in the parameters and are therefore difficult to invert algebraically.

To see how to proceed, let us reconsider the notion of an inverse model of the plant. Rather than defining an inverse model as a particular transformation from plant outputs to plant inputs, let us define an inverse model as any transformation that when placed in series with the plant yields the *identity transformation*. That is, an inverse model is any system that takes an input $\mathbf{y}^*[n+1]$ (at time n) and provides a control signal to the plant such that the plant output (at time $n+1$) is equal to $\mathbf{y}^*[n+1]$. This implicit definition of an inverse model recognizes that there may be more than one inverse model of the plant. Moreover, this definition suggests an alternative approach to training an inverse model. Suppose that we consider the controller and the plant together as a single composite system that transforms a desired plant output into an actual plant output. An indirect approach to training the controller is to train this composite system to be the identity transformation.

Stated in this manner, this indirect approach seems unrealizable, because learning algorithms require access to the internal structure of the system that they are training, and internal structure is precisely what is lacking in the case of the unknown physical plant. There is a way out, however, which involves using an internal forward model of the plant rather than the plant itself. This is the essence of the distal supervised learning approach, as illustrated diagrammatically in Figure 2.26. There are two interwoven processes depicted in the figure. One process involves the acquisition of an internal forward model of the plant. The forward model is a mapping from states and inputs to predicted plant outputs and it is trained using the *prediction error* ($\mathbf{y}[n] - \hat{\mathbf{y}}[n]$). The second process involves training

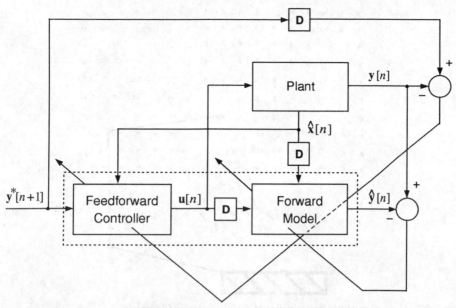

Figure 2.26. *The distal supervised learning approach. The forward model is trained using the prediction error* ($\mathbf{y}[n] - \hat{\mathbf{y}}[n]$).*The subsystems in the dashed box constitute the composite learning system. This system is trained by using the performance error* ($\mathbf{y}^*[n] - \mathbf{y}[n]$) *and holding the forward model fixed. The state estimate* $\hat{\mathbf{x}}[n]$ *is assumed to be provided by an observer (not shown).*

the controller. This is accomplished in the following manner. The controller and the forward model are joined together and are treated as a single *composite learning system*. Using a nonlinear supervised learning algorithm, the composite system is trained to be an identity transformation. That is, the entire composite learning system (the system inside the dashed box in the figure) corresponds to the box labeled 'Learner' in Figure 2.17. During this training process, the parameters in the forward model are held fixed. Thus the composite learning system is trained to be an identity transformation by a constrained learning process in which some of the parameters inside the system are held fixed. By allowing only the controller parameters to be altered, this process trains the controller indirectly.[11]

Let us consider the second component of this procedure in more detail. At any given time step, a desired plant output $\mathbf{y}^*[n + 1]$ is provided to the controller and an action $\mathbf{u}[n]$ is generated. These signals are delayed by one time step before being fed to the learning algorithm, to allow the desired plant output to be compared with the actual plant output at the following time step. Thus the signals utilized by the learning algorithm (at time n) are the delayed desired output $\mathbf{y}^*[n]$ and the delayed

---

[11]It has been suggested (Miall *et al.*, 1993) that the distal supervised learning approach requires using the backpropagation algorithm of Rumelhart, Hinton and Williams (1986). This is not the case; indeed, a wide variety of supervised learning algorithms is applicable. The only requirement of the algorithm is that it obey an 'architectural closure' property: a cascade of two instances of an architecture must itself be an instance of the architecture. This property is satisfied by a variety of algorithms, including the Boltzmann machine (Hinton and Sejnowski, 1986) and decision trees (Breiman *et al.*, 1984).

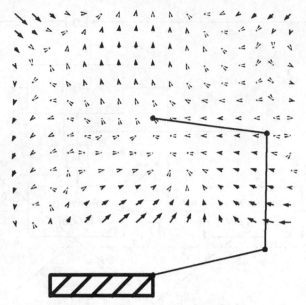

Figure 2.27. *Near-asymptotic performance of distal supervised learning.*

action $\mathbf{u}[n-1]$. The delayed action is fed to the forward model, which produces an internal prediction ($\hat{\mathbf{y}}[n]$) of the actual plant output.[12] Let us assume, temporarily, that the forward model is a perfect model of the plant. In this case, the internal prediction ($\hat{\mathbf{y}}[n]$) is equal to the actual plant output ($\mathbf{y}[n]$). Thus the composite learning system, consisting of the controller and the forward model, maps an input $\mathbf{y}^*[n]$ into an output $\mathbf{y}[n]$. For the composite system to be an identity transformation these two signals must be equal. Thus the error used to train the composite system is the *performance error* ($\mathbf{y}^*[n] - \mathbf{y}[n]$). This is a sensible error term – it is the observed error in motor performance. That is, the learning algorithm trains the controller by correcting the error between the desired plant output and the actual plant output. Optimal performance is characterized by zero error. In contrast to the direct inverse modeling approach, the optimal least-squares solution for distal supervised learning is a solution in which the performance errors are zero.

Figure 2.27 shows the results of a simulation of the inverse kinematic learning problem for the planar arm. As is seen, the distal supervised learning approach avoids the nonconvexity problem and finds a particular inverse model of the arm kinematics. (For extensions to the case of learning multiple, context-sensitive, inverse models, see Jordan, 1990.)

Suppose finally that the forward model is imperfect. In this case, the error between the desired output and the predicted output is the quantity ($\mathbf{y}^*[n] - \hat{\mathbf{y}}[n]$), the *predicted performance error*. Using this error, the best the system can do is to

---

[12]The terminology of *efference copy* and *corollary discharge* may be helpful here (see, for example, Gallistel, 1980). The control signal ($\mathbf{u}[n]$) is the efference, thus the path from the controller to the forward model is an efference copy. It is important to distinguish this efference copy from the internal prediction $\hat{\mathbf{y}}[n]$, which is the output of the forward model. (The literature on efference copy and corollary discharge has occasionally been ambiguous in this regard.)

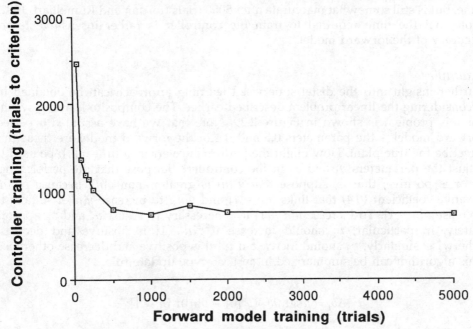

Figure 2.28. *Number of trials required to train the controller to an error criterion of 0.001 as a function of the number of trials allocated to training the forward model.*

acquire a controller that is an inverse of the forward model. Because the forward model is inaccurate, the controller is inaccurate. However, the predicted performance error is not the only error available for training the composite learning system. Because the actual plant output ($\mathbf{y}[n]$) can still be measured after a learning trial, the true performance error ($\mathbf{y}^*[n] - \mathbf{y}[n]$) is still available for training the controller.[13] This implies that the output of the forward model can be discarded; the forward model is needed only for the structure that it provides as part of the composite learning system (see below for further clarification of this point). Moreover, for the purpose of providing internal structure to the learning algorithm, an exact forward model is not required. Roughly speaking, the forward model need only provide coarse information about how to improve the control signal based on the current performance error, not precise information about how to make the optimal correction. If the performance error is decreased to zero, then an accurate controller has been found, regardless of the path taken to find that controller. Thus an accurate controller can be learned even if the forward model is inaccurate. This point is illustrated in Figure 2.28, which shows the time required to train an accurate controller as a function of the time allocated to training the forward model. The accuracy of the forward model increases monotonically as a function of training

---

[13]This argument assumes that the subject actually performs the action. It is also possible to consider 'mental practice' trials, in which the action is imagined but not performed (Minas, 1978). Learning through mental practice can occur by using the predicted performance error. This makes the empirically testable prediction that the efficacy of mental practice should be closely tied to the accuracy of the underlying forward model (which can be assessed independently by measuring the subject's abilities at prediction or anticipation of errors).

time, but is still somewhat inaccurate after 5000 trials (Jordan and Rumelhart, 1992). Note that the time required to train the controller is rather insensitive to the accuracy of the forward model.

Example

Further insight into the distal supervised learning approach can be obtained by reconsidering the linear problem described earlier. The composite learning system for this problem is shown in Figure 2.29. Note that we have assumed a perfect forward model – the parameters 0.5 and 0.4 in the forward model are those that describe the true plant. How might the performance error ($y^*[n] - y[n]$) be used to adjust the parameters v_1 and v_2 in the controller? Suppose that the performance error is positive; that is, suppose that $y^*[n]$ is greater than $y[n]$. Because of the positive coefficient (0.4) that links $u[n-1]$ and $y[n]$, to increase $y[n]$ it suffices to increase $u[n-1]$. To increase $u[n-1]$ it is necessary to adjust v_1 and v_2 appropriately. In particular, v_1 should increase if $\hat{x}[n-1]$ is positive and decrease otherwise; similarly, v_2 should increase if $y^*[n]$ is positive and decrease otherwise. This algorithm can be summarized in an LMS-type update rule:

$$\Delta v_i = \mu \operatorname{sgn}(w_2)(y^*[n] - y[n])z_i[n-1]$$

where $z_1[n-1] \equiv \hat{x}[n-1]$, $z_2[n-1] \equiv y^*[n]$, and $\operatorname{sgn}(w_2)$ denotes the sign of w_2 (negative or positive), where w_2 is the forward model's estimate of the coefficient linking $u[n-1]$ and $y[n]$ (cf. equation 43).

Note the role of the forward model in this learning process. The forward model is required in order to provide the sign of the parameter w_2 (the coefficient linking $u[n-1]$ and $\hat{y}[n]$). The parameter w_1 (that linking $\hat{x}[n-1]$ and $\hat{y}[n]$) is needed only during the learning of the forward model to ensure that the correct sign is obtained for w_2. A very inaccurate forward model suffices for learning the controller – only the sign of w_2 needs to be correct. Moreover, it is likely that the forward model and the controller can be learned simultaneously, because the appropriate sign for w_2 will probably be discovered early in the learning process.

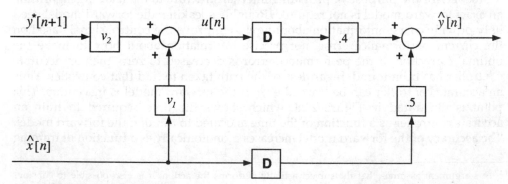

Figure 2.29. *The composite learning system (the controller and the forward model) for the first-order example. The coefficients* v_1 *and* v_2 *are the unknown parameters in the controller. The coefficients 0.4 and 0.5 are the parameters in the forward model.*

9 REFERENCE MODELS

Throughout this chapter we have characterized controllers as systems that invert the plant dynamics. For example, a predictive controller was characterized as an inverse model of the plant – a system that maps desired plant outputs into the corresponding plant inputs. This mathematical ideal, however, is not necessarily realizable in all situations. One common difficulty arises from the presence of constraints on the magnitudes of the control signals. An ideal inverse model moves the plant to an arbitrary state in a small number of time steps, the number of steps depending on the order of the plant. If the current state and the desired state are far apart, an inverse model may require large control signals, signals that the physical actuators may not be able to provide. Moreover, in the case of feedback control, large control signals correspond to high gains, which may compromise closed-loop stability. A second difficulty is that the inverses of certain dynamical systems, known as 'nonminimum phase' systems, are unstable (Åström and Wittenmark, 1984). Implementing an unstable inverse model is clearly impractical, thus another form of predictive control must be sought for such systems.[14]

As these considerations suggest, realistic control systems generally embody a compromise between a variety of constraints, including performance, stability, bounds on control magnitudes and robustness to disturbances. One way to quantify such compromises is through the use of a *reference model*. A reference model is an explicit specification of the desired input–output behavior of the control system. A simple version of this idea was present in the previous section when we noted that an inverse model can be defined implicitly as any system that can be cascaded with the plant to yield the identity transformation. From the current perspective, the identity transformation is the simplest and most stringent reference model. An identity reference model requires, for example, that the control system respond to a sudden increment in the controller input with a sudden increment in the plant output. A more forgiving reference model would allow the plant output to rise more smoothly to the desired value. Allowing smoother changes in the plant output allows the control signals to be of smaller magnitude.

Although reference models can be specified in a number of ways, for example as a table of input–output pairs, the most common approach is to specify the reference model as a dynamical system. The input to the reference model is the *reference signal*, which we now denote as $r[n]$, to distinguish it from the reference model output, which we denote as $y^*[n]$. The reference signal is also the controller input. This distinction between the reference signal and the desired plant output is a useful one. In a model of speech production, for example, it might be desirable to treat the controller input as a linguistic 'intention' to produce a given phoneme. The phoneme may be specified in a symbolic linguistic code that has no intrinsic articulatory or acoustic interpretation. The linguistic intention $r[n]$ would be tied to its articulatory realization $u[n]$ through the controller and also tied to its (desired)

---

[14]A discussion of nonminimum phase dynamics is beyond the scope of this chapter, but an example would perhaps be useful. The system $y[n + 1] = 0.5y[n] + 0.4u[n] - 0.5u[n - 1]$ is a nonminimum phase system. Solving for $u[n]$ yields the inverse model $u[n] = -1.25y[n] + 2.5y^*[n + 1] + 1.25u[n - 1]$, which is an unstable dynamical system, due to the coefficient of 1.25 that links successive values of u.

acoustic realization $y^*[n]$ through the reference model. (The actual acoustic realization $y[n]$ would of course be tied to the articulatory realization $u[n]$ through the plant.)

Example

Let us design a model-reference controller for the first-order plant discussed earlier. We use the following reference model:

$$y^*[n + 2] = s_1 y^*[n + 1] + s_2 y^*[n] + r[n] \tag{45}$$

where $r[n]$ is the reference signal. This reference model is a second-order difference equation in which the constant coefficients s_1 and s_2 are chosen to give a desired dynamical response to particular kinds of inputs. For example, s_1 and s_2 might be determined by specifying a particular desired response to a step input in the reference signal. Let us write the plant dynamical equation at time $n + 2$:

$$y[n + 2] = 0.5y[n + 1] + 0.4u[n + 1]$$

We match up the terms on the right-hand sides of both equations and obtain the following control law:

$$u[n] = \left(\frac{s_1 - 0.5}{0.4}\right) y[n] + \frac{s_2}{0.4} y[n - 1] + \frac{1}{0.4} r[n - 1] \tag{46}$$

Figure 2.30 shows the resulting model-reference control system. This control system responds to reference signals ($r[n]$) in exactly the same way as the reference model in equation 45.

Note that the reference model itself does not appear explicitly in Figure 2.30. This is commonly the case in model-reference control; the reference model often exists only in the mind of the person designing or analyzing the control system. It serves as a guide for obtaining the controller, but it is not implemented as such as part of the control system. On the other hand, it is also possible to design model-reference control systems in which the reference model does appear explicitly in the control system. The procedure is as follows. Suppose that an inverse model for a plant has

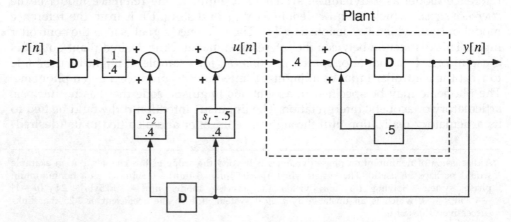

Figure 2.30. *The model-reference control system for the first-order example.*

already been designed. We know that a cascade of the inverse model and the plant yields the identity transformation. Thus a cascade of the reference model, the inverse model and the plant yields a composite system that is itself equivalent to the reference model. The controller in this system is the cascade of the reference model and the inverse model. At first glance this approach would appear to yield little net gain because it involves implementing an inverse model. Note, however, that despite the presence of the inverse model, this approach provides a solution to the problem of excessively large control signals. Because the inverse model lies after the reference model in the control chain, its input is smoother than the reference model input, thus it will not be required to generate large control signals.

Turning now to the use of reference models in learning systems, it should be clear that the distal supervised learning approach can be combined with the use of reference models. In the section on distal supervised learning, we described how an inverse plant model could be learned by using the identity transformation as a reference model for the controller and the forward model. Clearly, the identity transformation can be replaced by any other reference model and the same approach can be used. The reference model can be thought of as a source of input–output pairs for training the controller and the forward model (the composite learning system), much as the plant is a source of input–output pairs for the training of the forward model. The distal supervised learning training procedure finds a controller that can be cascaded with the plant such that the resulting composite control system behaves as specified by the reference model.

It is important to distinguish clearly between forward and inverse models on the one hand and reference models on the other. Forward models and inverse models are internal models of the plant. They model the relationship between plant inputs and plant outputs. A reference model, on the other hand, is a specification of the desired behavior of the control system, from the controller input to the plant output. The signal that intervenes between the controller and the plant (the plant input) plays no role in a reference model specification. Indeed, the same reference model may be appropriate for plants having different numbers of control inputs or different numbers of states. A second important difference is that forward models and inverse models are actual dynamical systems, implemented as internal models 'inside' the organism. A reference model need not be implemented as an actual dynamical system; it may serve only as a guide for the design or the analysis of a control system. Alternatively, the reference model may be an actual dynamical system, but it may be 'outside' the organism and known only by its inputs and outputs. For example, the problem of learning by imitation can be treated as the problem of learning from an external reference model. The reference model provides only the desired behavior; it does not provide the control signals needed to perform the desired behavior.

10 CONCLUSIONS

If there is any theme that unites the various techniques that we have discussed, it is the important role of internal dynamical models in control systems. The two varieties of internal models – inverse models and forward models – play complementary roles in the implementation of sophisticated control strategies. Inverse models are the basic module for predictive control, allowing the system to precompute an appropriate control signal based on a desired plant output. Forward models have several roles: they provide an alternative implementation of feed forward controllers, they can be used to anticipate and cancel delayed feedback, they are the basic building block in dynamical state estimation, and they play an essential role in indirect approaches to motor learning. In general, internal models provide capabilities for prediction, control and error correction that allow the system to cope with difficult nonlinear control problems.

It is important to emphasize that an internal model is not necessarily a detailed model, or even an accurate model, of the dynamics of the controlled system. In many cases, approximate knowledge of the plant dynamics can be used to move a system in the 'right direction'. An inaccurate inverse model can provide an initial push that is corrected by a feedback controller. An inaccurate forward model can be used to learn an accurate controller. Inaccurate forward models can also be used to provide partial cancellation of delayed feedback, and to provide rough estimates of the state of the plant. The general rule is that partial knowledge is better than no knowledge, if used appropriately.

These observations would seem to be particularly relevant to human motor control. The wide variety of external dynamical systems with which humans interact, the constraints on the control system due to delays and limitations on force and torque generation, and the time-varying nature of the musculoskeletal plant all suggest an important role for internal models in biological motor control. Moreover, the complexity of the systems involved, as well as the unobservability of certain aspects of the environmental dynamics, make it likely that the motor control system must make do with approximations. It is of great interest to characterize the nature of such approximations. Although approximate internal models can often be used effectively, there are deep theoretical issues involved in characterizing how much inaccuracy can be tolerated in various control system components. The literature on control theory is replete with examples in which inaccuracies lead to instabilities, if care is not taken in the control system design. As theories of biological motor control increase in sophistication, these issues will be of increasing relevance.

ACKNOWLEDGEMENTS

I wish to thank Elliot Saltzman, Steven Keele and Herbert Heuer for helpful comments on the manuscript. Preparation of this paper was supported in part by a grant from ATR Auditory and Visual Perception Research Laboratories, by a grant from Siemens Corporation, by a grant from the Human Frontier Science Program, by a grant from the McDonnell-Pew Foundation and by grant N00014-90-J-1942 awarded by the Office of Naval Research. Michael Jordan is an NSF Presidential Young Investigator.

REFERENCES

Anderson, B. D. O. and Moore, J. B. (1979). *Optimal Filtering*. Englewood Cliffs, NJ: Prentice-Hall.

Åström, K. J. and Wittenmark, B. (1984). *Computer Controlled Systems: Theory and Design*. Englewood Cliffs, NJ: Prentice-Hall.

Åström, K. J. and Wittenmark, B. (1989). *Adaptive Control*. Reading, MA: Addison-Wesley.

Atkeson, C. G. (1990). Using local models to control movement. In D. S. Touretzky (Ed.), *Advances in Neural Information Processing Systems*, vol. 2 (pp. 316–324). San Mateo, CA: Morgan Kaufmann.

Atkeson, C. G. and Reinkensmeyer, D. J. (1988). Using associative content-addressable memories to control robots. *IEEE Conference on Decision and Control*. San Francisco, CA.

Bernstein, N. (1967). *The Coordination and Regulation of Movements*. London: Pergamon.

Breiman, L., Friedman, J. H., Olshen, R. A. and Stone, C. J. (1984). *Classification and Regression Trees*. Belmont, CA: Wadsworth.

Carlton, L. G. (1981). Processing visual feedback information for movement control. *Journal of Experimental Psychology: Human Perception and Performance*, **7**, 1019–1030.

Duda, R. O. and Hart, P. E. (1973). *Pattern Classification and Scene Analysis*. New York: John Wiley.

Friedman, J.H. (1990). Multivariate adaptive regression splines. *Annals of Statistics*, **19**, 1–141.

Galliana, H. L. and Outerbridge, J. S. (1984). A bilateral model for central neural pathways in the vestibuloocular reflex. *Journal of Neurophysiology*, **51**, 210–241.

Gallistel, C. R. (1980). *The Organization of Action*. Hillsdale, NJ: Erlbaum.

Geman, S., Bienenstock, E. and Doursat, R. (1992). Neural networks and the bias/variance dilemma. *Neural Computation*, **4**, 1–59.

Goodwin, G. C. and Sin, K. S. (1984). *Adaptive Filtering Prediction and Control*. Englewood Cliffs, NJ: Prentice-Hall.

Haken, H., Kelso, J. A. S. and Bunz, H. (1985). A theoretical model of phase transitions in human hand movements. *Biological Cybernetics*, **51**, 347–356.

Hinton, G. E. (1989). Connectionist learning procedures. *Artificial Intelligence*, **40**, 185–234.

Hinton, G. E. and Sejnowski, T. J. (1986). Learning and relearning in Boltzmann machines. In D. E. Rumelhart and J. L. McClelland (Eds), *Parallel Distributed Processing*, vol. 1 (pp. 282–317). Cambridge, MA: MIT Press.

Hogan, N. (1984). An organising principle for a class of voluntary movements. *Journal of Neuroscience*, **4**, 2745–2754.

Hollerbach, J. M. (1982). Computers, brains and the control of movement. *Trends in Neuroscience*, **5**, 189–193.

Jordan, M.I. (1990). Motor learning and the degrees of freedom problem. In M. Jeannerod (Ed.), *Attention and Performance*, vol. XIII. Hillsdale, NJ: Erlbaum.

Jordan, M. I. (1992). Constrained supervised learning. *Journal of Mathematical Psychology*, **36**, 396–425.

Jordan, M. I. and Jacobs, R. A. (1992). Hierarchies of adaptive experts. In J. Moody, S. Hanson and R. Lippmann (Eds), *Advances in Neural Information Processing Systems*, vol. 4 (pp. 985–993). San Mateo, CA: Morgan Kaufmann.

Jordan, M. I. and Rosenbaum, D. A. (1989). Action. In M. I. Posner (Ed.), *Foundations of Cognitive Science*. Cambridge, MA: MIT Press.

Jordan, M. I. and Rumelhart, D. E. (1992). Forward models: Supervised learning with a distal teacher. *Cognitive Science*, **16**, 307–354.

Kawato, M. (1990). Computational schemes and neural network models for formation and control of multijoint arm trajectory. In W. T. Miller, III, R. S. Sutton and P. J. Werbos (Eds), *Neural Networks for Control*. Cambridge, MA: MIT Press.

Kawato, M., Furukawa, K. and Suzuki, R. (1987). A hierarchical neural-network model for control and learning of voluntary movement. *Biological Cybernetics*, **57**, 169–185.

Keele, S. and Posner, M. (1968). Processing of visual feedback in rapid movements. *Journal of Experimental Psychology*, **77**, 155–158.

Kelso, J. A. S. (1986). Pattern formation in speech and limb movements involving many degrees of freedom. *Experimental Brain Research*, **15**, 105–128.

Koh, K. and Meyer, D. E. (1991). Function learning: Induction of continuous stimulus–response relations. *Journal of Experimental Psychology: Learning, Memory, and Cognition*, **17**, 811–837.

Kuperstein, M. (1988). Neural model of adaptive hand–eye coordination for single postures. *Science*, **239**, 1308–1311.

Lindblom, B., Lubker, J. and Gay, T. (1979). Formant frequencies of some fixed-mandible vowels and a model of speech motor programming by predictive simulation. *Journal of Phonetics*, **7**, 147–161.

Miall, R. C., Weir, D. J., Wolpert, D. M. and Stein, J. F. (1993). Is the cerebellum a Smith predictor? *Journal of Motor Behavior*, **25**, 203–216.

Miller, W. T. (1987). Sensor-based control of robotic manipulators using a general learning algorithm. *IEEE Journal of Robotics and Automation*, **3**, 157–165.

Minas, S. C. (1978). Mental practice of a complex perceptual motor skill. *Journal of Human Movement Studies*, **4**, 102–107.

Misawa, E. A. and Hedrick. J. K. (1989). Nonlinear observers: A state-of-the-art survey. *ASME Journal of Dynamic Systems, Measurement, and Control*, **111**, 344–352.

Poggio, T. and Girosi, F. (1990). Regularization algorithms for learning that are equivalent to multilayer networks. *Science*, **247**, 978–982.

Robinson, D. A. (1981). The use of control system analysis in the neurophysiology of eye movements. *Annual Review of Neuroscience*, **4**, 463–503.

Rosenblatt, F. (1962). *Principles of Neurodynamics*. New York: Spartan.

Rumelhart, D. E., Hinton, G. E. and Williams, R. J. (1986). Learning internal representations by error propagation. In D. E. Rumelhart and J. L. McClelland (Eds), *Parallel Distributed Processing*, vol. 1 (pp. 318–363). Cambridge, MA: MIT Press.

Saltzman, E. L. (1979). Levels of sensorimotor representation. *Journal of Mathematical Psychology*, **20**, 91–163.

Schmidt, R. A. (1975). A schema theory of discrete motor skill learning. *Psychological Review*, **82**, 225–260.

Smith, O. J. M. (1959). A controller to overcome dead time. *ISA Journal*, **6**, 28–33.

Specht, D. F. (1991). A general regression neural network. *IEEE Transactions on Neural Networks*, **2**, 568–576.

Turvey, M. T., Shaw, R. E. and Mace, W. (1978). Issues in the theory of action: Degrees of freedom, coordinative structures and coalitions. In J. Requin (Ed.), *Attention and Performance*, vol. VII. Hillsdale, NJ: Erlbaum.

Wahba, G. (1990). *Spline Models for Observational Data*. Philadelphia, PA: SIAM.

Werbos, P. (1974). Beyond regression: New tools for prediction and analysis in the behavioral sciences. Unpublished doctoral dissertation, Harvard University.

Widrow, B. and Hoff, M. E. (1960). Adaptive switching circuits. *Institute of Radio Engineers, Western Electronic Show and Convention, Convention Record*, Part 4 (pp. 96–104).

Widrow, B. and Stearns, S. D. (1985). *Adaptive Signal Processing*. Englewood Cliffs, NJ: Prentice-Hall.

Chapter 3

Coordination

Herbert Heuer

Institut für Arbeitsphysiologie an der Universität Dortmund, Germany

When we speak or eat, ride a bike or drive a car, walk or jump – in almost any activity of everyday life – we have to coordinate simultaneous movements of different parts of the body. In addition to the obvious coordinative requirements there are more hidden ones. For example, when we reach for an object, the movement of the arm produces a shift of the center of mass of the body which has to be compensated to maintain equilibrium.

To a large extent coordination depends on the purpose of an action. Mostly, however, the purpose does not specify the required coordination uniquely. Also, some kinds of coordination are difficult or even impossible to achieve. Thus, in addition to voluntary constraints there are structural limitations, and within the range of possible coordinative patterns left by voluntary constraints and structural limits a choice has to be made. This general perspective on coordination will be outlined first. Thereafter the effects of voluntary constraints and the choice problem will be considered, followed by an extended discussion of structural constraints. Models of coordination will then be presented and the chapter will end with a consideration of lateral asymmetries and the coordination of purposeful movement with posture.

1 GENERAL CONSIDERATIONS

1.1 Voluntary and Structural Constraints

Many tasks require particular coordinations of different limbs or segments of a limb. For example, the two arms are coordinated differently when we open a bottle, swaddle a baby or reach for two objects simultaneously. It is obvious that coordination is primarily determined by the purpose of voluntary actions and by the objects toward which they are directed (Klatzky *et al.*, 1987).

Although coordination is largely under voluntary control, there are limitations. For example, Peters (1977) found no one among 100 students who could concurrently recite a nursery rhyme and tap a 1–3–123 rhythm. Another example of an almost impossible task is to draw a circle and a rectangle simultaneously with the two hands. In such tasks structural constraints on coordination become evident.

Handbook of Perception and Action, Volume 2
ISBN 0-12-516162-X

Structural constraints can be of a 'hard' type and make performance of a task impossible; in this case they impose limitations on voluntary coordination. Together with task constraints and the constraints imposed by the environment they usually define a set of movement patterns rather than a unique pattern. The fact that different movement patterns are possible to achieve a particular purpose is generally referred to as *motor equivalence*. From the very existence of motor equivalence it follows that task constraints and structural limitations are not sufficient to account for a particular coordination that can be observed.

Structural constraints can also be 'soft': they need not impose limitations but rather can induce preferences for one or the other coordinative pattern among the equivalent ones. For example, consider simultaneous rapid aiming movements of different amplitudes to targets of different sizes, the larger amplitude being associated with the smaller target. When performed in isolation, such movements have different durations according to Fitts' law (Fitts, 1954; Fitts and Peterson, 1964; Hancock and Newell, 1985; Meyer et al., 1988). However, durations become almost identical when the movements are performed simultaneously (Corcos, 1984; Kelso, Putnam and Goodman, 1983; Kelso, Southard and Goodman, 1979; Marteniuk and MacKenzie, 1980; Marteniuk, MacKenzie and Baba, 1984). This result has been obtained when subjects were instructed to perform both movements simultaneously without saying anything in particular about identical or different durations; with the instruction to use both hands independently the tendency towards identical durations is weaker but still present (Keele, 1986).

The similarity of the movement times of simultaneous aiming movements certainly does not mean that simultaneous movements with different durations cannot be performed; by way of trying it one can convince oneself that they can. However, to produce different durations seems to be more difficult than to produce identical ones. Thus some structural constraints appear to exist which favor movements of identical rather than different durations, although they can be overcome with some effort.

The above considerations can be conceptualized in terms of cost functions that are defined on the set of equivalent movements that are possible given the task constraints and the structural limitations (Heuer, 1991b). For example, when we reach for an object, its position in space usually does not uniquely specify the particular shoulder, elbow and wrist angles that we end up with. Many combinations are possible but only a small set of these is chosen, probably because they are associated with minimal costs. According to Cruse (1986) the final joint angles can be predicted from cost functions defined on each single joint (Figure 3.1) under the assumption that total costs are minimized (see Sections 2.2 and 4.2.1).

Two fundamental points about motor coordination will be emphasized that follow from the distinction between task constraints and structural constraints. The first one is that coordination is largely determined by the purpose (or intended outcome) of an action, but usually not uniquely so. Structural constraints of the 'harder' or 'softer' variety contribute to the choice of the particular coordinative pattern that is actually produced. The second point is that coordinative relations are fairly loose in general. They can be modified with some effort or through practice and can also be variable in their appearance. This follows from the operation of 'soft' structural constraints which induce stronger or weaker preferences for one or the other kind of coordinative pattern. The looseness of most coordinative relations

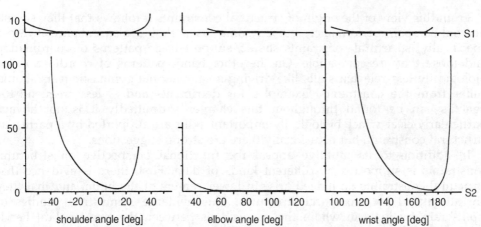

Figure 3.1. *Static costs (arbitrary units) as a function of shoulder, elbow and wrist angles for two subjects (S1, S2). Cost functions were estimated to predict the static joint angles chosen in reaching to targets in different locations. [After Cruse, 1986.]*

is captured by von Holst's (1939) term 'relative coordination', which refers to intermediate states between independence and rigid mutual interdependencies (absolute coordination).

1.2 The Origin of Structural Constraints

The benefits of task constraints on coordination can easily be appreciated: they allow us to perform the particular task at hand. The *raison d'être* of structural constraints, in contrast, is less obvious. Of course, they could be ascribed to an imperfect design of the human brain, neglecting the obvious mechanical constraints. However, this 'deficit perspective' can probably be replaced by a more functional perspective, similar to the view that attentional limitations serve a function rather than represent a deficit (Neumann, 1987).

It can be conjectured that structural constraints are some kind of evolutionary inheritance which have evolved to simplify or solve some basic motor problems. Human motor systems are not general-purpose systems designed for 'arbitrary' tasks like typing, driving a car or playing the piano, but rather they have evolved slowly in the face of some fairly constant requirements for survival and reproduction such as locomotion, stance, eating, etc. In addition, they have been developed by building higher layers of the central nervous system on top of lower ones, thus increasing behavioral flexibility by way of modulating lower systems rather than by replacing them. This suggests the hypothesis that even the most advanced human skills still exploit evolutionary old networks in the midbrain, brainstem or spinal cord that subserve more or less complex reflex patterns (Easton, 1976). The originally highly specialized lower systems could be the source of structural constraints on voluntary behavior.

From this view of the origin of structural constraints it follows that they should not only impair performance, but on some tasks should also enhance it. More specifically, structural constraints should support basic patterns of coordination and those that are compatible. On the other hand, patterns of coordination for biologically less relevant skills like driving a car or some gymnastic feats should suffer from the constraints. Examples for detriments and – less frequently – benefits can be found throughout this chapter. Admittedly it is not always particularly clear which biologically important skills are supported by a particular structural constraint, but occasionally there are strong suggestions.

In addition to its intuitive appeal the functional perspective on structural constraints is supported by different kinds of data. First, there is evidence that structural constraints do indeed arise in lower centers of the brain, and that they are attenuated by neocortical structures. This evidence stems from studies of 'split-brain' patients in whom the connections between the two cerebral hemispheres are (partially) cut.

The task used by Preilowski (1972) required his subjects to control the x–y position of a pen using two cranks: the left hand controlled the position on the y-axis and the right hand that on the x-axis. Subjects had to move the pen as fast as possible along a narrow track of width 2.5 mm and length 155 mm without touching the sidelines. The track had different orientations: a 90° orientation (vertical) required movement of the left hand only, a 180° orientation (horizontal) required movement of the right hand. With a 135° orientation both cranks had to be rotated with identical rates, while for an orientation of 112.5° the left hand had to be faster and for 157.5° the right hand had to be faster.

Two patients with anterior commissures and anterior parts of the corpus callosum sectioned performed this task worse than normal and epileptic control subjects. Figure 3.2 presents records from four consecutive trials of a patient and a control subject who closed their eyes after half the distance had been traversed. The immediate effect of visual occlusion was that the two hands tended to be moved with identical rates in the patient, but not in the control subject; in Figure 3.2 the tendency toward identical rates can be seen as the deviation in the orientation of the path from 157.5° toward 135°. The deviation occurred in consecutive trials although the subject was informed about the error after each of them. Thus, intact communication lines between the cerebral hemispheres appear to be important for overcoming the coupling of the two hands.

Compatible results have been found in studies of normal development. Under the functional perspective, structural constraints on coordination should become weaker as more complex skills are developed in the course of maturation. This is exactly what has been observed. For example, using essentially the same task as Preilowski (1972), Fagard (1987) found that from 5 to 9 years of age children became more proficient in producing a slanted line which required different rates of rotation of the two cranks. In addition, when rates were identical, it made a difference for children of 5 and 7 years, but not for 9-year-olds, whether the cranks had to be rotated in identical directions (parallel movements) or in opposite directions (mirror movements), the latter being easier (see Section 3.2.2). In more general terms, one could hypothesize that motor development is mainly the elimination of 'primitive' structural constraints that result in the mass action typical for newborns (cf. Basmajian, 1977).

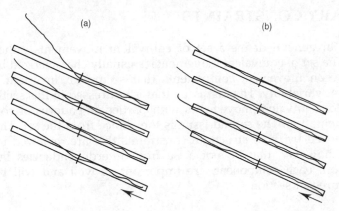

(a)　　　　　　　　　　　(b)

Figure 3.2. *The effect of closing the eyes on the control of* x−y *position using different rates of rotation of two cranks. Paths from four consecutive trials (from top to bottom) are shown for: (a) a patient with a partial commissurotomy, and (b) a control subject. The cursor had to be moved from right to left. [After Preilowski, 1972.]*

A third line of evidence in favor of the functional perspective on structural constraints is found in demonstrations of reflex modulations contingent upon the state of superordinate movement patterns. A well-known example is the reflex reversal in the spinal walking cat (Forssberg *et al.*, 1976). When the dorsum of the paw is stimulated mechanically or electrically, the response is increased extensor activity during the stance phase, but increased flexor activity during the swing phase (accompanied by increased extensor activity in the contralateral leg). The function of this reflex modulation is quite obvious: normally, stimulation of the dorsum of the paw indicates an obstacle that has to be resisted during stance but can be overstepped during swing. Similar reflex modulation during cyclic movements of intact humans has been reported by Belanger and Patla (1987; Patla and Belanger, 1987).

Finally, there is evidence that reflexes can be exploited to support voluntary action. Hellebrandt *et al.* (1956) had their subjects repeatedly lift a load by way of extending or flexing the wrist in pace with a metronome. After some time this task becomes strenuous and the amplitudes of successive lifts decline. Hellebrandt *et al.* observed that their subjects then adopted particular head positions spontaneously: with flexor contractions the face was turned away, but it was turned toward the moving hand when extensor contractions were required. When head position was instructed, orientation away from the working hand enhanced the amplitude of flexions and reduced that of extensions as compared with a condition in which the face was turned toward the working hand. These results correspond to the pattern of the tonic neck reflex which can be observed quite easily in newborns: when the head is turned to one side, extensor tonus is enhanced on this side and flexor tonus on the opposite side. This reflex pattern could also cause a difficulty in early stages of learning to drive a car. According to casual observations, when the head is turned to look back over one's own shoulder, this movement is accompanied by a tendency to turn the steering-wheel.

2 VOLUNTARY CONSTRAINTS

Task constraints in general define a set of equivalent movements rather than a unique pattern. The set of equivalent movements is usually characterized by certain covariations between movement components that secure an invariant outcome despite component variability. The first issue that is addressed in this section is the existence of sets of equivalent movements with particular patterns of covariation and their implementation. The second issue is the choice from the set. This choice is certainly influenced by those structural constraints that are reviewed in Section 3. Other factors, however, that do not arise from interdependencies but rather independently from each component, are important as well and will be briefly discussed in the present section.

2.1 Motor Equivalence

An early report of motor equivalence is that by Stimpel (1933). His subjects had to throw an ivory ball to hit a target at 50 cm distance by way of swinging the arm forward and up from a hanging position. They were trained to release the ball upon touching a horizontal string that was connected to a switch. A platform at the same height as the string was equipped with contact strips to measure distance and duration of the throw. Equations for the ballistic flight were used to determine the initial flight angle and the initial velocity from distance and duration. For a certain distance of a ballistic flight, initial velocity is minimal when the initial flight angle is 45°, and velocity has to be larger whenever the angle deviates from the optimum. To test whether such a relationship did exist in the spontaneous variability of series of (usually 20) throws, Stimpel computed rank correlations between initial velocity and the absolute deviation of the initial flight angle from 45°. The median correlations for 14 or 15 such series were 0.37, 0.30, 0.26 and 0.14 for the four subjects.

Stimpel interpreted the correlations as indicating the subordination of the components (velocity and angle) to the whole as determined by the purpose to throw a certain distance. Being associated with the largely forgotten Leipzig school of 'Ganzheitspsychologie' and its small group of students of motor behavior headed by Otto Klemm, he took his results as support for the notion of a 'movement Gestalt'. This notion, however, does not go much beyond the observation that components of a movement are related to each other in a way that is more or less dictated by the desired outcome. Nonetheless, the concept of a movement Gestalt is strongly reminiscent of the modern concept of a coordinative structure (Kelso, 1981; Turvey, 1977).

A more recent example for covariations of components of a movement has been reported by Hughes and Abbs (1976). Figure 3.3 presents the final positions of upper lip, lower lip and jaw during repeated utterances of a vowel in a context of consonants. While the position of the upper lip remained almost constant, compensatory covariation between the positions of lower lip and jaw can be seen, keeping the lip aperture about constant across repetitions. This was the most frequently found pattern of coordination. A less typical pattern is illustrated in the right half of Figure 3.3. During the first four utterances the compensatory covariation between

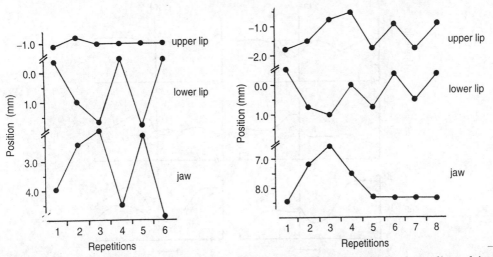

Figure 3.3. *Final positions (as deviations from resting positions) of upper lip, lower lip and jaw during repeated production of a vowel. Two series of repetitions are shown. [After Hughes and Abbs, 1976.]*

lower lip and jaw can again be seen, accompanied, however, by variable positions of the upper lip. During the last four utterances the jaw position remained constant while the positions of lower and upper lip covaried in a compensatory manner.

It is fairly obvious that neural networks that implement covariations between components of a motor pattern must be task specific because the task (or the intended outcome) determines which covariations are required. A second characteristic of task-induced covariations is that they are at least partly afference-based, that is, the underlying neural networks use afferent information on the state of the different components (e.g. articulator positions in speech). This follows from the observation of rapid remote corrections upon perturbation of the movement of one articulator (for review, see Abbs, Gracco and Cole, 1984).

Both the characteristics of task specificity and afferent influences are demonstrated in a study by Kelso *et al.* (1984). The subject repeated the utterance 'a /baeb/ again' or 'a /baez/ again'. The positions of the jaw, the upper lip and the lower lip were recorded continuously. In randomly selected trials a load was applied to the jaw for 1.5 s or 50 ms when the jaw moved upward from its low position during the vowel. Figure 3.4 presents the position–time curves for loaded trials (1.5 s) and control trials. The load was sufficient to depress the jaw; at the same time lower lip position was raised. The response of the lower lip was probably passive; it was not accompanied by an electromyographic response. A remote correction in the upper lip was only observed when the jaw moved upwards toward the final lip closure in /baeb/, but not when the jaw moved upwards toward the final frication in /baez/, in which the tongue rather than the lip aperture is critically involved.

Compensatory covariations seem to be a fairly general phenomenon that can be observed even in simple uniarticular aimed movements (Darling and Cooke, 1987; Garland and Angel, 1971). They are a straightforward adaptation to task requirements: components of the motor pattern are subordinated to a goal-related variable such as the distance of a throw, the aperture of the lips or the amplitude of an

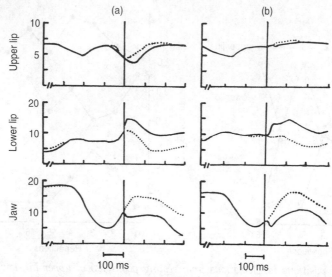

Figure 3.4. *Mean position–time curves for upper lip, lower lip and jaw during repeated perturbed (solid lines) and unperturbed (broken lines) productions of a vowel in: (a)* /baeb/, *and (b)* /baez/. *[After Kelso et al., 1984.]*

aimed movement. How is this subordination achieved? With respect to the formal representation of motor equivalence the answer can be based on a simple principle. This is exploited in the 'task-dynamic approach' (Saltzman, 1986; Saltzman and Kelso, 1987), which is described in more detail in Section 4.1.1. The simple principle is that of coordinate transforms.

Consider a planar movement of the hand from one position to another. This movement can be described in a Cartesian coordinate system in which one axis (the 'reach axis') runs through the start and target positions and the other one is orthogonal to it. Independent equations of motion can be specified for the two axes of this 'task space'. The first transform is that into 'body space', again a Cartesian coordinate system, but centered on the body (e.g. one axis running through the shoulders and the other orthogonal to it). As a consequence of this transform, in particular of the rotation of the coordinate system, the movements along both axes are no longer independent. Coordinate transforms serve to introduce not only interdependencies but also motor equivalence; that is, a set of different movements within a certain coordinate system that all correspond to a particular movement in task space. What is needed for this is an increased number of dimensions, e.g. in transforming the two-dimensional body space into a three-dimensional joint space. Such transforms in general have no unique solution; however, all possible solutions correspond to the unique movement in body space or task space, and the set of possible solutions exhibits the compensatory covariations that serve to fulfill the task requirements.

The task-dynamic approach applies formal charactericts of coordinate transforms to account for compensatory covariations. This, of course, does not solve the problem of implementation in a nervous system. It is noteworthy that compensatory covariations could be achieved using a well-known design principle: that of reciprocal inhibition (Rosenbaum, 1991, ch. 9). To take afferent influences into account, each of, say, two articulators could be inhibited by afferent signals from the other one. Different patterns of covariation could be obtained through the adjustment of gain factors in the inhibitory pathways.

Compensatory covariations serve to obtain stable values of a goal-related variable (e.g. lip aperture). However, they are not the only possible solution. Stable values of goal-related variables could also be obtained by way of using independent stable components instead of interdependent unstable ones. Thus one might suspect that certain advantages result from a system designed with compensatory covariations between component variables. One such advantage becomes obvious when speaking is considered. Phonemes are not characterized by particular articulator positions; rather, articulator positions depend on preceding and subsequent phonemes in addition to the current one (Chapter 9). It seems that such coarticulation is facilitated by compensatory covariations. They permit that some articulators can maintain previous positions or anticipate future ones; the behavior of the other articulators will compensate the context-dependent variations in such a way that the purpose of the gesture will be achieved. A second advantage of a design using compensatory covariations arises as soon as these are at least partly afference-based. In this case the covariations serve to prevent or at least to diminish the propagation of failures or disturbances in components to the system output, the goal-related variable, to the extent that the disturbances can be registered.

2.2 Choosing from Equivalent Movements

The examples of motor equivalence described in the preceding section show spontaneous variability which, however, does certainly not exhaust the set of equivalent movements. The assumption appears reasonable that the movements that are actually performed are chosen because they minimize some kind of costs (cf. Heuer, 1991b). This assumption, of course, poses the question as to the nature of these costs.

As described in Section 1, the final joint angles of the arm in reaching for an object can be predicted from the minimum of the sum of cost functions defined on each single joint (Cruse, 1986; cf. Figure 3.1). It should be noted that the cost functions in Figure 3.1 were not assessed independently but were fitted to predict the observed combinations of joint angles as accurately as possible. Cruse and Brüwer (1987) examined whether the principle of minimizing the sum of static cost functions could be extended to account for trajectories and not only the static situation. They found that the minimization of total static costs had to be supplemented by other principles; the final model produced some compromise between minimization of static costs, straight path of the end-effector, avoidance of non-monotonic joint movements and equal contribution of all joints to the movement (see Section 4.1.2).

In Cruse's (1986; Cruse and Brüwer, 1987) model, cost functions were estimated from performance data. It would be preferable, however, to have independent predictors. Several criteria have been suggested for this purpose (Nelson, 1983; Flash and Hogan, 1985; Wann, Nimmo-Smith and Wing, 1988). However, these are concerned with the trajectory of the end-effector (e.g. hand) and not with the trajectories of the various joints involved in the movement. An exception is the minimum torque-change criterion suggested by Uno, Kawato and Suzuki (1989). According to this criterion, multijoint movements are performed such that the integral of the sum of the first derivatives of torque at the joints involved is minimized. From this criterion smooth trajectories ensue for each joint.

A simple solution to the problem of choosing from a set of equivalent movements can be observed in young children who make their early attempts to use a pen for drawing or writing. Rather than optimizing the contributions of the various joints of the arm to the resulting movement of the pen by some criterion for costs, they 'freeze' the distal joints and by this reduce the set of equivalent movements considerably. The same strategy has been observed in right-handed adults when they attempt to write with their left hand (Newell and van Emmerik, 1989). Even in normal writing something of this strategy seems to be present, but instead of the distal finger and wrist joints the more proximal elbow and shoulder joints are more or less frozen.

Factors like the static costs in the model of Cruse (1986) or the torque change in the model of Uno, Kawato and Suzuki (1989) are defined independently for each joint, that is, for each component of the motor pattern. In addition to such component-specific factors the choice of a movement from the set of equivalent ones seems also to be determined by structural constraints on the relationship between components. An example can be seen in the task to perform two aiming movements simultaneously, as described in Section 1. To these softer or harder structural constraints on coordination I shall turn next.

3   STRUCTURAL CONSTRAINTS

Structural constraints can be inferred from the preferred modes of coordination. They can also be evidenced from errors in the production of certain coordinative patterns or even complete failures. In general, they can be described in terms of relationships between component movements, which again can be attributed to some kind of 'coupling' – a central concept for the following discussion.

In a very general way, structural constraints on coordination can be characterized by two opposing tendencies as described by von Holst (1939). The first tendency is some kind of attraction between simultaneous movements, called the 'magnet effect' (Magneteffekt). It is opposed by a tendency for each movement to maintain its own characteristics, called the 'maintenance tendency' (Beharrungstendenz). The compromise between these two tendencies captures the softer or harder nature of structural constraints. The general description in terms of a compromise between opposing tendencies has to be supplemented with a list of variables for which the compromise results in different strengths of coupling.

As a first example, consider some results reported by Gunkel (1962). Her experiments were modeled after von Holst's (1939) studies of fish. The different oscillations of fins, however, were replaced by oscillations of arms and legs of human subjects. Gunkel's report is only a rather brief summary of her studies on 134 subjects, and all the examples presented are from simultaneous oscillations of the arms. Nonetheless, they illustrate a variety of phenomena to which structural constraints on coordination can give rise.

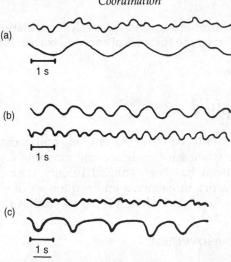

Figure 3.5. *Three pairs of position–time curves for the two arms which illustrate different effects of structural constraints on simultaneous oscillations. (a) Superposition of the slow oscillation on the fast oscillation; (b) the amplitude of the fast oscillation is modulated with the frequency of the slow oscillation; (c) essentially alternating movements of the two arms. See text for details. [After Gunkel, 1962.]*

Figure 3.5 presents position–time curves in which upward deflection of the upper trace represents a forward movement of the one arm while upward deflection of the lower trace represents a backward movement of the other arm. In Figure 3.5a a superposition of the slow oscillation on the fast one can be seen. The phase of the slow oscillation of the one arm relative to its superposition on the fast oscillation of the other arm is noteworthy: when the one arm moves forward, the other one moves backward. Also, there appears to be an integer ratio of 5:1 between the periods of the two oscillations. Finally, a single intrusion of the fast oscillation into the slow one can be seen; similar intrusions have been found by Duncan (1979, experiment 3) in a periodic tapping task.

In Figure 3.5b the amplitude of the fast oscillation is modulated with the frequency of the slow one. When the slowly moving arm is moved backward, the simultaneous backward movement of the faster moving arm is shorter than when the slowly moving arm is moved forward. Again, the periods of the two arms are related by an integer ratio (2:1). Finally, Figure 3.5c shows essentially alternating movements of the two arms. The slowly moving arm stays in a constant position while fast oscillation is produced by the other arm; when the slowly moving arm is moved, the faster arm exhibits a slow intrusion instead of its own oscillation which ends with a larger-amplitude first cycle of the fast oscillation.

Faced with the variety of phenomena that result from structural constraints on coordination, the question arises as to how these can be captured by a small set of principles or even a single comprehensive model. To my knowledge neither the one nor the other exists. What follows is an attempt to outline some major principles without the claim of completeness. These principles are related to the surface characteristics of structural constraints rather than to the generative mechanisms which will be addressed in Section 4. By 'surface characteristics' I mean observables such as the frequency, amplitude and phase of oscillations, while the term 'generative mechanisms' refers to theoretical control structures like motor programs or oscillators.

3.1 Temporal Coupling

Temporal coupling appears to be the most obvious and most pervasive phenomenon that we experience when we coordinate one movement with another or with external stimuli. Formally it has been studied mainly with rapid aiming movements, continuous oscillatory movements and sequences of discrete finger-taps. I shall review the findings from the different types of studies in turn.

3.1.1   Nonrepetitive Movements

As described in Section 1.1, simultaneous rapid aiming movements of different amplitudes to targets of different widths exhibit a striking tendency toward identical durations, even when movement times are vastly different for the movements performed in isolation and the movements are in different directions (Keele, 1986). This finding is supplemented by results on the spontaneous variability of durations when the required amplitudes of left-hand and right-hand movements are identical. Across trials the durations of the movements of the two hands have been found to be highly correlated (Schmidt *et al.*, 1979). However, temporal coupling in rapid aiming movements does not mean that movement times become identical; they only become highly similar, indicating a compromise between the magnet effect and the maintenance tendency which strongly favors the first of these.

Simultaneous aiming movements have simple paths that are identical for the two hands except for displacement and rotation in space. Nonrepetitive movements which differ in their geometric properties have hardly been studied. Casual observations suggest a potential reason: movements with different paths (like a circle and a triangle) are impossible or extremely difficult to produce simultaneously. It seems that one can only succeed when one chooses highly particular temporal structures (like one full circle for each straight line of the rectangle). This again suggests that it might be not so much the difference in geometric forms that makes the task so difficult but rather the difference in temporal structures. Spatial and temporal aspects of a movement are systematically related to each other (Derwort, 1938), although the exact nature of this relationship is somewhat debated (Thomassen and Teulings, 1985; Viviani, 1986; Wann, Nimmo-Smith and Wing, 1988). Temporal coupling, therefore, might prevent the simultaneous production of different temporal structures and, as a consequence, of different geometric forms.

Nevertheless, because temporal coupling is less than perfect, it is worthwhile exploring the limits for the simultaneous production of movements with different geometric forms and different temporal structures. It is likely that the results obtained for such a task will be quite variable; different strategies could be adopted to make the temporal structures compatible such that both movements can be performed simultaneously and task requirements be met as closely as possible. High variability has indeed been reported by Swinnen, Walter and Shapiro (1988) for the combination of a single rapid aiming movement of the left arm and a 'double-reversal movement' of the right arm. (The latter movement had to change direction twice on the way to the target.) Although the subjects were instructed to perform the movements concurrently and within 500 ms, one of the strategies to deal with the task was to somewhat delay the start of one movement relative to the other. This 'staggered initiation' represents a clear deviation from the tendency toward synchronization of movement onsets that has been found in other tasks (Section 3.2). Otherwise a highly variable picture emerged when acceleration of the one hand was plotted as a function of acceleration of the other hand. The rules that hold for the combination of different temporal structures such that they can be produced simultaneously have still to be discovered. (A tentative candidate for such a rule could be temporal alignment of peak accelerations, although this was not an invariant feature of the data.)

3.1.2 Oscillatory Movements

An oscillation of a limb around a certain position can be approximated as:

$$x(t) = C + A\sin(\omega t + \phi)$$

From the examples of Figure 3.5 it is apparent that simultaneous oscillations with different frequencies are possible. However, some effects of one oscillation on another can be evidenced. In the case of superposition the average position (C) of the fast oscillation is temporally coupled to the position x of the slow oscillation, and in the case of amplitude modulation it is the amplitude parameter A.

In most studies of oscillatory movements phenomena like superposition or amplitude modulation have been neglected; rather, the focus has been on frequencies. The outcome of combining two movements with different frequencies depends on the difference between them. A second factor appears to be the mode of control of at least one of the movements, that is, whether it is controlled voluntarily or automatically.

First, consider the coordination of a voluntary repetitive movement with breathing. Wilke, Lansing and Rogers (1975) had their subjects tap in synchrony with every fifth pacing signal; by having to count signals subjects were distracted from breathing, the recording of which was justified as a measure of relaxation. Initially the frequency of the pacing signals was adjusted such that tapping had the same frequency as breathing. When the frequency of tapping was speeded up or slowed down, the breathing rate followed as long as the required change was no larger than about two breaths per minute. The synchronization is illustrated in Figure 3.6a; although there is some phase variability, the taps are uniformly located in the early expiratory phase. Fluctuations in the periods of breathing and tapping covary so that a longer intertap interval is accompanied by a longer breathing cycle and a shorter intertap interval by a shorter breathing cycle. This synchronization is most likely an involuntary phenomenon because an attempt to match tapping and breathing frequencies voluntarily results in a quite irregular breathing pattern as shown in Figure 3.6b.

Another example for synchronization in the case of a small frequency difference has been reported by Kelso *et al.* (1981). The task of the subjects was to oscillate the forefingers with a freely chosen 'comfortable' speed. In isolated performance the

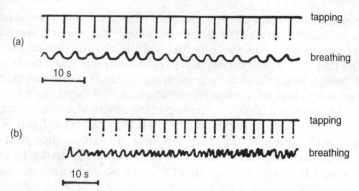

Figure 3.6. *(a) Involuntary synchronization of tapping and breathing; and (b) an attempt at voluntary synchronization. [After Wilke, Lansing and Rogers, 1975.]*

mean frequencies were 1.973 cycles per second for the left and 2.001 cycles per second for the right hand. In concurrent performance the frequencies became almost identical (1.996 and 1.995 cycles per second). Although both oscillations in this study were voluntarily controlled in principle, the small frequency difference was probably not under voluntary control; the increased similarity in bimanual performance was probably unnoticed by the subjects.

Results quite different from those of Kelso *et al.* (1981) were reported by Turvey *et al.* (1986). The subjects had to swing pendulums with the two hands. Even when highly similar 'comfortable' frequencies had been chosen for the two hands in isolation, the frequency of bimanual performance was outside the range of uni-manual frequencies, usually slower. Turvey *et al.* ascribed this new frequency to a 'virtual pendulum' that emerges from the two physical pendulums that had to be swung simultaneously. However, the subjects of this study were also instructed to swing the two pendulums in synchrony. It is not known which factor determines whether the bimanual frequency is a compromise between the unimanual ones or lies outside their range.

When periodic movements with a larger difference between frequencies are combined, one of three different types of outcome can be observed. First, the two oscillations or sequences of discrete movements can be performed essentially independently of each other. Second, the two sequences are combined into a single more complex one; and third, their concurrent production is impossible.

Independence of simultaneous periodic movements with different frequencies seems to be a rare phenomenon that is restricted to particular conditions. For example, Wilke, Lansing and Rogers (1975) observed that the synchronization of tapping and breathing broke down abruptly and was replaced by independence when the difference was larger than about two cycles per minute. In this case one of the periodic movements was clearly involuntary. Muzzie, Warburg and Gentile (1984) found a few subjects who were able to simultaneously walk and clap their hands with different frequencies that were not related to each other by an integer ratio. Again, one of the periodic movements was highly automated and probably subserved by specialized structures of the central nervous system. It is tempting to speculate that independence of periodic movements might be limited to situations where at least one of them is 'special', like breathing and walking; another factor that could contribute towards independence could be the difference between effector systems (McLeod, 1977).

The other two outcomes of combining periodic movements with different frequencies complement each other: either the two sequences can be integrated into a single one with more or less success, or their concurrent production is impossible. The data that support this generalization are from studies of sequences of discrete responses.

3.1.3 Sequences of Discrete Responses

From a series of experiments in which different combinations of rhythms had to be tapped with the two hands, Klapp (1979) concluded that performance strongly deteriorates as soon as the periods of the rhythms are not harmonically related, that is, by an integer ratio. While harmonic rhythms can easily be mapped on a repeated basic time interval and thus become integrated into a single 'combined rhythm', this is not the case for polyrhythms (nonharmonic rhythms). As illustrated in Figure 3.7a, in the harmonic case the basic time interval is given by the period of the faster rhythm, and the end of each interval is associated with a response by either one or both hands. For polyrhythms, in contrast, the basic time interval is not defined by any of the two concurrent rhythms directly, but is the largest common submultiple of the two period durations. Further, as illustrated in Figure 3.7b, in addition to time intervals that end in a unimanual or bimanual response there are time intervals that end in no response.

Deutsch (1983) studied the accuracy of the production of various combinations of rhythms with the same and different periods. The rhythms were produced with the left and right hands and were paced by tones presented to the two ears. The performance measure was the temporal variability of taps around the tones. Simple rhythms were produced more accurately than polyrhythms, and within the set of

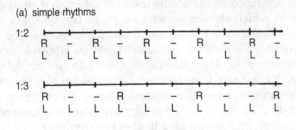

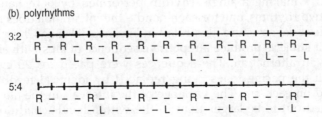

Figure 3.7. *Mapping of (a) simple rhythms, and (b) polyrhythms on a repeated basic time interval; R and L mark responses of the right and left hands.*

simple rhythms there were only small performance differences. These mainly replicated the known result that smaller time intervals are produced with less variability (Peters, 1989; Wing and Kristofferson, 1973). Interestingly, when a rhythm with a certain period was combined with rhythms of progressively shorter (harmonically related) periods, the accuracy of its production increased.

Polyrhythms were produced not only with less accuracy than simple rhythms but also, within the set of polyrhythms, large performance differences were observed. While accuracy was still fairly high for a 3:2 rhythm (the rhythms were paced and the subjects were musically trained), it was close to or at chance level when the ratios between the periods were 5:4, 5:3 or 4:3. Deutsch (1983) noted that the rank order of the polyrhythms with respect to accuracy could be fairly well predicted from a count of the number of subintervals in the kind of representation shown in Figure 3.7 which is mn for an m:n rhythm.

The data on the accuracy of the production of simple rhythms and polyrhythms are suggestive but less than conclusive evidence for the integrated rather than separate control of simultaneous rhythms with different periods. A more convincing approach has been pursued by Klapp et al. (1985, experiment 3). They studied the production of a 3:2 rhythm that was paced by two sequences of tones. The main experimental manipulation concerned the difference in pitch between these two sequences. The difference was either large (300 versus 3500 Hz) or small (300 versus 350 Hz, or 3000 versus 3500 Hz). Large and small frequency differences result in different perceptions of the two sequences. With a large difference in pitch, perception is 'streamed', that is, two separate sequences of tones are perceived. In contrast, with a small difference in pitch a unitary sequence is perceived which consists of high-pitch and low-pitch tones ('integrated'). The rationale for this experimental manipulation is that, if timing control for the two hands is integrated, it should be better served by the integrated than by the streamed pacing signals, while the reverse should be the case if timing for each hand were separately controlled.

Klapp et al. (1985) produced evidence in favor of integrated timing control. The proportion of cycles in which the sequence of taps of the two hands was correct was higher with integrated than with streamed pacing tones, and for correct cycles temporal accuracy was higher as well. The advantage of integrated over streamed pacing signals was replicated by Jagacinski et al. (1988). While the subjects of Klapp et al. (1985) had no particular musical training, Jagacinski et al.'s subjects had six or more years of practice on the piano. (To my knowledge the evidence on integrated timing control contrasts with the belief of professional or semiprofessional pianists that the two hands operate independently in the 3:2 rhythm.)

Although the available evidence strongly suggests integrated timing control for the two hands – making a single rhythm performed by both hands from what appears to be two rhythms, one for each hand – the integration does not necessarily have the simple serial structure illustrated in Figure 3.7. Wing, Church and Gentner (1989) had their subjects produce a repetitive sequence of taps with either one hand or both hands in alternation. The sequences were paced for 20 cycles and then continued with the pacing tones being replaced by identical feedback tones that were presented on each tap. The variance of the intervals in the alternating-hands condition turned out to be larger than in the within-hands condition. In addition the covariance between adjacent intervals, which is negative in general, had an even larger negative value in the between-hands condition. Thus bimanual tapping is not just 'unimanual tapping with both hands'. The same conclusion follows from the finding of Klapp *et al.* (1985, experiment 2) that tapping a polyrhythm, presented by lights and tones, with one hand is more accurate than with two hands. However, the difference between unimanual and bimanual tasks could originate at a rather peripheral level of control rather than at a central level, as pointed out by Wing *et al.*

More complex models of timing control (see Chapter 4) have been examined by Jagacinski *et al.* (1988). The evidence consistently favored integrated models in which controlled time intervals were defined not only within but also between hands. However, the exact nature of integrated timing control remains to be determined. An alternative to the model of a repeated basic time interval as illustrated in Figure 3.7, for example, has been proposed by Summers and Kennedy (1991). According to this alternative model the faster rhythms provide the basic time frame, and the taps of the slower rhythms are inserted into the appropriate intervals.

The rhythms combined can require a degree of complexity of an integrated control structure that exceeds the capacity of the subjects. Tasks that are impossible to perform can easily be found, and persons who are asked to perform such tasks usually refuse to do it from the very start or after a brief unsuccessful first attempt. The limits for producing two different periodic movements are clearly noticed; the performance breakdown is relatively abrupt and contrasts with the 'graceful decline' that can be observed in most tasks when the performance limits are approached.

3.1.4   The Pervasiveness of Temporal Coupling

The section on temporal coupling should not come to an end without noting its pervasiveness. From what has been said, the difficulty in producing two different rhythms simultaneously has much to do with establishing integrated control and relatively little with what is controlled. According to Klapp *et al.* (1985), it is almost as difficult to tap in synchrony with two different rhythms presented visually and auditorily using one hand (tap on each signal) as it is using both hands (one hand assigned to the visual signals, the other to the auditory signals). Similarly, Klapp (1981) obtained for a combination of periodic voice articulation and finger-tapping qualitatively the same results as in his previous study (Klapp, 1979) with right-hand and left-hand tapping. It appears that even mental arithmetic can be speeded up or slowed down by concurrent periodic manual activity (Bornemann, 1942).

Temporal coupling can also be evidenced when a periodic movement is combined with a periodic sequence of external events rather than with another self-produced movement. Casual observation proves that it is difficult to dance a waltz when the marching-band plays. These sensory influences suggest that temporal coupling is not only a motoric phenomenon, but a perceptual phenomenon as well (Klapp *et al.*, 1985, experiment 1). Consistent with this view is a brief remark of Gunkel (1962), according to which passive oscillations of a limb produced essentially the same effects on the other limb as did active oscillations. Such observations appear to support the more general conjecture that timing is a process that is common not only to movements of different limbs but also to perception (Keele *et al.*, 1985).

3.2 Phase Coupling

In the formal approximation of an oscillatory movement as a sine function:

$$x(t) = C + A \sin(\omega t + \phi)$$

the parameter ϕ is called the phase. It represents the position of the movement in time relative to some temporal reference. A particular value can be specified in three different ways, all of which are shown in this chapter. First, the argument of a trigonometric function can be used with radians or degrees as units. Specified in this way, phase can vary between 0 and 2π radians or between 0 and 360°. Second, a particular phase can be expressed as a proportion of the period; then it is a dimensionless number between 0 and 1.

Instead of specifying phase relative to a fixed temporal reference, it can also be specified relative to another movement. Then the term 'relative phase' will be used in this chapter. The term 'phase coupling' refers to a particular relative phase that is adopted when two periodic movements are performed simultaneously and cannot be changed easily. In addition, the term can be used somewhat loosely to designate the tendency to synchronize particular segments of concurrent movements even when they are not periodic; for example, the tendency to synchronize the onsets of simple discrete movements with different limbs (Haferkorn, 1933; Kelso, Southard and Goodman, 1979) can be characterized as phase coupling.

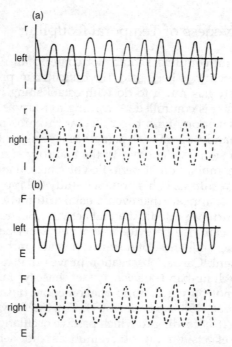

Figure 3.8. *Arbitrary mapping of oscillatory movements on real numbers. In (a) higher ordinate values indicate movements to the right, and the relative phase is about 180°; in (b) higher values on the ordinate indicate flexions, and the relative phase is about 0°.*

Some problems with the concept of relative phase are illustrated in Figure 3.8. Consider the two hands oscillating in a horizontal plane. The mapping of the position–time curves on real numbers is ambiguous. When the right–left dimension is mapped onto the number continuum (Figure 3.8a), the relative phase is approximately 0.5 (180 degrees, π radians), but when the flexion–extension dimension is used (Figure 3.8b), the relative phase is 0 (0 degrees, 0 radians). This, clearly, is an arbitrary choice. Also from Figure 3.8 it is apparent that the relative phase is not a constant as soon as it is determined not only at an absolute temporal reference (like the parameter of a trigonometric function) but also continuously over time.

Given the problems with the concept of phase coupling, other terms are more useful occasionally which do not refer to parameters of mathematical approximations. Two such terms will be used in this chapter: 'muscular coupling' (with 'homologous' and 'antagonistic' coupling as two variants) and 'spatial coupling'. Both these terms denote particular kinds of phase coupling. However, some of the phenomena that are subsumed under these concepts cannot be characterized in terms of phase coupling in any obvious way; on the other hand, there are varieties of phase coupling that cannot be characterized as muscular or spatial coupling.

3.2.1 Preferred Relative Phases

A preferred relative phase – von Holst (1939) used the term 'Koaktionslage' – can be observed in almost any pair of periodic movements. A well-studied problem has been the phase coupling of two periodic movements performed by the left and right hands which I shall consider first.

Yamanishi, Kawato and Suzuki (1980) studied the production of different relative phases between two sequences of finger-taps. The intertap interval was 1000 ms, and the relative phase was 0, 0.1, 0.2, ..., 1.0, so that each tap of the hand followed a tap of the other hand by 0, 100, 200, ..., 1000 ms. Beginning each trial, visual pacing signals for the two sequences were presented and subjects started by synchronizing their taps; measurements were made only in the continuation phase after the end of the pacing signals. The data, however, come out very similar when the pacing signals are continued during the measurements (Schöner and Kelso, 1988a).

Figure 3.9 presents the mean constant errors and mean variable errors (individual standard deviations) of the temporal placement as a function of the instructed relative phase. These data are from unskilled subjects; the results obtained with skilled pianists were qualitatively the same, but the effects were smaller. The variable errors were minimal at relative phases of 0 (synchronous taps) and 0.5 (alternating taps) and higher at the intermediate relative phases. The constant errors were almost zero at the same relative phases. In addition, they were almost zero at relative phases 0.2 and 0.7, but here interindividual variability was large: some subjects had positive constant errors, others had negative constant errors, and the mean values of approximately zero came about through averaging. At the other relative phases the constant errors were either positive or negative. The biases of temporal placement were toward relative phases 0 and 0.5, whichever was closer. Thus there are two stable phase relations. The production of all other relative phases was less stable, and they were biased towards the stable ones.

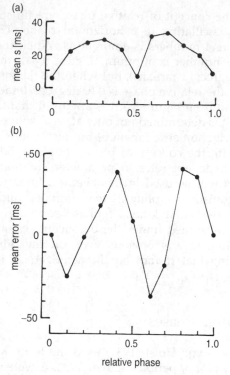

Figure 3.9. *(a) Mean variable error, and (b) mean constant error of temporal placement in bimanual tapping as a function of relative phase. [After Yamanishi, Kawato and Suzuki, 1980.]*

Yamanishi, Kawato and Suzuki (1980) discuss their results in terms of two coupled oscillators (see Section 4.3.2). However, their findings can also be viewed from a quite different perspective, namely that of integrated temporal control as discussed above. Viewed from this perspective, the question arises whether it makes a difference when the taps are performed with a single hand rather than with both hands. Summers, Bell and Burns (1989) studied the production of relative phases 1/12, 2/12, ..., 6/12 using a period of 1200 ms. In addition to the two-hands condition there were two single-hand conditions. In one of them the subjects used two different fingers, in the other only a single finger. Summers *et al.* considered the mean ratios between the two parts of each period; target values of these ratios were 1:11, 2:10, ..., 6:6. No reliable differences between the three response conditions were found. Thus the constant errors were not affected by whether two separate limbs were used to produce the taps or only a single one. In addition the differences between the three response conditions with respect to intraindividual variability (variable errors) were not reliable. These findings cast some doubts on an interpretation in terms of coupled oscillators and support the integrated-timing control perspective.

Unfortunately Summers, Bell and Burns (1989) did not only fail to find differences between the three response conditions, but also failed to replicate the biases observed by Yamanishi, Kawato and Suzuki (1980) as well as the particular dependency of the intraindividual variability on the instructed relative phase. In particular, when instructed relative phases were small (1/12 to 3/12), the bias was not toward synchronous responses but rather toward a relative phase of 4/12 which divides the total period in a 1 : 2 ratio. Similarly, when the instructed relative phase was 5/12, the bias was again toward 4/12 rather than 6/12 (alternating taps). It should be noted that these findings were also obtained when both hands were used to produce the taps; for sequences of taps produced by a single limb the bias toward a 1 : 2 ratio had been noted before (Povel, 1981).

It is unknown what exactly caused the difference between the findings of Yamanishi, Kawato and Suzuki (1980) and Summers, Bell and Burns (1989). Summers *et al.* mention a number of procedural differences which could have played a role, like the amount and type of practice given to the subjects, the modality (visual versus auditory) of the pacing signals and the presence or lack of auditory feedback signals after the end of the pacing signals. No matter what induces them, however, the discrepancy of the findings does strongly suggest that there are at least two different strategies that can be used to produce two sequences of responses that are out of phase. The particular kind of phase coupling depends on which strategy has been chosen. The choice again may depend on how the task is conceived, as the production of a single sequence of responses which happen to be performed by different limbs or as the production of two different sequences that have to be related in a particular way. According to Summers and Burns (1990), the integrated-control strategy could be adopted as a means to overcome the coupling of lower-level oscillators.

It should be noted that the evidence for different strategies of control in out-of-phase movements casts some doubts on the generality of the conclusion that polyrhythms are controlled in an integrated manner. There could be conditions that induce other control strategies for polyrhythms as well which, however, have not been experimentally realized so far.

A variety of phase couplings has been found with periodic movements other than sequences of taps. For example, Wilke, Lansing and Rogers (1975) observed that, in synchronized tapping and breathing, taps occurred mostly in the first 300 ms of the expiratory phase. Expiration thus might induce a tendency to flex a finger, which could also underly the finding that simple reaction time is particularly fast during the expiratory part of the breathing cycle (Buschbaum and Callaway, 1965). Muzzie, Warburg and Gentile (1984), in their study on simultaneous walking and hand-clapping, observed that in most subjects claps were synchronized with heel strikes; as mentioned above, however, some subjects did not exhibit a stable relative phase.

A variety of phase couplings has also been observed in different skills with nonperiodic component movements. Frequently these appear to be more or less dictated by the task. For example, Zimmermann (1980) found unusual phase relationships between different articulators in stutterers. It is possible that stuttering occurs as soon as a particular range of relative phases is left which is a prerequisite for normal speech. Another example which has been studied in some detail is walking. It is characterized by various phase relationships between the different body parts involved (Craik, Herman and Finley, 1975). Not all of them, however, remain constant when the speed of walking is varied.

Relative phases among movements of various joints change in the course of development (see, for example, Williams, 1987, for the forward role; Roberton and Halverson, 1988, for the hop). There seems to be a trend that in older children the tendency toward synchronization becomes weaker. This is consistent with the hypothesis that structural constraints on coordination are generally relaxed in the course of development (see Section 1.2). For example, Williams (1987) found that 5-year-old children have a higher amount of temporal overlap between extensions of various joints in the forward role than do 9-year-old children. It is an interesting question whether such developmental changes result from different age-dependent strategies for performing a particular task, chosen for whatever reasons, or whether such strategies (at least partly) result from relaxed structural constraints.

3.2.2   Muscular Coupling

Some varieties of phase coupling can be described as tendencies to coactivate particular muscle groups. This description can also be applied to data that are not easily subsumed under the notion of phase coupling. The most obvious coactivation tendency is 'homologous coupling': the human body is more or less symmetric, and the term 'homologous coupling' denotes the tendency to coactivate corresponding muscle groups of its two halves. The obvious benefit from this kind of coactivation is that it tends to stabilize the lateral position of the center of mass. (This advantage might not apply to finger movements because the masses are too small; however, homologous coupling between fingers of the two hands might be the result of a generalized coactivation tendency that produces benefits in many other instances.)

Homologous coupling has been most extensively studied using a task that was introduced by Cohen (1971). His subjects had to oscillate their wrists in a horizontal plane; later studies also used oscillations of the forefingers. The movements were performed symmetrically (simultaneous flexions and extensions) or asymmetrically (simultaneous leftward or rightward movements). Cohen used frequencies of 2–4 cycles per second. For symmetric movements be found a higher cross-correlation between the position–time curves of the two hands than for asymmetric movements. In addition he analyzed the temporal variability of the reversals of direction, more specifically the variability of time intervals between corresponding reversals of the two hands. Consistent with the cross-correlational data, he found larger variability in asymmetric movements. Finally, Cohen observed that his subjects sometimes switched involuntarily from asymmetric movements to symmetric ones, but never in the reverse direction.

Cohen's findings were extended by Kelso and associates. In particular, the transition from asymmetric to symmetric movements – that can be observed when the frequency of the oscillations is gradually increased – was studied extensively. One can easily convince oneself by trying it that to produce asymmetric movements is easy as long as the oscillations are slow, but essentially impossible with high-frequency oscillations. Kelso (1984) reported that, when the frequency was increased, the shift from asymmetric to symmetric movements occurred at 1.3 times the preferred frequency for asymmetric movements. This ratio was relatively constant across subjects with different preferred frequencies. It remained constant when friction was added to the manipulanda operated by the two hands, although both the preferred frequency and the transition frequency declined.

The transition from asymmetric to symmetric movements is relatively abrupt; nonetheless, it is preceded by some characteristics of the (still) asymmetric movements that have been reviewed by Kelso and Scholz (1985). Figure 3.10 presents continuous estimates of the relative phase where 180° designates asymmetric

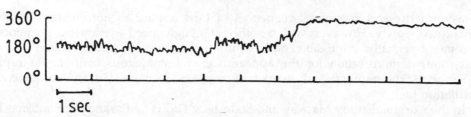

Figure 3.10. *Relative phase as a function of time before and after a transition from asymmetric (180°) to symmetric (360°) oscillations. [After Kelso and Scholz, 1985.]*

movements (periodic adductions/abductions of the forefingers). High-frequency fluctuations can be seen as well as lower-frequency fluctuations. The latter are particularly strong immediately before the transition. Thus, when the relative phase drifts away from its target value (180°), the return becomes more difficult. In addition, corresponding to Cohen's (1971) original findings, variability of the relative phase in high-frequency asymmetric movements before the transition is larger than in the even higher-frequency symmetric movement after the transition. In short, the target phase relation of 180° becomes unstable briefly before the transition occurs.

The findings on simultaneous oscillations of the two hands have been related to changes in gait patterns that can be observed when the speed of locomotion is increased (Kelso, 1984). This certainly does not mean that people start to hop with higher speeds; the phase relations in different gait patterns are more complex than homologous coupling. In addition to this triviality the formal characteristics of speed dependency in locomotion and in the simultaneous-oscillation task are different: while speeding up produces a change of the coordinative pattern in both tasks, slowing down produces a change in the preferred mode of coordination only in locomotion. Finally, at a certain speed different modes of locomotion are associated with different amounts of energy consumption, and the gait pattern appears to be chosen so as to minimize these costs; the minimization results in the choice of different gait patterns at different speeds because the speed dependency of energy consumption is different for different patterns (Hoyt and Taylor, 1981). Such energy considerations seem to play a minimal role at best in the simultaneous oscillation task. Taken together, it is fairly unclear what the relationship between the two tasks really is. Rather than being a paradigmatic task for the study of transitions between different types of coordination which permits the development of general theories for such phenomena, the simultaneous oscillation task might just demonstrate that homologous coupling is not effective in slow oscillations or movement sequences, but only in fast ones. There is other evidence that supports this more modest generalization.

MacKay and Soderberg (1971) have introduced a task on which corresponding observations can be made. This task has received considerably less experimental and theoretical attention than Cohen's (1971) task, probably because it lends itself less easily to an analysis in terms of coupled oscillators. Subjects have to tap simultaneously with the four fingers of each hand in sequence from left to right or from right to left (asymmetric sequences). Although MacKay and Soderberg (1971) did not study symmetric sequences in which homologous fingers of the two hands tap simultaneously, this is obviously an easier task. The difference in the difficulty of asymmetric and symmetric sequences of taps is hard to note when they are performed slowly. However, with a sufficiently high speed asymmetric sequences become essentially impossible and symmetric sequences are produced. As a classroom demonstration for the appearance of homologous coupling in rapid movements the tapping task works as well as Cohen's (1971) simultaneous oscillation task.

In their original study MacKay and Soderberg (1971) had asked their subjects to produce asymmetric sequences as rapidly as possible. A frequent type of error was called 'homologous intrusions'. Such errors consisted of simultaneous taps with homologous fingers of the two hands (note that in correctly performed asymmetric sequences there is no pair of taps that involves homologous fingers). Mostly in one hand the same finger was used twice, one of the two taps coinciding with a tap of the homologous finger of the other hand. Less frequently the sequence of fingers was reversed in the one hand.

The frequency of homologous intrusions depended on various factors. MacKay and Soderberg (1971) found that it was smaller in the dominant hand than in the nondominant one. When subjects were instructed to focus attention on one or the other hand, the frequency of homologous intrusions was reduced in the attended hand and increased in the other one. Finally, for sequences running from little finger to index finger homologous intrusions were less frequent than for sequences running from index finger to little finger. This difference appears to be related to biomechanical factors: sequences of taps from little to index fingers are much more readily performed in terms of 'rolling the hand' than sequences of taps in the reverse direction.

Evidence for homologous coupling can also be found in nonperiodic continuous movements like writing and drawing. According to casual observations, mirror writing with the left hand is relatively easy when one writes with both hands simultaneously. Further, anatomists who work a noticeable part of their lifetime with symmetric parts of the body have been highly skilled in producing bimanual symmetric blackboard illustrations during lectures (this skill could have suffered from an increased use of transparencies, but it certainly existed some 20 years ago).

More formally mirror writing has been studied by Jung and Fach (1984). They found an advantage for the left hand even in unimanual writing. It showed up in right-handers and in left-handers who used the right hand for writing; the latter group of subjects was even more proficient in mirror writing with the left hand than in normal writing with the right one. Only left-handers who wrote with the left hand had no opposite-hand advantage for mirror writing, but some subjects reported that right-handed mirror writing was subjectively easier than left-handed mirror writing. Although the factors that underlie the findings of Jung and Fach are not particularly clear, the results do clearly indicate that homologous coupling is not due to bilateral innervation (Preilowski, 1975) or other kinds of lower-level interactions that are bound to actual muscle activation.

Finally, evidence for homologous coupling has been found in a variety of studies in which discrete rapid movements were used. For example, Rabbitt, Vyas and Fearnley (1975) found faster choice reaction times for simultaneous key presses of homologous fingers of the two hands than for nonhomologous fingers. Wakelin (1976), in an experiment on the psychological refractory period in which the response to the first signal was a key press with index or middle finger of the one hand and the response to the rapidly following second signal a key press with index or middle finger of the other hand, found faster reaction times when the two successive responses were performed with homologous fingers rather than non-homologous ones. Finally, Rabbitt and Vyas (1970) found that errors on a serial choice reaction time task were more frequently performed by a finger that was homologous to the finger of the other hand used for the preceding correct response than by a nonhomologous finger. In anticipation of the discussion of Section 3.4.2, it should be noted that in all tasks described in this paragraph quick decisions as to which finger(s) to use were required.

Although evidence for homologous coupling has been found in a manifold of tasks, this type of muscular coupling is not universal. An exception can be seen when both arms are swung in forward–backward directions as illustrated by Gunkel's (1962) data (Figure 3.5). In this situation extensor activity in one arm tends to be accompanied by flexor activity in the other arm. 'Antagonistic coupling' here is apparently related to the normal walking pattern. Also, it appears to serve balance in that it tends to hold the position of the center of mass constant on the forward–backward axis.

3.2.3 Spatial Coupling

There are some structural constraints on coordination that cannot be described in terms of a preference for the coactivation of particular groups of muscles. Instead, a simple description requires the adoption of a spatial frame of reference. Only a few examples of this kind of coordination exist. One of them has been described by Baldissera, Cavallari and Civaschi (1982). Their sitting subjects had to produce concurrent periodic up-and-down movements with the hands and feet, and their basic result is easily accessible to self-observation. No matter whether the hands were held in a prone or a supine position, the task was easiest when hands and feet moved up and down in synchrony. Similar to Cohen (1971), Baldissera *et al.* observed involuntary shifts to the easier mode of coordination. When one tries the task with increasing frequency of the oscillations it seems difficult to avoid the shift.

Faced with the varieties of coupling, one wonders whether there might be a single principle that underlies homologous, antagonistic and spatial coupling. At least from the tasks studied it appears that these different kinds of coupling might be related to the main axes of the body: homologous coupling is found for movements that normally extend mainly on the right–left axis, antagonistic coupling is associated with movements mainly along a forward–backward axis, and spatial coupling with mainly vertical movements. At least homologous coupling on the right–left axis and antagonistic coupling on the forward–backward axis appear to serve equilibrium. Such a stabilizing function, however, is not apparent for simultaneous up-and-down movements. Thus the functional perspective on structural constraints, as outlined in Section 1.2, is somewhat wanting here.

In concluding the discussion of muscular and spatial coupling, a word of caution is necessary. I have described some observations as resulting from muscular and others as resulting from spatial coupling. This is justified as far as the major influence is concerned. Minor influences of the other kind of coupling, however, have been neglected. For example, differences could exist in the simultaneous oscillation task depending on whether the oscillations are performed in a horizontal or vertical plane. In the horizontal plane coactivation of homologous muscle groups is associated with different spatial directions, but in the vertical plane it can also be associated with same directions. There seems to be a lack of studies in which spatial and muscular relationships are systematically varied. Finally, it should be noted that things become more complicated when simultaneous movements are related to external stimuli; in this case it is not only the relationship between movements that matters, but in addition the relationship between stimuli and that between stimuli and movements (Alluisi and Warm, 1990).

3.3 Force Coupling

With respect to the question of whether forces developed by different limbs in concurrent movements are independent or not, the available evidence is mixed. On the one hand there are clear indications of independence, but on the other hand there are equally clear indications of force coupling. Fortunately the discrepant findings are from different kinds of task.

Evidence for independent force control for the two arms stems from studies of discrete movements, bimanual aiming movements in particular. Although Schmidt et al. (1979) reported a high correlation between the durations of simultaneous left-hand and right-hand movements (computed across series of movements), they found only a negligible correlation between the amplitudes which, for a given duration, are determined by the forces. Similarly, the temporal similarity of bimanual aiming movements of different amplitudes is accompanied by an increased difference in peak acceleration as compared with unimanual movements (Kelso, Southard and Goodman, 1979). This increased dissimilarity, of course, is a consequence of the temporal similarity, given that the amplitudes conform to task requirements.

The different findings on timing and forces in bimanual aiming movements are consistent with the view that timing and force control are separate processes. This hypothesis corresponds to a suggestion of von Holst (1939), and it is in line with generalized motor program theory according to which overall force level and duration are determined by different parameters (Schmidt, 1985). Other evidence in favor of separate temporal and force control is the constant time needed to draw figures of different size (Derwort, 1938; Kern, 1933), provided that the accuracy requirements decline when size increases (Hacker, 1974). According to von Holst (1939), constant durations are achieved by way of an isolated variation of forces, leaving the timing constant.

Evidence for force coupling stems from studies of periodic movements. One can easily convince oneself that it is difficult or impossible, in bimanual sequences of taps, to stress a tap of only one hand. This phenomenon has been studied more formally by Kelso, Tuller and Harris (1983). Their subjects had to oscillate a finger and at the same time repeat the syllable 'stock'. In one condition every second syllable had to be stressed while the frequency and amplitude of finger oscillations had to be maintained. Subjects were not successful in performing this task in that stressed syllables were accompanied by larger-amplitude finger oscillations. In the second condition the task was reversed. Here voluntarily increased finger amplitudes were accompanied by stronger stresses. These observations have been confirmed by Chang and Hammond (1987). In addition they observed a suggestive but unreliable tendency that the effect of the stressed syllable on the amplitude of right-hand finger oscillations is stronger than on the amplitude of left-hand finger oscillations.

What causes the discrepant findings with discrete and periodic movements? A hint toward an answer can be found in a study of Denier van der Gon and Thuring (1965). Their subjects had to write sequences of letters 'e' or 'l' of different sizes. While the forces increased with size, the duration remained essentially constant. This conforms to the early observations of Kern (1933) and Derwort (1938) mentioned above. However, the results were different for the letters 'e' and 'l' in alternation (in cursive writing these are essentially the same forms but of different size). Here the timing for smaller and larger letters became different. This finding suggests that different rules may hold for changing the overall size of a pattern and for the variation of size within a pattern.

One can easily verify that in simultaneous aiming movements, although forces are independent for isolated pairs of movements, coupling does exist when movement sequences are performed. It is difficult or impossible to produce concurrent sequences of constant-amplitude aiming movements with the one hand and alternating small-and-large amplitude movements with the other hand. A prerequisite for the difficulty of this task is that the time intervals between successive bimanual movements are sufficiently small. Therefore, the basic difference between tasks that give evidence for force independence on the one hand and force coupling on the other hand appears to have to do with 'overall differences' in force levels (or different gains) versus 'within-pattern variations' (or different force patterns). As long as the force levels of simultaneous movements can be selected in advance of movement execution, evidence for force independence will be observed. In contrast, when force levels have to be adjusted during execution of one of the movements, these changes will be reflected in simultaneous movements of another limb.

Such considerations suggest the hypothesis that parameters for force control are independent in the steady state, but coupled during transitions. Thus, force coupling is likely to be a transient phenomenon. As long as the transient states of adjusting the force parameters are temporally separated from movement execution, no evidence for force coupling will be found in simultaneous movements. Force coupling will become visible, however, when force parameters are modified during an ongoing movement.

3.4 Structural Constraints During Motor Preparation

So far evidence for various kinds of structural constraints on coordination has been reviewed that can be found in studies of simultaneous movements. However, with respect to motor control a movement begins before a limb changes its position and even before electric signals from the muscles can be recorded. Such preparatory activity has been tapped with different methodologies. In animals, single-cell recordings from various regions of the brain have revealed patterns of activity that are related to characteristics of a forthcoming movement, for example to its direction (Georgopoulos *et al.*, 1989). In people, movement-related slow potentials have been recorded from the surface of the skull which depend, for example, on whether the movement will be performed by the left or the right hand (for review, see Brunia, Haagh and Scheirs, 1985). Finally, on a behavioral level reaction time has been found to depend on some of the characteristics of the response, such as the number of its components (for review, see Rosenbaum, 1985).

Given the evidence for the existence of preparatory processes that precede the open onset of a movement, the question arises whether structural constraints on the simultaneous execution of two movements also apply to their simultaneous preparation. In other words: do structural constraints come into existence only with the onset of the open movements or with the onset of their preparation? This question can receive an 'early' as answer on the tentative assumption that there is no qualitative difference between processes during preparation and execution but rather some kind of continuity so that the actual onset of the movement is not a particularly distinguished event in terms of motor control (Heuer, 1985; Näätänen and Merisalo, 1977).

The tentative answer to the question of the existence of structural constraints during motor preparation is supported by the results of several choice reaction time experiments that have been reviewed by Heuer (1990a). The basic rationale of these experiments is quite simple, although the details have been a matter of debate (Heuer 1988a; Rosenbaum, Barnes and Slotta, 1988). Suppose that upon presentation of a response signal the subject has to perform a left-hand or a right-hand response as rapidly as possible. On each trial only one response is executed, namely the one indicated by the response signal. Preceding the presentation of the response signal, however, and probably for some time thereafter until its full identification, subjects do not know which of the two responses they will have to perform. It would thus be a good strategy for them to prepare both of the alternative responses simultaneously as thoroughly as possible when they aim at really fast reaction times.

The extent to which different left-hand and right-hand movements can be prepared simultaneously should depend on structural constraints. Without the effects of structural constraints it should be possible to prepare two different movements simultaneously to a full extent. Thus, motor preparation should be as good as in a control condition in which the same movements are assigned to the left and right hands, and choice reaction time should not differ between conditions. However, when structural constraints are in effect, the simultaneous preparation of different movements should be impaired. As a consequence, choice reaction time should be longer than in the control condition.

From the rationale of the choice reaction time experiments one would expect their results to converge with those obtained in studies of simultaneous movements. Such convergence was in fact observed, at least for those varieties of coupling that have been studied. The evidence for each type of coupling will be reviewed in turn. It should be noted that the convergence of results from choice reaction time experiments and simultaneous movement studies suggests that the various kinds of coupling originate at a central level of motor control which is already involved in motor preparation, and are not caused by overflow of muscle innervation or similar processes that are bound to movement execution.

3.4.1 Temporal Coupling

Temporal coupling of simultaneous movements is probably the most conspicuous type of coupling. As reviewed in Section 3.1.1, it is almost impossible to perform two movements with different spatiotemporal patterns simultaneously. Evidence for this structural constraint has also been found in choice reaction time experiments.

Heuer (1982a, b) studied two simple finger movements, the one being an up-and-down movement of the forefinger or thumb (called 'tapping'), and the other a mainly horizontal to-and-fro movement between two keys with only a small vertical component (called 'alternating'). Although both movements had a single reversal of direction, they had clearly different spatiotemporal characteristics, and most people find it difficult or even impossible to perform them simultaneously.

When subjects had to choose between left-hand and right-hand responses, reaction time depended on whether same (tapping-tapping, alternating-alternating) or different movements (tapping-alternating, alternating-tapping) were assigned to the two hands. In different-movements conditions mean reaction time was longer. In addition, the trial-to-trial variability of reaction times was larger than in same-movement conditions, and choice accuracy (percentage of responses with the correct hand) was higher. Although the longer mean reaction time in different-movements conditions was accompanied by higher choice accuracy, the difference between conditions could not be explained simply in terms of a speed–accuracy tradeoff (Heuer, 1983).

Follow-up experiments (Heuer, 1984a) revealed that the three effects on mean reaction time, reaction time variability and choice accuracy could also be obtained when tapping responses of different durations were used or tapping and alternating responses of identical rather than different durations. In this experiment tapping responses of different durations also differed in relative timing: longer durations were mainly achieved by increasing the duration of the reversal phase of the movement, while the up-and-down strokes were scarcely affected. Similar findings, at least as far as mean reaction time is concerned, have been reported by Zelaznik, Shapiro and Carter (1982) when key presses of different durations were assigned to the two hands.

Less conspicuous evidence for temporal coupling than in the simultaneous production of different spatiotemporal patterns has been observed in studies of simultaneous rapid aiming movements (cf. Section 3.1.1). Corresponding to these results, choice reaction time experiments have revealed an increase of reaction time when aimed movements of different durations rather than same durations were assigned to the two hands (Heuer, 1986a). Interestingly, the increase in reaction time was small compared with that found in the 'tapping-alternating' experiments, and no effects were observed for intraindividual variability and choice accuracy. In view of the different findings it is suggestive to hypothesize that temporal coupling might not be a unitary phenomenon. Differences, for example, could exist between the coupling of overall durations of essentially the same temporal patterns and the coupling of temporal patterns.

3.4.2   Homologous Coupling

Despite the evidence for homologous coupling as reviewed in Section 3.2.2, choice reaction time experiments initially failed to reveal differences between conditions with same and different fingers assigned to the two hands (Heuer, 1982a, b, c; Rosenbaum and Kornblum, 1982; Zelaznik, Shapiro and Carter, 1982). However, closer scrutiny revealed the reasons for this failure.

As discussed in Section 3.2.2, evidence for homologous coupling comes from tasks in which rapid decisions about which finger to use are required. In contrast, when there is sufficient time first to decide which finger to use and only thereafter to activate it, no evidence for homologous coupling appears to be visible. In the choice reaction time experiments which failed to produce evidence for homologous coupling, the assignment of fingers to hands was constant over blocks of trials. Thus the decision about which finger of each hand to use was probably made well in advance of actually using the finger. Under such circumstances homologous coupling should not show up, according to the observations made with simultaneous movements. However, evidence for homologous coupling should emerge as soon as the selection of the appropriate finger and its activation are not sufficiently separated in time.

Heuer (1986b) tested this expectation by means of two different procedures that were intended to avoid the temporal separation of selection and activation of fingers. The mean reaction times obtained with one of these procedures are presented in Figure 3.11. In this experiment each response signal was preceded by a precue. Forefingers and middle fingers of the two hands rested on keys. The precue consisted of two light-emitting diodes from a row of four. It indicated those two fingers from which a rapid choice had to be made upon presentation of the response signal, which was a single light-emitting diode from a second row of four.

When the precue comes up simultaneously with the response signal, reaction time should not benefit from it. Consequently reaction time was long at the precuing interval of 0 ms and not different between conditions with same and different fingers assigned to the two hands (as instructed by the precue). When the precue precedes the response signal by a relatively long time interval, reaction time should be faster overall because the response signal specifies one of two rather than one of four potential responses. However, again no difference between same-fingers and different-fingers conditions should exist because finger selection can be finished well in advance of the response signal. Corresponding results are shown in Figure 3.11 for precuing intervals of 800 and 2000 ms. Between the precuing intervals of 0 and 800 ms, however, time intervals should exist where finger specification is not yet finished when the response signal is presented. Here the longer time needed to specify nonhomologous fingers (different fingers of the two hands) as compared with homologous fingers (same fingers of the two hands) should become visible as an increased reaction time. In Figure 3.11 this is the case at the precuing interval of 250 ms.

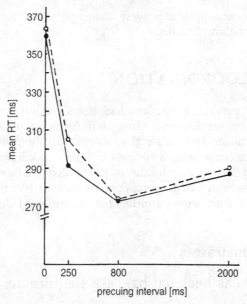

Figure 3.11. *Choice reaction time with same (homologous, ●——●) and different (nonhomologous, ○——○) fingers assigned to the two hands as a function of the time interval between precue and response signal. RT, reaction time. [After Heuer, 1986b.]*

The results of this as well as of the second experiment of Heuer (1986b) support the notion of homologous coupling as a transient phenomenon, similar to force coupling in this respect (see Section 3.3). Homologous coupling exists only during the transient states of specifying muscle groups to be activated, not for the steady states after specification has been finished. This hypothesis is not only consistent with the choice reaction time data, but also with the finding that simultaneous movement sequences or periodic movements which require coactivation of non-homologous muscle groups are easy as long as they are slow, but become progressively more difficult and finally impossible when speeded up. Speeding them up probably reduces the temporal separation of specification and activation so that activation finally coincides with the transient states, making them visible in overt behavior. Interestingly, transient homologous coupling can also generate the shift from asymmetric to symmetric movements in the simultaneous oscillation task when frequency is increased (Heuer, 1993).

3.4.3 Force Coupling

As argued in Section 3.3, it is likely that force coupling is a transient phenomenon like homologous coupling. However, the relevant reaction time data to support this hypothesis are missing. What is available, however, are data that support force independence for steady states of movement specifications and which correspond to the results obtained with simultaneous aiming movements of different ampli-tudes. Heuer (1986a) found no reliable increase of reaction time when aiming movements with different amplitudes were assigned to the left and right hand as compared with the same amplitudes.

4 MODELS OF COORDINATION

The emphasis of the preceding section has been on surface characteristics of coordination. The present section, in contrast, will focus on generative mechanisms. It deals with theoretical models rather than empirical phenomena and generalizations. Models of motor coordination address different problems: the subordination of coordinative patterns to task requirements, the choice of a particular pattern from a set of equivalent ones, and phenomena that are caused by structural rather than voluntary constraints. I shall review models for the different domains in turn.

4.1 Voluntary Constraints

4.1.1 Coordination as Dictated by Task Requirements

As exemplified in Section 1.2.1, components of a movement often covary in such a way that the task requirements are met with only little variation despite higher variability of the components. In general terms, the 'parts' are organized as a coordinative structure or as a movement Gestalt. A formal model for the transformation of task requirements into the appropriate covariations has been proposed by Saltzman and Kelso (1987; Saltzman, 1986). The principle of coordinate transforms on which this model is based has been briefly described in Section 1.2.1; this will be completed with a more comprehensive presentation of the model here. As an example, consider a movement that is aiming in a horizontal plane and that is performed using the elbow, the shoulder and the wrist.

The model starts with the definition of a 'task space'. This is a Cartesian coordinate system which, for the task at hand, is centered on the target, the 'reach axis' (t_1) running through the start position (Figure 3.12a). Equations of motion are defined for both axes with a common mass coefficient and separate damping and stiffness coefficients. The initial values are 0 for accelerations and velocities; for positions they are 0 for the normal axis and equal to the start position for the reach

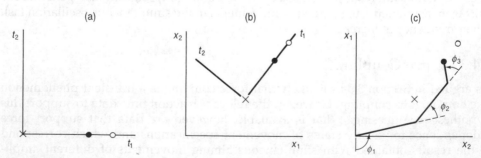

Figure 3.12. (a) Task space, (b) body space, and (c) articulator space for discrete reaching. Target position is indicated by a cross, start position by an open circle, and 'task-mass' position by a closed circle. [After Saltzman, 1986.]

axis. The task-space part of the model is thus a simple mass-spring model (Cooke, 1980) that can be rejected when tested against real movements (Darling and Cooke, 1987). In Saltzman's model, however, the simple mass-spring model is applied to a virtual mass that has no physical existence. The parameters and variables are abstract and cannot be identified with measurable quantities.

The next step in the model is to locate the task space in 'body space', which for the reach is a Cartesian coordinate system centered in the shoulder (Figure 3.12b). In this step the coordinate system is usually transposed and rotated. As a result of the rotation the motions on the two dimensions x_1 and x_2 are no longer independent; 'coordination' is thus introduced in a basically very simple manner.

The second transform is from body space into 'articulator space' (Figure 3.12c). In this step the positions, velocities and accelerations on the two dimensions of body space are expressed in terms of angular accelerations, angular velocities and angles of the shoulder, elbow and wrist (ϕ_1, ϕ_2, ϕ_3). This transform is indeterminate, that is, there is no unique solution. The indeterminateness results from the fact that the body space is two-dimensional, but the joint space three-dimensional, and it corresponds to the phenomenon of motor equivalence; there are many different joint configurations for a certain position of the finger in a plane. To obtain a unique solution more or less arbitrary decisions have to be made, the results of which affect the relative contributions of the three joints to the movement. In addition to defining a pattern of covariations among the different joint movements, the transform into articulator space also defines time-varying parameters for their equations of motion. Thus, although the parameters are constant in task space, they are no longer so in articulator space.

The concepts of task space, body space and articulator space refer to an abstract model arm. Therefore a final step is needed which links the behavior of the model arm to that of a real arm. However, as far as the problem of coordination is concerned, this link to the real world is of little relevance; it is designed such that the behavior of the real arm matches that of the model arm as closely as possible.

The task-dynamic approach, as the class of models has been called that start with the specification of movement dynamics in task space and run through the series of transforms described above, provides a straightforward formal description of the subordination of movement components to task requirements as well as of the genesis of sets of equivalent movements. However, the problem of choosing from the set of equivalent movements is left to essentially arbitrary decisions about the elements of a weighting matrix that is needed to obtain a unique solution for the transform from body space into joint space. Both problems – that of coordination as enforced by task requirements and that of choosing between equivalent movements – are also addressed by a model of Bullock and Grossberg (1988), which, however, originated from a quite different general approach.

Although coordination is not the central problem addressed by Bullock and Grossberg's (1988) model, its relevant features will be briefly reviewed. The basic structure of a single channel of the model (more accurately, a lumped channel for an antagonistic pair of muscles) is illustrated in Figure 3.13 (Heuer, 1991a). Essentially, it is a closed-loop system in which the difference between the target position (T) and the current position (P) is first low-pass filtered and then integrated. A linear closed-loop system of this kind, however, exhibits some characteristics which deviate from those of human movements. For example, its output starts with peak velocity when the target position is shifted stepwise, while

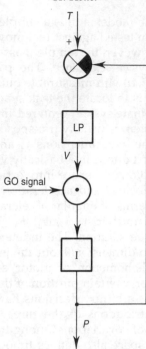

Figure 3.13. *Diagram of a channel (lumped channel for an antagonistic pair of muscles) of the model of Bullock and Grossberg (1988). LP, low-pass filter; I, integrator.*

a human aiming movement starts with a gradual increase of velocity (and also of acceleration). Undesirable characteristics are eliminated through the introduction of the GO signal which multiplies the low-pass filtered error V. It is equivalent to a time-dependent gain factor (or time constant) of the integrator. When the gain factor is gradually increased after a stepwise shift of the target position, the model produces output that is highly similar to human aimed movements.

Coordination is addressed by the model when the variables T, P and V are treated as vectors rather than scalars, that is, when multiple channels rather than a single one are considered. The vector components and thus the channels are related to the various muscles involved in the movement. At time zero the current-position vector **P** specifies their start lengths and the target-position vector **T** their intended final lengths. The difference vector **V** specifies the contribution of each muscle to the movement and by this not only the movement's amplitude but also its direction. While the variables **T**, **P** and **V** are vectors, the GO signal is a scalar in principle. Otherwise its application would modify the relative magnitudes of the **V** components and thus the direction of the movement.

As presented by Bullock and Grossberg (1988, 1991) the model neglects the problem that, although the target position for a reach uniquely determines the amplitude and the direction of the movement, it does not generally specify a unique target vector **T**, that is, intended final muscle lengths. Thus the model does not tackle the static aspect of motor equivalence, the fact that a particular static position of an end-effector can be achieved by way of different static lengths of the various muscles involved. Implicitly, however, it recognizes the phenomenon of motor equivalence.

In contrast, the model offers a solution for the dynamic aspect of motor equivalence once the static target-position vector has been determined. Formally this solution is contained in the scalar GO signal. The operation of the GO signal has the effect that all muscles involved in the movement work in synchrony. Different length changes of different muscles are achieved through different velocities rather than different durations. Although Bullock and Grossberg (1988) consider synchronous activity of the muscles of a synergy as a fundamental characteristic of motor control, they also recognize that muscle contractions do not always start in strict synchrony. One of the model's characteristics is that, when the components of the target-position vector change at variable times after the start of the GO signal, termination of the activity of the various muscles will be more in synchrony than initiation. This results from the fact that for later-starting muscles the large initial components of the difference vector **V** are multiplied by larger values of the increasing GO signal, thus producing increased initial velocities as compared with an earlier start where the initially large components of **V** are multiplied with the earlier and smaller values of the GO signal.

The solution of the dynamic aspect of motor equivalence which is adopted in Bullock and Grossberg's (1988) model can be characterized in a very simple manner: all components (muscles) are driven by a single signal, the GO signal. To accommodate different distances, it is multiplied by different time-dependent factors (the **V** components). Whether or not this simple scheme provides a valid description for coordination in principle appears to depend on how the components are defined. Bullock and Grossberg (1988, 1991) conceive of them as representing different muscles (rather than, for instance, joint angles or dimensions of external space). Soechting and Lacquaniti (1981) presented data on the electromyographic activity of muscles acting on the shoulder and the elbow during a reach. These activity patterns appear not to correspond to the characteristics of model-muscle length changes (Soechting and Lacquaniti, 1981, Figs 7–9).

4.1.1 Choosing from Equivalent Movements

Models for the choice from a set of equivalent movements have been briefly discussed in Sections 1.1 and 2.1. For planar reaching movements, Cruse's (1986) model predicted terminal joint configurations in terms of cost functions which were defined on static joint angles (Figure 3.1). These cost functions, however, turned out not to be predictive for the dynamic aspect of motor equivalence (Cruse and Brüwer, 1987). A model for the choice of movement trajectories rather than terminal joint configurations required additional assumptions.

Cruse and Brüwer (1987) developed a stepwise approximation of the model to human trajectories by way of adding further assumptions to the minimization of static costs. The first additional assumption was that of straight paths (Morasso, 1981). A second additional assumption was that of equal contributions to the movement of the various joints. It is fairly obvious that the three criteria – minimization of static costs, straight path and equal joint contributions – may conflict with each other. Thus a compromise had to be envisaged, which was implemented by Cruse and Brüwer (1987) in the following way.

A small change in one of the joint angles is accompanied by a small shift of the position of the end-effector that can be represented by a vector (dx, dy); the shift in the position of the end-effector which results from simultaneous incremental changes of all three joints is given by the sum of three such vectors. The conditions of straight paths and equal joint contributions (as far as possible) were met by calculating the incremental changes such that the squared vector lengths were minimized. Static costs were taken into account by weighting the vector lengths with the corresponding costs before minimization. In this stage of development the model provided a reasonable qualitative fit to the joint movements observed when the end-effector moved along a straight path. However, Cruse and Brüwer observed not only straight paths, but curved ones as well (Atkeson and Hollerbach, 1985).

To account for curved paths, Cruse and Brüwer (1987) suggested a tendency to avoid extreme nonlinearities in the relationships between the movements of different joints, that is, extreme nonlinearities in the functions which relate one joint angle to another one. Formally this hypothesis was implemented through a compromise between a straight path of the end-effector and linear relationships between joint angles. To the incremental changes in joint angles computed as outlined above, were added incremental changes derived from separate mass-spring models (Cooke, 1980) for the three joints.

The complete model of Cruse and Brüwer (1987) chooses trajectories according to a fairly complex mixture of different types of costs. Several of the solutions adopted in the model appear somewhat arbitrary, and it is not fully clear to what extent its fit is the result of its essential characteristics or simply its many degrees of freedom. Also, the nature of static costs remains vague. Cruse (1986) suggested that they might be determined physiologically as well as strategically. For example, it is apparent that extreme joint positions are more uncomfortable than the middle range; in addition, they are strategically bad choices because they are associated with a restricted range of potential movements. Thus it is at least plausible that static cost functions defined on joint angles should be U-shaped (see Figure 3.1).

The choice process described by Cruse and Brüwer (1987) is considerably more complex than that of Bullock and Grossberg's (1988) model, which rests on only a single principle for the dynamic aspect of motor equivalence, namely that of a common GO signal. However, the two models are not really rival models because they refer to different types of components of a movement, to joint angles and muscle lengths, respectively.

Even for joint angles simpler models for motor choice have been proposed that are based on the minimization of other kinds of costs. One such model is the minimum torque-change model of Uno, Kawato and Suzuki (1989) which is a modification of the minimum jerk model (Flash and Hogan, 1985; Hogan, 1984). Instead of minimizing the time integral of the sum of squared third derivatives with respect to time of the Cartesian coordinates of the end-effector, it minimizes the time integral of the sum of the squared third derivatives of joint angles (for a constant moment of inertia); more correctly, it is the torque change that is considered rather than the derivative of angular acceleration. In intuitive terms, movements performed in line with this criterion are maximally smooth; as far as possible, forces remain constant or are modulated in a very gentle manner. In the mimimum torque-change model this criterion is applied to individual joints, and in the minimum jerk model it is applied to resulting forces at the end-effectors.

Uno, Kawato and Suzuki (1989) did not present the joint movements generated by the model, but only the trajectories of the end-effector in Cartesian coordinates. Thus it is not fully clear what patterns of joint coordination are chosen according to the minimum torque-change criterion. Whatever these are, however, the resulting trajectories of the end-effector correspond fairly well to those of human arms. In particular, they mimicked the changes in human trajectories when movements were performed in different parts of the workspace; for example, movements between two points approximately in front of the trunk have straight paths, while movements that start with an almost laterally extended arm and end in front of the trunk are curved. Such changes in trajectories across the workspace are inconsistent with the minimum jerk model, which invariably predicts straight paths. In contrast to the minimum torque-change model the minimum jerk model is neutral with respect to the component movements that together produce the movement of the end-effector.

4.2 Structural Constraints

As stressed repeatedly, patterns of coordination are largely dictated by the task requirements, but often the task requirements do not specify a unique pattern. Models for the subordination of movement patterns to task requirements and for the choice among the potential movements that fulfill the requirements have been reviewed in the preceding section. In this section I shall turn to models of structural constraints on coordination. Such constraints impose limits on the varieties of coordination that can be adopted voluntarily.

4.2.1 Common and Specific Parameters of Control

According to everyday observations, movements differ qualitatively as well as quantitatively. This distinction between two types of differences has been captured by the notion of generalized motor programs (Heuer, 1990b; Schmidt, 1975; for review, see Summers, 1989). Generalized motor programs are thought of as central structures that are suited to control a particular class of movement. Which particular movement of the class is actually performed depends on the values of parameters that have to be set before the movement is initiated.

A major issue for generalized motor program theory is the distinction between invariant characteristics of movements that are determined by the program and variable characteristics that depend on the parameters. It has been suggested that relative forces and relative timing are among the invariant characteristics, while average force level and total duration depend on parameters (Schmidt, 1980, 1985). This hypothesis essentially holds that a generalized motor program specifies a force–time profile, the axes of which are scaled by the parameters. It should be noted that this is a simple kind of parameterization which corresponds to that of a sine function, but which cannot claim particularly high plausibility *a priori*.

Given the notion of different parameters for generalized motor programs, it is a fairly straightforward assumption that some parameters, the specific ones, can be set independently for the two hands, while other parameters, the common ones, apply to movements of both hands simultaneously. This view is illustrated in Figure 3.14, which, in addition, implies that only one program is used for bimanual movements. With respect to bimanual aiming, Schmidt *et al.* (1979) argued from their correlational data on durations and amplitudes (see Sections 3.1.1 and 3.3) that duration parameters are common to both hands while force parameters are specific.

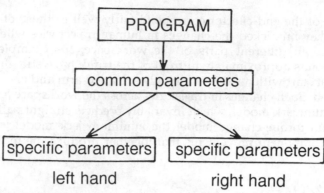

Figure 3.14. *The distinction between common and specific parameters of a generalized motor program. [After Schmidt et al., 1979.]*

This hypothesis has been supported by the results of choice reaction time experiments (Heuer, 1986a; and see Sections 3.4.1 and 3.4.3).

The conceptualization of structural constraints on coordination in terms of common programs and common and specific parameters has some virtues. For example, generalized motor program theory clearly distinguishes between a temporal pattern and its overall duration. Under the assumption that only one program at a time can be applied to both hands, it is a straightforward prediction that it should be impossible to produce two different temporal patterns simultaneously. This may not be exactly so but the statement is a reasonable approximation (see Section 3.1). Although overall duration is postulated to be determined by common parameters, there could be differences between tasks that require the production of different overall durations (different parameters) or different temporal patterns (different programs). Such differences have been observed in choice reaction time experiments (Heuer, 1986a; and see Section 3.4.1); in simultaneous performance, in addition, the one kind of task appears to be more difficult than the other one. Finally, the distinction between common and specific parameters permits a simple conceptualization of findings according to which some characteristics of movements are independent for the two hands, while others are more or less tightly coupled.

Despite the virtues, closer scrutiny reveals several weaknesses of generalized motor program theory as far as coordination is concerned. For example, some varieties of coupling appear to be transient phenomena; no distinction between transient and steady states of parameters, however, is made in the theory. Also, the distinction between common and specific parameters is categorical, while structural constraints on coordination are a matter of degree; therefore the model is unable to capture the basic compromise between the magnet effect and the maintenance tendency in simultaneous movements. More basic than these weaknesses are the uncertainties about which movement characteristics are actually defined by programs or by parameters. For example, the hypothesis that relative timing is an invariant characteristic might not be tenable (Gentner, 1982, 1987; Heuer, 1984b); even if it were tenable (Heuer, 1988a), there is evidence that it is a strategic movement characteristic rather than a mandatory one as required by generalized motor program theory (Heuer, 1988b; Heuer and Schmidt, 1988).

4.2.2 Coupled Oscillators

The notion of central oscillators has been invoked to model the generation of periodic movements. Central oscillators can be thought of as particular generalized motor programs (Cruse *et al.*, 1990). Structural constraints on simultaneous movements can be captured through couplings between two or more such oscillators. Thus, models of coupled oscillators are somewhat limited in scope, but formally they are the best developed models on structural constraints. I shall consider three different approaches.

Mechanical Analogues

Figure 3.15 presents two mechanical analogues that have been described by von Holst (1939, 1955). These devices had actually been built, and they produced traces that exhibited characteristics of coordination as observed, for example, in fin movements of fishes. The exact formal characteristics of these mechanical models appear fairly complicated. They need not be known, however, to gain an intuitive understanding of their operation and of the 'soft' nature of structural constraints on coordination as implemented by them.

The device shown in Figure 3.15a consists of a double pendulum hinged at D with weight G. This represents the first oscillator which drives the 'limb' (more accurately, the pen) H_1. The second oscillator consists of the vertical axis supported by bearings F, that is rotated using a string and weight L. It produces oscillations of the pen H_2. The two oscillators are coupled through a viscous liquid in the container B that is attached to the pendulum. The vertical axis ends with an eccentric ball K that is located in the liquid. Thus, lateral motion of the container

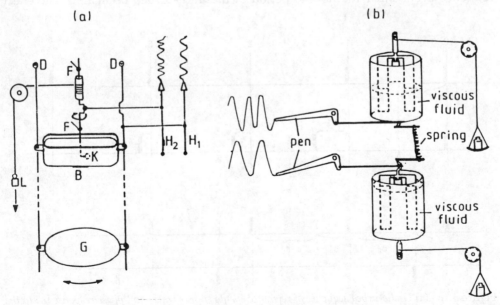

Figure 3.15. *Two mechanical analogues for coupled oscillators: coupling is viscous in (a) and viscoelastic in (b). See text for details. [After von Holst, 1939, 1955.]*

will affect the rotation of the vertical axis in different ways depending on the current position, velocity and acceleration of the eccentric ball; also, rotary motion of the eccentric ball will modify the lateral motion of the container. These mutual influences are 'soft' and depend on the resistance of the viscous fluid (which was treacle) to the relative motion between the container and the eccentric ball.

The device of Figure 3.15b is of a later date. It is simpler, and to figure out its operation will be left to the mechanical reasoning of the reader. The coupling between the two oscillators, in this case, is viscoelastic rather than viscous.

Phase Transition Curves and Phase Response Curves

Yamanishi, Kawato and Suzuki (1980) studied the simultaneous production of two sequences of taps, using two hands, with different relative phases. Their experimental results have been discussed at some length in Section 3.2.1. These were modeled in terms of coupled oscillators as described below. However, the formal treatment of Yamanishi *et al.* is more a particular kind of analysis of the coupling of two oscillators than a model that specifies the equations that govern the coupling. Thus, as long as the assumptions implied by the analysis are met, the 'model' cannot be wrong. Its main virtue appears to be that it provides a more theoretically oriented description of the experimental data.

The analysis of Yamanishi, Kawato and Suzuki (1980) makes use of two basic concepts: the phase transition curve and the phase response curve. These concepts will be explained first (Yamanishi, Kawato and Suzuki, 1979). Consider a sequence of arbitrarily defined reference events in a periodic movement like key presses; such a sequence is shown in Figure 3.16a (upper part). Suppose that at phase ϕ (in terms of the 'normal' period) a disturbance occurs, marked by the arrow in Figure 3.16a (lower part). Phase ϕ here is defined as t/τ, where t is the time since the last reference event and τ the normal period of the undisturbed oscillation. The effect

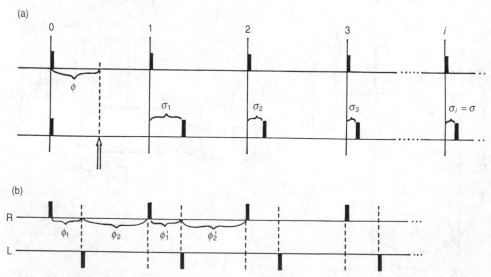

Figure 3.16. (a) Undisturbed sequence of reference events (upper trace) and phase response (σ) to the disturbance marked by arrow (lower trace). (b) Two oscillators R and L which mutually disturb each other. See text for details. [After Yamanishi, Kawato and Suzuki, 1979, 1980.]

of the disturbance is shown as a delay of the subsequent reference events i. In terms of time this delay is $\Delta t(i)$, which is the difference between the normal time of occurrence of the event i and its time of occurrence when a disturbance has been introduced before; thus $\Delta t(i)$ is negative in the case of a delay and positive in the case of temporal advance. Instead of the temporal shift $\Delta t(i)$, the phase shift $\sigma_i = \Delta t(i)/\tau$ can be used.

For each reference event i after the disturbance, the phase shift σ_i in general will depend in a particular way on the phase ϕ at which the disturbance was introduced. As i moves towards infinity, however, the disturbed oscillator will achieve a stable period again, and σ_i will become independent of i. The limit of σ_i as i approaches infinity is σ, and its relationship to the phase of the disturbance, $\sigma(\phi)$, is called the *phase response curve*. When the phase of the disturbance is added to the phase response curve, one obtains the *phase transition curve $\phi + \sigma(\phi) = \phi'$*. In this curve the phase shift can be seen as deviation from the main diagonal.

Instead of a single oscillator and a single disturbance Yamanishi, Kawato and Suzuki (1980) considered two oscillators R and L which disturb each other mutually and repeatedly. The two oscillators are assumed to have identical periods; their phase transition curves are $\phi + \sigma_L(\phi)$ and $\phi + \sigma_R(\phi)$. In addition, they are assumed to recover quickly to their normal period so that the phase shift is already stable at the first reference event after the disturbance. For this situation, consider the relationships that hold for the various phases shown in Figure 3.16b.

Phase ϕ_1 is the phase of the initial disturbance of R by L. As a result of the disturbance, the second R event is delayed by $\sigma_R(\phi_1)$ so that $\phi_2 = 1 - \phi_1 - \sigma_R(\phi_1)$ instead of $1 - \phi_1$. By the same token $\phi_1' = 1 - \phi_2 - \sigma_L(\phi_2)$ where $\sigma_L(\phi_2)$ is the delay caused by the initial disturbance of the oscillator L by the R event. In a steady state, phases ϕ_1 and ϕ_1' are identical. Therefore, for the steady state one obtains:

$$\phi_2 = 1 - \phi_1 - \sigma_R(\phi_1)$$
$$\phi_1 = 1 - \phi_2 - \sigma_L(\phi_2)$$

The first equation can be rearranged as $\phi_1 = 1 - \phi_2 - \sigma_R(\phi_1)$. Thus it can be seen that a steady state requires that $\sigma_R(\phi_1) = \sigma_L(\phi_2)$. Only when this condition is fulfilled will a particular value of ϕ_1 result in a value of ϕ_2 that again results in ϕ_1.

Figure 3.17 shows ϕ_2 plotted as a function of ϕ_1 (continuous line) and ϕ_1 as a function of ϕ_2 (broken line). These curves were constructed from phase transition curves measured in a single subject of Yamanishi, Kawato and Suzuki's (1980) experiment. It is clear that steady states exist only at values of ϕ_1 and ϕ_2 where the two curves cross: only here does one go from a particular ϕ_1 to a particular ϕ_2 (via the continuous line) and back again to the same ϕ_1 (via the broken line). This is not the case for other values of ϕ_1 and ϕ_2.

Figure 3.17 depicts four steady states, but these have different characteristics. Only the ones close to relative phases 0.5 and 1.0 are stable, while the other two are unstable. This becomes obvious when small deviations from the steady states are considered. For example, move upward from ϕ_1 close to 0.5 to the continuous line which gives ϕ_2; then move back to ϕ_1 via the broken line: the slopes of the curves around the stable steady states are such that, after a random deviation, relative phase is brought back to the steady state. This is quite different for unstable steady states. For example, move upward from ϕ_1 close to 0.7 to the continuous line which

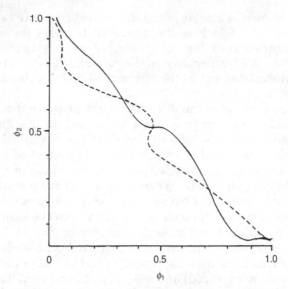

Figure 3.17. ——, *Relative phase ϕ_2 as a function of ϕ_1*; - - - -, *relative phase ϕ_1 as a function of ϕ_2. Symbols ϕ_1 and ϕ_2 as shown in Figure 3.16b. [After Yamanishi, Kawato and Suzuki, 1980.]*

gives ϕ_2; moving back via the broken lines leads to a value of ϕ_1 that deviates even more from the steady state than the initial value. After a while this process will end at one of the two stable states. Thus, in the long run, these are the only states that the system can adopt.

At first glance the analysis in terms of two coupled oscillators provides a convincing redescription of Yamanishi, Kawato and Suzuki's (1980) experimental results. A second glance, however, reveals that the analysis is incomplete. A system of two coupled oscillators with phase transition curves as experimentally determined would produce only relative phases of about 0 and 0.5, the stable steady states, and no others. Human subjects, in contrast, can produce other relative phases as well; these are only biased and more variable than the steady states. Therefore, if one does not adopt a completely different theoretical interpretation, for example in terms of an integrated timing control, the coupled oscillators model has to be completed. Yamanishi *et al.* envisage superordinate centers of control that maintain the instructed relative phases against the autonomous behavior of the oscillators.

Synergetic Models

Synergetic models, in general, deal with the question of how a large number of elements come to behave in an organized manner without the 'command level' of an organizing agent. They are applicable to a variety of different problems, and the treatment that they receive here is very limited. I shall first present a model proposed by Haken, Kelso and Bunz (1985) for the phase transition that can be observed when simultaneous asymmetric movements of the two hands are speeded up (see Section 3.2.2); this finding indicates a loss of the stable relative phase of 0.5 with higher-frequency oscillations. Thereafter an extension of the model (Schöner and Kelso, 1988a, b) will be briefly sketched that includes the 'superordinate control' that enables human performance away from the stable relative phases of 0 and 0.5.

The model of Haken, Kelso and Bunz (1985) consists of two parts. The first part deals with the collective behavior of the two oscillating limbs as characterized by their relative phase. The second part of the model is a derivation of the collective behavior described in the first part from a particular kind of coupling between two oscillators. For the sake of mathematical simplicity the presentation here will be limited to the first part of the model.

How can one describe the experimental observation of two stable relative phases with low-frequency oscillations? One way is to consider $\dot{\phi}$, the first derivative of relative phase ϕ with respect to time, as a function of the relative phase. For stable values of ϕ its first derivative should not only be zero, but it should also be negative for values of ϕ slightly above the stable state and positive for values slightly below; in this case small random deviations of the relative phase ϕ will tend to be reduced over time.

Rather than considering $\dot{\phi}(\phi)$, Haken, Kelso and Bunz (1985) defined a potential $V(\phi)$ with the characteristic $\dot{\phi} = -(dV/d\phi)$. From the potential V not only $\dot{\phi}$ is apparent (as the negative slope), but it also has intuitive appeal as will become clear below.

The analytic expression for the potential was chosen in a somewhat arbitrary manner to be consistent with the experimental results (in addition to being periodic and symmetric). A simple equation that fulfills the requirements is the sum of two cosine functions with a frequency ratio of $1:2$,

$$V = -(a \cos \phi + b \cos 2\phi)$$

Figure 3.18 illustrates this function for the range $-\pi \leqslant \phi \leqslant +\pi$ and different ratios b/a. It also illustrates the intuitive appeal of a potential which, in this application, is essentially a cost function defined on relative phase. Imagine a ball rolling on the curve. It will be in a stable steady state only when it is in a valley. At a minimum of the potential, $\dot{\phi}$ is negative for larger and positive for smaller values of ϕ; this is the requirement for a stable steady state. The ball will also be in a steady state on top of a hill ($\dot{\phi} = 0$), but a small random fluctuation would cause it to roll down into the next valley; thus the maxima represent unstable steady states.

As is evident from Figure 3.18, the potential function has minima at 0 and $\pm\pi$, corresponding to stable steady states at relative phases 0 and 0.5 (180°). However, when the ratio b/a is reduced, the minima at $\pm\pi$ vanish. In the extreme case of $b = 0$ the potential becomes $-(a \cos \phi)$ with the only minimum at $\phi = 0$. In fact, the minima at $\pm\pi$ vanish when $|b|$ becomes smaller than $0.25|a|$. Thus, the ratio b/a is suited to model the loss of the stable steady state at the relative phase 0.5 when the frequency of oscillations is increased.

The link between the ratio b/a and the frequency of oscillation (ω) is the second important step in the model next to the definition of the potential; again, it is somewhat arbitrary. Based on the experimental observation that the amplitudes of the oscillations decline when their frequency is increased, the parameter b is expressed in terms of a ratio of the amplitude $r(\omega)$ and a critical value r_c: $b = 0.25a(r(\omega)/r_c)^2$. Thus the critical value b_c at which the phase shift occurs is reached when $(r(\omega)/r_c)^2 < 1$.

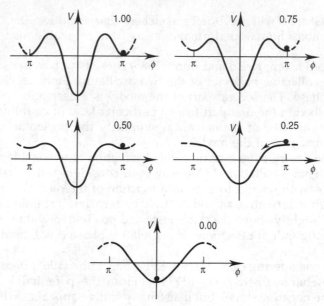

Figure 3.18. *Potentials V(ϕ) as weighted sums of two cosine functions with frequency ratio 1:2 for different ratios of weights (weight of higher-frequency function/weight of lower-frequency function). [After Haken, Kelso and Bunz, 1985.]*

The model of Haken, Kelso and Bunz (1985) permits oscillatory movements with two stable relative phases when the frequency is low; when the frequency is high only one stable relative phase remains. For the experimental data which are the intended domain of the model this is sufficient because subjects were only instructed to produce relative phases of 0 and 0.5. But if requested, subjects can also produce other relative phases. This ability is beyond the scope of the model of Haken *et al.*, as was the case with the model of Yamanishi, Kawato and Suzuki (1980). However, Haken *et al.*'s model has been extended to deal with the production of other relative phases as well.

In line with the model of Haken, Kelso and Bunz (1985), the extension of Schöner and Kelso (1988a, b) also consists of two parts. The first one again deals with the 'collective behavior' as described by the relative phase, and the second with the derivation of the collective behavior from the characteristics of component oscillators. Again, the presentation here will be limited to the first part.

Schöner and Kelso (1988a) take Haken, Kelso and Bunz's (1985) potential function as a characterization of the intrinsically determined behavior of the coupled oscillators. In addition, a tendency is introduced to minimize the deviation between the current relative phase ϕ and the instructed phase ψ. This tendency is captured by a third term in the potential function which drives ϕ towards ψ. The new potential function therefore becomes:

$$V = -(a \cos \phi + b \cos 2\phi + c \cos 0.5(\phi - \psi))$$

Illustrative examples for this function are shown in Figure 3.19 for different values of ψ. The new term distorts the 'intrinsic potential' as specified by Haken,

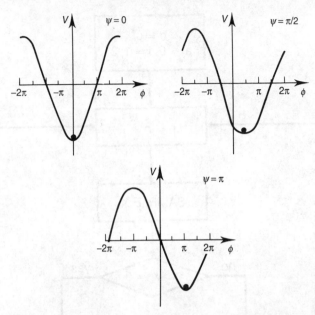

Figure 3.19. *Potentials V(φ) with weights equal one and a third component being added (weight 20) which is a cosine function of the difference between relative phase φ and instructed phase ψ; the location of the minimum depends on the instructed phase (0, π/2 and π), but is biased at instructed phases unequal to 0 or π. [After Schöner and Kelso, 1988a.]*

Kelso and Bunz (1985); it produces a unique minimum in the range $\pm\pi$ at a relative phase which approximates the instructed phase. However, whenever the instructed phase differs from the location of the minima of the 'intrinsic potential' (0, $\pm\pi$), the minimum is broad and shifted away from ψ towards one of the intrinsic minima. At such values of ψ there is some kind of rivalry between the intrinsic characteristics of the oscillators and the task requirement to produce a particular relative phase; the outcome of the conflict varies depending on the choice of the parameters a, b and c.

It should be noted that in terms of performance a broader minimum corresponds to a higher variability of relative phase, and the shift away from the instructed relative phase to a bias in production; thus the predictions of the model are consistent with the experimental data of Yamanishi, Kawato and Suzuki (1985; and see Section 3.2.1).

4.2.3 Simultaneous Preparatory Processes

Structural constraints on simultaneous movements are apparent not only when the movements are actually performed, but also when they are both prepared simultaneously. As reviewed in Section 3.4, structural constraints on the simultaneous preparation of movements can be evidenced from reaction times when a rapid choice has to be made between a left-hand and a right-hand response. In particular, reaction time is increased when the movements assigned to the two hands differ in

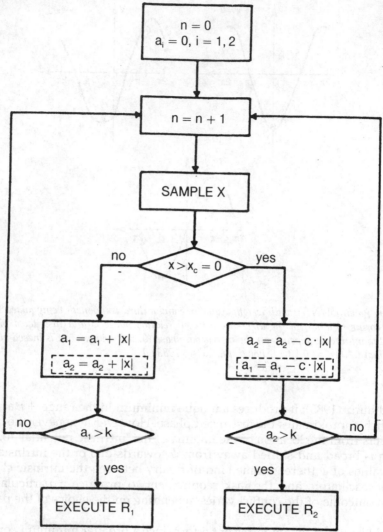

Figure 3.20. *Flow diagram of a modified accumulator model with inhibitory coupling of the accumulators (framed by broken lines). [After Heuer, 1987.]*

a characteristic with respect to which intermanual coupling exists. Two different types of model have been proposed to account for such effects.

The first type of model is a variant of the movement precuing rationale (Rosenbaum, 1980, 1983) which is supplemented with the distinction between common and specific parameters, taken from generalized motor program theory. The outcome is a simple and straightforward hypothesis: when the movements that are assigned to the two hands differ in a characteristic that is controlled by specific parameters, both movements can be prepared in advance of the response signal. This, however, is not possible when the movements differ in a characteristic that is controlled by common parameters (or require different programs). Therefore, at the time of the response signal, preparation is more advanced in the first case than in the second, and only in the second case will reaction time be increased as compared with a control condition in which the same movements are assigned to the two hands.

The alternative type of model is a variant of accumulator models that have been developed for sensory discrimination (Vickers, 1979). A flow diagram of one such model (Heuer, 1987) is shown in Figure 3.20. During each time interval Δt information on which of the alternative response signals is presented becomes available. This is modeled as the sampling of a sensory variable X (e.g. position of the signal). Depending on whether the sampled value x is smaller or larger than a criterion value x_c, this is taken as evidence for the presentation of one or the other signal. So far the process corresponds to the scheme of the theory of signal detection. However, the decision here is assumed to depend on more than one sample. Therefore the sampled value is added to one of two accumulators, and a reponse is triggered when the first of them reaches a threshold.

The notion of an 'accumulator' is fairly abstract. When a tight link between perceptual evidence for the presentation of one or the other signal and preparation of the corresponding response is assumed, the accumulators can be taken to represent the current state of preparation for the alternative responses. Structural constraints on simultaneous preparation can then be modeled in terms of inhibitory coupling of the two accumulators. Specifically, in the model of Figure 3.20 each value added to the one accumulator is also subtracted from the other one, but only after multiplication with the 'coupling constant' which can vary between 0 and 1. The choice of this particular kind of inhibitory coupling was based on formal considerations. It provides a continuous transition between accumulator models ($c = 0$) and random-walk models ($c = 1$) that traditionally have been treated as categorically distinct types of model (Heath, 1984).

Monte-Carlo simulations of the model of Figure 3.20 revealed that variation of the coupling parameter c produces a triad of effects (Heuer, 1987): when c is larger, the number of cycles, each with duration Δt, required to reach the threshold of an accumulator is increased. This corresponds to a longer mean reaction time. In addition the variability of the number of cycles is increased, and the frequency of choice errors is reduced. This is exactly the triad of effects that has been observed when movements with different spatiotemporal patterns were assigned to the two hands rather than same movements (see Section 3.4.1). However, when different durations of aimed movements were used, only an increase of mean reaction time relative to that of the control condition was found. The latter finding is inconsistent with the type of model illustrated in Figure 3.20; it is consistent, however, with the model based on the movement precuing rationale. Thus, as argued by Heuer (1988a, 1990a), both types of model described in this section may have their respective merits; the only problem is to know when this is the case for the one or the other.

4.3 Differences and Commonalities

It is fairly commonplace to complain about the fragmentary nature of psychological models. The review of phenomena and models of coordination could drive one to chime in with such complaints. There is no such thing as a unitary theory of coordination from which formal models for the various phenomena could be derived. This is so despite some claims to the contrary. This section will end with an attempt to bring some order into the variety of models. For this purpose some major differences and commonalities will be delineated.

Major differences are obvious with respect to the general domain, the level and the 'language'. Regarding general domains, it seems indeed difficult to unify models for task-imposed coordination, motor equivalence and structural constraints. The notion of different levels is somewhat vague. However, different levels are made explicit in synergetic models. On the one hand they refer to variables like relative phase, which characterize coordination, and on the other hand they refer to certain kinds of couplings between oscillators that generate the higher-level relationships specified for relative phase. Similarly, generalized motor program theory can be said to refer to a higher level than, for example, the coupled accumulators model; the one makes global statements about coupled and independent hypothetical control parameters, while the other specifies a mechanism for coupling and is not concerned to which movement characteristics it can or cannot be applied.

Probably the most important differences exist with respect to 'language', that is, with respect to concepts and formal tools that are used. While models for different general domains or at different levels are not really rivals – one only wants them to be consistent with each other – models that employ different 'languages' and often represent different approaches compete for approval. They are competitors not in the sense that the one might turn out to be right and the other to be wrong, but the criterion for the judgement is usefulness which, for example, refers to the range and importance of phenomena that can be dealt with. Thus, evaluation of the different approaches represented by the models that I have reviewed should probably be delegated to the future.

More important than the differences may be the commonalities of different models for a particular general domain. Regarding the structural constraints on coordination, some such commonalities are apparent. A major distinction can be drawn between theoretical positions that claim 'unification' of concurrent movements in terms of control and positions that claim coupling of separate control structures. From the data on phase coupling (see Section 3.2.1) it appears that both claims have their respective validity. The claim of coupling between separate control structures is a theme that is shared by many models, however different their representations of control structures (generalized motor programs, central oscillators, accumulators) and however different their representations of coupling (verbal statement of coupled/independent, dynamic nonlinear coupling of oscillators, static coupling of accumulators). As coupling appears to be at the heart of coordination, the attempt to delineate basic types, which could have different particular formulations in different models, could be a worthwhile effort which could help to bind together models for different phenomena.

5   RIGHT–LEFT ASYMMETRIES

Humankind is distinguished from the rest of the animal kingdom (with very few exceptions) by its population preference for the right hand. This preference is probably related to another distinguishing characteristic: the mastery of language (Annett, 1985). Although many animals have individual preferences for right or left limbs, these are about equally frequent in the population. Our closest kinship, monkeys and apes, exhibits only very weak and task-specific population preferences, if at all (MacNeilage, Studdert-Kennedy and Lindblom, 1987). The human preference for the right hand is accompanied not only by a higher level of skill in almost all unimanual tasks, but also by a typical assignment of different functions in bimanual activity. This functional specialization of the hands appears to be supported by asymmetric structural constraints.

Many bimanual tasks require holding and manipulating. Right-handers typically use the left hand for holding and the right hand for manipulations. An example for this assignment of functions is threading. Casual observations show that some people hold the needle in the left hand and the thread in the right hand, while others do the reverse. Nonetheless there is an invariant characteristic in that the right hand is moved relative to the left one. When the thread is held in the right hand, it is moved toward the needle, and when the needle is held in the right hand, the needle is moved toward the thread. The particular assignment of functions is apparently not only a matter of convenience; at least according to subjective experience the reverse assignment is more difficult.

A more detailed analysis of bimanual performance has been provided by Guiard (1987). He identified three aspects of functional specialization. The first and most obvious aspect is this: in right-handers the left hand provides the spatial reference for movements of the right hand, as is evident from holding-and-manipulating tasks. The difference can also be seen in tasks like batting where neither of the two hands is stationary: then the left hand usually provides a moving pivot around which the lever (bat) is rotated by the right hand.

The other two aspects of the functional specialization follow from the first one. The movements of the two hands differ in temporal and spatial scales, the left one producing movements of lower frequencies and smaller amplitudes than the right. Also, the left hand should establish the reference before right-hand movements relative to it are initiated. Therefore Guiard (1987) postulated a left-hand precedence in action.

Why is it that right-handers exhibit the particular functional specialization of the two hands in bimanual tasks? It seems that some benefits accrue from this assignment of functions rather than the reverse. Probably these have to do with different performance characteristics of the two hands. In right-handers neuromotor noise appears to be smaller in the right hand than in the left. This can be evidenced from faster aiming movements, in particular when accuracy requirements are high (Annett *et al.*, 1979; Todor and Cisneros, 1985), and from faster and less variable repetitive tapping (Peters, 1980; Peters and Durding, 1979). The superior temporal and spatial precision of the right hand makes the functional specialization of the two hands in bimanual tasks appear quite natural. It is tempting to speculate that the superiority is related to the tighter link of the right hand to the left cerebral hemisphere, which is also critically involved in the control of the delicate articulator movements in speech.

Although the functional specialization in bimanual tasks is likely to be induced by the different performance characteristics of the left and right hand in unimanual tasks, it seems also to be supported by asymmetric structural constraints. The very nature of the normal cooperation suggests a hypothesis on this asymmetry. Movements of the right hand relative to a reference provided by the left one can be subdivided into two components. One of them is the common component that is defined by the motion of the reference. The other is the specific right-hand component which in general will contain higher frequencies than the common component. This subdivision of movements is similar to the vectorial decomposition of motion in perceptual analysis (Börjesson and von Hofsten, 1972). From the existence of a common component, defined by movements of the left hand as the reference, and a specific right-hand component in addition one would expect that the right hand should be coupled to the left hand. This would support it in following the reference. In contrast, the specific right-hand movements, usually in a higher frequency range, should not affect the left hand. Several studies support this hypothesis in a general way, although none has been explicitly designed to test it. (A good illustration of the hypothesis is the asymmetric superposition of Figure 3.5a in which only the low-frequency oscillation is added to the fast one, but not vice versa, corresponding to the addition of the low-frequency movements of the reference to the higher-frequency manipulatory movements.)

Gunkel (1962), in her brief report, mentioned that right-handers exhibited a higher degree of independence of simultaneous rhythms when the slow one was performed by the left hand and the faster one by the right hand. Similarly, Peters (1981) found that simultaneous paced and rapid tapping is easier when paced tapping is assigned to the left hand and maximally fast tapping to the right hand than vice versa. More specifically, when paced tapping is speeded up, an abrupt breakdown of performance can be observed: subjects frequently refuse to continue the task. The breakdown occurs at a higher frequency of paced tapping when this is performed by the left hand rather than by the right.

Related to Peters' observation is the 'rhythm dominance' reported by Ibbotson and Morton (1981). When a steady beat and a more complex rhythm are to be tapped simultaneously, the task is easier when the steady beat is assigned to the left hand rather than to the right. (Asymmetries have also been found for hand–foot pairings.) Interestingly, and contrary to what one would expect from the notion of hand dominance, the performance breakdown typically consisted of the right hand giving up the steady beat and taking over the rhythm assigned to the left hand.

Although these results appear consistent with the hypothesis on the nature of asymmetric structural constraints outlined above, there is an alternative interpretation available (Peters, 1981). According to this interpretation attention is focused on the right hand during bimanual activities. Thus, the asymmetry would be one between attended and unattended hand instead of left and right. It follows that it should be possible to reverse the asymmetry by directing attention to the left hand. In fact, Peters and Schwartz (1989) found that a $3:2$ polyrhythm was produced more accurately when attention was directed to the faster rhythm, no matter whether this was assigned to the left or the right hand. To manipulate attention, the subjects had to count one of the two rhythms aloud. It is not fully clear whether this is indeed only a manipulation of attention. Counting aloud can have quite other effects. Given the evidence for integrated timing control in polyrhythms (see Section 3.1.3) it is possible that the rhythm that is emphasized by counting constitutes the basic time frame. In any case, the attentional theory makes one wonder why asymmetric structural constraints can be observed at all; people should be able to direct their attention voluntarily to whichever hand has higher demand and not accept poorer performance when it can be easily improved by redirecting attention to the other hand.

So far left-handers have been neglected in this section on asymmetric structural constraints. In general, left-handers are not just mirror images of right-handers, and the same is true with respect to asymmetric coupling. Although left-handers tend to have the reverse asymmetries, these are less strong than in right-handers (Ibbotson and Morton, 1981; Peters, 1981).

A final point that should be briefly mentioned is related to the tighter link of the right hand to the left cerebral hemisphere and thus the centers involved in the control of speech. The difference between the two hands with respect to their anatomical link to the (left) speech hemisphere has given rise to a considerable number of studies which show that speaking interferes more with simultaneous movements of the right hand than with those of the left hand (for review, see Summers, 1990). Unfortunately, these studies typically employed global perform-ance measures which make it impossible to obtain a more detailed picture of the differences between the relationships of speech to left-hand and right-hand move-ments. One exceptional experiment by Chang and Hammond (1987) revealed no clear hand differences with respect to force coupling (see Section 3.3).

6 MOVEMENT AND POSTURE

The final section of this chapter is devoted to a particular kind of coordination that goes unnoticed in many motor patterns. Usually we are aware of the movements that serve our particular intentions (e.g. in throwing, reaching for an object, etc.) but we are only little or not at all aware of the consequences that these intended movements have at remote body parts. Movements that serve an action's purpose frequently shift the position of the center of mass of the body. Therefore they have to be accompanied by adequate postural responses. In general, remote activity in the legs is required to maintain an upright stance.

The available evidence suggests that maintenance of posture is an integrated part of voluntary movement. It might be difficult or even impossible to find differences between the principles that govern the coordination of different component move-ments that are directly related to the purpose of the action (see Section 2) and those principles that govern the coordination of voluntary and postural activity. Three such principles will be discussed.

The first principle is that postural activity is basically nonreflexive. It is related to the predictable consequences of purposeful movements (Paulignan *et al.*, 1989), and it is not a set of reflexes that are triggered by a loss of equilibrium or by afferent signals which indicate a threat to balance. The nonreflexive nature of postural activity can be most clearly seen when it precedes voluntary movement. For example, Cordo and Nashner (1982) had their subjects pull a hand-held lever in response to an auditory signal. The postural electromyographic (EMG) activity of the gastrocnemius started about 40 ms earlier than that of the biceps which had to contract to actually pull the lever. Similarly, Zattara and Bouisset (1986) found longer latencies for voluntary arm raising than for postural support; the more the voluntary movements were a threat to balance (bilateral, unilateral, unilateral with additional weight), the longer was their latency, while the latency of the measured postural responses remained constant. In addition, Dufossé *et al.* (1983) described two different patterns of postural response in the cat, one of them being associated with 'voluntary' lifting of a paw (as a conditioned response) and the other with 'unexpected' loss of support (e.g. reflexive lifting of a paw).

Although postural activity is adapted to the expected consequences of voluntary movements, it is also afference based. It exhibits rapid remote corrections similar to

those discussed in Section 2. One example for such corrections can be seen in Figure
3.21a, b. In this experiment of Marsden, Merton and Morton (1983) the subject had
to pull a string by flexing the thumb. The other end of the string was attached to a
torque motor. Initially flexion had to be performed against a certain resistance, but
during the movement this was abruptly increased, reduced or the movement was
even halted. The upper traces in Figure 3.21a, b present integrated EMG activity
from a thumb flexor; the curves diverge after the different conditions (load, halt,
release) have been introduced. The same divergence can also be seen in remote
muscles: the pectoralis major of the shoulder and the gastrocnemius and soleus of
the lower leg. These remote responses were only slightly delayed (about 20 ms)
relative to the responses of the pulling muscle.

Finally, support activity is highly task-specific. For example, when the subjects
of Cordo and Nashner (1982) leaned against a padded cross-brace that prevented
them from falling when they pulled the lever, no early postural activity in leg
muscles could be seen. Instead the biceps EMG activity started about 25 ms earlier
as compared with the condition with active rather than passive support.

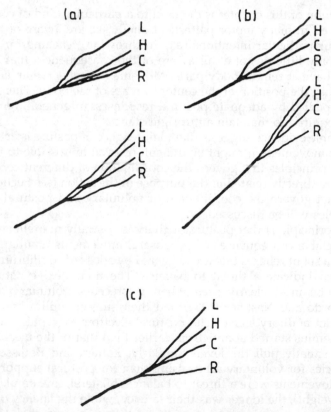

Figure 3.21. *Integrated electromyographic activity (EMG) in different muscles while pulling a string
against a constant resistance (C); in some trials load was added (L), the string was released (R) or
halted (H). The string was attached to the thumb, and integrated EMG of a thumb flexor is shown
in the upper traces of (a) and (b). Lower traces show: integrated EMG of (a) a shoulder muscle, and
(b) ankle extensors. In (c) the integrated EMG of an elbow extensor involved in support is shown.
[After Marsden, Merton and Morton, 1983.]*

Figure 3.21c illustrates task specificity of remote corrections. In this experiment of Marsden, Merton and Morton (1983) subjects pulled the string with the hand held in the median plane, while the other arm grasped a platform that was located in front of the subject. Integrated EMG activity of the biceps of the holding arm is shown. With increased load on the string, which pulled the trunk forward, biceps activity increased to stabilize the stance, and with reduced load it decreased. The remote responses could only be seen when the arm was actually used to support equilibrium, but not otherwise. With a sufficiently awkward posture (the subject kneels in front of the platform, leans slightly forward, and uses the pad of a thumb, pressed against the platform at head height, to support this posture) rapid remote responses can even be elicited in a thumb muscle that in normal life essentially never serves a postural function. Thus, while the coordination of component movements that are directly related to the purpose of an action is probably induced by this purpose, it is highly unclear what information establishes the appropriate coordinative patterns between voluntary movements and postural activity, even for highly unusual postures. In short, how does the thumb know that it is needed for support, and how does it know what to do in this situation?

ACKNOWLEDGEMENTS

I am grateful to S. Keele and J. Summers for extensive comments on an earlier version of this chapter. Parts of it were written while I enjoyed the hospitality of the Netherlands Institute for Advanced Study in the Humanities and Social Sciences, Wassenaar, The Netherlands.

REFERENCES

Abbs, J. H., Gracco, V. L. and Cole, K. J. (1984). Control of multi-movement coordination: sensorimotor mechanisms in speech motor programming. *Journal of Motor Behavior*, **16**, 195–232.

Alluisi, E. A. and Warm, J. S. (1990). Things that go together: A review of stimulus–response compatibility and related effects. In R. W. Proctor and T. G. Reeve (Eds), *Stimulus–Response Compatibility: An Integrated Perspective* (pp. 3–30). Amsterdam: North-Holland.

Annett, J., Annett, M., Hudson, P. T. W. and Turner, A. (1979). The control of movement in the preferred and non-preferred hands. *Quarterly Journal of Experimental Psychology*, **31**, 641–652.

Annett, M. (1985). *Left, Right, Hand and Brain: The Right Shift Theory*. Hillsdale, NJ: Erlbaum.

Atkeson, C. G. and Hollerbach, J. M. (1985). Kinematic features of unrestrained vertical arm movements. *Journal of Neuroscience*, **5**, 2318–2320.

Baldissera, F., Cavallari, P. and Civaschi, P. (1982). Preferential coupling between voluntary movements of ipsilateral limbs. *Neuroscience Letters*, **34**, 95–100.

Basmajian, J. V. (1977). Motor learning and control: A working hypothesis. *Archives of Physical Medicine and Rehabilitation*, **58**, 38–41.

Belanger, M. and Patla, A. E. (1987). Phase-dependent compensatory responses to perturbations applied during walking in humans. *Journal of Motor Behavior*, **19**, 434–453.

Börjesson, E. and von Hofsten, C. (1972). Spatial determinants of depth perception in two-dot motion patterns. *Perception and Psychophysics*, **11**, 263–268.

Bornemann, E. (1942). Untersuchungen über den Grad der geistigen Beanspruchung. *Arbeitsphysiologie*, **12**, 142–192.

Brunia, C. H. M., Haagh, S. A. V. M. and Scheirs, J. G. M. (1985). Waiting to respond: Electrophysiological measurements in man during preparation for a voluntary movement. In H. Heuer, U. Kleinbeck and K.-H. Schmidt (Eds), *Motor Behavior. Programming, Control, and Acquisition* (pp. 36–78). Berlin: Springer.

Bullock, D. and Grossberg, S. (1988). Neural dynamics of planned arm movements: Emergent invariants and speed–accuracy properties during trajectory formation. *Psychological Review*, **95**, 49–90.

Bullock, D. and Grossberg, S. (1991). Adaptive neural networks for control of movement trajectories invariant under speed and force rescaling. *Human Movement Science*, **10**, 3–53.

Buschbaum, M. and Callaway, E. (1965). Influences of respiratory cycle on simple reaction time. *Perceptual and Motor Skills*, **20**, 961–966.

Chang, P. and Hammond, G. R. (1987). Mutual interactions between speech and finger movements. *Journal of Motor Behavior*, **19**, 265–274.

Cohen, L. (1971). Synchronous bimanual movements performed by homologous and non-homologous muscles. *Perceptual and Motor Skills*, **32**, 639–644.

Cooke, J. D. (1980). The organization of simple, skilled movements. In G. E. Stelmach and J. Requin (Eds), *Tutorials in Motor Behavior* (pp. 199–212). Amsterdam: North-Holland.

Corcos, D. M. (1984). Two-handed movement control. *Research Quarterly for Exercise and Sport*, **55**, 117–122.

Cordo, P. J. and Nashner, L. M. (1982). Properties of postural adjustments associated with rapid arm movements. *Journal of Neurophysiology*, **47**, 287–302.

Craik, R., Herman, R. and Finley, F. R. (1975). Human solutions for locomotion. II: Interlimb coordination. In R. M. Herman, S. Grillner, P. S. G. Stein and D. G. Stuart (Eds), *Neural Control of Locomotion* (pp. 51–64). New York: Plenum Press.

Cruse, H. (1986). Constraints for joint angle control of the human arm. *Biological Cybernetics*, **54**, 125–132.

Cruse, H. and Brüwer, M. (1987). The human arm as a redundant manipulator: the control of path and joint angles. *Biological Cybernetics*, **57**, 137–144.

Cruse, H., Dean, J., Heuer, H. and Schmidt, R. A. (1990). Utilization of sensory information for motor control. In O. Neumann and W. Prinz (Eds), *Relationships between Perception and Action: Current Approaches* (pp. 43–79). Berlin: Springer.

Darling, W. G. and Cooke, J. D. (1987). A linked muscular activation model for movement generation and control. *Journal of Motor Behavior*, **19**, 333–354.

Denier van der Gon, J. J. and Thuring, J. P. (1965). The guiding of human writing movements. *Kybernetik*, **2**, 145–148.

Derwort, A. (1938). Untersuchungen über den Zeitablauf figurierter Bewegungen beim Menschen. *Pflügers Archiv für die gesamte Physiologie*, **240**, 661–675.

Deutsch, D. (1983). The generation of two isochronous sequences in parallel. *Perception and Psychophysics*, **34**, 331–337.

Dufossé, M., Macpherson, J. M., Massion, J. and Polit, A. (1983). Maintenance of equilibrium during movement. In A. Hein and M. Jeannerod (Eds), *Spatially Oriented Behavior* (pp. 15–33). Berlin: Springer.

Duncan, J. (1979). Divided attention: The whole is more than the sum of its parts. *Journal of Experimental Psychology: Human Perception and Performance*, **5**, 216–228.

Easton, T. A. (1976). Reflexes and fatigue: New directions. In E. Simonson and P. C. Weiser (Eds), *Psychological Aspects and Physiological Correlates of Work and Fatigue* (pp. 55–105). Springfield, IL: Thomas.

Fagard, J. (1987). Bimanual stereotypes: Bimanual coordination in children as a function of movements and relative velocity. *Journal of Motor Behavior*, **19**, 355–366.

Fitts, P. M. (1954). The information capacity of the human motor system in controlling the amplitude of movement. *Journal of Experimental Psychology*, **47**, 381–391.

Fitts, P. M. and Peterson, J. R. (1964). Information capacity of discrete motor responses. *Journal of Experimental Psychology*, **67**, 103–112.

Flash, T. and Hogan, N. (1985). The coordination of arm movements: an experimentally confirmed mathematical model. *Journal of Neuroscience*, **5**, 1688–1703.

Forssberg, H., Grillner, S., Rossignol, S. and Wallén, P. (1976). Phasic control of reflexes during locomotion in vertebrates. In R. M. Herman, S. Grillner, P. S. G. Stein and D. G. Stuart (Eds), *Neural Control of Locomotion* (pp. 647–674). New York: Plenum Press.

Garland, H. and Angel, R. W. (1971). Spinal and supraspinal factors in voluntary movement. *Experimental Neurology*, **33**, 343–350.

Gentner, D. R. (1982). Evidence against a central control model of timing in typing. *Journal of Experimental Psychology: Human Perception and Performance*, **8**, 793–810.

Gentner, D. R. (1987). Timing of skilled motor performance: Tests of the proportional duration model. *Psychological Review*, **94**, 255–276.

Georgopoulos, A. P., Lurito, J. T., Petrides, M., Schwartz, A. B. and Massey, J. T. (1989). Mental rotation of the neuronal population vector. *Science*, **243**, 234–236.

Guiard, Y. (1987). Asymmetric division of labor in human skilled bimanual action: The kinematic chain as a model. *Journal of Motor Behavior*, **19**, 486–517.

Gunkel, M. (1962). Über relative Koordination bei willkürlichen menschlichen Glieder-bewegungen. *Pflügers Archiv für die gesamte Physiologie*, **275**, 472–477.

Hacker, W. (1974). Anforderungen an Regulation und Zeitbedarf bei geführten Bewegungen: Zur Gültigkeit des Derwort – von Weizsäckerschen Gesetzes der konstanten Figurzeit. *Zeitschrift für Psychologie*, **182**, 307–337.

Haferkorn, W. (1933). Über die zeitliche Eingliederung von Willkürbewegungen. *Neue Psychologische Studien*, **9**, 37–63.

Haken, H., Kelso, J. A. S. and Bunz, H. (1985). A theoretical model of phase transitions in human hand movements. *Biological Cybernetics*, **51**, 347–356.

Hancock, P. A. and Newell, K. M. (1985). The movement speed–accuracy relationship in space–time. In H. Heuer, U. Kleinbeck and K.-H. Schmidt (Eds), *Motor Behavior: Programming, Control, and Acquisition* (pp. 153–188). Berlin: Springer.

Heath, R. A. (1984). Random-walk and accumulator models of psychophysical discrimination: A critical evaluation. *Perception*, **13**, 57–65.

Hellebrandt, F. A., Houtz, S. J., Partridge, M. J. and Walters, C. E. (1956). Tonic neck reflexes in exercises of stress in man. *Journal of Physical Medicine*, **35**, 144–159.

Heuer, H. (1982a). Binary choice reaction time as a criterion of motor equivalence. *Acta Psychologica*, **50**, 35–47.

Heuer, H. (1982b). Binary choice reaction time as a criterion of motor equivalence: Further evidence. *Acta Psychologica*, **50**, 48–60.

Heuer, H. (1982c). Choice between finger movements of different and identical forms: The effect of relative signal frequency. *Psychological Research*, **44**, 323–342.

Heuer, H. (1983). Reaktionszeit und Genauigkeit bei der Wahl zwischen formgleichen und formverschiedenen Bewegungen beider Hände. *Psychologische Beiträge*, **25**, 532–556.

Heuer, H. (1984a). Binary choice reaction time as a function of the relationship between durations and forms of responses. *Journal of Motor Behavior*, **16**, 392–404.

Heuer, H. (1984b). On re-scaleability of force and time in aiming movements. *Psychological Research*, **46**, 73–86.

Heuer, H. (1985). Intermanual interactions during simultaneous execution and programming of finger movements. *Journal of Motor Behavior*, **17**, 335–354.

Heuer, H. (1986a). Intermanual interactions during programming of aimed movements: Converging evidence for common and specific parameters of control. *Psychological Research*, **48**, 37–46.

Heuer, H. (1986b). Intermanual interactions during programming of finger movements: Transient effects of 'homologous coupling'. In H. Heuer and C. Fromm (Eds), *Generation and Modulation of Action Patterns* (pp. 87–101). Berlin: Springer.

Heuer, H. (1987). Visual discrimination and response programming. *Psychological Research*, **49**, 91–98.

Heuer, H. (1988a). Advance specification and programming interactions: A reply to Rosenbaum, Barnes, and Slotta (1988). *Psychological Research*, **50**, 63–68.

Heuer, H. (1988b). Adjustment and readjustment of the relative timing of a motor pattern. *Psychological Research*, **50**, 83–93.

Heuer, H. (1988c). Testing the invariance of relative timing: Comment on Gentner (1987). *Psychological Review*, **95**, 552–557.

Heuer, H. (1990a). Rapid responses with the left or right hand: Response–response compatibility effects due to intermanual interactions. In R. W. Proctor and T. G. Reeve (Eds), *Stimulus–Response Compatibility. An Integrated Perspective* (pp. 311–342). Amsterdam: North-Holland.

Heuer, H. (1990b). Psychomotorik. In H. Spada (Ed.), *Lehrbuch Allgemeine Psychologie* (pp. 495–559). Berne: Huber.

Heuer, H. (1991a). Some characteristics of VITE. *Human Movement Science*, **10**, 55–64 .

Heuer, H. (1991b). A note on limitations and strategies in movement production. In R. Daugs, H. Mechling, K. Blischke and N. Olivier (Eds), *Sportmotorisches Lernen und Techniktraining, Bd 1* (pp. 117–131). Schorndorf: Hofmann.

Heuer, H. (1991c). Structural constraints on bimanual movements. *Psychological Research/ Psychologische Forschung*, **55**, 83–98.

Heuer, H. and Schmidt, R. A. (1988). Transfer of learning among motor patterns with different relative timing. *Journal of Experimental Psychology: Human Perception and Performance*, **14**, 241–252.

Hogan, N. (1984). An organizing principle for a class of voluntary movements. *Journal of Neuroscience*, **4**, 2745–2754.

Hoyt, D. F. and Taylor, C. R. (1981). Gait and the energetics of locomotion in horses. *Nature*, **292**, 239–240.

Hughes, O. M. and Abbs, J. H. (1976). Labial–mandibular coordination in the production of speech: Implications for the operation of motor equivalence. *Phonetica*, **33**, 199–221.

Ibbotson, N. R. and Morton, J. (1981). Rhythm and dominance. *Cognition*, **9**, 125–138.

Jagacinski, R. J., Marshburn, E., Klapp, S. T. and Jones, M. R. (1988). Tests of parallel versus integrated structure in polyrhythmic tapping. *Journal of Motor Behavior*, **20**, 416–442.

Jung, R. and Fach, C. (1984). Spiegelschrift und Umkehrschrift bei Linkshändern und Rechtshändern: Ein Beitrag zum Balkentransfer und Umkehrlernen. In L. Spillmann and B. R. Wooten (Eds), *Sensory Experience, Adaptation, and Perception. Festschrift for Ivo Kohler* (pp. 377–399). Hillsdale, NJ: Erlbaum.

Keele, S. W. (1986). Motor control. In K. R. Boff, L. Kaufman and J. P. Thomas (Eds), *Handbook of Perception and Human Performance*, vol. II: *Cognitive Processes and Performance* (pp. 30.1–30.60). Chichester: John Wiley.

Keele, S. W., Pokorny, R. A., Corcos, D. M. and Ivry, R. (1985). Do perception and motor production share common timing mechanisms: a correlational analysis. *Acta Psychologica*, **60**, 173–191.

Kelso, J. A. S. (1981). Contrasting perspectives on order and regulation of movement. In J. Long and A. Baddeley (Eds), *Attention and Performance*, vol. IX (pp. 437–457). Hillsdale, NJ: Erlbaum.

Kelso, J. A. S. (1984). Phase transitions and critical behavior in human bimanual coordination. *American Journal of Physiology: Regulatory, Integrative, and Comparative*, **246**, R1000–R1004.

Kelso, J. A. S., Holt, K. G., Rubin, P. and Kugler, P. N. (1981). Patterns of human interlimb coordination emerge from the properties of nonlinear limit cycle oscillatory processes: Theory and data. *Journal of Motor Behavior*, **13**, 226–261.

Kelso, J. A. S, Putnam, C. A. and Goodman, D. (1983). On the space–time structure of human interlimb co-ordination. *Quarterly Journal of Experimental Psychology*, **35A**, 347–375.

Kelso, J. A. S and Scholz, J. P. (1985). Cooperative phenomena in biological motion. In H. Haken (Ed.), *Complex Systems: Operational Approaches in Neurobiology, Physical Systems and Computers* (pp. 124–149). Berlin: Springer.

Kelso, J. A. S., Southard, D. L. and Goodman, D. (1979). On the coordination of two-handed movements. *Journal of Experimental Psychology: Human Perception and Performance*, **5**, 229–238.

Kelso, J. A. S., Tuller, B. and Harris, K. S. (1983). A 'dynamic pattern' perspective on the control and coordination of movement. In P. F. MacNeilage (Ed.), *The Production of Speech* (pp. 137–173). Berlin: Springer.

Kelso, J. A. S., Tuller, B., Vatikiotis-Bateson, E. and Fowler, C. A. (1984). Functionally specific articulatory cooperation following jaw perturbation during speech: Evidence for co-ordinative structures. *Journal of Experimental Psychology: Human Perception and Performance,* **10,** 812–832.

Kern, G. (1933). Motorische Umreißung optischer Gestalten. *Neue Psychologische Studien,* **9,** 65–104.

Klapp, S. T. (1979). Doing two things at once: The role of temporal compatibility. *Memory and Cognition,* **7,** 375–381.

Klapp, S. T. (1981). Temporal compatibility in dual motor tasks. II: Simultaneous articulation and hand movements. *Memory and Cognition,* **9,** 398–401.

Klapp, S. T., Hill, M., Tyler, J., Martin, Z., Jagacinski, R. and Jones, M. (1985). On marching to two different drummers: Perceptual aspects of the difficulties. *Journal of Experimental Psychology: Human Perception and Performance,* **11,** 814–828.

Klatzky, R. L., McCloskey, B., Doherty, S., Pellegrino, J. and Smith, T. (1987). Knowledge about hand shaping and knowledge about objects. *Journal of Motor Behavior,* **19,** 187–213.

MacKay, D. G. and Soderberg, G. A. (1971). Homologous intrusions: An analogue of linguistic blends. *Perceptual and Motor Skills,* **32,** 645–646.

MacNeilage, P. F., Studdert-Kennedy, M. G. and Lindblom, B. (1987). Primate handedness reconsidered. *Behavioral and Brain Sciences,* **10,** 247–303.

Marsden, C. D., Merton, P. A. and Morton, H. B. (1983). Rapid postural reactions to mechanical displacement of the hand in man. In J. E. Desmedt (Ed.), *Motor Control Mechanisms in Health and Disease* (pp. 645–659). New York: Plenum Press.

Marshall, R. N., Wood, G. A. and Jennings, L. S. (1989). Performance objectives in human movement: A review and application to the stance phase of normal walking. *Human Movement Science,* **8,** 571–594.

Marteniuk, R. G. and MacKenzie, C. L. (1980). A preliminary theory of two-hand co-ordinated control. In G. E. Stelmach and J. Requin (Eds), *Tutorials in Motor Behavior* (pp. 185–197). Amsterdam: North-Holland.

Marteniuk, R. G., MacKenzie, C. L. and Baba, D. M. (1984). Bimanual movement control: Information processing and interaction effects. *Quarterly Journal of Experimental Psychology,* **36A,** 335–365.

McLeod, P. (1977). A dual-task response modality effect: Support for multiprocessor models of attention. *Quarterly Journal of Experimental Psychology,* **29,** 651–667.

Meyer, D. E., Abrams, R. A., Kornblum, S., Wright, C. E. and Smith, J. E. K. (1988). Optimality in human motor performance: Ideal control of rapid aimed movements. *Psychological Review,* **95,** 340–370.

Morasso, P. (1981). Spatial control of arm movements. *Experimental Brain Research,* **42,** 223–227.

Muzzie, R. A., Warburg, C. L. and Gentile, A. M. (1984). Coordination of the upper and lower extremities. *Human Movement Science,* **3,** 337–354.

Näätänen, R. and Merisalo, A. (1977). Expectancy and preparation in simple reaction time. In S. Dornic (Ed.), *Attention and Performance,* vol. VI (pp. 115–138). Hillsdale, NJ: Erlbaum.

Nelson, W. L. (1983). Physical principles for economies of skilled movements. *Biological Cybernetics,* **46,** 135–147.

Neumann, O. (1987). Beyond capacity: A functional view of attention. In H. Heuer and A. F. Sanders (Eds), *Perspectives on Perception and Action* (pp. 361–394). Hillsdale, NJ: Erlbaum.

Newell, K. M. and van Emmerik, R. E. A. (1989). The acquisition of coordination: Preliminary analysis of learning to write. *Human Movement Science.* **8,** 17–32.

Patla, A. E. and Belanger, M. (1987). Task-dependent compensatory responses to perturbations applied during rhythmic movements in humans. *Journal of Motor Behavior*, **19**, 454–475.

Paulignan, Y., Dufossé, M., Hugon, M. and Massion, J. (1989). Acquisition of co-ordination between posture and movement in a bimanual task. *Experimental Brain Research*, **77**, 337–348.

Peters, M. (1977). Simultaneous performance of two motor activities: The factor of timing. *Neuropsychologia*, **15**, 461–465.

Peters, M. (1980). Why the preferred hand taps more quickly than the nonpreferred hand: Three experiments on handedness. *Canadian Journal of Psychology*, **34**, 62–71.

Peters, M. (1981). Attentional asymmetries during concurrent bimanual performance. *Quarterly Journal of Experimental Psychology*, **33A**, 95–103.

Peters, M. (1989). The relationship between variability of intertap intervals and interval duration. *Psychological Research*, **51**, 38–42.

Peters, M. and Durding, B. (1979). Left-handers and right-handers compared on a motor task. *Journal of Motor Behavior*, **11**, 103–111.

Peters, M. and Schwartz, S. (1989). Coordination of the two hands and effects of attentional manipulation in the production of a bimanual 2:3 polyrhythm. *Australian Journal of Psychology*, **41**, 215–224.

Povel, D.-J. (1981). Internal representation of simple temporal patterns. *Journal of Experimental Psychology: Human Perception and Performance*, **7**, 3–18.

Preilowski, B. (1972). Possible contribution of the anterior forebrain commissures to bilateral motor coordination. *Neuropsychologia*, **10**, 267–277.

Preilowski, B. (1975). Bilateral motor interaction: Perceptual-motor performance of partial and complete 'split-brain' patients. In K. J. Zülch, O. Creutzfeldt and G. G. Galbraith (Eds), *Cerebral Localization* (pp. 115–132). Berlin: Springer.

Rabbitt, P. M. A. and Vyas, S. M. (1970). An elementary preliminary taxonomy for some errors in laboratory choice RT tasks. In A. F. Sanders (Ed.), *Attention and Performance*, vol. III. (pp. 56–76). Amsterdam: North-Holland.

Rabbitt, P. M. A., Vyas, S. M. and Fearnley, S. (1975). Programming sequences of complex responses. In P. M. A. Rabbitt and S. Dornic (Eds), *Attention and Performance*, vol. V (pp. 395–417). London: Academic Press.

Roberton, M. A. and Halverson, L. E. (1988). The development of locomotor coordination: Longitudinal change and invariance. *Journal of Motor Behavior*, **20**, 197–241.

Rosenbaum, D. A. (1980). Human movement initiation: Specification of arm, direction, and extent. *Journal of Experimental Psychology: General*, **109**, 444–474.

Rosenbaum, D. A. (1983). The movement precuing technique: Assumptions, applications, and extensions. In R. A. Magill (Ed.), *Memory and Control of Action* (pp. 231–274). Amsterdam: North-Holland.

Rosenbaum, D. A. (1985). Motor programming: A review and a scheduling theory. In H. Heuer, U. Kleinbeck and K.-H. Schmidt (Eds), *Motor Behavior. Programming, Control, and Acquisition* (pp. 1–33). Berlin: Springer.

Rosenbaum, D. A. (1991). *Human Motor Control*. New York: Academic Press.

Rosenbaum, D. A., Barnes, H. J. and Slotta, J. D. (1988). In defense of the advance specification hypothesis for motor control. *Psychological Research*, **50**, 58–62.

Rosenbaum, D. A. and Kornblum, S. (1982). A priming method for investigating the selection of motor responses. *Acta Psychologica*, **51**, 223–243.

Saltzman, E. (1986). Task dynamic coordination of the speech articulators: A preliminary model. In H. Heuer and C. Fromm (Eds), *Generation and Modulation of Action Patterns* (pp. 129–144). Berlin: Springer.

Saltzman, E. and Kelso, J. A. S. (1987). Skilled actions: A task-dynamic approach. *Psychological Review*, **94**, 84–106.

Schmidt, R. A. (1975). A schema theory for discrete motor skill learning. *Psychological Review*, **82**, 225–260.

Schmidt, R. A. (1980). On the theoretical status of time in motor-program representations. In G. E. Stelmach and J. Requin (Eds), *Tutorials in Motor Behavior* (pp. 145–165). Amsterdam: North-Holland.

Schmidt, R. A. (1985). The search for invariance in skilled movement behavior. *Research Quarterly for Exercise and Sport*, **56**, 188–200.

Schmidt, R. A., Zelaznik, H. N., Hawkins, B., Frank, J. S. and Quinn, J. T. (1979). Motor-output variability: A theory for the accuracy of rapid motor acts. *Psychological Review*, **86**, 415–451.

Schöner, G. and Kelso, J. A. S. (1988a). A synergetic theory of environmentally-specified and learned patterns of movement coordination. I: Relative phase dynamics. *Biological Cybernetics*, **58**, 71–80.

Schöner, G. and Kelso, J. A. S. (1988b). A synergetic theory of environmentally-specified and learned patterns of movement coordination. II: Component oscillator dynamics. *Biological Cybernetics*, **58**, 81–89.

Soechting, J. E. and Lacquaniti, F. (1981). Invariant characteristics of a pointing movement in man. *Journal of Neuroscience*, **1**, 710–720.

Stimpel, E. (1933). Der Wurf. *Neue Psychologische Studien*, **9**, 105–138.

Summers, J. J. (1989). Motor programs. In D. H. Holding (Ed.), *Human Skills*, 2nd edn (pp. 49–69). Chichester: John Wiley.

Summers, J. J. (1990). Temporal constraints on concurrent task performance. In G. R. Hammond (Ed.), *Cerebral Control of Speech and Limb Movements* (pp. 395–417). Amsterdam: North-Holland.

Summers, J. J., Bell, R. and Burns, B. D. (1989). Perceptual and motor factors in the imitation of simple temporal patterns. *Psychological Research*, **51**, 23–27.

Summers, J. J. and Burns, B. D. (1990). Timing in human movement sequences. In R. A. Block (Ed.), *Cognitive Models of Psychological Time* (pp. 181–206). Hillsdale, NJ: Erlbaum.

Summers, J. J. and Kennedy, T. M. (1991). Strategies in the production of a 5:3 polyrhythm. *Human Movement Science*, **11**, 101–112.

Swinnen, S., Walter, C. B. and Shapiro, D. C. (1988). The coordination of limb movements with different kinematic patterns. *Brain and Cognition*, **8**, 326–347.

Thomassen, A. J. W. M. and Teulings, H.-L. (1985). Size and shape in handwriting: Exploring spatio-temporal relationships at different levels. In J. A. Michon and J. L. Jackson (Eds), *Time, Mind, and Behavior* (pp. 253–263). Berlin: Springer.

Todor, J. I. and Cisneros, J. (1985). Accommodation to increased accuracy demands by the left and right hands. *Journal of Motor Behavior*, **17**, 355–372.

Turvey, M. T. (1977). Preliminaries to a theory of action with reference to vision. In R. Shaw and J. Bransford (Eds), *Acting and Knowing: Toward an Ecological Psychology* (pp. 211–265). Hillsdale, NJ: Erlbaum.

Turvey, M. T., Rosenblum, L. D., Kugler, P. N. and Schmidt, R. C. (1986). Fluctuations and phase symmetry in coordinated rhythmic movements. *Journal of Experimental Psychology: Human Perception and Performance*, **12**, 564–583.

Uno, Y., Kawato, M. and Suzuki, R. (1989). Formation and control of optimal trajectory in human multijoint arm movement: Minimum torque-change model. *Biological Cybernetics*, **61**, 89–101.

Vickers, D. (1979). *Decision Processes in Visual Perception*. New York: Academic Press.

Viviani, P. (1986). Do units of motor action really exist? In H. Heuer and C. Fromm (Eds), *Generation and Modulation of Action Patterns* (pp. 201–216). Berlin: Springer.

von Holst, E. (1939). Die relative Koordination als Phänomen und als Methode zentralner-vöser Funktionsanalyse. *Ergebnisse der Physiologie*, **42**, 228–306.

von Holst, E. (1955). Periodisch-rhythmische Vorgänge in der Motorik. 5. *Conference of the Society for Biological Rhythms* (pp. 7–15). Stockholm, Sweden.

Wakelin, D. R. (1976). The role of the response in psychological refractoriness. *Acta Psychologica*, **40**, 163–175.

Wann, J., Nimmo-Smith, I. and Wing, A. M. (1988). Relation between velocity and curvature in movement: Equivalence and divergence between a power law and a minimum-jerk model. *Journal of Experimental Psychology: Human Perception and Performance*, **14**, 622–637.

Wilke, J. T., Lansing, R. W. and Rogers, C. A. (1975). Entrainment of respiration to repetitive finger tapping. *Physiological Psychology*, **3**, 345–349.

Williams, K. (1987). The temporal structure of the forward roll: Inter- and intra-limb coordination. *Human Movement Science*, **6**, 373–387.

Wing, A. M., Church, R. M. and Gentner, D. R. (1989). Variability in the timing of responses during repetitive tapping with alternate hands. *Psychological Research*, **51**, 28–37.

Wing, A. M. and Kristofferson, A. B. (1973). The timing of interresponse intervals. *Perception and Psychophysics*, **13**, 455–460.

Yamanishi, J., Kawato, M. and Suzuki, R. (1979). Studies on human finger tapping neural networks by phase transition curves. *Biological Cybernetics*, **33**, 199–208.

Yamanishi, J., Kawato, M. and Suzuki, R. (1980). Two coupled oscillators as a model of the coordinated finger tapping by both hands. *Biological Cybernetics*, **37**, 219–225.

Zattara, M. and Bouisset, S. (1986). Chronometric analysis of the posturo-kinetic programming of voluntary movement. *Journal of Motor Behavior*, **18**, 215–223.

Zelaznik, H. N., Shapiro, D. C. and Carter, M. C. (1982). The specification of digit and duration during motor programming: A new method of precuing. *Journal of Motor Behavior*, **14**, 57–68.

Zimmermann, G. (1980). Articulatory behaviors associated with stuttering: A cinefluorographic analysis. *Journal of Speech and Hearing Research*, **23**, 108–121.

Chapter 4

Modeling Variability and Dependence in Timing

Dirk Vorberg* and Alan Wing[†]

*Institut für Psychologie der TUB, Braunschweig, Germany and
[†]MRC Applied Psychology Unit, Cambridge, UK

1 INTRODUCTION

Many actions involve sequences of movements whose elements must not only be in the correct order, but whose relative timing is also a crucial component to successful attainment of the goal. As illustration of this point, consider the simulation of handwriting described by Vredenbregt and Koster (1971) and shown in Figure 4.1. Two orthogonally mounted sets of opposed pairs of electric motors were used to move a pen across paper. One pair of motors produced movements in the horizontal direction, the other pair resulted in vertical movement. At any point in time only one motor in each pair was functioning. The amplitude of a pen 'stroke' in a given direction was determined by the duration of the voltage applied to one motor and the interval allowed before the opposing motor in the pair was switched on. Letters of the alphabet could be produced with this system by a sequence of commands specifying which motor to activate or inactivate and the time at which to take the action.

An insightful observation of the authors was that natural variation evident in handwritten letters could be simulated by the variation in the timing of the motor commands. Changes in letter shape could be produced by disturbance in just the onset time of one motor. This would upset the relative timing even – as shown in Figure 4.1 – to the extent that one letter-form might be changed qualitatively into another. In contrast, a simultaneous change of all times, leaving the proportional durations of the component intervals unchanged, would scale the overall size of a letter but leave shape invariant. This example thus illustrates the need in studying the control of serial action to consider not only the amount but also the form of timing variability. In this chapter we provide a tutorial approach to quantitative models of the origin and nature of temporal *variability* in movement sequences.

Sometimes, psychologists appear to approach behavior with the aim of explaining variability away (Wing, 1992). Our approach to timing mechanisms differs in that we take variability of timing to be a feature of interest in its own right. In particular, we wish to focus attention on departures from random variability evident in intervals defined by psychologically significant events or *responses* occurring in sequences of movement. We consider that patterns of statistical

Handbook of Perception and Action, Volume 2
ISBN 0-12-516162-X

(a)

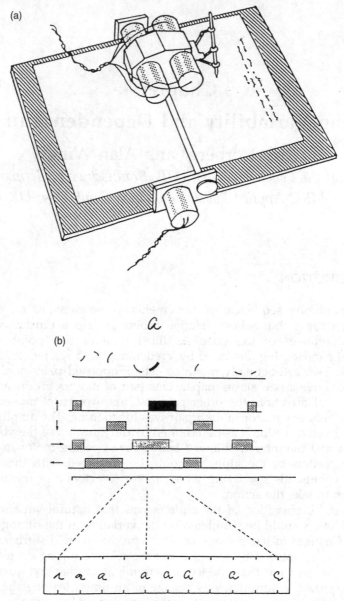

(b)

Figure 4.1. *The Vredenbregt and Koster (1971) handwriting simulator. (a) Two pairs of orthogonally mounted electric motors drive a pen over paper in vertical and horizontal directions. (b) An error in the time of application of just one in the series of force pulses driving the pen distorts the resulting letter shape.*

dependence in the interresponse intervals can provide important clues to the functional arrangement of a number of underlying independent processes, each contributing a degree of variability. Our approach is based on intervals between discrete events; we do not consider oscillator-based models of timing behavior (see Chapter 3). One problem with these nonlinear models is that they do not admit closed-form solutions of the kind that we develop here. We shall not argue that the linear timing models we are going to discuss are more appropriate than the more complex nonlinear models. We do believe, however, that a rewarding strategy is to study simple models first because very often a simple model can provide a useful first-order approximation, even though it turns out not to be correct in every detail. Such seems to be the case with the two-level timing model proposed by Wing and Kristofferson (1973b) for timing in tapping tasks. In this chapter, we shall try to show that the model provides a powerful theoretical framework for the study of timing mechanisms in many quite complex situations.

A cornerstone in our approach is an idea raised by two founding fathers of modern studies of motor control: Bernstein and Lashley. In treating serial action, both Bernstein (1967) and Lashley (1951) suggested that successive elements of an activity may be centrally linked without regard to the occurrence of the overt peripheral motor event to which they give rise. That is, Bernstein and Lashley both hypothesized that recognition of the completion of each movement component in a sequence (for example via feedback) is neither a necessary nor a desirable stage in the generation of the next element in the sequence. In the approach we present below we interpret this view in terms of a dichotomy between central processes involved in maintaining timekeeping, and execution processes that are directly responsible for motor events. Given a series of repeated responses with intervals between them that exhibit variability around some period, we show that this simple dichotomy predicts characteristic dependence patterns between successive intervals in the series.

In Sections 2 and 3 we set out the basic framework based on a two-level partitioning of variability in timing which distinguishes between central timing processes and mechanisms involved in the execution of movement. At this stage we also introduce certain tools of probability and statistics that are needed in deriving the properties of the models we consider and in relating their predictions to data. Section 4 discusses statistical issues of estimation and testing the model.

The basic model does not include feedback. Nonetheless our ability, for example, to synchronize responses with a pacing stimulus implies that the model should admit feedback correction under certain circumstances. In Section 5 we illustrate how a simple feedback scheme for phase correction may be developed within the basic model. In Section 6 we generalize the basic model to allow more complex forms of central timekeeping. We then illustrate these in the following two sections on motor programming (Section 7) and rhythm (Section 8). The penultimate Section 9 may be seen as bringing together the ideas of the previous two sections; there, we propose the rhythm program as a new theoretical concept in accounting for timing in rhythmic performance, as in music.

2   TIMING REPETITIVE MOVEMENT

It has long been recognized that the timing of even the simplest of movements is variable. More than one hundred years ago, Stevens (1886) described a task in which subjects attempted to tap a lever repetitively at a fixed rate for a minute or so. This rate, which was set by a metronome at the beginning of the trial, was varied over trials between 360 and 1500 ms. Stevens provided a graph of the raw data from

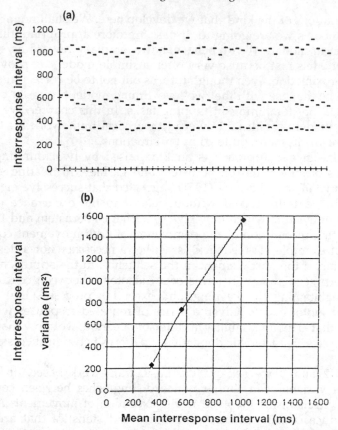

Figure 4.2. *Interresponse interval data from Stevens (1886). (a) Data from three trials for a professional musician producing interresponse intervals at three different target intervals: 400, 600 and 1000 ms. (b) Variance computed from the data above as a function of the mean interval.*

a number of such trials in the form shown in Figure 4.2a. The individual curves there show that the subject was able both to adjust the response rate according to the beat provided by the metronome and to maintain it over an extended period. There is evident variability in performance and this variability increases with the interval (Figure 4.2b).

One focus of Stevens' work was the size and direction of the discrepancy between the target interval and the mean of the intervals produced by the subject, which he noted typically remained within about 5% of the standard. However, Stevens was also interested in the form of the variability evident in the inter-response intervals. On the basis of visual inspection of the data he observed that the variability comprised both short-term fluctuations and longer-term drift. The former he described as a 'constant zig-zag' such that 'two sequent variations in the same direction' were rather rare. The latter he characterized as 'larger and more primary waves' extending over much of the sequence.

From our perspective it is particularly significant that Stevens' examination of timing variability led him to speculate on the nature of the underlying mechanisms; the thesis of this chapter is also that timing variability provides a hallmark for the underlying control mechanisms. Moreover, Stevens' account included another idea that we develop, namely, that of two distinct levels of control in timing. However, Stevens' view was that the nature of the variability implied that the levels must be linked through a process of active error correction. In contrast we show below that negative correlation between successive interresponse intervals (consistent with their zig-zag values) can arise from a two-level timing mechanism without any need to assume active correction. Nonetheless, Stevens' insight remains. The variability of timing in repetitive movement sequences is not purely random. There is often pronounced structure to the fluctuations in interresponse intervals and it is the nature of that structure and the implications of such structure for our understanding of the control of timing to which we now turn.

2.1 Sources of Variance in Timing

Stevens' (1886) data clearly demonstrate variability in the timing of movement. However, they also point to a remarkable degree of temporal control, in the sense that his subjects were able to adjust the interval between their responses to match any of a wide range of target intervals and then maintain the mean interval within a few percent of the target. This kind of flexibility encourages the concept of a timekeeping process in the central nervous system that is subject to voluntary influences. Such a timekeeper might serve not only the regulation of timing of a series of movements but also, for example, the interposition of an arbitrary delay between some external event and a subsequent response. It might even be that time judgements, such as discriminating differences in the duration of two stimuli, make use of the same timekeeping process so that the latter might therefore be thought of as a 'central clock'. The hypothesis of a single module subserving clock-like functions would, for example, be consistent with the observation that, in certain neurological patients with damage to the cerebellum, deficits in time perception and production are associated (Ivry and Keele, 1989).

The variability in the timing of movement will in part reflect the operation of the timekeeper. However, it will also reflect neural transmission delays intervening between the triggering of the motor command and the observable events at the periphery by which we identify a response. A model based on this idea was proposed by Wing and Kristofferson (1973a) and is shown in Figure 4.3.

The upper line depicts a series of intervals generated with some mean and variance by a central timekeeper; the lower line shows the corresponding intervals between observable responses. It is assumed that there are delays in the execution of movement so that each response lags behind its timekeeper trigger. If these motor delays are variable, the interresponse interval variability will reflect both timekeeper interval and motor delay variability. Although neither of these processes is open to direct observation, we show later how this model provides estimators for the variance of the motor delays and the timekeeper intervals in terms of the statistics derived from series of observable interresponse intervals (Wing and Kristofferson, 1973b). First we illustrate the potential of partitioning the variance of interresponse intervals into components by turning to an experiment on timing pairs of responses described by Rosenbaum and Patashnik (1980a, b).

On each trial in Rosenbaum and Patashnik's study subjects produced a brief time interval by making two key-press responses, first with the left index finger then with the right. The required interval ranged from 0 ms (the two keys were to be

D. Vorberg and A. Wing

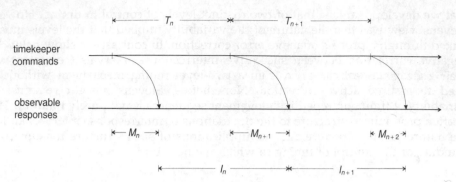

Figure 4.3 *Intervals generated in a central timekeeper can be observed only through the movements with which they are associated after delays that arise in the execution of each movement.*

pressed simultaneously) to 1050 ms and was kept constant over a block of trials. Their measures included the variance of the intervals between left- and right-hand responses. This was lowest when the interresponse interval was 0 ms. In this condition we may suppose a motor command could be passed simultaneously to left- and right-motor systems with no contribution required of the timekeeper. Any variability in interresponse interval may therefore be attributed to random fluctuations in left and right motor delays introducing chance departures from perfect synchrony (Ulrich and Stapf, 1984; see also Section 6.2).

With nonzero target intervals between responses, Rosenbaum and Patashnik found the left–right interresponse interval variance increased linearly with the mean. Since the movements required of the subject did not change over the different target intervals, the variability of motor execution delays may be assumed to have stayed constant. The variance increase may therefore be attributed to increased demands placed on the timekeeper by having to generate longer intervals of time.

The linearity of the increase in variance with mean interval deserves comment. The finding is consistent with a timekeeper that waits until a predetermined count of random neural events is attained (Creelman, 1962; Gibbon, Church and Meck, 1984). In the literature it is sometimes reported that it is the standard deviation of interresponse intervals (and not their variance) that increases linearly with the mean (Kristofferson, 1976). A linear relationship between standard deviation and mean represents a greater increase of variance than would be predicted by the counter-model; however, it does correspond to Weber's law for perceptual judgements. At present it is not clear under what circumstances one or the other relationship holds. Therefore, some researchers (e.g. Killeen, 1992) permit the variance to be a second-degree polynomial of the mean, as we will do in Section 9.

The idea that two sources of variability contribute to interresponse interval variance is clearly equally applicable to movement sequences comprising more than just two responses. Moreover, when it is applied to longer sequences, the idea can account for what Stevens described as the zig-zag nature of successive interresponse intervals. For an intuitive account of this phenomenon, we need only note in Figure 4.3 the implication of the common event demarcating successive intervals I_n and I_{n+1}, namely, the response delay M_{n+1}. Suppose the clock were absolutely regular so that any observed interresponse interval variability is attributed to the response delays (such a case has been considered by McGill, 1962). Then it is clear that chance fluctuation in any delay will affect two adjacent interresponse intervals.

If, for example, M_{n+1} is longer than average, this will have the effect of increasing I_n but, at the same time, decreasing I_{n+1} by the same amount. Thus adjacent interresponse intervals might be expected to fluctuate in opposite directions with respect to the mean. However, two factors operate to make such alternation less than perfectly reliable. The first is that the peripheral response delays M_n and M_{n+2} may, by chance, fluctuate in ways that cancel the alternation. The second is that any variability in the timekeeper intervals will also tend to reduce the apparent alternation of fluctuations around the mean. Before we provide a more formal derivation of these properties, we first present some necessary tools drawn from the language of probability and random variables.

2.2 Covariance Defined

In order to derive the predictions of the model depicted in Figure 4.3, we first provide some basic definitions. Covariance is a measure of the linear association between two random variables X and Y, and is defined by:

$$\text{cov}(X, Y) = E\{[X - E(X)][Y - E(Y)]\} \tag{1}$$

The size and sign of the covariance reflect the strength of the dependence between two variables and its direction; covariances (as well as the correlation, see below) equal zero if the variables are stochastically independent of each other. Note that the constancy of one or both variables also implies zero covariance (since $E(X) = c$ if $X = c = $ constant). By the definition, covariances are symmetric, i.e. $\text{cov}(X, Y) = \text{cov}(Y, X)$ for all random variables X and Y.

It is important to note that the variance, defined by:

$$\text{var}(X) = E\{[X - E(X)]^2\} \tag{2}$$

can be seen as a special kind of covariance, namely, the covariance of a variable with itself, i.e. $\text{var}(X) = \text{cov}(X, X)$. For this reason, we will often use the terms 'covariance' and 'covariance structure' to refer to variances and covariances at the same time.

2.2.1 Distributivity

Covariance predictions for models with theoretical variables linearly related to the observable ones can be derived in a straightforward manner if use is made of the *distributivity* of covariances. Distributivity refers to the fact that covariances of linear combinations behave analogously to products of sums, e.g. $(a + b)(c + d) = ac + ad + bc + bd$. Let W, X, Y and Z denote random variables, and a, b, c and d constants. Consider the random variables defined by $U = aW + bX$ and $V = cY + dZ$. By distributivity, the covariance between these linear combinations is given as:

$$\text{cov}(U, V) = \text{cov}(aW + bX, cY + dZ)$$

$$= ac \cdot \text{cov}(W, Y) + ad \cdot \text{cov}(W, Z)$$

$$+ bc \cdot \text{cov}(X, Y) + bd \cdot \text{cov}(W, Z) \tag{3}$$

Example
As an illustration, we apply distributivity in deriving the variance of the difference
of two random variables, X and Y. Noting that $X - Y = (+1)X + (-1)Y$ leads to:

$$\text{var}(X - Y) = \text{cov}(X - Y, X - Y)$$
$$= \text{cov}(X, X) - \text{cov}(X, Y) - \text{cov}(Y, X) + \text{cov}(Y, Y)$$
$$= \text{var}(X) - 2\text{cov}(X, Y) + \text{var}(Y)$$

2.2.2   Covariance and Correlation

The covariance bears a simple relation to the product–moment correlation. The
correlation between two random variables equals the covariance normalized by
their variance,

$$\rho(X, Y) = \text{cov}(X, Y)/[\text{var}(X)\,\text{var}(Y)]^{1/2} \tag{4}$$

Because of this normalization, correlations are bounded by $+1$ and -1, and the
degree of linear dependence between the variables is directly expressed by the size
of the correlation coefficient, which is not the case with covariances. There are
theoretical advantages, however, for using covariances rather than correlations.
Since distributivity holds for covariances (but not for correlations), the derivation
of covariance predictions for linear models is straightforward. Once the covariances
and variances have been obtained for a given model, it is a simple matter to convert
to correlations via equation (4) if desired.

3   THE TWO-LEVEL TIMING MODEL

A formal statement of the two-level timing notion embodied in Figure 4.3 was given
by Wing and Kristofferson (1973b). For a sequence of responses, we define the
interval I_n as the interresponse interval that is bounded by response n and response
$n + 1$. According to the model, each I_n is given by the algebraic sum of three
independent random variables: the current timer interval (T_n), plus the response
delay (M_{n+1}) leading to the response that terminates I_n, minus the delay (M_n) in the
response initiating the I_n:

$$I_n = T_n + M_{n+1} - M_n \qquad n = 1, N \tag{5}$$

It will be noted that this equation constitutes a *linear* model in the following sense.
The observable variable, I_n, is additively related to the underlying theoretical
variables, T_n and M_n; changes in any one or more of the underlying variables are
related to the resulting change in the observed variable in a linear fashion.

Wing and Kristofferson (1973b) assumed independence between as well as
within the timekeeper and the motor subsystems. This means that all timekeeper
intervals and motor delays are mutually uncorrelated, i.e. $\text{cov}(T_m, M_n) = 0$ for all m,

n and $\mathrm{cov}(T_m, T_n) = \mathrm{cov}(M_m, M_n) = 0$ for $m \neq n$. Let us look at the amount of dependence between interresponse intervals predicted by the model.

By the defining equation of the model (equation 5), the covariance between any two interresponse intervals j steps apart can be written as:

$$\mathrm{cov}(I_n, I_{n+j}) = \mathrm{cov}(T_n + M_{n+1} - M_n, T_{n+j} + M_{n+j+1} - M_{n+j})$$

By distributivity:

$$\mathrm{cov}(I_n, I_{n+j}) = \mathrm{cov}(T_n, T_{n+j}) + \mathrm{cov}(M_{n+1}, M_{n+j+1}) - \mathrm{cov}(M_{n+1}, M_{n+j})$$
$$- \mathrm{cov}(M_n, M_{n+j+1}) + \mathrm{cov}(M_n, M_{n+j})$$

as all covariances between timer intervals and motor delays are zero. Wing and Kristofferson further assumed that the variances stay constant with n, i.e. $\mathrm{var}(T_n) = \sigma_T^2$ and $\mathrm{var}(M_n) = \sigma_M^2$. This yields the following predictions for the dependence to be expected:

for $j = 0$:

$$var(I_n) = \mathrm{cov}(T_n, T_n) + \mathrm{cov}(M_{n+1}, M_{n+1}) + \mathrm{cov}(M_n, M_n)$$
$$= \mathrm{var}(T_n) + \mathrm{var}(M_n) + \mathrm{var}(M_{n+1})$$
$$= \sigma_T^2 + 2\sigma_M^2 \tag{6a}$$

for $j = 1$:

$$\mathrm{cov}(I_n, I_{n+1}) = -\mathrm{cov}(M_{n+1}, M_{n+1})$$
$$= -\mathrm{var}(M_{n+1})$$
$$= -\sigma_M^2 \tag{6b}$$

for $j > 1$:

$$\mathrm{cov}(I_n, I_{n+j}) = 0 \tag{6c}$$

This expression shows the significant role of motor delay variance. Not only does it increase the variance of the interresponse intervals beyond that resulting from imprecision in the timekeeper, but it also generates a *negative dependence between successive intervals*. Note that according to the model the covariance between intervals separated by at least one intervening interval should be zero.

3.1 Autocovariance Function and Autocorrelation Function

The dependence structure within the sequence of random variables $\{I_n\}$ has thus been described in terms of the mutual covariances between all pairs of variables. Consider $\mathrm{cov}(I_n, I_{n+j})$, which indicates the dependence between two particular variables of the sequence $\{I_n\}$ j steps apart; the difference in the indices, j, is called the *lag*. The sequence is said to be *stationary* (in the second moments) if $\mathrm{cov}(I_n, I_{n+j})$ depends only on the lag, j, but not on the position in the sequence, n. The statistical structure of a stationary sequence is conveniently summarized by its *autocovariance function (acvf)*, defined as:

$$\gamma_I(j) \equiv \text{cov}(I_n, I_{n+j})$$

The acvf expresses the linear dependence between any two variables j steps apart; at lag $j = 0$, the acvf equals $\text{var}(I_n)$. Note that acvf.s are symmetric around zero, i.e. $\gamma_I(-j) = \text{cov}(I_n, I_{n-j}) = \text{cov}(I_{n-j}, I_n) = \gamma_I(j)$.

This allows equation (6) to be rewritten as:

$$\gamma_I(j) = \begin{cases} \sigma_T^2 + 2\sigma_M^2 & j = 0 \\ -\sigma_M^2 & j = 1 \\ 0 & j > 1 \end{cases} \tag{7}$$

The covariance predictions of the Wing–Kristofferson model at different lags show that successive interresponse intervals are statistically dependent. This point is most clearly demonstrated in terms of the *autocorrelation function (acf)*, defined as the acvf normalized by the lag zero autocovariance, i.e. $\rho_I(j) \equiv \gamma_I(j)/\gamma_I(0)$; note that, trivially, $\rho(0) = 1$ for any acf. The model indicates that, in general, successive intervals will be negatively correlated, whereas intervals separated by one or more intervening intervals have a theoretical correlation of zero. From equation (7):

$$\rho_I(j) = \begin{cases} -1/[2 + \sigma_T^2/\sigma_M^2] & j = 1 \\ 0 & j > 1 \end{cases} \tag{8}$$

If the model holds, the lag-one autocorrelation is bounded by:

$$-1/2 \leqslant \rho_I(1) \leqslant 0 \tag{9}$$

which follows from equation (8). The value of $\rho_I(1)$ will be close to zero when σ_T^2 is much greater than σ_M^2. If, however, most of the variability is attributable to the motor system so that σ_T^2 is much smaller than σ_M^2, the lag-one autocorrelation will be close to $-1/2$.

Data supporting the lag one predictions of the model were reported by Wing and Kristofferson (1973b) based on a paradigm similar to that of Stevens (1886). Each trial commenced with the definition of a target interval by means of a series of repetitive tone pulses with which subjects attempted to synchronize finger-tapping responses. After 24 tone pulses, the pacing stimuli stopped and subjects were required to maintain the same rate of responding until, 31 responses later, another tone signaled the end of the trial. With these relatively short sequences it was found that subjects were able to produce consistent performance without excessive levels of fatigue or boredom.

Four subjects, none of whom had special musical skills, took part in the experiment. Target intervals, run in different blocks of trials, ranged from 180 to 350 ms. Autocovariance functions were estimated over the 30 interresponse intervals in the unpaced phase of each trial. The lag-one autocovariance at a given target interval was estimated separately for each trial and then averaged. (We return to issues in the estimation of autocovariance functions later in Section 4.) Figure 4.4

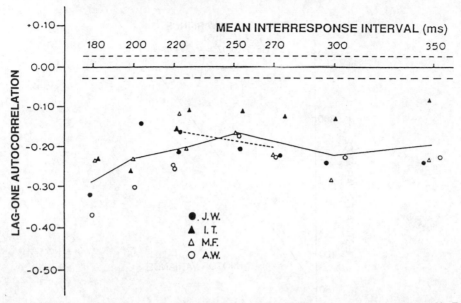

Figure 4.4. *Lag-one autocorrelations for each of four subjects (different symbols used for each). Data averaged over approximately 200 sequences for each data point. There are two lines showing the overall average; the dotted line is for targets of 220 and 270 ms that were run at a later date. The dashed lines on either side of zero are approximate confidence intervals (see Section 4.1). [Reproduced from Wing and Kristofferson, 1973a.]*

shows the results, transformed into correlations by normalizing the covariance estimates by the average variances. The correlations lie well within the theoretical bounds of 0 and $-1/2$, thus supporting the predictions of the two-level timing model.

3.1 Timekeeper and Motor Delay Variance

Given support for the two-level timing model in terms of the observed lag-one covariances (later we present data supporting the prediction of zero dependence at larger lags), it is interesting to use the model to determine the variability of the timekeeper intervals and the response delays. This may be done by rearranging equation (7):

$$\sigma_M^2 = -\gamma_I(1) \tag{10a}$$

$$\sigma_T^2 = \gamma_I(0) + 2\gamma_I(1) \tag{10b}$$

Average data from four subjects in an experiment (Wing, 1980) in which the target interval was varied in steps of 30 ms between 220 and 490 ms are shown in Figure 4.5. Each subject's data followed the form of the average in that timekeeper variance estimates increased more or less linearly, whereas motor delay variance remained in the region of 20 ms². Moreover, individual differences in regularity of

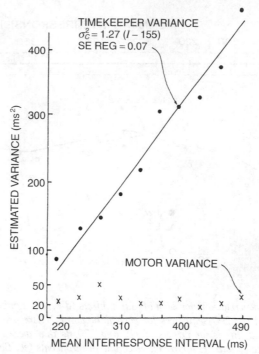

Figure 4.5. *The differential effect of target interval on estimates of timekeeper and response delay variance. [Reproduced from Wing, 1980].*

tapping were associated with timekeeper interval variance. Motor delay variance estimates were relatively constant over subjects.

The dissociation of the effects of target duration on the variability estimates of the component delays of the model may be seen as support for the timing model. It strengthens the assumption that the component delays arise in distinct processes since they are susceptible to different influences. A demonstration of double dissociation between estimates of timekeeper interval variance and response delay variance within a single study has been presented by Ivry, Keele and Diener (1988) based on observations of contrasting effects of neurologic damage to the cerebellum. Their report comprised case study analyses of seven patients with focal damage of the cerebellum, four of whom had lesions that were primarily lateral, the other three having medially located lesions. Each patient provided a number of runs of 31 tapping responses both with the impaired hand (ipsilateral to the lesion) and the uninvolved, contralateral hand. At the beginning of each trial a series of synchronization tones was used to set the target interval at 550 ms. The data of interest came from the unpaced tapping.

Every patient was found to have increased tapping variability when using the hand ipsilateral to the lesion. Decomposing tapping variability into timekeeper and motor delay components (via equations 10a and 10b) gave a more differentiated picture: the poor performance of patients with lateral damage could be attributed to increased timekeeper variance, whereas that of patients with medial lesions was associated with increased variance of the motor delays. This result is clearly consistent with the two-process model of timing. It also suggests that the lateral cerebellum is a component of the timekeeper. However, it should be observed that the result does not exclude the possibility that other structures within the central nervous system are also contributing to timekeeping. For example, in a single-case study of a patient with asymmetric signs of Parkinson's disease, which is a movement disorder stemming from lesions in the basal ganglia, Wing, Keele and Margolin (1984) observed selective effects on timekeeper interval variance.

4 STATISTICAL ISSUES OF AUTOCOVARIANCE ESTIMATION

In this section we consider some technical matters relating to the estimation of autocovariance functions predicted by timing models. We first define an estimator and then consider the problem of estimation bias and the consequences of nonstationarity.

4.1 Estimator Definition

We denote the data by $\{i_{n,s}; n = 1,N; s = 1,S\}$; they consist of S sequences each of length N. If the $i_{n,s}$ are independent realizations of the random variables I_n, all of which are assumed to follow the same distribution, a *serial* estimator can be computed *within* each sequence:

$$\hat{\gamma}_{I,s}(j) = \sum_{n=1}^{N-j} (i_{n,s} - \hat{\mu}_{.,s})(i_{n+j,s} - \hat{\mu}_{.,s})/(N - j) \tag{11}$$

where

$$\hat{\mu}_{.,s} = \sum_{n=1}^{N} i_{n,s}/N$$

This covariance estimator is the analog to the standard autocorrelation estimator frequently used in time series analysis (see Huitema and McKean, 1991, for a comparison of alternative autocorrelation estimators and their statistical properties). Table 4.1 illustrates the computation of the lag-one autocovariance from a sequence $\{i_{n,s}; n = 1,N\}$. Note that the second line is the same sequence shifted one place to the left; the bold-faced rectangle gives the pairs $(i_{n,s}, i_{n+1,s})$ *within* sequence s that enter the calculation. The estimators per sequence can be combined by

Table 4.1. *Arrangement of interresponse interval data for the calculation of the serial covariance estimator $\hat{\gamma}(1)$ for repeating events*

$i_{1,s}$	$i_{2,s}$	$i_{3,s}$	$\cdots$	$i_{n-1,s}$	$i_{n,s}$	$i_{n+1,s}$	$\cdots$	$i_{N-1,s}$	$i_{N,s}$
$i_{1,s}$	$i_{2,s}$	$i_{3,s}$	$\cdots$	$i_{n-1,s}$	$i_{n,s}$	$i_{n+1,s}$	$\cdots$	$i_{N-1,s}$	$i_{N,s}$

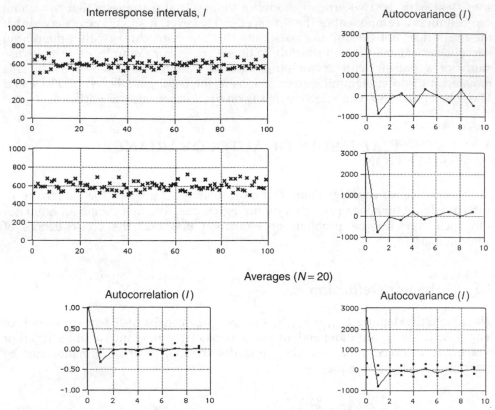

Figure 4.6. *Simulation of the two-level model; values for* T *and* M *were drawn from uniformly distributed rv.s with range* 50 ms. *(Top, middle): two sequences of 100 interresponse intervals are shown on the left with their autocovariance as a function of lag on the right. (Bottom): averaged autocorrelation (left) and autocovariance (right) functions over 20 independent sequences. The points on either side of zero at each lag are confidence intervals given by two standard errors about zero.*

averaging across sequences; their standard deviation is useful for calculating approximate confidence intervals of the estimates.

Figure 4.6 shows two sets of simulated data from the Wing–Kristofferson model and corresponding estimates of the autocovariance functions. Note the amount of statistical error that is involved at lags $j > 1$ when the acvf is estimated from a single sequence of $N = 100$ interresponse intervals; 20 such sequence estimates were included in the average function on the right, the shape of which resembles the theoretical acvf quite closely. As expected, the average acvf is close to zero except at lag one.

4.2 Bias

In testing a model, it is necessary to consider the *bias* problem that arises when quantitative predictions from a model are compared with empiric estimates computed from samples. When small samples are used, discrepancies between the estimate and the theoretical value are to be expected by chance, even if the underlying model is correct. If these discrepancies cancel each other in the long run, then the estimator is said to be *unbiased*. An estimator is called *biased* if its expected value differs from the theoretical value it is supposed to estimate. The acvf estimators given above (equation 11) are biased; depending on sample size, i.e. sequence length N, the bias may be severe. Contrary to what is often believed, the bias is not removed when $(N - j - 1)$ rather than $(N - j)$ is used as the denominator in equation (11).

For a model that is specified in terms of its acvf, the bias can be derived and corrected for. Let $\gamma(j) = \text{cov}(I_n, I_{n+j})$ denote the acvf of a stationary model, and $\hat{\gamma}(j)$ the corresponding estimator as given by equation (11). The estimator's expectation can be obtained by standard procedure (e.g. Anderson, 1971); it is:

$$E[\hat{\gamma}(j)] = \gamma(j) - 2 \sum_{i=1}^{N-j} \sum_{k=1}^{N} \gamma(i - k)/[N(N - j)]$$

$$+ \sum_{i=1}^{N} \sum_{k=1}^{N} \gamma(i - k)/N^2 \qquad (12)$$

Equation (12) holds for any distribution of the variables $\{I_n\}$, in contrast to corresponding derivations for acf estimators (which are usually derived under normal distributional assumptions; see Huitema and McKean, 1991).

The important point to note about equation (12) is that the expected value of the estimates depends not only on the 'true' acvf value at lag j, $\gamma(j)$, but on those at all other lags from 0 onwards to $N - 1$ as well. Although the bias vanishes as N tends to infinity, it is sizeable at values in the region of 20 or so that are often used in tapping experiments. If due allowance is not made this can create serious problems for quantitative tests of models (Vorberg, 1978).

Example

We use the Wing–Kristofferson two-level model to give an impression of the distortion of covariance estimates. With $\sigma_T^2 = 81$ and $\sigma_M^2 = 25$, the model predicts $\text{var}(I) = 81 + (2 \times 25) = 131$ and $\text{cov}(I_n, I_{n+1}) = -25$. The estimators $\hat{\gamma}(0)$ and $\hat{\gamma}(1)$, however, when used on response sequences with $N = 20$ intervals, yield long-run estimates of 126.8 and -29.1, respectively. If these are translated back into estimators of the theoretical variances via equation (10), values of $\hat{\sigma}_T^2 = 68.7$ and $\hat{\sigma}_M^2 = 29.05$ are obtained, which means that the timer variance is underestimated by 15.2%, at the cost of the motor delay variance which is overestimated by 16.2%.

Equation (12) can be used to predict the bias of acvf estimators for lags larger than 1. A naive test of the two-level model might check whether the estimates at larger lags are equal to zero except for sampling error, rejecting the model if nonzero values show up. Inserting $\gamma(j) = 0, j > 1$, into equation (12) gives the expectations of the acvf estimators:

$$E[\hat{\gamma}(j)] = -(1/N)\gamma(0) - (2/N)\{1 - j/[N(N - j)]\}\gamma(1) \quad j > 1 \qquad (13)$$

which differ from zero for the larger lags, in contrast to the theoretical acvf. For the parameters of the previous example and for sequence length $N = 20$, equation (13) gives -4.06, -4.07, -4.08 and -4.09 as the expected values of the estimators at lags $j = 2$ through $j = 5$, respectively.

4.2.1   Unbiased Lag-0 and Lag-1 Estimators

For the two-level model, we construct unbiased estimators $G(0)$ and $G(1)$ of the acvf at lags 0 and 1 as follows. If the model holds, the theoretical acvf equals zero at lags $j > 1$; from equation (12), the expectations of the lag-0 and lag-1 estimators are:

$$E[\hat{\gamma}(0)] = a\gamma(0) + b\gamma(1)$$
$$E[\hat{\gamma}(1)] = c\gamma(0) + d\gamma(1)$$

where $a = (N - 1)/N$, $b = -2(N - 1)/N^2$, $c = -1/N$, $d = 1 - \{1 - 1/[N(N - 1)]\}$ $(2/N)$. We define the new estimators by:

$$G(0) \equiv [d\hat{\gamma}(0) - b\hat{\gamma}(1)]/(ad - bc) \tag{14}$$
$$G(1) \equiv [c\hat{\gamma}(0) - a\hat{\gamma}(1)]/(bc - ad) \tag{15}$$

It is not difficult to show that these estimators are unbiased, i.e. $E[G(0)] = \gamma(0)$ and $E[G(1)] = \gamma(1)$.

An appropriate test of the model's independence prediction for *nonadjacent* interresponse intervals is to test for a difference of the acvf statistics at lags $j > 1$ from their corresponding bias predictions (equation 13). In practice, this involves estimating the model's parameters via $G(0)$ and $G(1)$ and obtaining the predictions for larger lags by inserting the estimates into equation (13).

4.2.2   Other Models

Note that the bias in estimator equation (11) as given by equation (12) holds for any stationary model, whereas equations (13) to (15) hold under the restriction $\gamma(j) = 0$, $j > 1$ only. Therefore, the estimators $G(0)$ and $G(1)$ will not be unbiased unless the two-level model is valid. For models with different acvf.s (e.g. the synchronization model discussed later in Section 5) these estimators cannot be used. In general, the estimator bias problem becomes more severe the slower the theoretical acvf $\gamma(j)$ tends to zero as $j \rightarrow \infty$. Figure 4.7 gives a realistic impression of the discrepancies between the theoretical acvf and the expected empirical acvf that have to be dealt with even for moderately long sequences. The graph compares the acvf of the synchronization errors predicted by the synchronization model (Section 5) with the expected values of the biased acvf estimates. It is clear that tests of the model will be totally misleading if the bias problem is ignored.

Constructing unbiased acvf estimators becomes quite messy for more complex models. Moreover, when several models are to be compared against one set of data, this requires computing different acvf estimates for each model. For evaluating models by how well they predict the dependence structure of the interresponse

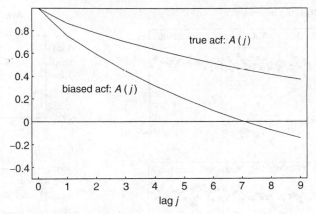

Figure 4.7. *Estimation bias in acvf. Theoretical (true) and expected empiric (biased) acf of synchronization errors, as predicted from the synchronization model (Section 5). (Parameters: $\sigma_T = 12$, $\sigma_M = 5$, $\alpha = 0.1$, and $N = 30$.)*

intervals (or any other time series), a different approach is preferable:

(1) Estimate the uncorrected empiric acvf $\hat{\gamma}(j)$ via estimator equation (11).
(2) For the model under consideration, compute the theoretical acvf $\gamma(j)$ from appropriate parameter values.
(3) Compute the (biased) expected values of the empiric acvf, $E[\hat{\gamma}(j)]$, by inserting the numeric $\gamma(j)$ into equation (12).
(4) Evaluate the goodness-of-fit of the model by comparing empiric and predicted acvf.s.

4.3 Nonstationarity

A crucial assumption underlying acvf estimation is *stationarity* of the interresponse intervals, that is, constancy of $E(I_n)$, $\text{var}(I_n)$ and $\text{cov}(I_n, I_{n+j})$ for all n. This precludes drifts in tempo, which are likely to occur when subjects are to produce long response sequences. In general, violating stationarity will give distorted acvf estimates. To gain intuition, we provide some examples. Figure 4.8 shows Monte Carlo simulations of the two-level model that result when there is a trend in the mean interresponse intervals. Inspection of the average acvf.s shows that such a trend raises the covariances everywhere.

The consequences of trend in the mean can be worked out analytically. Assume stationarity in the variances and covariances, but let the interval means depend on the response index, i.e. $E(I_n) = \mu_n$. The expected value of the acvf estimator (equation 11) differs from that under complete stationarity by the amount:

$$\sum_{n=1}^{N-j} (\mu_n - \mu_.)(\mu_{n+j} - \mu_.)/(N-j) \tag{16}$$

where

$$\mu_. = \sum_{n=1}^{N} \mu_n/N$$

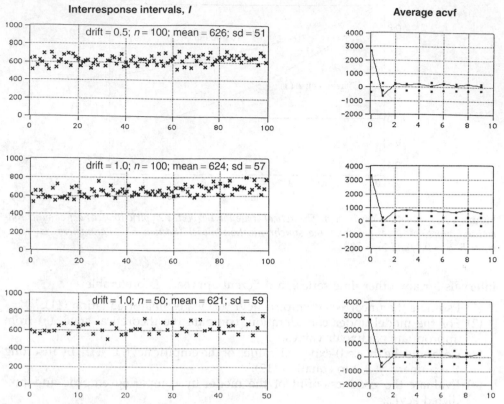

Figure 4.8. *Simulation of effects of linear drift. Single runs are shown on the left, acvf.s averaged over 20 runs on the right. Moderate drift of 0.5 ms per response results in a nonzero autocovariance at larger lags (top). This becomes more pronounced for a larger drift of 1.0 ms per response (middle); however, the problem is reduced for shorter sequences (bottom).*

The sum equals zero if $\mu_n = \mu$ for all n, as it should. Note that equation (16) is just the acvf estimator applied to the expected intervals (rather than their realizations) which permits some inferences about the effects of different tempo drifts for sufficiently long response sequences. For $j \ll N$, the sum in equation (16) is positive for all lags if the means μ_n are either monotonically increasing or decreasing with n. However, even with quadratic trends in the means the acvf is likely to be overestimated at small lags.

Example Continued

Let us examine the distortions created by linear trend in the means on the parameter estimates of the two-level timing model with parameters $\sigma_T^2 = 81$ and $\sigma_M^2 = 25$. Table 4.2 shows the values of the acvf estimators to be expected for sequences of $N = 30$ or $N = 100$ interresponse intervals.

The second column indicates the size of the linear trend assumed, decreasing from 2 ms change per interval to 0.1 ms change. For example, a slope of 1 ms may stand for a drift in which the intervals within a sequence of $N = 30$ increase linearly from 300 to 330 ms, or decrease from 400 to 370 ms; note that neither the absolute tempo nor the trend's direction have differential effects on the estimators. For

Table 4.2. *Effects of nonstationarity in the means on the expected variance and lag-one covariance for the Wing–Kristofferson model. Top row: theoretical values to be expected given stationarity*

		$E[\hat{\gamma}(0)]$	$E[\hat{\gamma}(1)]$	$E[\hat{\gamma}(1)]/E[\hat{\gamma}(0)]$
		131.00	−25.00	−0.191
$N = 30$	Slope = 2	460.67	254.00	0.551
	1	205.95	44.75	0.217
	0.5	149.73	−7.56	−0.051
	0.2	134.00	−22.21	−0.166
	0.1	131.75	−24.30	−0.184
$N = 100$	Slope = 2	3464.00	3240.67	0.936
	1	964.25	791.42	0.821
	0.5	339.31	179.10	0.528
	0.2	164.33	7.66	0.047
	0.1	139.33	−16.84	−0.121

$N = 100$, a trend of 0.2 ms per interresponse interval (a tempo change of 20 ms within about half a minute) has disastrous effects: in the long run, the interresponse interval variance will be overestimated by 25.4%; the average lag-one covariance estimate is not even negative, but differs from the 'true' value of −25 by more than 130%. For shorter sequences, the situation is better; here, the estimators are more robust and less affected by trends in the means. Therefore, collecting the data by several moderately sized sequences is preferrable to one long sequence.

Recommendations

Guarding against nonstationarity is of utmost importance, as acvf estimates may otherwise be totally misleading. We recommend two approaches: experimental control and data screening. Experimental control for stationarity might include: e.g. providing a synchronization phase, trial-to-trial knowledge of results possibly with pretraining. Data screening might include: e.g. filtering out a small percentage of deviant sequences identified by graphical and statistical procedures (possibly with replication of defective sequences).

If it is not possible to ensure stationarity, analysis of the residuals after removal of linear trend seems preferable to the risk of acvf distortion by drift in the mean. Preliminary Monte Carlo results have shown that linear trends in the mean can safely be removed by regression techniques without introducing additional distortions of the 'true' acvf. Whether this holds for more complex kinds of trend as well remains an open question, however.

5 ERROR CORRECTION IN SYNCHRONIZATION

So far, we have assumed that tapping proceeds without any correction mechanism by which the subject adjusts the timekeeper for inaccurate interresponse intervals. In this section, which is largely theoretical, we modify the two-level timing model to include such a mechanism. Our aim is to give some insight into the dynamics of error correction as well as to demonstrate useful analysis tools.

The assumption that in tapping there is no feedback from the interresponse intervals to the timing level seems a good approximation, as the empiric success of the Wing–Kristofferson model demonstrates. Nevertheless, there are situations in which subjects must exert some kind of error correction. An example is the synchronization phase of the task used by Stevens (1886) and Wing and Kristofferson (1973a). In order to get subjects to tap at a given rate, the subjects had to start responding in synchrony with a metronome that produced an isochronous train of clicks. Keeping synchrony requires error correction, as otherwise the responses will drift away from the metronome with probability 1 except for a timekeeper with zero variance. This is so even if the timekeeper is set perfectly to the target interval and the subject starts off tapping in perfect synchrony.

Subjects do not seem to have difficulty in keeping synchrony. Also, as described earlier, there is strong evidence that the timekeeper does, in fact, have sizeable variance. On logical grounds, therefore, mechanisms must exist that lock the subject's response to the metronome.

Experimental studies on synchronization go back to Dunlap (1910) and Woodrow (1932). Recent theoretical work, inspired by the influential papers of Michon (1967) and Voillaume (1971), has focused on the task of tracking a metronome with variable intervals (Hary and Moore, 1987a, b). For details and reviews of the literature, the reader is referred to Schulze (1992) and Vos and Helsper (1992).

Surprisingly, theoretical work on synchronization has ignored the two-level timing model and the evidence put forward for it. For example, the models proposed by Schulze (1992) and Vos and Helsper (1992) do not distinguish between a central level of timing control and a peripheral level at which responses are observed. However, synchronization models are tested by how successful they are in predicting the dependence structure of sequences of interresponse intervals and synchronization errors. Hence, dependence due to the two-level nature of timing should be taken into account in addition to dependence caused by error correction.

In the following, we consider the simplest synchronization task, that of isochronous tapping in synchrony with a perfect metronome. As will be shown below, for this situation, *phase correction* strategies, which compensate only for phase differences between the responses and the metronome without adjusting the timekeeper period, are sufficient for maintaining synchrony. Our extension of the Wing–Kristofferson model to synchronization assumes a first-order linear feedback mechanism that adjusts for phase differences.

To account for synchronization performance in situations in which the metronome period undergoes systematic variations, such as drifts or abrupt tempo changes, *period correction* mechanisms are needed which require the subject to adjust the internal clock to the period changes of the metronome (Hary and Moore, 1987a; Vorberg, 1992). Clearly, the model sketched here is no competitor to the more complex models proposed for such situations by Hary and Moore (1987a, b). We see several advantages in our approach, however.

One is that, contrary to the Hary–Moore models, our model includes the Wing–Kristofferson model as a limiting case which might enable us to account for continuation and synchronization performance within the same framework. Another advantage is that the model allows for the derivation of predictions in closed form, thus admitting more decisive empiric tests than models amenable to computer simulation only. Moreover, the model is easily generalized to more challenging situations such as synchronization with a variable metronome (Vorberg and Schulze, submitted) or even to synchronization between two subjects (Vorberg, unpublished). The analysis techniques as well as most results carry over to these more complex versions of the model.

5.1 Synchronization with a Metronome

Our analysis focuses on the *synchronization errors* or *asynchronies*, A_n, defined as the difference in the occurrence of the n-th metronome click and the corresponding response; by convention, negative synchronization errors stand for anticipations. Let π denote the fixed period of the metronome. The interresponse intervals, $\{I_n\}$, are related to the synchronization errors, $\{A_n\}$, by the basic equation:

$$I_n = \pi + A_{n+1} - A_n \tag{17}$$

Note that this important relationship, which can be verified from Figure 4.9, holds for any model as it follows from the very definitions of the observables.

As usual, we start from the two-process assumption and express the interresponse intervals as a linear combination of timekeeper and motor delay components:

$$I_n = T_n^* + M_{n+1} - M_n \tag{18}$$

The central component, T_n^*, consists of an interval generated by the timekeeper, T_n, and a correction term. We assume that the metronome's period π is known to the subject such that the timekeeper mean is well set and need not be adjusted. The subject corrects for phase differences by subtracting a fixed proportion, α, of the last synchronization error from the interval T_n generated by the timekeeper:

$$T_n^* = T_n - \alpha A_n \tag{19}$$

Admittedly, this proportional-error assumption is an approximation to more realistic models where large (e.g. suprathreshold) synchronization errors are treated differently from smaller (e.g. subthreshold) errors. This simplification allows full analysis of the model, however, in contrast to models based on nonlinear threshold assumptions.

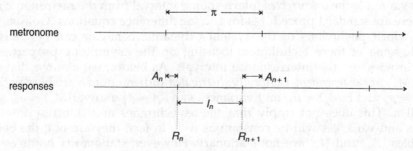

Figure 4.9. *Synchronization with a metronome. Relating asynchronies, metronome and interresponse intervals.*

5.1.1 Monte Carlo Simulation of the Model

Before analysing the model in detail, we illustrate its behavior by way of Monte Carlo simulations. Figure 4.10 shows sequences of interresponse intervals, $\{I_n\}$, and asynchronies, $\{A_n\}$, with estimates of the acvf.s as would be obtained if the model holds. In each figure, the top left-hand graph shows the interresponse interval sequence, the graph below that of the asynchronies; the graph in the middle displays the acvf estimate from the corresponding sequence. The right-hand graphs show the average acvf estimated from 20 independent runs of the model.

Note that the interresponse intervals and the asynchronies fluctuate around a constant mean; this is so even if the timekeeper mean, $E(T_n)$, differs systematically from the metronome period (Figure 4.10b). Again, there is considerable noise in the acvf estimates based on a single sequence, as the comparison with the average estimates makes evident. Figure 4.11 shows the average acvf.s for a range of values of the correction factor α.

Note the shape of the acvf.s: depending on the value of α, the asynchrony acvf may show positive dependences for nonadjacent responses. The interresponse interval acvf, however, looks remarkably similar to the predictions for continuation made by the original two-level model, with the characteristic dip at lag 1, although the value falls below the theoretical bound of -0.5. At lags larger than 1, dependence shows up for larger values of α only. By studying the model analytically, we can determine the conditions under which the interresponse interval acvf will have the same shape for synchronization as for continuation.

5.1.2 Characteristic Difference Equation

As a first step in the analysis of the model, we combine equations (17) to (19). This gives a first-order (stochastic) difference equation for the synchronization errors:

$$A_{n+1} = (1 - \alpha)A_n + (T_n + M_{n+1} - M_n) - \pi \qquad (20)$$

which fully characterizes the dynamic properties of the model.

Equation (20) states how the upcoming asynchrony is determined by the effects of the n-th and the $(n + 1)$-th response events. Note that $(T_n + M_{n+1} - M_n)$ corresponds to what the interresponse interval I_n would be without error correction; this means that each asynchrony is equal to a constant fraction of the previous one plus the deviation of the *uncorrected* interresponse interval from the metronome interval.

There are standard procedures for solving difference equations (Goldberg, 1958), from which predictions of the system's dynamic behavior can be derived. We sketch some of these techniques, focusing on the asymptotic properties of the asynchronies and the interresponse intervals. As before, we assume that the $\{T_n\}$ and $\{M_n\}$ are *independent identically distributed* (iid) random variables with means $E(T_n) = \mu_T$ and $E(M_n) = \mu_M$ and variances $\text{var}(T_n) = \sigma_T^2$ and $\text{var}(M_n) = \sigma_M^2$, constant for all n. This does not imply that the asynchronies and interresponse interval means and variances will be constant as well. In fact, they are not; the observable variables $\{A_n\}$ and $\{I_n\}$ are not stationary. However, stationarity holds asymptotically if the correction factor α lies in the right range. In that case, means, variances and covariances will tend toward limiting values. We will show how to obtain these limits.

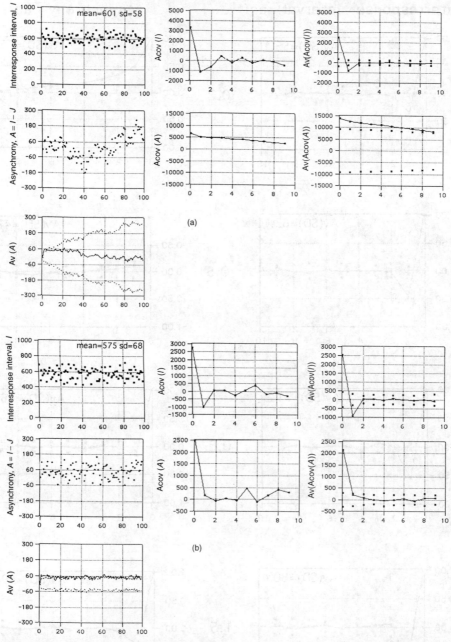

Figure 4.10. *Simulation of synchronization with a metronome with constant period $E(J) = 600$ ms. (a) Timekeeper mean matching the metronome ($E(I) = E(J)$) but no feedback correction ($\alpha = 0$). On the left (top, middle) are shown the interresponse intervals and the asynchrony between the metronome and the responses. The average (solid line) and variance (broken line) of 20 such sequences is shown below. Observe the linear increase in variance with the index number of the interval. On the right, estimates of the autocovariance (Acov) for lags 0 through 9 are shown for single sequences and averages over 20 sequences. (b) Feedback correction with timekeeper set at 575 ms. Despite the 25 ms mismatch between timekeeper and metronome, feedback correction ($\alpha = 0.5$) produces reasonable synchronization.*

Interresponse interval acf   Asynchrony acf

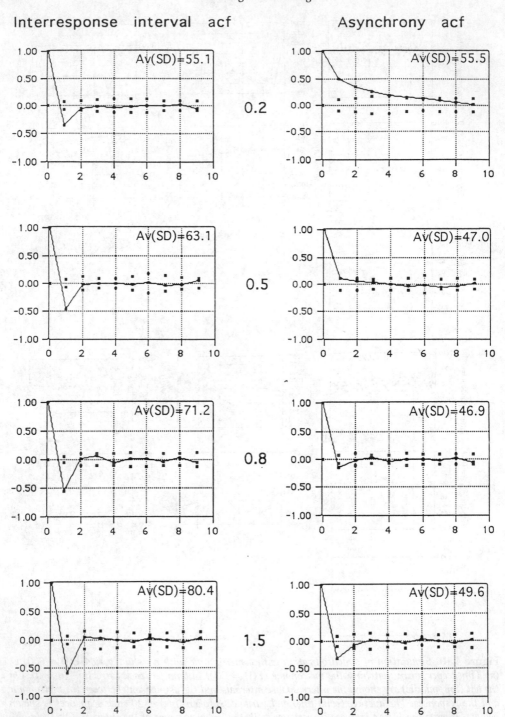

Figure 4.11. *Simulation of synchronization with varying degrees of feedback correction. Empiric acf.s for interresponse intervals (left) and asynchronies (right) for various values of the correction factor, α, computed from 20 independent samples of* N = 100 *responses.*

5.2 Asymptotic Stationarity

Without error correction, the responses will drift out of phase from the metronome sooner or later. Will the error correction scheme (equation 19) prevent this? Let us look at the mean asynchronies first.

5.2.1 Asymptotic Stationarity of the Asynchrony Mean

Taking expectations on both sides of equation (20) leads to:

$$E(A_{n+1}) = (1 - \alpha)E(A_n) + E(T_n + M_{n+1} - M_n) - \pi$$
$$= (1 - \alpha)E(A_n) + \mu_T - \pi$$

Simplifying by setting $E(A_n) = \mu_n$ and $c = \mu_T - \pi$ gives another difference equation:

$$\mu_{n+1} = (1 - \alpha)\mu_n + c \qquad n > 0 \tag{21}$$

which describes how the expected asynchrony changes with time.

Let us look at the means of the first few asynchronies:

$$\mu_2 = (1 - \alpha)\mu_1 + c$$
$$\mu_3 = (1 - \alpha)\mu_2 + c$$
$$= (1 - \alpha)[(1 - \alpha)\mu_1 + c] + c$$
$$= (1 - \alpha)^2\mu_1 + [1 + (1 - \alpha)]c$$
$$\mu_4 = (1 - \alpha)\mu_3 + c$$
$$= (1 - \alpha)[(1 - \alpha)^2\mu_1 + [1 + (1 - \alpha)]c] + c$$
$$= (1 - \alpha)^3\mu_1 + [1 + (1 - \alpha) + (1 - \alpha)^2]c$$

Hence, we guess:

$$\mu_n = (1 - \alpha)^{n-1}\mu_1 + [1 + (1 - \alpha) + (1 - \alpha)^2 + \cdots + (1 - \alpha)^{n-2}]c$$

which, by induction, can be proven for all $n > 0$. Reducing the geometric series yields the solution:

$$\mu_n = (1 - \alpha)^{n-1}\mu_1 + \frac{c}{\alpha}[1 - (1 - \alpha)^{n-1}] \tag{22}$$

For $-1 < 1 - \alpha < 1$, the first term approaches 0 as n tends to infinity, while the bracketed term on the right tends to 1. Therefore, for a correction factor obeying $0 < \alpha < 2$, the expected asynchrony converges to the limit $E(A) \equiv \lim_{n \to \infty} E(A_n)$ which is given by:

$$E(A) = [\mu_T - \pi]/\alpha \tag{23}$$

Hence, the asynchrony mean will stabilize for any value of α in this range. For $\alpha < 1$, the limit is approached in a monotonic fashion; for $1 < \alpha < 2$ (which corresponds to overcompensating for the last synchronization error) the approach to the asymptote is oscillatory. For values of the correction factor outside this range, stable performance cannot be achieved, and the mean phase difference from the metronome will increase forever. Table 4.3 shows the predicted behavior of the asynchrony mean for selected values of α.

It is remarkable how robust the phase correction scheme is. In general, non-stationarity obtains when the mean interresponse interval does not match the metronome period (i.e. $\mu_T \neq \pi$). However, correcting by subtracting a fixed fraction of each asynchrony will keep the mean synchronization error within bounds and produce stationarity even when the timekeeper mean is but a rough approximation of the metronome rate.

Often, an *anticipation bias*, i.e. a negative asynchrony mean, is reported (see Vos and Helsper, 1992), although there are exceptions (e.g. Schulze, 1992). The model is neutral in this regard: depending on the timekeeper parameter μ_T, positive or negative mean asynchronies can be predicted. There seems no good reason, however, for predicting a negative rather than a positive bias. This situation changes if optimality considerations are taken into account. For any value of the correction factor $0 < \alpha < 2$, it can be shown that the optimal timekeeper mean is $\mu_T < \pi$ (which from equation (23) implies anticipation) whenever: (1) the subject tries to minimize the expected squared error, $E(A^2)$; and (2) the variance of the timekeeper, σ_T^2, increases monotically with the mean, μ_T (Vorberg and Schulze, submitted). The reason for this is the same as in statistical estimation where biased estimators are often used for gaining efficiency: because $E(A^2) = E^2(A) + \text{var}(A)$, risking a small error in the mean may reduce the contribution of the variance to the total cost. If small timekeeper means go with small variances, the gain in the variance reduction may outweigh the loss due to the timekeeper's bias for anticipation.

It is not clear yet whether these arguments are sufficient to account for the amount of anticipation reported in the literature; it seems likely that additional explanations are needed, such as differences in the perceptual feedback delays (Aschersleben and Prinz, 1995; Fraisse, 1980; Prinz, 1992). However, they serve to

Table 4.3. *Expected initial and asymptotic asynchronies for selected values of the correction factor, α*

α	n						
	1	2	3	4	5	10	∞
−0.2	−10	−22	−36.4	−53.7	−74.4	−259.6	−∞
0.2	−10	−18	−24.4	−29.5	−33.6	−44.6	−50.0
0.6	−10	−14	−15.6	−16.2	−16.5	−16.7	−16.7
1.0	−10	−10	−10.0	−10.0	−10.0	−10.0	−10.0
1.4	−10	−6	−7.6	−7.0	−7.2	−7.1	−7.1
1.8	−10	−2	−8.4	−3.3	−7.4	−5.0	−5.6
2.2	−10	2	−12.4	4.9	−15.9	23.6	±∞

show an important implication of the robustness of the phase correction scheme: if anticipation bias is *intended* because it is in some sense optimal (e.g. Koch, 1992), rather than being due to incorrect parameter setting, most period correction schemes will be inadequate, as they drive the timekeeper's period toward that of the metronome and hence prevent optimality. This supports our earlier observation that phase correction is likely to underlie synchronization with a constant metronome, while period correction becomes more appropriate whenever systematic tempo changes have to be coped with.

5.2.2 Asymptotic Stationarity of the Asynchrony Variance

The informal derivation above served two different goals: proving asymptotic stationarity and deriving the limit itself. An alternative derivation of equation (23) can be given that illustrates a useful 'quick-and-dirty' method for obtaining limits. We start by assuming that there is an asymptotic limit. For n sufficiently large, $\mu_{n+1} = \mu_n = \mu_A$, *given that the limit exists*. Replacing both μ_n and μ_{n+1} in equation (21) by μ_A leads to:

$$\mu_A = (1 - \alpha)\mu_A + c$$

solving for μ_A immediately gives solution (23).

We use this heuristic method for finding the asymptotic variance of the asynchronies, $\text{var}(A) \equiv \lim_{n \to \infty} \text{var}(A_n)$, which forms the basis for all other variance and covariance predictions. Note that asymptotic stationarity needs to be established by other methods, which is more involved for the variance than for the mean. It can be proven (Vorberg and Schulze, submitted) that the asynchronies $\{A_n\}$ and the interresponse intervals $\{I_n\}$ do, in fact, obey asymptotic stationarity in the second moments (i.e. including means, variances and covariances) if $0 < \alpha < 2$.

For the derivations, it is helpful to introduce the auxiliary variable I'_n corresponding to the interresponse intervals without the correction term, i.e.

$$I'_n = T_n + M_{n+1} - M_n$$

This permits rewriting equation (20) as:

$$A_{n+1} = (1 - \alpha)A_n + I'_n - \pi \tag{24}$$

Taking the variance of this recursion gives:

$$\begin{aligned}
\text{var}(A_{n+1}) &= \text{var}[(1 - \alpha)A_n + I'_n - \pi] \\
&= \text{var}[(1 - \alpha)A_n + I'_n] \\
&= (1 - \alpha)^2 \text{var}(A_n) + \text{var}(I'_n) + 2(1 - \alpha)\text{cov}(A_n, I'_n)
\end{aligned}$$

Given asymptotic stationarity, $\text{var}(A_n) = \text{var}(A_{n+1}) = \text{var}(A)$; inserting and solving for $\text{var}(A)$ yields:

$$\text{var}(A) = [\text{var}(I'_n) + 2(1 - \alpha)\text{cov}(A_n, I'_n)]/[1 - (1 - \alpha)^2]$$

From its definition and the assumptions above,

$$\text{var}(I_n') = \sigma_T^2 + 2\sigma_M^2$$

For the derivation of $\text{cov}(A_n, I_n')$, we apply recursion (24) once more:

$$\text{cov}(A_n, I_n') = \text{cov}[(1 - \alpha)A_{n-1} + I_{n-1}' - \pi, I_n']$$
$$= (1 - \alpha)\,\text{cov}(A_{n-1}, I_n') + \text{cov}(I_{n-1}', I_n')$$

The auxiliary variable I_n' is independent of asynchrony A_{n-1}, as it is constituted of T_n, M_n and M_{n+1} which, by assumption, are independent of events preceding the n-th response. The remaining covariance term corresponds to the lag-one autocovariance of the original Wing–Kristofferson model; therefore,

$$\text{cov}(A_n, I_n') = \text{cov}(I_{n-1}', I_n') = -\sigma_M^2$$

Putting these results together shows that, for $0 < \alpha < 2$, the asynchrony variance approaches the limiting value:

$$\text{var}(A) = [\sigma_T^2 + 2\alpha\sigma_M^2]/[1 - (1 - \alpha)^2] \tag{25}$$

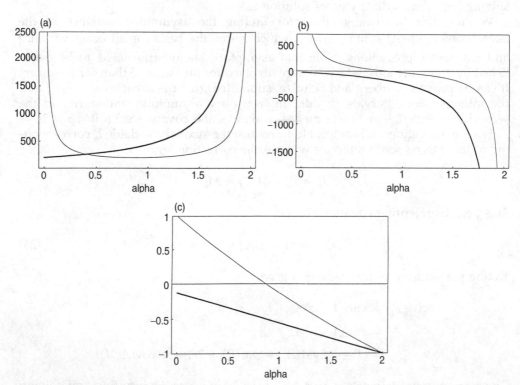

Figure 4.12. *Asymptotic variability and lag-1 dependence of interresponse intervals (bold) and asynchronies (thin), as predicted by the synchronization model. (Parameters: $\sigma_T = 12$, $\sigma_M = 5$ and $\alpha = 0.1$.) (a) Variances var(I) and var(A); (b) acvf.s $\gamma_I(1)$ and $\gamma_A(1)$; (c) acf.s $\gamma_I(1)/\gamma_I(0)$ and $\gamma_A(1)/\gamma_A(0)$.*

Figure 4.12a shows how the asynchrony variance changes as the correction factor α varies between 0 and 2. Note that var(A) tends to infinity at either end of the admissable interval. In general, var(A) achieves a single minimum in the interior of the interval if $\sigma_T^2 > 0$, except for a perfect timekeeper with $\mu_T = \pi$ and $\sigma_T^2 = 0$, where var(A) is smallest at $\alpha = 0$, i.e. without error correction. In Section 5.4, we look at the model's behavior when α is chosen such that var(A) is minimized.

5.3 Autocovariance Functions

5.3.1 Autocovariance Function of the Asynchronies

With these results, the asymptotic acvf of the asynchronies can be obtained in an analogous way, starting from:

$$\text{cov}(A_n, A_{n+j}) = \text{cov}[A_n, (1-\alpha)A_{n+j-1} + I'_{n+j-1} - \pi]$$
$$= (1-\alpha)\,\text{cov}(A_n, A_{n+j-1}) + \text{cov}(A_n, I'_{n+j-1})$$
$$= (1-\alpha)\,\text{cov}(A_n, A_{n+j-1})$$

for $j > 1$ by the argument above. For $j = 1$,

$$\text{cov}(A_n, A_{n+1}) = (1-\alpha)\,\text{cov}(A_n, A_n) + \text{cov}(A_n, I'_n)$$
$$= (1-\alpha)\,\text{var}(A_n) + \text{cov}(A_n, I'_n)$$
$$= (1-\alpha)\,\text{var}(A_n) - \sigma_M^2$$

by the derivation for $\text{cov}(A_n, I'_n)$ above.

Figure 4.12b shows the covariance between adjacent asynchronies as a function of the correction factor α. Note that, depending on the value of α, positive or negative dependence will be predicted. This also holds if the degree of dependence is expressed by correlation rather than covariance (see Figure 4.12c).

Taking the limit gives $\gamma_A(j) = \lim\limits_{n\to\infty} \text{cov}(A_n, A_{n+j})$; thus, for $j > 1$, the acvf obeys the difference equation:

$$\gamma_A(j) = (1-\alpha)\gamma_A(j-1)$$

which has solution:

$$\gamma_A(j) = (1-\alpha)^{j-1}\gamma_A(0) \qquad j > 1$$

Combining these results shows that, asymptotically, the dependence structure among the asynchronies is described by the acvf:

$$\gamma_A(j) = \begin{cases} \text{var}(A) & j = 0 \\ (1-\alpha)^{j-1}[\text{var}(A)(1-\alpha) - \sigma_M^2] & j > 0 \end{cases} \tag{26}$$

with var(A) given by equation (25). Except at $j = 0$, the acvf is a geometric function of lag j; hence, asynchronies from nonadjacent responses may be correlated. Figure 4.13a displays the acvf predicted for $\alpha = 0.5, 0.7, 0.9, 1.1, 1.3$ and 1.5. Clearly, values of $\alpha > 1$ produce oscillatory behavior of the acvf.

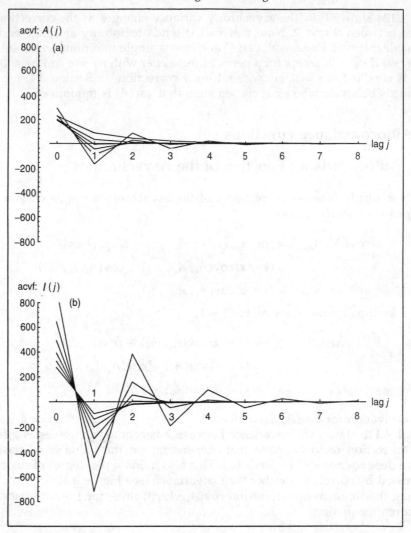

Figure 4.13. *Acvf predictions of the synchronization model, for* $\sigma_T = 12$, $\sigma_M = 5$ *and* $\alpha = 0.5, 0.7,$
0.9, 1.1, 1.3 and 1.5. (a) Asynchrony acvf; (b) interresponse interval acvf. At lag 1, the acvf.s decrease
monotonically with increasing α.

5.3.2 Autocovariance Function of the Interresponse Intervals

Knowing the acvf of the asynchronies is sufficient for determining that of the
interresponse intervals, $\gamma_I(j)$. By equation (17):

$$
\begin{aligned}
\text{cov}(I_n, I_{n+j}) &= \text{cov}(\pi + A_{n+1} - A_n, \pi + A_{n+j+1} - A_{n+j}) \\
&= \text{cov}(A_{n+1} - A_n, A_{n+j+1} - A_{n+j}) \\
&= \text{cov}(A_{n+1}, A_{n+j+1}) - \text{cov}(A_n, A_{n+j+1}) \\
&\quad - \text{cov}(A_{n+1}, A_{n+j}) + \text{cov}(A_n, A_{n+j})
\end{aligned}
$$

At asymptote, then,

$$\gamma_I(j) = \begin{cases} 2\gamma_A(0) - 2\gamma_A(1) & j = 0 \\ 2\gamma_A(j) - \gamma_A(j-1) - \gamma_A(j+1) & j > 0 \end{cases} \tag{27}$$

Figure 4.13b shows the acvf of the interresponse intervals for selected values of α.

Again, values of $\alpha > 1$ produce an oscillatory acvf. In general, error correction creates dependence between nonadjacent interresponse intervals, in contrast to the Wing–Kristofferson model which predicts dependence for adjacent intervals only.

For comparison with the model without error correction, we present the variance and the lag-one autocovariance of the interresponse intervals:

$$\gamma_I(0) = \frac{2}{2-\alpha} [\sigma_T^2 + (2+\alpha)\sigma_M^2] \tag{28a}$$

$$\gamma_I(1) = -\frac{1}{2-\alpha} [\alpha\sigma_T^2 + (2+\alpha+\alpha^2)\sigma_M^2] \tag{28b}$$

Figures 4.12 illustrates how $\mathrm{var}(I_n) = \gamma_I(0)$ and $\mathrm{cov}(I_n, I_{n+1}) = \gamma_I(1)$ vary as a function of α. The variance as well as the covariance attain their smallest values for $\alpha = 0$ which equal those of the original model without error correction (see equation 7). Thus, error correction has its costs on the interresponse interval variance. Because each adjustment adds to the central variance above that already contributed by the timekeeper, the interresponse interval variance always exceeds the variance obtainable without error correction. Of course, error correction cannot be dispensed with if the goal is to remain synchronized.

The dependence between adjacent interresponse intervals becomes more pronounced the larger the correction factor α; this holds both for covariance and correlation as dependence measure. Figure 4.12 shows the lag-one autocorrelation of the interresponse intervals as a function of α. In general, error correction makes adjacent interresponse intervals more negatively correlated than they would be by the two-level architecture alone. This can also be seen from the bounds on the lag-one autocorrelation which follow from equation (28):

$$-\frac{1}{2}\left[1 + \frac{\alpha^2}{2+\alpha}\right] \leqslant \rho \leqslant -\frac{\alpha}{2} \tag{29}$$

For $\alpha > 0$, the bounds lie below those predicted for the original model (see equation 8).

5.4 Optimal Error Correction

Which choice of the correction factor α is best? Clearly, the answer depends on the performance goal that the subject is trying to optimize. It is not possible to minimize the asymptotic asynchrony mean, $E(A)$, its variance, $\mathrm{var}(A)$, and the response time variance, $\mathrm{var}(I)$, at the same time. We have already seen (equation 23) that, for an imprecisely set timekeeper, $E(A)$ will be smallest if α is set close to 2. Values of $\alpha > 1$ are in conflict with variance minimization, however. In fact, they are not admissable in the sense that var(I) and var(A) can both be reduced by lowering α. Focusing on the variances only leads to a similar conflict. Response interval variance and asynchrony variance cannot be minimized together either: as can be verified from Figure 4.12, there is a range $0 < \alpha < \alpha'$ within which var(I) increases while var(A) decreases with α. Rather than minimizing a weighted function of the two variances, let us look at the value of the correction factor that produces the smallest asynchrony variance. In the following, we use 'optimal' to refer to a strategy that optimizes this goal.

Intuitively, the optimal α should reflect the causes of synchronization errors. Lapses due to a variable central timer have consequences different from those caused by variable motor delays. Look at an extreme case, a perfect subject (with $\sigma_T^2 = \sigma_M^2 = 0$) tracking a metronome with known period. Assume that a single asynchrony occurs. If it was caused by a deviant timer interval, it has to be corrected for. Otherwise, the subsequent responses will be shifted away from the metronome as well. To do nothing is the best strategy, however, if the cause was an irregular motor delay: without any correction, all future responses will be in synchrony again.

In general, the optimal value of α should reflect the relative contributions of the timekeeper and motor delay variances. This is, in fact, the case. By forming the derivative of equation (25) and setting it equal to zero, the minimum variance can be shown to be achieved whenever $\alpha = \alpha'$, with α' given by:

$$\alpha' = \begin{cases} 1 & \sigma_M^2 = 0 \\ [r(2 + r)]^{1/2} - r & \sigma_M^2 > 0 \end{cases} \tag{30}$$

where $r = \sigma_T^2/2\sigma_M^2$. The optimal correction factor depends on the ratio of the timekeeper and the motor delay variances only. As expected, correcting by subtracting a small fraction of the preceding asynchrony is indicated when the motor delays contribute most of the variance, whereas α should be selected close to 1 if the variance is mostly due to the timekeeper. Note that $\alpha' \leqslant 1$ holds in general; hence, overcompensating ($\alpha > 1$) is suboptimal with respect to the asynchrony variance.

Optimal phase correction has striking consequences for the dependence structure of the asynchronies and the interresponse intervals: surprisingly, adjacent asynchronies are uncorrelated if $\alpha = \alpha'$; this can be verified from equation (26) as well as from Figure 4.12b. Moreover, by its geometric shape, the asynchrony acvf vanishes everywhere if it vanishes at lag one. Thus, $\gamma_A(j) = 0$ for all $j > 0$ whenever var(A) is minimal.

By equation (27), $\gamma_I(j)$ is completely determined by $\gamma_A(j)$. If the subject minimizes var(A) by setting $\alpha = \alpha'$, then

$$\gamma_I(j) = \begin{cases} 2\gamma_A(0) = 2\,\text{var}(A) & j = 0 \\ -\gamma_A(1) = -\text{var}(A) & j = 1 \\ 0 & j > 1 \end{cases} \tag{31}$$

Hence, optimal phase correction produces an interresponse interval acvf that is nonzero for adjacent interresponse intervals only. Its shape is the same as that of the Wing–Kristofferson model for continuation tapping.

Strictly speaking, the model predicts identical interresponse interval avcf.s for synchronization and for continuation only if $\alpha = \alpha'$. However, as Figure 4.11 shows, the prediction is quite robust. Therefore, we should expect the statistical structure of the interresponse intervals to be quite similar for synchronization and for continuation if the subject selects a value of α not too far from the optimal value α'. Vorberg (1992) has noted some striking similarities between synchronization and continuation data. Our optimality considerations may provide an explanation for these puzzling findings.

Despite the acvf shape similarities predicted for near-optimal α, the model predicts that the amount of dependence should differ between synchronization and continuation. For synchronization with optimal error correction, equation (31) implies a correlation $\rho_I(1) = -1/2$ between adjacent interresponse intervals, equal to the lower bound ever attainable without error correction (see equation 9).

This illustrates an important point. In general, the action of online error correction in synchronization is bound to create dependence above that due to the two-level architecture. Although there are good reasons why synchronization and continuation data might look similar, we should expect more dependence for synchronization. Applying the original Wing–Kristofferson model to synchronization data, without regard to the likely existence of error correction, need not lead to its rejection. However, such an approach is at risk of producing variance estimates that systematically distort the relative contributions of timekeeper and motor delay variability.

5.5 Additional Considerations

An important function of a model is to guide the analysis and interpretation of data, even if the model turns out to be incorrect in some of the details. The statistics of synchronization experiments are notoriously difficult to understand without a model. We close this section with two examples illustrating our point.

Which aspects of synchronization data can be taken as evidence for the operation of an error correction mechanism? One might try to diagnose online error correction from the dependence between successive synchronization errors, hoping that online error correction will reveal itself by a negative dependence (*conjecture 1*). Alternatively, it might seem a good idea to look at how the size and sign of the current synchronization error influences the timing of the upcoming response. For example, in a scatterplot showing the regression of I_n on A_n, a systematic tendency for large positive synchronization errors to be followed by shorter than average interresponse intervals, and vice versa, might be taken as evidence for error correction (*conjecture 2*). Both conjectures can be found in the recent literature. It turns out that the underlying intuitions are incorrect, showing the need for a formal analysis.

We have already shown that conjecture 1 is wrong: for our model, the correlation between adjacent synchronization errors may take on any value between -1 and $+1$ (see Figure 4.12). Paradoxically, a zero correlation implies $\alpha = \alpha' > 0$, i.e. optimal error correction. In the framework of the model, conjecture 1 is therefore not valid, although models are conceivable for which it holds.

In contrast, conjecture 2 can be rejected for *any* model. By the basic relationship (17), we have:

$$\text{cov}(A_n, I_n) = \text{cov}(A_n, \pi + A_{n+1} - A_n)$$

$$= \text{cov}(A_n, \pi) + \text{cov}(A_n, A_{n+1}) - \text{cov}(A_n, A_n)$$

$$= \text{cov}(A_n, A_{n+1}) - \text{var}(A_n)$$

$$= -(1/2)\,\text{var}(I_n)$$

$$< 0 \tag{32}$$

where the last substitution follows from equation (27). Because equations (17) and (27) follow from the very definition of synchronization errors, they hold for any model. Therefore, the current interresponse interval will always be negatively dependent on the preceding synchronization error, irrespective of whether there is online error correction or not – a result difficult to predict on intuitive grounds.

These examples show that, in general, inferences from data to underlying mechanisms are dangerous if they are not based on an explicit theoretical framework. We see the main advantage of the two-level timing model with phase correction in that it provides such a framework. It remains to be seen whether it is as successful in accounting for synchronization data as the original model is for continuation; some promising empirical tests of the model have already been reported (Vorberg and Schulze, submitted).

6   GENERALIZED TWO-LEVEL TIMING MODELS

Despite its simplicity, the Wing–Kristofferson model has proved successful in describing interresponse interval data in unpaced tapping. Essentially, this is because of its two-level architecture, while the details of the timekeeper and motor delay assumptions seem less important. In the following sections of this chapter, we shall study various extensions of the basic two-level model in which we relax the strong assumption that the intervals produced by the timekeeper are independent and identically distributed and, likewise, that the series of motor delays are independently and identically distributed. Permitting these variables to have richer statistical structure, but retaining the two-level notion as a theoretical framework, we show how considerably more complex timing structures can be analyzed.

The generalized two-level timing model can be summarized by the following three assumptions:

A1: *Two-level representation.* For all n,

$$I_n = T_n + M_{n+1} - M_n$$

A2: *Independence between systems.* For all m and n,

$$\text{cov}(T_m, M_n) = 0$$

A3: *Order preservation.* The order of responses set up by the timing system is not altered by the motor system, that is,

$$P(T_n + M_{n+1} - M_n > 0) = 1 \quad \text{for all } n$$

Some comment on the assumptions is in order. Assumption A1 restates the Wing–Kristofferson model. Assumption A2 states that independence holds *between* systems only, whereas arbitrary dependence is permitted among the variables *within* each system. It is conceivable that this assumption might be violated. For example, suppose successive motor delays are correlated. If the degree of that correlation depends on how closely in time two responses follow each other, then the variability of the timekeeper intervals might affect the dependence structure of the motor delays and therefore violate independence between systems. For tapping at medium or slower tempos where interresponse intervals are sufficiently below maximum response rates, the problem should be negligible.

Assumption A3 is essential for any two-level model and was implicitly assumed in the Wing–Kristofferson model. If order preservation does not hold, responses might be sequenced in an order that differs from the corresponding commands, violating the interresponse interval representation as stated in assumption A1 (see Figure 4.14). For example, if the n-th command is delayed so much that its response comes later than that triggered by the $(n + 1)$-th command, the standard two-level representation will no longer apply and has to be changed into $I_n = T_n + M_n - M_{n+1}$. Order preservation will hold if the variability of the difference between successive motor delays, $\text{var}(M_{n+1} - M_n)$, is small compared with the mean interresponse interval, $E(T_n + M_{n+1} - M_n)$. From the findings sketched above, A3 is almost certainly true.

By assumptions A1 to A3, any covariance between interresponse intervals can be decomposed as:

$$\text{cov}(I_n, I_{n+j}) = \text{cov}(T_n, T_{n+j}) + \text{cov}(M_{n+1} - M_n, M_{n+j+1} - M_{n+j}) \quad (33)$$

In deriving predictions, we will use this property of the two-level framework extensively because it permits us to analyze the contributions of the timekeeper structures separately. Adding the motor delay contributions is then straightforward.

The covariance between two interresponse intervals $j \geq 0$ steps apart equals the covariance of the corresponding timer intervals plus that of the motor delay *differences*. By distributivity, the latter can be expressed as a sum of the covariances

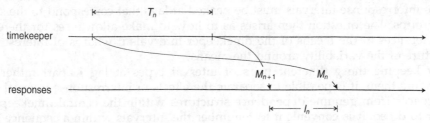

Figure 4.14. *Order preservation violated.*

between the motor delays separated by $j - 1$, j and $j + 1$ steps, respectively, since:

$$\text{cov}(M_{n+1} - M_n, M_{n+j+1} - M_{n+j}) = \text{cov}(M_{n+1}, M_{n+j+1}) - \text{cov}(M_{n+1}, M_{n+j})$$
$$- \text{cov}(M_n, M_{n+j+1}) + \text{cov}(M_n, M_{n+j}) \quad (34)$$

If the $\{M_n\}$ are independent with $\text{var}(M_n) = \sigma^2_{M,n}$, this equals:

$$\text{cov}(M_{n+1} - M_n, M_{n+j+1} - M_{n+j}) = \begin{cases} \sigma^2_{M,n} + \sigma^2_{M,n+1} & j = 0 \\ -\sigma^2_{M,n+1} & j = 1 \\ 0 & j > 1 \end{cases} \quad (35)$$

For dependent motor delays with autocovariance function $\gamma_M(j)$, the contribution to the interresponse interval covariance is:

$$\text{cov}(M_{n+1} - M_n, M_{n+j+1} - M_{n+j}) = 2\gamma_M(j) - \gamma_M(j-1) - \gamma_M(j+1) \quad (36)$$

6.1 Serial Covariances for Grouped Responses

So far our analysis of two-level timing has assumed equal intervals through the series. However, this is not a prerequisite of the generalized model. Suppose there are systematic differences in the timekeeper intervals, which is likely if the subject groups the successive responses. For example, consider the effect of a group of size two operating such that alternate intervals have values μ_1 and μ_2 (as, for example, in a two-element rhythm with a short–long interval pattern). The sequence of timekeeper intervals would then appear as $\mu_1, \mu_2, \mu_1, \mu_2, \ldots$, with overall mean $\mu = (\mu_1 + \mu_2)/2$ assuming N is even. The lag-j autocovariance for such a sequence will be based on pairs (μ_1, μ_2) and (μ_2, μ_1) if j is odd, and pairs (μ_1, μ_1) and (μ_2, μ_2) if j is even. The autocovariance is based on summing products of deviations of the variables with respect to the overall mean, μ. For j even, the sign of the product will be positive, for j odd, it will be negative. This means that the acvf $\gamma_T(j)$ will equal the variance among the two types of intervals if $j = 0, 2, 4, \ldots, N$ and -1 times this variance if $j = 1, 3, 5, \ldots, N - 1$ (assuming N is even).

For grouping g responses, there are g different types of interval with means $\mu_1, \mu_2, \ldots, \mu_g$. It can be shown that, in general, $\text{cov}(T_n, T_{n+g})$ equals the variance of the interval means, even if the intervals show random variability about those means. The end result is that, unless all the interval means are identical, the acvf of the interresponse intervals must be peaked at lags that correspond to the size of the groups. The question then arises as to how to make allowances for the effects of differences in the means of the timekeeper intervals if what is of interest is the structure of the variability around the means?

By keeping the g different pairs of interval types at lag j apart rather than averaging them, it is possible to separate the effects of interresponse interval mean differences from genuine dependence structures within the central timekeeper. In order to do so, it is convenient to renumber the intervals within a sequence using two indices: one (m) referring to the group, the other (i) to the interval within

Table 4.4. *Variance–covariance structure* $\mathbf{M}_m$ *contributed by the motor delays*

$$
\begin{pmatrix}
2\sigma_M^2 & -\sigma_M^2 & 0 & \cdots & 0 & 0 \\
-\sigma_M^2 & 2\sigma_M^2 & -\sigma_M^2 & \cdots & 0 & 0 \\
0 & -\sigma_M^2 & 2\sigma_M^2 & \cdots & 0 & 0 \\
\cdots & \cdots & \cdots & \cdots & \cdots & \cdots \\
0 & 0 & 0 & \cdots & 2\sigma_M^2 & -\sigma_M^2 \\
0 & 0 & 0 & \cdots & -\sigma_M^2 & 2\sigma_M^2
\end{pmatrix}
$$

groups. Thus, $I_{i,m}$ and $T_{i,m}$ correspond to the observed interresponse interval and the timekeeper interval, respectively, whose onset corresponds to the i-th response within the m-th group. (The original numbering can be recovered via $n = i + g(m - 1)$.) By analyzing what we will term the *periodic covariances* $\mathrm{cov}(I_{i,m}, I_{j,n})$ between all intervals within and between groups, any spurious correlation due to differences in the means will be eliminated.

As the most interesting aspect is the dependence structure within groups, we concentrate on the covariance matrix $\mathbf{I}_m = ((\mathrm{cov}(I_{i,m}, I_{j,m})))$. Generalizing equation (33) we have:

$$
\mathbf{I}_m = \mathbf{T}_m + \mathbf{M}_m \tag{37}
$$

where

$$
\mathbf{T}_m = ((\mathrm{cov}(T_{i,m}, T_{j,m})))
$$

and

$$
\mathbf{M}_m = ((\mathrm{cov}(M_{i+(m-1)g+1} - M_{i+(m-1)g}, M_{i'+(m-1)g+1} - M_{i'+(m-1)g+1})))
$$

If grouping leaves the peripheral motor delays unchanged, the matrix $\mathbf{M}_m$ has the form shown in Table 4.4, where $\mathrm{var}(M_n) = \sigma_M^2$ for all n.

6.2 Two-Hand Synchronous Timing Model

The original Wing–Kristofferson timing model assumed independence within as well as between the timekeeper intervals and the motor delays. With these assumptions relaxed in the generalized model we now turn to consider a procedure developed by Vorberg and Hambuch (1984) based on synchronous two-hand tapping that allows direct assessment of the amount of dependence within each subsystem. The central assumption is that a single central timekeeper structure controls both the left and the right hand. Thus, three subsystems are assumed: a timekeeping system, a left-hand and a right-hand motor subsystem (Figure 4.15).

As before, T_n stands for the n-th timekeeper interval. Let L_n and R_n denote the motor delays added by the left-hand and right-hand subsystems. Then the interresponse intervals produced by the right and the left hand, denoted by I_n and J_n,

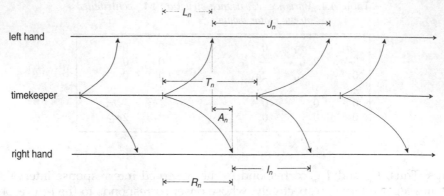

Figure 4.15. *Two-hand synchronized tapping: definition of variables.*

respectively, are given by:

$$I_n = T_n + R_{n+1} - R_n \tag{38}$$

$$J_n = T_n + L_{n+1} - L_n \tag{39}$$

Vorberg and Hambuch (1984) assumed mutual independence between the subsystems, such that $\mathrm{cov}(T_i, L_j) = \mathrm{cov}(T_i, R_k) = \mathrm{cov}(L_j, R_k) = 0$ for all i, j and k, whereas arbitrary dependence was permitted within each of the sequences $\{T_n\}$, $\{L_n\}$ and $\{R_n\}$. If these assumptions hold, it is possible to investigate the statistical structure of the subsystems in isolation, i.e. the timekeeper intervals uncontaminated by the motor delays, and vice versa.

6.2.1 Dependence Structure of the Timekeeping System

The two-hand model provides estimates of the timing system's acvf that do not depend on properties of the motor system. For this, the cross-covariance function (ccvf) between the right-hand and left-hand interresponse intervals is needed:

$$\begin{aligned}
\mathrm{cov}(I_n, J_{n+j}) &= \mathrm{cov}(T_n + L_{n+1} - L_n, T_{n+j} + R_{n+j+1} - R_{n+j}) \\
&= \mathrm{cov}(T_n, T_{n+j}) + \mathrm{cov}(L_{n+1} - L_n, R_{n+j+1} - R_{n+j}) \\
&= \mathrm{cov}(T_n, T_{n+j})
\end{aligned}$$

Thus, the covariance between intervals across hands directly reflects the dependence between the timer intervals that they have in common. By similar steps, $\mathrm{cov}(J_n, I_{n+j})$ may also be seen to equal $\mathrm{cov}(T_n, T_{n+j})$, which gives:

$$\mathrm{cov}(I_n, J_{n+j}) = \mathrm{cov}(T_n, T_{n+j}) = \mathrm{cov}(J_n, I_{n+j}) \tag{40}$$

Equation (40) has two important consequences in assessing the variability that two interresponse intervals at a given lag across hands have in common: (1) it gives a direct view of the dependence structure of the timekeeper intervals, and (2) it enables us to test hypotheses on underlying timing mechanisms, thus 'filtering out' the influences of the motor subsystems.

In general, ccvf.s are not symmetric. However, equation (40) states a testable condition that must hold if the model is valid: the ccvf has to be symmetric, i.e. the dependence between the current right-hand interresponse interval and a left-hand interresponse interval j steps later must be the same as that between the current left-hand interresponse interval and the corresponding later right-hand interresponse interval. From this it follows that, if the model holds, sample estimates of $cov(I_n, J_{n+j})$ and $cov(J_n, I_{n+j})$ differ from each other by sampling error only. Therefore, their average provides a reasonable estimator of the timer acvf:

$$\widehat{cov}(T_n, T_{n+j}) = [\widehat{cov}(I_n, J_{n+j}) + \widehat{cov}(J_n, I_{n+j})]/2 \tag{41}$$

6.2.2 Dependence Structure of the Motor Subsystems

Define A_n as the n-th *asynchrony* between hands, i.e. the time difference between the corresponding left-hand and right-hand responses, with positive sign indicating the right hand's lead. As both responses are assumed to be triggered by the same central command (Figure 4.15), this implies:

$$A_n = L_n - R_n \tag{42}$$

Therefore,

$$
\begin{aligned}
cov(A_n, A_{n+j}) &= cov(L_n - R_n, L_{n+j} - R_{n+j}) \\
&= cov(L_n, L_{n+j}) + cov(R_n, R_{n+j})
\end{aligned}
\tag{43}
$$

This shows that the acvf of the response asynchronies estimates the sum of the acvf.s of the right-hand and the left-hand motor delays, irrespective of the timer intervals.

Finally we note that equations (38) to (40) can be combined to yield the relationships:

$$var(I_n) - cov(I_n, J_n) = var(R_n) + var(R_{n+1}) - 2\,cov(R_n, R_{n+1}) \tag{44}$$

$$var(J_n) - cov(I_n, J_n) = var(L_n) + var(L_{n+1}) - 2\,cov(L_n, L_{n+1}) \tag{45}$$

which provide separate estimates of the right-hand and left-hand motor delay variances.

6.3 Findings on Two-Hand Tapping of Rhythms

Vorberg and Hambuch (1984) applied the above model to data from an experiment in which five highly trained subjects (one professional, four amateur musicians) produced simple rhythms with both hands in synchrony. Four rhythms were used, denoted by 2-4-2, 2-1-3-2, 3-1-2-2 and 2-2-2-2, respectively, where the numbers give the number of eighth notes per interval. The tempo was fixed at 175 ms per eighth note; thus, the cycles of intervals to be produced were 350-700-350, 350-175-525-350, 525-175-350-350 and 350-350-350-350. The data analysis kept the different intervals within the rhythmic groups separate, as outlined in Section 6.1. In a later section we will return to consider accounts of timekeeper structures in these rhythms; the present focus is on the application of the method and the implications for the generalized two-level timing model.

6.3.1   Test of the Symmetry Prediction

Vorberg and Hambuch computed all periodic cross-covariances for each condition and lags $1 \leqslant j \leqslant g$, where g is the number of intervals per cycle (group). Comparison of the estimates $\hat{\text{cov}}(I_n, J_{n+j})$ and $\hat{\text{cov}}(I_{n+j}, J_n)$ produced only a few significant deviations from equality for some lags and some subjects, and these did not form a discernible pattern. Altogether, no systematic differences were revealed when testing across conditions and/or across subjects, supporting the model's symmetry prediction of the ccvf of the interresponse intervals between hands.

6.3.2   Dependence Between Motor Delays

One advantage of the two-hand model is that it permits an assessment of the amount of dependence within the motor delays via the serial covariances of the response asynchronies, rather than assuming independence of the successive delays. For each of the g asynchronies within a rhythmic group, the serial covariances with lags 1, 2 and 3 were estimated separately and then averaged within the group. Table 4.5 shows these estimates, averaged across subjects, and expressed as correlations. By equation (43), they can be interpreted as the means of left-hand and right-hand autocorrelations of the motor delays at the different lags.

The data show that adjacent motor delays are correlated. Averaged across conditions, the correlation between adjacent motor delays is 0.076 only, however, and vanishes altogether for lags beyond 1. Thus, although not exactly correct, Wing and Kristofferson's (1973b) assumption of independent motor delays provides an excellent approximation. In fact, the consequences of ignoring the small dependence will be negligible under most circumstances. This is demonstrated by comparing the estimates of the motor delay variance: across conditions and hands, an estimate of 23.12 ms^2 results from equations (44) and (45), when independence is assumed, compared with a value of 24.81 ms^2, when the actual lag-one dependence is taken into consideration. In terms of standard deviations, the independence approximation amounts to an underestimation of the correct value by less than 0.2 ms.

Table 4.5. *Serial autocorrelations of the motor delays (see text)*

Rhythm	Lag 1	Lag 2	Lag 3
2-4-2	0.045	0.000	−0.013
2-1-3-2	0.092	−0.015	0.000
3-1-2-2	0.054	0.010	−0.015
2-2-2-2	0.114	−0.031	−0.010
Mean	0.076	−0.009	−0.010

Table 4.6. *Observed interresponse interval variances and estimates of the timer and motor delay variances*

Rhythm	$[\mathrm{var}(I) + \mathrm{var}(J)]/2$	var(L)	var(R)	var(T)
2-4-2	144.5	23.1	29.4	94.5
2-1-3-2	128.9	23.1	25.6	84.1
3-1-2-2	121.1	24.9	25.6	75.1
2-2-2-2	73.4	25.3	21.5	29.2

6.3.3 Timekeeper and Motor Delay Variances

Using equations (41), (44) and (45), the variances of the timer intervals and the motor delays can be estimated. Table 4.6 gives, averaged across the different intervals within rhythmic groups, the observed interresponse interval variances, the estimates of the variances of the timer intervals, var(T), and the left-hand and right-hand motor delays, var(L) and var(R), respectively. The estimates of var(L) and var(R) are corrected for the observed lag-one dependences (Table 4.5), assuming that the correlations are identical for the left-hand and the right-hand delays.

Across conditions, the motor delay variances are remarkably similar, as they should be. This stands in marked contrast to the timer variances, which are almost three times as large for the dotted rhythms (2-4-2, 2-1-3-2, 3-1-2-2) as for the isochronous condition (which is not simply because the dotted rhythms contain longer intervals, as was checked by comparing the estimated timekeeper variances for the medium-sized intervals only). This, then, is another example of the dissociation of the timing and the motor components reported for the basic model in Section 3.1. We may thus conclude that the generalized two-level timing model works well for data comprising repeating or periodic interval sequences produced in situations where timing is an explicit task focus. In the next section we consider the applicability of the model to tasks such as typing, in which timing is not an explicit requirement.

7 TIMING IN MOTOR PROGRAMS

It is often observed that overlearned skills like typing, handwriting or even walking exhibit highly regular timing. The relative durations of different phases within each activity appear to change rather little, even if the overall duration of the activity (or the rate of the events within the activity) changes considerably. Such *invariant relative timing* has been a key element in the hypothesis of the generalized motor program. The idea is that actions are represented in the central nervous system in quite general terms. Prior to the performance of an action it is assumed that effector-specific parameters must be selected that will determine the timing and amplitude of movements executed by a particular combination of effectors chosen to implement the action. Thus, for example, the central representation of an action might include the *relative* duration of intervals between key events in the sequence, and overall *rate* might be a parameter that is set, perhaps with some random error, separately on each trial.

A comprehensive introduction and overview of the motor programming literature may be found in Schmidt (1988). In this section we focus on the rate-setting aspect of the motor program hypothesis. We ask what are the implications of the generalized two-level model in evaluating the idea that invariant relative timing emerges from a rate-setting process under the motor program hypothesis?

Up to now, we have focused on timing in tasks, like isochronous synchronization and tapping, which can be characterized by their repeating nature. As we have seen, data collection and statistical tests of model predictions are relatively straightforward if the behavior can be broken down into a sequence of elements that are functionally equivalent. This allows the interresponse intervals to be treated as different realizations of the same underlying random variables. In skills such as typewriting and speech this is not possible; it does not seem reasonable to assume that the interresponse intervals – bounded by keystrokes or phoneme onsets – into which a typed or spoken word is decomposed, come from the same underlying distribution. Therefore, we distinguish between situations in which the events define *repeating* intervals (possibly defined over a repeating group) and those on which the events in the sequence do not recur exactly so that the intervals between them may be said to be *nonrepeating*.

7.1   Covariance Estimator for Nonrepeating Intervals

Earlier we defined an autocovariance estimator for repeating events where it could be assumed that the data $\{i_{n,s}; n = 1,N; s = 1,S\}$ comprised independent realizations of the random variables I_n, all of which were assumed to follow the same distribution. For the statistical analysis of nonrepeating events, replications of response sequences are needed, e.g. several typings of the same word by different subjects or, better, by the same subject on repeated occasions. Table 4.7 provides an illustrative layout. If it can be assumed that each $i_{n,s}$, $s = 1,S$ is an independent realization of the interresponse interval variable I_n, $n = 1,N$, then a reasonable estimator of the covariance between I_n and I_{n+j} is given by:

$$\widehat{\mathrm{cov}}(I_n, I_{n+j}) = \sum_{s=1}^{S} (i_{n,s} - \hat{\mu}_n)(i_{n+j,s} - \hat{\mu}_{n+j})/(S - 1) \qquad (46)$$

where

$$\hat{\mu}_n = \sum_{s=1}^{S} i_{n,s}/S$$

Table 4.7 demonstrates the computation of the estimator $\widehat{\mathrm{cov}}(I_n, I_{n+1})$; the bold-lined rectangle indicates which data pairs $(i_{n,s}, i_{n+1,s})$ *across* sequences enter its calculation.

With the covariance estimator given above, there is the danger that the statistical structure underlying skilled performance is obscured by uncontrolled differences in the rate with which it is executed. In the following, we look at the consequences of

Table 4.7. *Arrangement of interresponse interval data for nonrepeating events*

$i_{1,1}$	$i_{2,1}$	$\cdots$	$i_{n-1,1}$	$i_{n,1}$	$i_{n+1,1}$	$\cdots$	$i_{N-1,1}$	$i_{N,1}$
$i_{1,2}$	$i_{2,2}$	$\cdots$	$i_{n-1,2}$	$i_{n,2}$	$i_{n+1,2}$	$\cdots$	$i_{N-1,2}$	$i_{N,2}$
$\cdots$	$\cdots$	$\cdots$	$\cdots$	$\cdots$	$\cdots$	$\cdots$	$\cdots$	$\cdots$
$i_{1,s}$	$i_{2,s}$	$\cdots$	$i_{n-1,s}$	$i_{n,s}$	$i_{n+1,s}$	$\cdots$	$i_{N-1,s}$	$i_{N,s}$
$\cdots$	$\cdots$	$\cdots$	$\cdots$	$\cdots$	$\cdots$	$\cdots$	$\cdots$	$\cdots$
$i_{1,S}$	$i_{2,S}$	$\cdots$	$i_{n-1,S}$	$i_{n,S}$	$i_{n+1,S}$	$\cdots$	$i_{N-1,S}$	$i_{N,S}$

rate variability when the rate acts like a variable multiplier. This raises the question as to how the rate variation is engendered and we discuss particular models that have been proposed for multiplicative rate variation. However, first we cover a particularly useful tool for models with multiplicatively related variables, namely *conditional expectation*.

7.2 Conditional Expectation

Let X, Y and Z be random variables such that the (conditional) expectations $E(X|Z = z)$, $E(Y|Z = z)$, $var(X|Z = z)$ and $cov(X, Y|Z = z)$ exist for all values of Z. Define $E(X|Z)$ as the random variable that takes on value $E(X|Z = z)$ whenever Z takes on z, and correspondingly for $E(Y|Z)$, $var(X|Z)$ and $cov(X, Y|Z)$. For conditional expectation as a random variable, expected value, variance and covariance are defined in the usual way. It can be shown (Ross, 1988) that the following identities hold:

$$E(X) = E[E(X|Y)] \tag{47}$$

$$cov(X, Y) = E[cov(X, Y|Z)] + cov[E(X|Z), E(Y|Z)] \tag{48}$$

$$var(X) = E[var(X|Z)] + var[E(X|Z)] \tag{49}$$

Note that any random variable may be used for conditioning, including those that appear before the conditioning bar. This is the main technique for deriving variances and covariances of multiplicatively related random variables, because variables which are used to condition by can be 'factored out', e.g.:

$$E(XZ|Z) = Z\,E(X|Z)$$

which holds because $E(XZ|Z = z) = E(Xz|Z = z) = zE(X|Z = z)$. That is, given the condition $Z = z$, Z behaves like a constant. Similarly,

$$cov(XZ, YZ|Z) = Z^2\,cov(X, Y|Z)$$

since $cov(XZ, YZ|Z = z) = z^2\,cov(X, Y|Z = z)$.

Example

To illustrate the power of conditional expectation techniques, we derive the variance of a product of independent random variables, A and B:

$$\begin{aligned} \text{var}(AB) &= \text{E}[\text{var}(AB \mid B)] + \text{var}[\text{E}(AB \mid B)] \\ &= \text{E}[B^2 \, \text{var}(A \mid B)] + \text{var}[B\text{E}(A \mid B)] \\ &= \text{E}[B^2 \, \text{var}(A)] + \text{var}[B\text{E}(A)] \\ &= \text{var}(A)\text{E}(B^2) + \text{E}^2(A) \, \text{var}(B) \end{aligned} \tag{50}$$

By using the identity $\text{var}(X) = \text{E}(X^2) - \text{E}^2(X)$ in substituting for $\text{E}(X^2)$, this can be further developed into:

$$\text{var}(AB) = 2 \, \text{var}(A) \, \text{var}(B) + \text{E}^2(B) \, \text{var}(B) + \text{E}^2(A) \, \text{var}(B).$$

(Note that equation (50) gives the exact variance of a product, in contrast to the approximation by Taylor series expansion often used, e.g. Jagacinski *et al.*, 1988.)

7.3 Multiplicative Rate Effects on the Covariance Structure

In principle, the effects of rate variability are the same, whether due to individual differences between subjects, or to rate fluctuation from one trial to the next in the case of single-subject studies. To understand its action, consider the covariance between interresponse intervals I_n and I_{n+j}. Using conditional expectations, we may write:

$$\text{cov}(I_n, I_{n+j}) = \text{E}[\text{cov}(I_n, I_{n+j} \mid R)] + \text{cov}[\text{E}(I_n \mid R), \text{E}(I_{n+j} \mid R)] \tag{51}$$

where R stands for the rate variable.

As an example, consider typewriting and take R to be the rate at which different subjects type a particular word. Equation (51) says that the covariance, estimated across subjects, equals the mean within-subject covariance, $\text{E}[\text{cov}(I_n, I_{n+j} \mid R)]$, plus a second term which equals the covariance of the mean interresponse intervals, $\text{E}(I_n \mid R)$ and $\text{E}(I_{n+j} \mid R)$, between subjects. The second term vanishes if all subjects type at the same rate; realistically, it has to assumed to be nonzero, however. Due to the between-subjects term, any estimate of the covariance between interresponse intervals, $\text{cov}(I_n, I_{n+j})$, will be shifted upwards, possibly to such an extent that positive dependence is obtained even though I_n and I_{n+j} covary negatively within each subject. This is so because both I_n and I_{n+j} will, on average, tend to be large for slow subjects and small for fast subjects. Thus, there is the danger of confounding the average dependence *within* subjects with that of the dependence of the interresponse interval means *between* subjects. More generally, covariances estimated across sequences risk confounding the average dependence within fixed rates with that of the means across rates.

It is possible to work out the effects of rate variability in more detail if we assume that the current rate acts as a *multiplicative* transformation of the intervals. Let $\{I_n\}$ represent the interresponse intervals as predicted by some arbitrary model given a constant rate, and $\{I_n^*\}$ the corresponding intervals after contamination by a variable rate. We distinguish between the cases where the rate combines multiplicatively with: (1) the observable interresponse intervals; or (2) the intervals produced by a central timekeeper.

If rate variability directly affects the observable interresponse intervals we may write:

$$I_n^* = I_n R \tag{52}$$

where R is a rate variable with mean μ_R and variance σ_R^2; R is assumed to be constant within but to vary between sequences. The crucial assumption is that R is independent of the $\{I_n\}$. Applying the conditional expectation techniques described above gives:

$$\begin{aligned}
\mathrm{var}(I_n^*) &= \mathrm{E}[\mathrm{var}(RI_n \,|\, R)] + \mathrm{var}[\mathrm{E}(RI_n \,|\, R)] \\
&= \mathrm{E}[R^2 \,\mathrm{var}(I_n \,|\, R)] + \mathrm{var}[R\mathrm{E}(I_n \,|\, R)] \\
&= \mathrm{E}(R^2)\,\mathrm{var}(I_n) + \sigma_R^2 \mathrm{E}^2(I_n)
\end{aligned}$$

due to the independence assumption. Using $\sigma_R^2 = \mathrm{E}(R^2) - \mu_R^2$ yields:

$$\mathrm{var}(I_n^*) = [\sigma_R^2 + \mu_R^2]\,\mathrm{var}(I_n) + \sigma_R^2 \mathrm{E}^2(I_n) \tag{53}$$

and, by analogous steps,

$$\mathrm{cov}(I_n^*, I_{n+j}^*) = [\sigma_R^2 + \mu_R^2]\,\mathrm{cov}(I_n, I_{n+j}) + \sigma_R^2 \mathrm{E}(I_n)\mathrm{E}(I_{n+j}) \tag{54}$$

These equations show how the covariance structure of the interresponse intervals is altered by rate variability; the variances and covariances do not faithfully reflect the 'true' structure, as they depend on the interval *means* as well. Equations (53) and (54) show that the variance–covariance predictions derived from arbitrary models need to be modified if there is multiplicative rate variability.

It may be more plausible to assume that rate variability acts not on the observable but on the central timing level, as Heuer (1988) has argued. For a general two-level model with nonrepeating events, assume that the timekeeper generates intervals:

$$T_n^* = T_n R \tag{55}$$

where the $\{T_n\}$ have arbitrary structure but are independent of the rate R. Let the timekeeper intervals be observable after some execution delay, M_n, which are themselves unaffected by the rate. Replacing the I_n^* and I_n in equations (53) and (54) by T_n^* and T_n, respectively, and adding the variance components due to the motor delays yields:

$$\text{var}(I_n^*) = (\sigma_R^2 + \mu_R^2)\,\text{var}(T_n) + \sigma_R^2 E^2(T_n) + \text{var}(M_n + M_{n+1}) \tag{56}$$

$$\text{cov}(I_n^*, I_{n+j}^*) = (\sigma_R^2 + \mu_R^2)\,\text{cov}(T_n, T_{n+j}) + \sigma_R^2 E(T_n)E(T_{n+j})$$

$$+ \text{cov}(M_{n+1} - M_n, M_{n+j+1} - M_{n+j}) \tag{57}$$

Again, rate variability raises variances and covariances and may mask the negative covariance between adjacent intervals that is characteristic for models with independent timekeeper intervals. However, as we note later, the two-level model would still predict that the covariance of adjacent intervals, even if not negative, should nonetheless be less than the covariance of nonadjacent intervals.

7.4   Statistical Aspects of Rate Variability

The identities given in the previous section can be used for a quantitative assessment of the distortion effects produced by uncontrolled rate variability. As an example, consider the lag-one covariance prediction of the generalized two-level timing model for a nonrepeating sequence with:

$$E(T_n) = 250 \text{ ms}, \qquad E(T_{n+1}) = 300 \text{ ms}$$
$$\text{var}(T_n) = 50 \text{ ms}^2, \qquad \text{var}(T_{n+1}) = 72 \text{ ms}^2$$
$$E(M_n) = E(M_{n+1}) = E(M_{n+2})$$
$$\text{var}(M_n) = \text{var}(M_{n+1}) = \text{var}(M_{n+2}) = 25 \text{ ms}^2$$

For these values, if there is no rate variability, interresponse intervals I_n and I_{n+1} will be negatively correlated:

$$\rho = \rho(I_n, I_{n+1}) = -25/[(50 + (2 \times 25))(72 + (2 \times 25))]^{1/2} = -0.226$$

When a variable rate affects the central level, with mean $E(R) = 1$ and variances as small as 0.005^2, 0.010^2, 0.015^2, 0.020^2, 0.025^2 or 0.030^2, the correlation of the contaminated intervals $\rho^* = \rho(I_n^*, I_{n+1}^*)$ changes into values of -0.206, -0.148, -0.064, $+0.036$, $+0.139$ or $+0.239$, respectively. (The predicted effects are virtually indistinguishable, with differences in the fourth place only, if the rate directly multiplies into the observable intervals.) These calculations show that reliable within-sequence negative dependence may be completely obscured by a fluctuating rate.

7.4.1   Effects of Rate Variability on Serial Estimates

Multiplicative rate variability mainly affects covariance estimates in situations with nonrepeating events, i.e. estimated across different response sequences (equation 46). For repeating events where serial estimates can be calculated per sequence and combined across sequences (equation 11), rate variability is much less of a problem, as the following example shows. Consider the basic two-level model with a variable rate affecting the timekeeper intervals only. An unbiased estimator of the acvf at lag j will, based on a sequence with rate $R = r$, estimate:

$$r^2 \operatorname{cov}(T_n, T_{n+j}) + \operatorname{cov}(M_{n+1} - M_n, M_{n+j+1} - M_{n+j})$$

For independent timekeeper intervals, all nonzero lag acvf estimators depend on the motor delay variances only; thus, the expected values of all acvf estimates at lags $j > 0$ will be constant for any rate value r. Averaging the estimates across sequences, i.e. taking the expectation with regard to R, therefore produces estimators uncontaminated by rate variability, except at lag 0, i.e. for the variance, which has expectation:

$$[\operatorname{var}(R) + E^2(R)] \operatorname{var}(T_n) + 2\operatorname{var}(M_n)$$

Even the rate distortion of the variance estimator is neglible, however. For $E(R) = 1$ and $\operatorname{var}(R) = 0.03^2$ (the largest value considered above), $\operatorname{var}(T_n) = \operatorname{var}(T_{n+1}) = 50 \text{ ms}^2$, and $\operatorname{var}(M_n) = \operatorname{var}(M_{n+1}) = 25 \text{ ms}^2$, the long-run estimate of $\operatorname{var}(I_n^*)$ deviates from $\operatorname{var}(I_n)$ by less than 0.045%, reducing the lag-1 correlation from $\rho = -0.25$ to $\rho^* = -0.2499$.

In studying the dependence structure of the interresponse intervals from non-repeating events, i.e. across sequences, there is the danger that the underlying dependences are obscured by uncontrolled rate differences. We now briefly discuss problems of some statistical techniques that have been proposed for coping with rate variability.

7.4.2 Statistical Rate Corrections

Since rate differences express themselves in differences in the total durations, D_s, of the response sequences, it might seem a good idea to 'normalize' the data by dividing each interresponse interval within a sequence by its corresponding total $D_s = \sum_{m=1}^{N} i_{m,s}$, and to perform the calculations on the transformed durations. Unfortunately, this has disastrous effects on the structure of the covariances. Normalizing makes the average covariance negative, no matter what the original covariance structure was.

Example
For a given set of interresponse intervals $I_n, n = 1, N$, construct the 'normalized' random variables $I_n^* = I_n/D$, where $D = \sum_{m=1}^{N} I_m$. Consider the sum of the covariances of a given I_n^* with all the other $I_m^*, m \neq n$. Due to normalizing, $\sum_{m=1}^{N} I_m^* = 1$; therefore:

$$\sum_{m \neq n} \operatorname{cov}(I_n^*, I_m^*) = \operatorname{cov}(I_n^*, \Sigma_{m \neq n} I_m^*)$$

$$= \operatorname{cov}(I_n^*, 1 - I_n^*)$$

$$= \operatorname{cov}(I_n^*, 1) - \operatorname{cov}(I_n^*, I_n^*)$$

$$= -\operatorname{var}(I_n^*)$$

implying that the sum of the covariances, and hence the average covariance of I_n^* with any other variable, must be negative. If $\text{var}(I_n^*) = \text{var}(I_m^*)$ for all m and n, the average correlation between any two normalized variables equals:

$$\rho(I_n^*, I_m^*) = -1/(N-1)$$

Thus, if the variance–covariance structure of the variables is of interest, normalizing must be avoided. This caveat holds also for the related procedure of limiting the statistical analysis to sequences of the sample with total duration closest to the sample mean. For empiric examples from speech timing, see Ohala (1975) and Ohala and Lyberg (1976), who discuss this and other statistical problems. Other transformations for handling rate variability, like the 'homothetic' by Viviani and Terzuolo (1982) and the 'proportional' by Gentner (1982), also suffer from the defect of distorting the variance–covariance patterns. For a critical evaluation of these procedures in the context of timing in typing, the reader is referred to Gentner (1982).

In this section we have provided illustrative calculations to show how misleading tests of models may be if rate variability is not taken into account. Having discussed pitfalls of attempts to cope with rate variability by statistical techniques, we turn to develop and test models that address rate variability explicitly.

7.5   Modeling Invariant Relative Timing

In the preceding sections, rate variability was considered as a kind of nuisance factor to be coped with. In the multiplicative rate models to be considered now, rate variability becomes itself of theoretical interest. Underlying these models is the notion of a generalized motor program. The timing of a highly overlearned skill like typing is assumed to be controlled via centrally stored patterns which specify the relative times of commands; the handwriting simulator of Vredenbregt and Koster (1971) discussed in the introduction of this chapter is a good example. Before the program is executed, an appropriate value of the rate parameter must be chosen; the actual time intervals are then generated from the stored pattern by multiplication of the relative components by the rate currently in effect. Intuitively, one expects ratios of durations to remain invariant across rate changes if these assumptions hold. The problem is how to test such a 'central control model of timing' or 'proportional duration model' in the face of random error.

In two remarkable papers, Gentner (1982, 1987) has given a careful statement of the problem and presented detailed analyses of timing in typewriting as well as in other domains of motor performance, with results not in favor of invariant relative timing. Similar negative results have been obtained for handwriting (Wann and Nimmo-Smith, 1990), speech (Löfquist, 1991) and gait (Burgess-Limerick, Neal and Abernethy, 1992). However, the issue is not settled; Heuer (1988) has questioned some of Gentner's conclusions in terms of limitations in the theoretical framework on which the analyses were based. A variety of models for invariant relative timing have been proposed (Gentner, 1982, 1987; Heuer, 1988; Viviani and Terzuolo, 1980). Except for Heuer's model, they do not distinguish between central timing and an observable response level. In the following, we sketch a generalized model embedded within the two-level framework which contains all the models proposed so far as special cases, and derive testable predictions.

Let I_n denote the interresponse interval bounded by responses n and $n + 1$. As before, we assume that the I_n are composed of timekeeper and motor delay intervals, i.e. $I_n = T_n + M_{n+1} - M_n$. The multiplicative rate is assumed to affect the timekeeper level only; for the moment, we focus on the timekeeping components, and add the motor delay contributions later. We assume that the motor program for, say, typing a particular word contains a set of parameters which specify relative durations, $\{S_n\}$. The intervals controlling the delay between commands n and $n + 1$ are computed by multiplying these relative durations by the current value of a rate parameter, R. We allow the intervals actually generated by the timekeepers to differ by an error variable, E_n, from those computed, such that:

$$T_n = S_n R + E_n \tag{58}$$

(Equation (58) represents a serial version of the model; in the next section, it will be contrasted with a parallel version.)

Let the $\{S_n\}$ and $\{E_n\}$ be sequences of independent random variables with $E(S_n) = \mu_{S,n}$, $\text{var}(S_n) = \sigma_{S,n}^2$ and $\text{var}(E_n) = \sigma_{E,n}^2$; they are independent of the rate variable, R, which has $\text{var}(R) = \sigma_R^2$. In contrast to the assumptions made by other authors, we permit the pattern components S_n to be random variables rather than constants. This means that the intervals computed from the central patterns may be masked by additive as well as by multiplicative 'temporal noise'. Writing $S_n = S_n' + \mu_{S,n}$, where S_n' is an error variable with zero mean, makes this more obvious; equation (58) then becomes:

$$T_n = (S_n' + \mu_{S,n})R + E_n = R\mu_{S,n} + RS_n' + E_n$$

The models proposed by Gentner (1982, 1987), Heuer (1988) and Viviani and Terzuolo (1980) differ mainly in the kind of random errors that they permit. The analysis of the generalized model will show that the covariance structures of the models all share a property useful for testing. Note that the predictions hold whatever the distributions of the random variables are.

By independence, we obtain from equation (58):

$$\text{cov}(T_j, T_k) = \text{cov}(S_j R, S_k R) + \text{cov}(E_j, E_k) \tag{59}$$

where $\text{cov}(E_j, E_k)$ equals $\sigma_{E,j}^2$ if $j = k$, and zero otherwise. We use conditional expectation techniques again to derive the first term on the right. Combining results and adding the motor delay contributions yields the predicted covariance structure of the interresponse intervals:

$$\text{cov}(I_j, I_k) = \begin{cases} \mu_{S,j}^2 \sigma_R^2 + \sigma_{S,j}^2(\sigma_R^2 + 1) + \sigma_{E,j}^2 + \sigma_{M,j}^2 + \sigma_{M,j+1}^2 & k = j \\ \mu_{S,j}\mu_{S,k}\sigma_R^2 - \sigma_{M,k}^2 & k = j + 1 \\ \mu_{S,j}\mu_{S,k}\sigma_R^2 & k > j + 1 \end{cases} \tag{60}$$

For convenience, we have set $E(R) = 1$.

Equation (60) shows that multiplicative rate variability creates positive dependence in the timekeeper intervals (which would be independent if $\sigma_R^2 = 0$), and hence in the interresponse intervals. Note that the covariance between timekeeper intervals ($j \neq k$) depends on their means and the rate variance, but not on the variability of the additive and multiplicative errors.

We now take up three implications: the first comprises a general test for the multiplicative model; the second concerns parameter estimation given the model; and the third concerns the expected value of the covariance of nonadjacent interresponse intervals.

7.5.1 Multiplicativity

The characteristic feature of multiplicative rate models is the *multiplicativity* of their covariance structure, i.e. the fact that, for nonadjacent interresponse intervals, the covariances are proportional to the product of the means. Heuer (1988) observed this to be the case for models with constant central components; equation (60) shows that multiplicativity holds in general. A straightforward test of the multiplicativity prediction is to compute the so-called *tetrad difference* and check whether it differs from zero. For any four responses j, k, l and m with $\max(j, l) + 1 < \min(k, m)$, the model predicts:

$$\mathrm{cov}(I_j, I_k)\,\mathrm{cov}(I_l, I_m) - \mathrm{cov}(I_j, I_m)\,\mathrm{cov}(I_l, I_k) = 0 \qquad (61)$$

This prediction must hold for all quadruples of nonadjacent responses, which requires at least five interresponse intervals, i.e. sequences of $N = 6$ or more responses. Note that testing this crucial prediction neither requires distributional assumptions nor knowledge of the model's parameters. Heuer (1988) has reported simulation results on the sampling distributions of the tetrad difference, showing it to be distributed with mean zero when the model holds. Unfortunately, none of the many existing timing data sets has yet been subjected to this test.

7.5.2 Identifying the Parameters

The model has more free mean and variance parameters than can be identified from data; noting multiplicativity gives a cue which parameters are identifiable. If the model holds, the following functions of the parameters can be identified from the covariance structure:

$$b_j = \sigma_R \mu_{S,j}$$
$$c_j = \sigma_{S,j}^2(\sigma_R^2 + 1) + \sigma_{E,j}^2$$
$$d_j = \sigma_{M,j}^2$$

Rewriting equation (60) in terms of the identifiable parameter functions makes the multiplicative structure of the variance–covariance matrix more salient:

$$\mathrm{cov}(I_j, I_k) = \begin{cases} b_j^2 + c_j + d_j + d_{j+1} & k = j \\ b_j b_k - d_k & k = j + 1 \\ b_j b_k & k > j + 1 \end{cases} \qquad (62)$$

If the serial model is to hold for a set of sequences with $N + 1$ responses, nonnegative values of b_j, c_j and d_j, must exist for all j such that equation (62) fits the empirical variance–covariance matrix. Hence, the motor delay variances are fully identifiable (except for $\sigma_{M,1}^2 = d_1$). The contributions of the two kinds of random errors cannot be separated from each other, however, since only their weighted sums $c_j = \sigma_{S,j}^2(\sigma_R^2 + 1) + \sigma_{E,j}^2$ can be identified. This shows that *models with additive random errors are equivalent to models with multiplicative errors*, as far as the co-variance structure is concerned. On the basis of variance–covariance data, it is not possible to decide whether the central pattern intervals are jittered additively or multiplicatively.

In general, the variance of the rate parameter, σ_R^2, cannot be determined unless further assumptions are imposed on the means of the additive random errors and the motor delays. If $\mu_{E,j} = 0$ and $\mu_{M,j} = \mu_M$ for all j, the mean interresponse intervals can be used to estimate the parameters $\mu_{S,j}$, which allows determination of the rate variance by $\sigma_R = b_j/\mu_{S,j}$. Note, however, that the assumption of equal motor delay means has been considered unrealistic by Heuer (1988).

7.5.3 Covariance Predictions for Lags Larger than 1

A weaker prediction following from equation (60) is that all nonadjacent interresponse intervals should be positively correlated. Gentner (1982, 1987) has carefully tested this prediction for typewriting, and reports average correlations in the order of 0.20, at most, with the majority of the correlations not significantly different from zero. Can the serial multiplicative rate model account for these findings?

Equation (60) can be used for an educated guess about the correlation to be expected under realistic conditions. At medium rates of tapping, say, with $\mu_{S,j} = 250$ ms, Wing and Kristofferson (1973b) obtained serial estimates of the timekeeper and motor delay variances in the order of 100 and 25 ms^2, respectively (see Section 3.1). Using these values as conservative estimates of the (multiplicative or additive) random error and the motor delay variance in equation (53), we predict correlations of 0.040, 0.143, 0.273, 0.400 and 0.510 for values of the rate standard deviation, σ_R, as small as 0.01, 0.02, 0.03, 0.04 and 0.05, respectively. Thus, if our estimates are realistic, the correlations should, in fact, be much larger than those found by Gentner, which casts severe doubt on the appropriateness of the multiplicative rate model for typewriting. This conclusion is also in agreement with the results of the regression analyses performed by Gentner (1982, 1987), although the latter have been criticized for methodological problems by Heuer (1988). For a description of the regression methods and their problems, the reader is referred to the original papers.

7.6 Parallel Versus Serial Models

Viviani and Terzuolo (1980) have contrasted serial and parallel control of timing. In a *serial* version of the central control model, the time of each response is specified from the previous response, whereas in *parallel* models the central pattern gives the times as measured from a common origin. Thus, serial models control the nonoverlapping intervals between responses, and parallel models control the response times in an overlapping fashion (Figure 4.16).

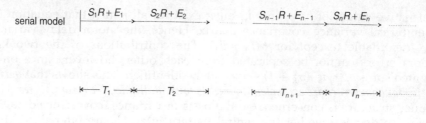

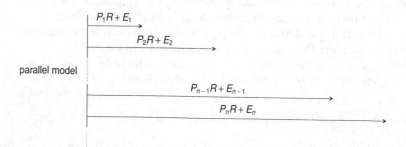

Figure 4.16. *Serial and parallel motor programs.*

Clearly, equation (58) characterizes a serial model. We now look at the predictions of the corresponding parallel model; surprisingly, parallel models also feature multiplicativity. This reflects a general problem of distinguishing serial from parallel models, closely related to the well-known problem of equivalence between serial and parallel information processing models in reaction time research (Townsend and Ashby, 1983; Vorberg and Ulrich, 1987).

Let T_n stand for the n-th *intercommand interval*, i.e. the time interval bounded by the n-th and the $(n + 1)$-th command. In a parallel model, it is assumed that the timekeeper (or a set of timekeepers) controls the response times in parallel by generating them from the overlapping $\{P_n\}$ in the central timing pattern (Figure 4.16). The occurrence time of command $n + 1$, as measured from command 1, equals $T_1 + T_2 + \cdots + T_n$; therefore,

$$T_1 + T_2 + \cdots + T_n = P_n R + E_n$$

Solving for the intercommand intervals, T_n, gives:

$$T_n = (P_n - P_{n-1})R + E_n - E_{n-1} \tag{63}$$

where, for convenience, we have defined $P_0 = E_0 = 0$. By independence:

$$\operatorname{cov}(T_j, T_k) = \operatorname{cov}[(P_j - P_{j-1})R, (P_k - P_{k-1})R] + \operatorname{cov}(E_j - E_{j-1}, E_k - E_{k-1})$$

By conditional expectation,

$$\text{cov}[(P_j - P_{j-1})R, (P_k - P_{k-1})R] = E(R^2)\,\text{cov}(P_j - P_{j-1}, P_k - P_{k-1})$$
$$+ \text{var}(R)E(P_j - P_{j-1})E(P_k - P_{k-1})$$

Note that for independent random variables $\{X_j\}$ with variances $\sigma_{X,j}^2$:

$$\text{cov}(X_j - X_{j-1}, X_k - X_{k-1}) = \begin{cases} \sigma_{X,j-1}^2 + \sigma_{X,j}^2 & k = j \\ -\sigma_{X,j}^2 & k = j+1 \\ 0 & k > j+1 \end{cases}$$

Therefore, the variance–covariance structure predicted by the parallel model is given by:

$$\text{cov}(I_j, I_k) = \begin{cases} (\mu_{P,j} - \mu_{P,j-1})^2\sigma_R^2 + \sigma_{P,j-1}^2(\sigma_R^2 + 1) + \sigma_{E,j-1}^2 + \sigma_{M,j}^2 \\ \quad + \sigma_{P,j}^2(\sigma_R^2 + 1) + \sigma_{E,j}^2 + \sigma_{M,j+1}^2 & k = j \\ (\mu_{P,j} - \mu_{P,j-1})(\mu_{P,k} - \mu_{P,k-1})\sigma_R^2 - \sigma_{P,j}^2(\sigma_R^2 + 1) - \sigma_{E,j}^2 - \sigma_{M,k}^2 & k = j+1 \\ (\mu_{P,j} - \mu_{P,j-1})(\mu_{P,k} - \mu_{P,k-1})\sigma_R^2 & k > j+1 \end{cases} \tag{64}$$

with $\mu_{P,n} = E(P_n)$ and $\sigma_{P,n}^2 = \text{var}(P_n)$.

7.6.1 Multiplicativity

From equation (64) we see that covariance multiplicativity is again predicted for nonadjacent interresponse intervals. Thus, the tetrad difference condition described above for the serial model must hold for the parallel model as well. For any set of data either both models will pass the tetrad test or both will fail. The tetrad test does not allow parallel timing control to be discriminated from serial control.

7.6.2 Identification of the Parameters

As before, the parameters of the parallel model are identifiable only up to some function, namely,

$$b_j = (\mu_{P,j} - \mu_{P,j-1})\sigma_R$$
$$d_j = \sigma_{P,j-1}^2(\sigma_R^2 + 1) + \sigma_{E,j-1}^2 + \sigma_{M,j}^2$$

leading to the simplified version:

$$\text{cov}(I_j, I_k) = \begin{cases} b_j^2 + d_j + d_{j+1} & k = j \\ b_j b_k - d_k & k = j+1 \\ b_j b_k & k > j+1 \end{cases} \tag{65}$$

Given parallel control, multiplicative and additive sources of error variance are confounded with motor delay variability; in the parallel case, unlike the serial model, it is not possible to estimate the $\sigma^2_{M,j}$ separately from the other error sources.

7.6.3   Can Serial Models be Distinguished from Parallel Models?

An important observation about multiplicative rate models comes from comparing the identifiable versions of the serial and the parallel model (equations 62 and 65). Consider a particular covariance structure to which we try to fit both models. Let $b_j^{(P)}$ and $d_j^{(P)}$ denote the parallel model's parameter estimates, and $b_j^{(S)}$, $c_j^{(S)}$ and $d_j^{(S)}$ that of the serial model. How do the parameter sets map on each other?

If the parallel model holds perfectly, then $b_j^{(P)} = b_j^{(S)}$, $d_j^{(P)} = d_j^{(S)}$ and $c_j^{(S)} = 0$ for all j, as is easily verified; this implies that the serial model also fits the data perfectly. However, the converse is not necessarily true: if the serial model holds with some of the $c_j^{(S)} > 0$, then parameters $\{b_j^{(P)}\}$ and $\{d_j^{(P)}\}$ do not exist that permit the parallel model to fit the covariance structure. Therefore, serial models of timing control may be said to be more general than parallel models, although both possess the same number of free parameters. Whenever a parallel model describes the data, an equally good description exists in terms of a serial model, but there may be data sets consistent with serial models that would reject any parallel model. In the language of identifiability theory (Restle and Greeno, 1970), the class of parallel timing models *implies* that of serial models.

What are the implications of these theoretical results? Obviously, determining which model is more adequate may not be decidable by experiment, because the serial model can never be worse than the parallel model. Only if we are lucky can we hope to arrive at a situation where the serial model succeeds whereas the parallel model fails. Note that this could only be found out by fitting the models to the data (i.e. by estimating the parameters), since both models would pass the hurdle set by the tetrad difference test for multiplicativity.

Using a different approach based on an analysis of the nonlinearly transformed keystroke times, Gentner (1982) concluded that his typewriting data support the serial and falsify the parallel model. On a closer look, it seems that his finding was not simply due to the implication relationship between the model classes, but requires a different interpretation.

Gentner did not use the two-level framework; moreover, he assumed additive random errors only, i.e. $\sigma^2_{S,j} = \sigma^2_{P,j} = \sigma^2_{M,j} = 0$ for all j. These restrictions impose different constraints on the parallel than on the serial model, however. For the simplified parallel model, the covariance predictions have the same structure as in equation (65), with $d_j = \sigma^2_{E,j-1}$, whereas the simplified serial model predicts $\mathrm{cov}(I_j, I_k) = b_j b_k$ for all $k \neq j$.

Thus, Gentner's parallel model reflects the covariance structure implied by the two-level framework, with the characteristically lowered covariances at lag 1, but his serial version does not. Nevertheless, the transform patterns simulated from the serial model resembled his data much more closely than those from the parallel model. This raises doubts about whether the two-level model is adequate at all as an explanation for timing in typewriting. Closely related is Gentner's finding that the average correlation between interstroke intervals did not increase if adjacent intervals were excluded.

These results could indicate that the distinction between timekeeper and motor delay levels is not equally appropriate for all motor skills. It might be necessary to distinguish explicit timing in skills for which temporal goals are of prime importance (as in tapping and synchronization, or in musical performance) from implicit timing in skills where one goal of timing control is to prevent the programmed serial order from being disturbed in the execution (as in typewriting). At present, this is speculation. We do not know of studies which have systematically compared timing control in these two types of task.

8 MULTILEVEL TIMING

In the previous section the application of the generalized two-level timing model to nonrepeating movement sequences involved a dichotomy between serial and parallel timing. We used the term 'serial' to refer to single-level timing with nonoverlapping, concatenated timekeeper intervals and parallel to imply multilevel timing in which timekeeper intervals overlap. In this section we extend our ideas about timekeeping structures to take in the yet more general concept of hierarchically organized timekeeping. In doing this, we return to interresponse interval data from repeating movement sequences and, in particular, move to experimental paradigms in which timing is once again an explicit focus of the task.

In Western music it is common to employ note durations and stress patterns to produce rhythmic figures that follow hierarchical rules (Martin, 1972). Larger units are subdivided into smaller units; the bar is divided into beats which in turn may be further subdivided into parts that are relatively simple fractions of the beat (Figure 4.17). An important psychological consequence of such rhythms is that, in listening to music, they induce perceptual groupings of notes (which are often enhanced by the performer adding differential stress at major junctures in the hierarchy).

There is a considerable psychological literature on the perception of rhythm including, for example, Longuet-Higgins' (1987) and Povel's (1985) work on

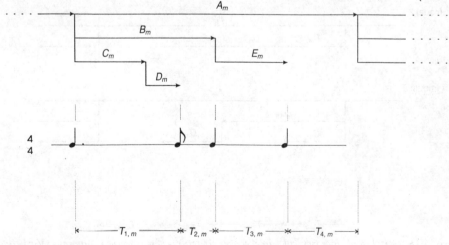

Figure 4.17. *Musical notation and tree-structure for a rhythm.*

hierarchical rules in active inferential processes in the perception of rhythm and meter. However, our focus on movement timing takes us down a different path, one suggested by Vorberg and Hambuch (1978). These authors proposed that a timekeeping mechanism that implements a rhythm which may be described in terms of hierarchical rules might itself be hierarchically organized. If so, they argued, it should be possible to see the consequences of the hierarchical timekeeper structure in the variances and covariances of the interresponse intervals.

In the following sections we outline a number of theoretical models for hierarchical timekeeping and then examine data from studies in which evidence was sought for hierarchical timing in terms of the stochastic structure of the interresponse intervals, over and above that implied by the generalized two-level timing model.

8.1   Hierarchical Timekeeper Structures

Suppose that, in repetitive tapping, subjects produce their responses in a series of groups. Then it might be imagined that a superordinate timekeeper regulates the long intervals taking in the whole group, while a set of lower-level timekeepers is responsible for timing the succession of short intervals within each group. Vorberg and Hambuch (1978) contrasted various hierarchical structures of this kind with a model in which a series of timekeepers works at a single level. They showed that these models make distinguishable predictions for the within-group structure of interresponse interval variability. As an illustration, consider three possible timekeeper organizations for group size $g = 4$.

For each model, four timekeepers are assumed which generate intervals $\{A_m\}$, $\{B_m\}$, $\{C_m\}$ and $\{D_m\}$ (Figure 4.18). The models differ with respect to the organiz-

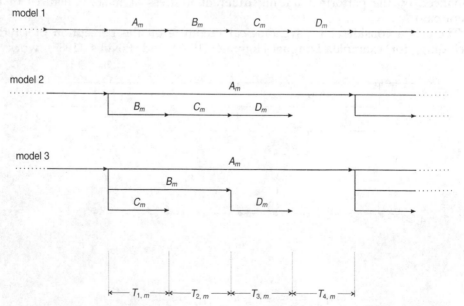

Figure 4.18. *Serial and hierarchical timekeeper structures for grouped tapping (Vorberg and Hambuch, 1978).*

ation of the timekeepers only. Model 1 illustrates a serial or chaining organization where each timekeeper triggers the next one after a delay. The last timekeeper in the chain restarts the first one, and the cycle is repeated. Model 2 illustrates a simple hierarchical organization of the timekeepers where the timekeeper at the top level controls the duration of groups, whereas the remaining timekeepers control the timing of the responses within groups in a chained fashion. Model 3 represents a fully hierarchical structure with timekeeper A controlling the duration of full groups, timekeeper B that of half groups, and C and D subdividing still further. Note that models 2 and 3 involve parallel timing, requiring the simultaneous control of overlapping intervals.

It is straightforward to derive the defining equations of the nonoverlapping *intercommand intervals* $T_{i,m}$, $i = 1, g$, which give the intervals between time points at which successive responses are initiated by the timekeeper system (Figure 4.18):

Model 1:

$$T_{1,m} = A_m, \quad T_{2,m} = B_m, \quad T_{3,m} = C_m, \quad T_{4,m} = D_m \tag{66}$$

Model 2:

$$T_{1,m} = B_m, \quad T_{2,m} = C_m, \quad T_{3,m} = D_m, \quad T_{4,m} = A_m - B_m - C_m - D_m \tag{67}$$

Model 3:

$$T_{1,m} = C_m, \quad T_{2,m} = B_m - C_m, \quad T_{3,m} = D_m, \quad T_{4,m} = A_m - B_m - D_m \tag{68}$$

The remarkable fact is that these structures leave their mark on the serial covariance structure of the intercommand intervals $T_{i,m}$, which makes it possible to infer the underlying structure from the serial covariance matrix of the interresponse intervals. For stochastic independence within and between the timekeepers, the covariance matrices $\mathbf{T}_m$ of the intercommand intervals are predicted as shown in Table 4.8, where a, b, c and d denote the variance of A_m, B_m, C_m and D_m, respectively.

In Table 4.8 it can be seen that the hierarchical timekeeper structures reveal themselves by: (1) negative dependence between some of the intercommand intervals; and (2) characteristic variance patterns for the different intervals within a group. Both effects are consequences of concurrent independent timing at several different levels. In contrast, independent serial timekeeper structures exhibit zero covariances between all the subintervals within a group; also, no particular variance pattern is predicted under serial timing control.

When the effects of the motor delays, $\mathbf{M}_m$, are added adjacent interresponse intervals become more negatively correlated. Nevertheless, the models can still be distinguished from each other by features (1) and (2) above. Moreover, although the models were developed for grouped tapping of isochronous intervals, they are also applicable to rhythmic tapping, i.e. the production of cyclically repeating intervals as in a dotted rhythm with means 600, 200, 400 and 400 ms, say. Thus, provided there is some timekeeper variability, timekeeper organization is revealed by the variance–covariance pattern of the interresponse intervals, $\mathbf{I}_m$.

So far we have only considered two specific hierarchical models of rhythmic grouping, but others are possible. To proceed further we provide a formal definition of a hierarchical timekeeper structure. Hierarchical structures which

Table 4.8. *Variance–covariance structures of the intercommand intervals for different timekeeper structures*

Model 1

a	0	0	0
	b	0	0
		c	0
			d

Model 2

b	0	0	$-b$
	c	0	$-c$
		d	$-d$
			a+b+c+d

Model 3

c	$-c$	0	0
	b+c	0	$-b$
		d	$-d$
			a+b+d

control a cycle of g intervals are defined in terms of the following properties:

(1) The structure contains g timekeepers.
(2) When started, a timekeeper generates an interval; when this expires, the timekeeper may start other timekeepers *on the same* or *on lower levels* of the hierarchy.
(3) A timekeeper is started by exactly one timekeeper (which may be itself if it is at the top level).
(4) The intervals generated by lower-level timekeepers are overlapped completely by those generated at higher levels.

Note that parallel models (Section 7.6) are included in this class of timekeeper structures, as well as serial models (e.g. model 1) which can be considered as special cases in which all g timekeepers operate at the same level.

There are many distinguishably different structures that satisfy conditions (1) to (4) above. For example, for $g = 3$ ($g = 4$), there exist 10 (31) different structures (some of which differ from each other only by a shift with respect to the onset of the cycle). Rather than investigating them all, Vorberg and Hambuch (1978) proposed a simple test for distinguishing the serial structure from any of the truly hierarchical ones. This test, called the *cycle variance test*, compares the timing precision of full cycles composed in different ways.

With g responses per group, there are g different ways of combining consecutive interresponse intervals into cycles, e.g. for $g = 4$:

$$G_{1,m} = I_{1,m} + I_{2,m} + I_{3,m} + I_{4,m}$$
$$G_{2,m} = \phantom{I_{1,m} + {}} I_{2,m} + I_{3,m} + I_{4,m} + I_{1,m+1}$$

$$G_{3,m} = \qquad I_{3,m} + I_{4,m} + I_{1,m+1} + I_{2,m+1}$$
$$G_{4,m} = \qquad I_{4,m} + I_{1,m+1} + I_{2,m+1} + I_{3,m+1}$$

For each cycle, the mean durations will clearly be identical: no matter which response we start with and regardless of the underlying timekeeper structure, the same mean total duration results. If the serial model holds, the cycle variance is also unchanged across different starting responses. However, this is not the case if the intervals are generated by hierarchically organized timekeepers. Given a hierarchical organization with a high-level timekeeper controlling the duration of the full group, the variance of the successive intervals will be smaller if they coincide with the boundaries of a group than if j of them are taken from one group and the remaining $g - j$ from the next one. In the latter case, the timing precisions of both groups contribute to the variance, whereas it is only that of one group in the former case.

As an example, consider the cycle variance predictions for model 2 above. As can be verified geometrically (Figure 4.18) or from equation (67):

$$
\begin{aligned}
G_{1,m} &= A_m & & & + M_{m+1} - M_m \\
G_{2,m} &= A_m - B_m & + B_{m+1} & & + M_{m+1} - M_m \\
G_{3,m} &= A_m - B_m - C_m & + B_{m+1} + C_{m+1} & & + M_{m+1} - M_m \\
G_{4,m} &= A_m - B_m - C_m - D_m & + B_{m+1} + C_{m+1} + D_{m+1} & & + M_{m+1} - M_m
\end{aligned}
$$

(For simplicity, we disregard the exact indexing of the motor delays.) This gives:

$$\text{var}(G_{1,m}) = \sigma_A^2 + 2\sigma_M^2$$
$$\text{var}(G_{2,m}) = \sigma_A^2 + 2\sigma_B^2 + 2\sigma_M^2$$
$$\text{var}(G_{3,m}) = \sigma_A^2 + 2\sigma_B^2 + 2\sigma_C^2 + 2\sigma_M^2$$
$$\text{var}(G_{4,m}) = \sigma_A^2 + 2\sigma_B^2 + 2\sigma_C^2 + 2\sigma_D^2 + 2\sigma_M^2$$

The predictions for model 3 are obtained analogously. In this way, the following ordering predictions result.

For σ_A^2, σ_B^2, σ_C^2, $\sigma_D^2 > 0$,

$$\text{var}(G_{1,m}) = \text{var}(G_{2,m}) = \text{var}(G_{3,m}) = \text{var}(G_{4,m}) \tag{69}$$

holds if the serial model (model 1) is true, while the orderings for the hierarchical models are:

$$\text{var}(G_{1,m}) < \text{var}(G_{2,m}) < \text{var}(G_{3,m}) < \text{var}(G_{4,m}) \tag{70}$$

for model 2, and

$$\text{var}(G_{1,m}) < \min[\text{var}(G_{2,m}), \text{var}(G_{3,m})]$$
$$\text{var}(G_{3,m}) < \text{var}(G_{4,m}) \tag{71}$$

for model 3 (Vorberg and Hambuch, 1978).

It should be obvious that the cycle variance test can be generalized to arbitrary rhythmic cycles with any number g of responses. For any timekeeper structures some of the cycle variances differ from the rest, unless the structure is serial which implies equal cycle variances. Hence, the test permits serial to be distinguished from (nonserial) hierarchical timing.

8.2   Findings on Timekeeping in Rhythm Production

Vorberg and Hambuch (1978) used a task that required subjects to depress a morse key repetitively at a constant rate which was set by having the subjects synchronize their initial responses with a train of brief tones. The purpose of the study was to see what happens when subjects group responses; to encourage grouping, there were tones with only every second, every third or every fourth response in the synchronization phase of some of the experimental conditions. This manipulation may be likened to the situation in music where, in order to produce a sequence of short notes, a performer divides an external beat into smaller units such as quarter notes. In a control condition, each response was associated with a tone in the synchronization phase. Data from three highly trained subjects were reported.

The control condition resulted in acvf.s in accord with the two-process model (i.e. the autocovariance was negative at lag one and zero at larger lags). In contrast, each of the grouping manipulations resulted in a marked positive peak in the acvf at a lag corresponding to the size of the experimenter-intended grouping (Figure 4.19).

Clearly the task of subdividing the interval during synchronization had induced a grouping of a kind. However, earlier (Section 6.1) we pointed out that differences in the mean interresponse intervals within groups will in themselves result in nonzero acvf.s at lag g. Controlling for spurious dependence by computing the periodic covariance estimators showed that systematic differences in interresponse interval means had, in fact, produced the peculiar acvf patterns evident in Figure 4.19.

With the periodic acvf procedure (equation 37), Vorberg and Hambuch found no evidence for hierarchical timekeeper structures. None of the empiric variance–covariance matrices contained any negative entries for interresponse intervals within and between neighboring groups, except for adjacent interval pairs (where negative dependence is to be expected due to the shared motor delays). Of course, this is contrary to what models 2 and 3 predict. The cycle variance test produced the same picture; no systematic differences among the cycle variances were observed. On the other hand, the variance–covariance predictions of serial model 1 were consistent with the data. So, Vorberg and Hambuch concluded that timing of grouped tapping is not controlled hierarchically, even though grouping was sufficient to make the interresponse intervals slightly unequal in the mean.

A later study revealed, however, that this conclusion holds for isochronous tapping only, whereas rhythmic tapping seems to be under hierarchical control (Vorberg and Hambuch, 1984). In their synchronous two-hand tapping experiment described in Section 6.3, five highly trained subjects produced dotted rhythms repetitively. The interval cycles to be produced were of the form 2-4-2, 2-1-3-2 or 3-1-2-2, where the numbers give the number of eighth notes per interval; even

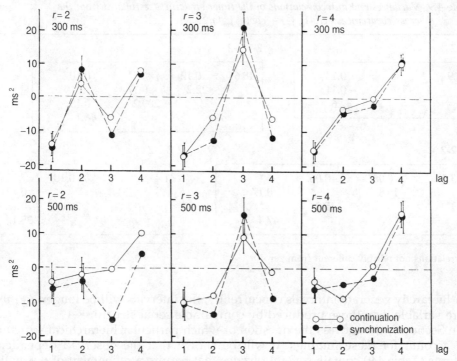

Figure 4.19. *Peaked acvf.s for three subjects at two response rates when tapping in groups of size* r = 2, 3 *or 4 (Vorberg and Hambuch, 1978).*

tapping (2-2-2-2) was also included. The tempo was fixed at 175 ms per eight note; thus, the cycles of intervals to be produced were 350-700-350, 350-175-525-350, 525-175-350-350 and 350-350-350-350.

The variance–covariance patterns of the intercommand intervals obtained for the different rhythms are displayed in Table 4.9. The variances and covariances were estimated from the mean cross-covariances $[\hat{cov}(I_m, J_n) + \hat{cov}(I_n, J_m)]/2$ (see equation 41) and thus directly reflect the stochastic structure of the timekeeper organization, uncontaminated by the motor delays. The variances of the intercommand intervals are given in the diagonal. The off-diagonal entries show the dependence in the timekeepers; for convenience, covariances have been normalized, with asterisks standing for correlations not reliably different from zero.

For the isochronous condition, no negative dependences were found. However, for each of the dotted rhythms, some entries did show reliable negative dependences which rejects serial timing structures; this conclusion was supported by an analysis of the cycle variances. Thus, there is evidence for hierarchical timing of rhythmic performance here. However, hierarchical timing seems to be involved in the control of genuine rhythmic patterns only, and not in isochronous tapping, even if grouped. It is instructive to compare the size of the timekeeper variances in Table 4.9: they are much smaller for isochronous tapping than for the rhythmic conditions. This is consistent with the interpretation of qualitatively different timing structures underlying rhythmic versus isochronous tapping: because timekeepers

Table 4.9. *Variances and autocorrelations of the timer structures, estimated from the cross-covariances* $[\hat{cov}(I_m, J_n) + \hat{cov}(I_n, J_m)]/2$

2-4-2

```
42.9        *        0.13
          195.9     -0.11
                     32.6
```

2-1-3-2

```
48.6    0.12      *        0.10
        22.2    -0.17       *
               209.2      0.13
                          46.1
```

3-1-2-2

```
183.8   -0.08   -0.06      *
         15.8     *       0.17
                45.3       *
                          47.4
```

2-2-2-2

```
31.4      *     0.10       *
        31.1     *        0.12
                30.0      0.13
                          25.1
```

*Correlations not reliably different from zero.

in a hierarchy generate intervals concurrently, the intervals will be longer and thus more variable than those produced by comparable serial structures.

In Section 9, we address the question of which particular hierarchical structures can account for these findings. It will be shown that the observed dependence patterns (Table 4.9) contain several puzzles that require a refinement of our notion of rhythmic timing.

8.3 Polyrhythms

In an intriguing paper, Jagacinski *et al.* (1988) have applied multilevel timing models to the study of polyrhythms. Two-handed performance of polyrhythms involves simultaneous tapping at different rates, for example tapping at a rate of two beats per second with the left against three beats per second with the right hand. Polyrhythmic tapping is quite difficult because the two rhythms involve intervals that are not integer subdivisions of each other. What type of motor organization do subjects use to accomplish bimanual coordination in this task? Jagacinski *et al.* approached this problem by developing and testing a set of alternative models for the timekeeper organization that underlies tapping three against two.

The authors contrasted *integrated* and *parallel* timekeeper organizations. Integrated models assume a single timekeeper structure controlling the timing of both hands, whereas parallel models assume separate structures for each hand. Figure 4.20 shows two examples of each type: (a) and (b) illustrate integrated, (c) and (d) parallel structures. For each model, A, B and C denote the intervals that are generated by the corresponding timekeepers. The dotted lines pointing upward (downward) indicate the departures of left-hand (right-hand) responses; we have left out the motor delays for simplicity. The bottom line shows how the intercommand intervals T_1, T_2 and T_3 within cycles are defined.

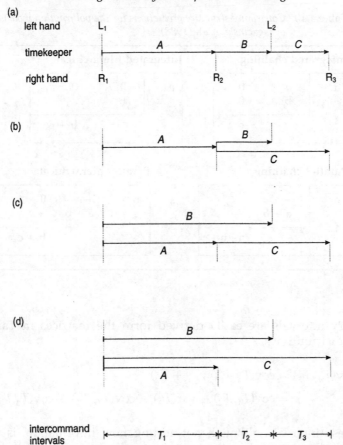

Figure 4.20. *Integrated (a, b) and parallel (c, d) timing models for polyrhythmic tapping (Jagacinski et al., 1988).*

The models differ by their timekeeper structures. All four models belong to the class defined in Section 8.1; the 'integrated chaining' (a) and the 'parallel hierarchical' model (d) correspond to the serial and the parallel models of Section 7, respectively. For the parallel models (c) and (d), with separate timing for the hands, some kind of coupling has to be assumed to keep the two timekeeper structures locked to each other. Jagacinski *et al.* (1988) tried to avoid this problem by excluding the last intercommand interval in each cycle from the analysis, assuming that most of the phase locking occurs there.

Under the assumption of independent timekeeper intervals, it is straightforward to derive the dependence structures of the intercommand intervals. Table 4.10 displays the results; for each model, the box gives the predicted variance–covariance matrix in which a, b and c stand for the variances of the timekeeper intervals A, B and C, respectively.

Jagacinski *et al.* considered two additional intervals (denoted T_4 and T_5) defined as the interval between the second and the third right-hand commands, and that between the first and second left-hand commands, respectively. Because $T_4 = T_2 + T_3$ and $T_5 = T_1 + T_2$, all variances and covariances involving these

Table 4.10. *Covariance structure predictions for the polyrhythm models of Jagacinski et al. (1988)*

Integrated chaining

a	0	0
	b	0
		c

Integrated hierarchical

a	0	0
	b	$-b$
		b + c

Parallel chaining

a	$-a$	a
	a + b	$-a-b$
		a+b+c

Parallel hierarchical

a	$-a$	0
	a + b	$-b$
		b + c

nonelementary intervals are easily derived form the matrices in Table 4.10; for example, by distributivity,

$$\text{cov}(T_4, T_5) = \text{cov}(T_2 + T_3, T_1 + T_2)$$
$$= \text{cov}(T_1, T_2) + \text{var}(T_2) + \text{cov}(T_1, T_3) + \text{cov}(T_2, T_3)$$

Including these intervals, although not adding new information, is nevertheless diagnostic, as will now be shown.

Jagacinski *et al.* (1988) compared the models by how successful they were in predicting $\text{cov}(I_1, I_3)$ and $\text{cov}(I_4, I_5)$. If all motor delay variances are equal, the predictions for the interresponse interval covariances are identical with those for the intercommand intervals; therefore, the predictions can be read off from Table 4.10. For each model the upper right 2×2 square encloses the terms making up $\text{cov}(I_4, I_5)$, and the top right entry gives $\text{cov}(I_1, I_3)$. Let us represent a model's predictions by the pair $[\text{cov}(I_4, I_5), \text{cov}(I_1, I_3)]$. By Table 4.10, the two integrated models can be seen to be characterized by the pairs $(b, 0)$ and $(0, 0)$, and the two parallel models by $(0, a)$ and $(0, 0)$.

Jagacinski *et al.* (1988) presented their results in this form, with correlations replacing covariances (Figure 4.21). The graph summarizes the performance of eight highly trained subjects (amateur pianists) who were required to tap two beats per cycle with the left hand against three with the right hand, at a rate of 1300 ms per cycle. Each point represents the correlation pair of one subject. By the analysis above, the points should cluster around the y-axis if the two hands are under parallel timing control, but cluster around the x-axis if an integrated structure underlies polyrhythmic tapping. Clearly, the results are consistent with the predictions of the integrated models but reject both parallel timekeeper structures.

Having eliminated the parallel timekeeper models, the authors proceeded to determine the most appropriate integrated model. The integrated chaining model

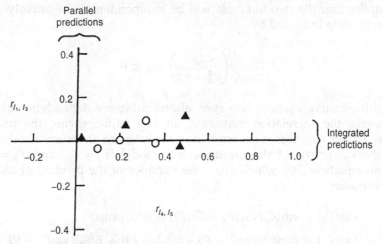

Figure 4.21. *Correlations between intervals 1, 3 and 4, 5 used by Jagacinski* et al. *(1988) in testing integrated versus parallel models for polyrhythmic tapping.*

(a) gives a better account of the data in Figure 4.21 than the integrated hierarchical model (b) as the latter predicts the data should cluster around the origin $(0, 0)$, which evidently is not the case. By quantitatively fitting the models to the complete variance–covariance matrices of all subjects, both integrated models turned out to fit rather badly, sometimes yielding uninterpretable parameter values (i.e. zero or negative variances). Remarkably, however, a variant of the integrated hierarchical model with correlated (rather than independent) timekeeper intervals B and C proved quite successful. Let us look at this model, called the *multiplicative* hierarchical by Jagacinski *et al.*

8.3.1 Multiplicative Versus Independent Hierarchical Models

Stochastic independence between all timekeeper intervals lies at the heart of the models originally proposed by Vorberg and Hambuch (1978). Jagacinski *et al.* (1988) considered the intriguing idea that concurrent timekeeping at different levels might lead to intervals that are dependent on each other because they are *ratio related*. Whereas B and C are produced by independent timekeepers in the original hierarchical model (Figure 4.20b), now it is assumed that B is constructed by its timekeeper as a fraction P of the interval C. Thus, interval B stands in a ratio relation to C:

$$B = PC \tag{72}$$

where the fraction $P, 0 \leqslant P \leqslant 1$ is a random variable which is independent of C. The main consequences of this modification of the hierarchical model will be on the dependence between the intercommand intervals T_2 and T_3. In the independent model, with $T_2 = B$ and $T_3 = C - B$,

$$\text{cov}(T_2, T_3) = -\text{var}(B)$$

which implies that the two intervals will be independent or negatively correlated, with correlation ρ bounded by

$$-\sqrt{\left(\frac{\sigma_B^2}{\sigma_B^2 + \sigma_C^2}\right)} \leqslant \rho \leqslant 0 \tag{73}$$

The multiplicative version, however, allows arbitrary dependence between the two intervals; the correlation may take on any value, giving the model more flexibility. To see why this is so, we derive the relevant covariance and variances.

By the assumptions of the multiplicative model, $T_2 = PC$ and $T_3 = (1 - P)C$. Thus, from equation (50), which gives the variance of the product of independent random variables,

$$\text{var}(T_2) = \text{var}(C)[\text{var}(P) + \text{E}^2(P)] + \text{E}^2(C)\,\text{var}(P) \tag{74}$$

$$\text{var}(T_3) = \text{var}(C)[\text{var}(1 - P) + \text{E}^2(1 - P)] + \text{E}^2(C)\,\text{var}(1 - P)$$

$$= \text{var}(C)[\text{var}(P) + \text{E}^2(1 - P)] + \text{E}^2(C)\,\text{var}(P) \tag{75}$$

By conditional expectation,

$$\text{cov}(T_2, T_3) = \text{cov}[PC, (1 - P)C]$$

$$= \text{E}[\text{cov}(PC, (1 - P)C\,|\,C)] + \text{cov}[\text{E}(PC\,|\,C), \text{E}((1 - P)C\,|\,C)]$$

$$= \text{E}[C^2\,\text{cov}(P, 1 - P)] + \text{cov}[CE(P), CE(1 - P)]$$

$$= -[\text{var}(C) + \text{E}^2(C)]\,\text{var}(P) + \text{E}(P)\text{E}(1 - P)\,\text{var}(C) \tag{76}$$

Two special cases suffice for showing that the dependence between T_2 and T_3 is not constrained by the ratio relationship of B to C. Setting $\text{var}(C) = 0$, $\text{E}(C) = c$ implies:

$$\text{var}(T_2) = \text{var}(T_3) = c^2\,\text{var}(P)$$

$$\text{cov}(T_2, T_3) = -c^2\,\text{var}(P)$$

and thus $\rho = -1$. On the other hand, setting $\text{var}(P) = 0$, $\text{E}(P) = p$ implies:

$$\text{var}(T_2) = p^2\,\text{var}(C)$$

$$\text{var}(T_3) = (1 - p)^2\,\text{var}(C)$$

$$\text{cov}(T_2, T_3) = p(1 - p)\,\text{var}(C)$$

and thus $\rho = 1$. Thus, as far as the covariance between the two intercommand intervals is concerned, the multiplicative must be superior to the independent hierarchical model.

For the interpretation of the model it is instructive to investigate the direction of the dependence in which the data force the multiplicative model to deviate from the independent model. When the parameter values reported by Jagacinski et al. (1988) for the six subjects for which the multiplicative model gave the best fit are inserted into equations (74) to (76), positive dependence between T_2 and T_3 results for one subject only; for the remaining five subjects, strong negative dependence is predicted with correlations ranging from -0.28 to -0.80. In four out of these five cases, the correlations lie below the lower bound of -0.43 attainable by the independent model; we computed this bound from equation (73) by inserting plausible estimates of var(B) and var(C) derived from Wing's (1980) variance-to-mean function (cf. Figure 4.5).

Thus, it seems that the multiplicative model surpassed the independent model at least partly because of the considerable negative dependence in the interresponse intervals which must have been much larger than observed by Vorberg and Hambuch (1978, 1984) in simpler rhythmic tasks (cf. Table 4.9). By itself, the multiplicative model does not give a reason why negative rather than positive dependence should result; deviations in both directions could be accounted for equally well by the multiplicative model, with direction determined by the relative size of fraction P's variance. Before accepting the notion of ratio-related timekeeper intervals as an explanation, alternative interpretations of the findings of Jagacinski *et al.* should therefore be considered.

Scrutinizing the experimental procedure used for studying polyrhythmic tapping suggests that the negative dependence may have had a different origin. Since polyrhythmic tapping is quite hard, the authors simplified the task by having the subject tap in synchrony with a three versus two tonal pattern that *went on throughout the sequence*; thus, the data were collected under synchronization rather than under continuation conditions. It is arguable whether applying continuation models to data from a synchronization task is appropriate. It may be true (as Jagacinski *et al.*, 1988, p. 420, suggest) that: 'with practice, a tapping pattern becomes a well-defined motor program in which the intertap intervals are primarily determined by central timekeeper intervals and motor delays. The auditory stimulus pattern is assumed to affect the entire pattern in a holistic or relational manner, rather than on a specific tap-by-tap or tone-by-tone basis.' Our analysis of the two-level timing model for synchronization (Section 5) suggests a different interpretation, however.

One of our main findings was that online phase correction makes the interresponse interval covariances more negative, although it may leave the shape of the acvf unchanged. Extrapolating from isochronous tapping to the more complex polyrhythmic situation, we expect that a continuation model may serve as a good approximation for synchronization data; however, the approximation is most likely to break down as far as the amount of negative correlation between intervals is concerned. Under most circumstances, error correction will produce more negative dependence than can be coped with by a model that does not contain a correction mechanism. Therefore, at this time, we consider the evidence put forward for the multiplicative hierarchical model as inconclusive, since the failure of the independent hierarchical model may have resulted from the subjects' use of synchronization strategies in the polyrhythmic task.

In summary then, the extension of hierarchical timing models to polyrhythmic performance by Jagacinski *et al.* (1988) has yielded convincing evidence for the integrated control of the two hands, and against separate timing, as formalized by parallel models. It remains to be seen whether the integrated hierarchical model with ratio-related timekeeper intervals holds up as well when synchronization is excluded. Despite our reservation in this regard, we believe that the notion of ratio-related intervals is extremely important. In fact, it forms the essence of the theoretical concept that we discuss in the remaining pages of the chapter. Paradoxically, however, we invoke this assumption to account for *positive* dependence between interresponse intervals.

9 THE RHYTHM PROGRAM HYPOTHESIS

As discussed in Section 8.2, differences in the cycle variances as well as negative entries in the covariance structures led Vorberg and Hambuch (1984) to reject serial and to infer hierarchical timing for rhythmic tapping. However, they were unable to identify the particular hierarchical structures responsible for the covariance patterns that they observed (see Table 4.9). As it turns out, models with stochastically independent timekeeper intervals are too limited to account for these data, for two reasons.

A look at the models in Table 4.8 shows that their covariance structures share an important property: all entries are either zero or negative, but never positive. In general, no timekeeper structure that obeys the hierarchy conditions 1–4 specified above (see Section 8.1) can predict positive covariances when the timekeeper intervals are stochastically independent. Vorberg and Hambuch's (1984) results in Table 4.9 violate this prediction. For isochronous as well as for rhythmic tapping, systematic positive dependences show up between the intercommand intervals.

A second problem of hierarchical models with independent timekeeper intervals is the particular pattern that they predict for the variances of the intercommand intervals within a rhythmic cycle. Whenever a succession of intervals is controlled by timekeepers on different levels, intercommand intervals that involve differences between overlapping timekeeper intervals will stand out as more variable. This leads to an inevitable 'piling up' of variance of intercommand intervals with progression through to the lowest levels in the hierarchy.

As examples, consider the covariance structures in Table 4.8. In model 2, the variance of the fourth interval in each cycle must exceed the sum of the three other interval variances. In the fully hierarchical model 3, the variance of the second and fourth intervals is predicted to exceed that of the first and third intervals, respectively; moreover, the three-level hierarchy is reflected in the ordering prediction $\mathrm{var}(T_{1,m} + T_{2,m}) < \mathrm{var}(T_{3,m} + T_{4,m})$ for higher-order intervals. Inspection of the patterns in Table 4.9 shows, however, that the predicted pile-up of the variances of intervals later in the cycle is not found in the data.

To account for these conflicting results, we propose an important modification to our notion of timekeeper structures (a second one will be introduced below). Our earlier discussion of the motor program as an abstract representation of the events in a movement sequence included the idea that event intervals be specified as adjustable parameters which are set prior to execution according to requirements of the context in which the action is to be performed. We now propose a related idea but one whose application we see as limited to situations with an explicit rhythmic timing component.

Our hypothesis is that for every rhythmic figure there is an underlying rhythm program that specifies a hierarchical structure (e.g. model 3 above). To generate the same rhythm across a range of tempi, we suppose the rhythm program is adjustable to the tempo requirements in the sense that its parameters, i.e. its timekeeper intervals, may be altered appropriately, while its structure remains invariant. This idea therefore leads us to distinguish *parameter specification* of the rhythm program, when particular interval targets are passed to the timekeepers, from its *execution*, when the timekeepers are set to run and generate intercommand intervals. So far, we have only recognized errors arising in execution, which means that central variability is caused by imprecision in the *production* of intervals by the time-keepers. In order to account for positive dependences, we now assume that there may be an additional source of error due to setting up of the program parameters, that is, in the *specification of the timekeeper targets* at a given tempo.

More specifically, we assume that the rhythm program is implemented as a hierarchy of adjustable timekeepers. Each of them, when triggered, generates an interval which depends on its current target value. To accommodate tempo changes, the timekeepers have to update their target values every cycle. Moreover, the timekeepers have to communicate information on their current targets. Information flow is determined by the hierarchical structure of the program, which has the effect that errors in the target specification arising at any level in the hierarchy propagate to all subordinate levels and produce positively correlated effects.

9.1 Target Specification and Interval Production of Timekeepers

We make these ideas explicit by an example. Consider the four-level hierarchy in Figure 4.17 as a possible model for the production of a dotted rhythm. The target duration of each timekeeper on levels 2–4 corresponds to half that of its super-ordinate timekeeper. Let A_m, B_m, C_m, D_m and E_m stand for the target durations of the timekeepers during the m-th execution of the rhythm program. We denote the intervals actually produced by A_m^*, B_m^*, C_m^*, D_m^* and E_m^*, respectively, and assume the following rule for their dependence on target duration.

9.1.1 Program Execution

A timekeeper with target duration $T_m = t$ produces intervals T_m^* with mean and variance given by:

$$E(T_m^* \mid T_m = t) = t \tag{77}$$

$$\text{var}(T_m^* \mid T_m = t) = p_0 + p_1 t + p_2 t^2 \tag{78}$$

On the average, performance reflects the target durations veridically, i.e. the interval mean equals the target. We assume that the interval variance is a second-order polynomial of the target value, which includes constant variance as well as Poisson- and Weber-type dependence of the variance on the mean (see Section 2.1) as special cases; using a general assumption permits us to focus on qualitative properties that hold for a large class of models.

As usual, we assume stochastic independence between intervals produced by different timekeepers *conditional on the target values*. Therefore,

$$\text{cov}(T_m^*, U_n^* \,|\, T_m = t, U_n = u) = 0 \tag{79}$$

for any pair of timekeepers T and U, and all m, n, t and u.

With target durations fixed, the covariance predictions are identical to those sketched in the preceding sections. This is no longer true if there is error in the specification of the targets.

9.1.2 Target Specification

We suppose the information about timekeeper targets flows down paths determined by the hierarchical organization. Thus, each timekeeper receives the information from its superordinate timekeeper, computes its own target value and then passes that value on down to the timekeeper(s) on the level below. The tree in Figure 4.22 shows how information would flow down the timekeeper hierarchy for the dotted rhythm in Figure 4.17.

To specify the targets, information on the current rate, R_m, is fed to the top timekeeper in the hierarchy. From this, target A_m is computed and passed down to timekeeper B, which uses it to compute the target value B_m, sends it to its subordinate timekeepers, and so on. In this way, each timekeeper can function as a separate module while achieving the proper subdivision of the target interval of the timekeeper on the level above. This scheme can control the performance of a rhythm in the face of tempo changes yet leave proportions intact, if we assume that proportionality holds on the average, e.g.

$$E(A_m \,|\, R_m = t) = at, \quad E(B_m \,|\, A_m = t) = bt \tag{80}$$

etc, where we use a, b, c, d and e to denote the proportionality constants at the corresponding level (cf. Figure 4.22). In our example, equal subdivision results if $b = c = d = e = 1/2$. As equation (83) below shows, these multiplicative parameters can be determined from the interval means. The value of a depends on the unit in which the rate variable R_m is expressed and may thus be set equal to 1 without loss of generality.

With the above scheme, not only the desired tempo, but also errors at any step in the target specification, propagate to all lower levels. Therefore, a crucial assumption is how variability in the target specification of a timekeeper depends on its input. As before, we assume that the conditional variance of a target interval is a second-degree polynomial of the mean:

$$\text{var}(B_m \,|\, A_m = t) = q_0 + q_1(bt) + q_2(bt)^2 \tag{81}$$

and analogously for the other timekeepers; the same (nonnegative) coefficients q_0, q_1 and q_2 apply on all levels of the hierarchy. Again, we assume stochastic independence of the target intervals for any two timekeepers *conditional on the input they have in common*, e.g.

$$\text{cov}(B_m, C_m \,|\, A_m = t) = 0 \tag{82}$$

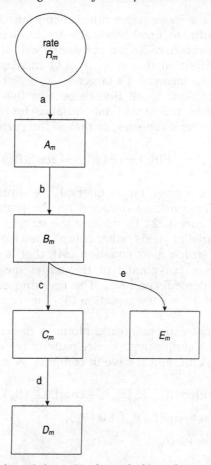

Figure 4.22. *Propagation of rate information down the hierarchy.*

9.2 Dependence Structure of the Target Intervals

What can we say about the variability of and the dependence between the target intervals when the timekeeper inputs are not known? By conditional expectation tools, we derive how the mean and the variance of a given target interval depend on the statistics of its superordinate timekeeper's target, e.g.

$$
\begin{aligned}
E(B_m) &= E[E(B_m \,|\, A_m)] \\
&= E[bA_m] \\
&= bE(A_m) \tag{83}
\end{aligned}
$$

$$
\begin{aligned}
\mathrm{var}(B_m) &= \mathrm{var}[E(B_m \,|\, A_m)] + E[\mathrm{var}(B_m \,|\, A_m)] \\
&= \mathrm{var}[bA_m] + E[q_0 + q_1(bA_m) + q_2(bA_m)^2] \\
&= b^2 \,\mathrm{var}(A_m) + q_0 + q_1 bE(A_m) + q_2 b^2 E(A_m^2) \\
&= (1 + q_2)b^2 \,\mathrm{var}(A_m) + q_0 + q_1 bE(A_m) + q_2 b^2 E^2(A_m) \tag{84}
\end{aligned}
$$

Equation (83) shows that the mean target interval computed by timekeeper B is a fixed fraction of superordinate timekeeper A's target, whatever that is at the moment. In general, the variance of B's target interval will depend on A's variance; errors in the target specification (i.e. $q_0, q_1, q_2 > 0$) increase B's variance by an amount that depends on the mean of A's target.

We can apply this technique to all timekeepers in the hierarchy. Doing this recursively, we can express the mean and variance for each timekeeper as a function of the top timekeeper's statistics, or that of the current rate, e.g.

$$\mathrm{E}(E_m) = e\,\mathrm{E}(B_m) = eb\,\mathrm{E}(A_m) = eba\,\mathrm{E}(R_m)$$

For finding the mean of a given target interval, we simply multiply the mean rate by the proportionality constants collected on the path up to the node that represents the rate (see Figure 4.22). Expressing the target variances as a function of the top timekeeper's statistics yields rather complicated expressions, all of which, however, have the same structure as equation (84), that is, each variance can be written as a second-degree polynomial of the target mean and variance of a timekeeper at a given superordinate level. The resulting equations are not very revealing, however; therefore, we use equation (84) for recursive numeric computations only (see below).

Applying the conditional expectation technique to the covariances shows that error propagation induces a simple dependence pattern. For example, by conditioning on the timekeeper which C and E have in common as input,

$$\begin{aligned}
\mathrm{cov}(C_m, E_m) &= \mathrm{E}[\mathrm{cov}(C_m, E_m \mid B_m)] + \mathrm{cov}[\mathrm{E}(C_m \mid B_m), \mathrm{E}(E_m \mid B_m)] \\
&= 0 + \mathrm{cov}[\mathrm{E}(cB_m), \mathrm{E}(e \mid B_m)] \\
&= ce\,\mathrm{var}(B_m)
\end{aligned}$$

Thus, the covariance between the target specifications of the timekeepers is proportional to the variance of the superordinate timekeeper's target.

Generalizing this idea provides an algorithm for determining the covariances from the tree that is induced by the hierarchy (see Figure 4.22): for any two timekeepers not on the same path, move upward until the first node in the tree that lies on both paths is reached; the covariance is then given by the target variance of that timekeeper times the product of all the multipliers on the paths traversed. For example,

$$\mathrm{cov}(D_m, E_m) = (dc)e\,\mathrm{var}(B_m) \tag{85}$$

An analogous rule holds for timekeepers that lie on the same path: the covariance equals the variance of the higher-level timekeeper times the product of the multipliers on the path, e.g.

$$\mathrm{cov}(A_m, E_m) = (eb)\,\mathrm{var}(A_m) \tag{86}$$

Thus, error propagation in the hierarchy induces positive dependence among the targets, because lower-order timekeepers are influenced by errors in target specifi-

Table 4.11. *Target interval variance–covariance structure induced by error propagation*

	A_m	B_m	C_m	D_m	E_m
A_m	$\text{var}(A_m)$	$b\,\text{var}(A_m)$	$cb\,\text{var}(A_m)$	$dcb\,\text{var}(A_m)$	$eb\,\text{var}(A_m)$
B_m		$\text{var}(B_m)$	$c\,\text{var}(B_m)$	$dc\,\text{var}(B_m)$	$e\,\text{var}(B_m)$
C_m			$\text{var}(C_m)$	$d\,\text{var}(C_m)$	$ce\,\text{var}(B_m)$
D_m				$\text{var}(D_m)$	$dce\,\text{var}(B_m)$
E_m					$\text{var}(E_m)$

cation on higher levels in the same way. The degree of dependence is attenuated the more steps the information has to pass from the source to the destinations.

Table 4.11 summarizes the target covariances for all pairs of timekeepers. Note the multiplicative structure in the off-diagonal cells which follows from the invariant proportion assumption of the target means.

9.3 Dependence Structure of the Timekeeper Intervals

When the program is executed, the timekeepers produce intervals which equal their target in the mean, since, by equation (77):

$$E(T_m^*) = E[E(T_m^* \mid T_m)] = E(T_m) \tag{87}$$

irrespective of the variability in the target intervals. On setting $a = 1$ and $b = c = d = e = 1/2$ and $E(R_m) = 1000$, the timekeepers in the example produce intervals with $E(A_m) = 1000$, $E(B_m) = 500$, $E(C_m) = E(E_m) = 250$ and $E(D_m) = 125$.

The variance–covariance structure of the intervals actually produced bears a simple relationship to that of their targets: for any timekeeper with target duration T_m, the produced intervals T_m^* have variance:

$$\text{var}(T_m^*) = (1 + p_2)\,\text{var}(T_m) + p_0 + p_1 E(T_m) + p_2 E^2(T_m) \tag{88}$$

while all covariances equal those of the target intervals, i.e.

$$\text{cov}(T_m^*, U_n^*) = \text{cov}(T_m, U_n) \tag{89}$$

Table 4.12. *Timekeeper interval variance–covariance structure*

	A_m^*	B_m^*	C_m^*	D_m^*	E_m^*
A_m^*	$\text{var}(A_m^*)$	$b\,\text{var}(A_m)$	$cb\,\text{var}(A_m)$	$dcb\,\text{var}(A_m)$	$eb\,\text{var}(A_m)$
B_m^*		$\text{var}(B_m^*)$	$c\,\text{var}(B_m)$	$dc\,\text{var}(B_m)$	$e\,\text{var}(B_m)$
C_m^*			$\text{var}(C_m^*)$	$d\,\text{var}(C_m)$	$ce\,\text{var}(B_m)$
D_m^*				$\text{var}(D_m^*)$	$dce\,\text{var}(B_m)$
E_m^*					$\text{var}(E_m^*)$

for any pair of timekeepers T and U, and all m, n. Table 4.12 summarizes these results.

To illustrate the mechanics of the error propagation model, let us look at some predictions for the dotted rhythm shown in Figure 4.17 when we insert hypothetical parameter values. Consider tapping at a rate of 1000 ms mean duration per cycle, i.e. $E(R_m) = 1000$. Let $a = 1$, $b = c = d = e = 1/2$; we arbitrarily set $\mathrm{var}(R_m) = 220$. Assume that variability due to target specification error is characterized by $q_0 = 5$ and $q_1 = q_2 = 0$. Equation (84) then leads to:

$$\mathrm{var}(A_m) = a^2 \, \mathrm{var}(R_m) + q_0 = 220 + 5 = 225$$

$$\mathrm{var}(B_m) = b^2 \, \mathrm{var}(A_m) + q_0 = 225/4 + 5 = 61.25$$

$$\mathrm{var}(C_m) = c^2 \, \mathrm{var}(B_m) + q_0 = 61.25/4 + 5 = 20.31 \text{ etc.}$$

The matrix at the top of Table 4.13 displays the target variances computed from these parameter values in the diagonal, and the covariances in the upper half. Clearly, error propagation produces positive dependence, with strength varying over almost the full range, from $\mathrm{corr}(D_m, E_m) = 0.09$ between timekeepers separated

Table 4.13. *Variance–covariance structures induced by error propagation and timekeeper variability within a hierarchy (see text)*

	A	B	C	D	E
A	**225**	112.5	56.3	28.1	56.3
B		**61.3**	30.6	15.3	30.6
C			**20.3**	10.2	15.3
D				**10.1**	1.3
E					**20.3**

	A*	B*	C*	D*	E*
A*	**435**	112.5	56.3	28.1	56.3
B*		**171.3**	30.6	15.3	30.6
C*			**80.3**	10.2	15.3
D*				**45.1**	1.3
E*					**80.3**

	T_1^*	T_2^*	T_3^*	T_4^*
T_1^*	**145.7**	−99.8	16.6	21.8
T_2^*		**225.1**	14.1	111.2
T_3^*			**80.3**	−54.7
T_4^*				**410.3**

by more than one step, to corr$(A_m, B_m) = 0.96$ between the targets of the top two timekeepers.

Running this hierarchical scheme with timekeeper variances governed by $p_0 = 10$, $p_1 = 0.2$ and $p_2 = 0$ (i.e. Poisson-type dependence plus constancy) produces timekeeper intervals which obey the covariance structure displayed in the middle section of Table 4.13. By equation (89), the off-diagonal covariances are identical to those of the targets, while the variances have increased, e.g.

$$\text{var}(B_m^*) = \text{var}(B_m) + p_0 + p_1 E(B_m)$$
$$= 61.25 + 10 + [0.2 \times 500]$$
$$= 171.25$$

Thus, these variances reflect both sources of variability, one due to imprecisely specified target durations, the other to accuracy losses in the generation of the actual time intervals, whereas the dependence among the intervals is due solely to variability in the target specification.

From here, it is straightforward to generate the covariance matrix predicted for the (nonoverlapping) intercommand intervals $T_{1,m}^*$, $T_{2,m}^*$, $T_{3,m}^*$ and $T_{4,m}^*$ (for reasons that will become clear below, we mark the intercommand intervals by asterisks here, as they represent actual time intervals). We use the defining equations (see Figure 4.17):

$$T_{1,m}^* = C_m^* + D_m^*$$
$$T_{2,m}^* = B_m^* - C_m^* - D_m^*$$
$$T_{3,m}^* = E_m^*$$
$$T_{4,m}^* = A_m^* - B_m^* - E_m^*$$

to derive, e.g.

$$\text{cov}(T_{1,m}^*, T_{3,m}^*) = \text{cov}(C_m^* + D_m^*, E_m^*)$$
$$= \text{cov}(C_m^*, E_m^*) + \text{cov}(D_m^* E_m^*)$$
$$= 15.3 + 1.3 = 16.6$$

The lower part of Table 4.13 shows the resulting variances and covariances of the intercommand intervals. Let us examine the dependence pattern of our example, keeping in mind the two problems for independent hierarchical models that were described in the beginning of this section.

The error propagation model is clearly able to generate dependence patterns consisting of negative and positive covariances. A comparison with the numeric prediction for the model without target specification error ($q_0 = \text{var}(R_m) = 0$) shows that negative entries are predicted at the same places by both models (cf. the upper and lower left matrices in Table 4.14). Hierarchical timekeeping reveals itself in the negative covariances of the interval pairs $(T_{1,m}^*, T_{2,m}^*)$, $(T_{3,m}^*, T_{4,m}^*)$ and $(T_{1,m}^* + T_{2,m}^*, T_{3,m}^* + T_{4,m}^*)$. Adding variability due to imprecise target specification leaves this pattern more or less unchanged but raises all zero covariances, thus solving the first puzzle posed by the results reported by Vorberg and Hambuch (1984).

Table 4.14. *Comparison of interresponse interval variance–covariance structures, induced by hierarchical or serial timer organization with (top) and without (bottom) error in target specification*

Hierarchical–hierarchical

146	−100	25	13
	225	14	−111
		80	−55
			410

Hierarchical–serial

146	−5	17	22
	55	14	−1
		80	5
			90

Serial–serial

136	10	21	21
	43	7	7
		79	14
			79

Hierarchical

95	−95	0	0
	205	0	−110
		60	−60
			380

Serial

85	0	0	0
	35	0	0
		60	0
			60

However, the second problem persists: the modified model, too, wrongly predicts a variance increase for the intercommand intervals late in the cycle. For example, the third and the fourth intercommand interval have equal means; however, the last interval's variance is predicted to be about five times as large as that of its predecessor. Our example illustrates what can be shown more generally: without additional modifications, the error propagation model is not capable of giving a satisfactory account of the data.

9.4   Serializing the Timekeeper Intervals

On logical grounds, timing control of rhythmic performance by serially organized timekeepers should be superior to hierarchical control for two reasons. One is that serial timekeepers do not risk disturbing the serial order of the behavior components set up by the program (Vorberg and Hambuch, 1978). The other reason is timing precision: if timekeeper variability increases with its mean, serial control via (nonoverlapping) short intervals will achieve better timing precision than hierarchical control via (overlapping) long intervals. These plausibility arguments provide a clue as to how to modify our rhythm program hypothesis.

We already made the distinction between the parameter specification and the production levels of the rhythm program, both contributing separable sources of variability (in addition to that of the motor delays). We sharpen this distinction by assuming that parameter specification is determined by the hierarchical structure of the target rhythm, whereas execution of the program is serial, thus affording the advantages for serial timekeeper structures pointed out above. To do so, new target intervals have to be computed from those set up in parameter specification before the program can be executed by a serial timekeeper structure. It is helpful to contrast the two versions of the rhythm program hypothesis for making the serialization assumption more precise.

In the original version parameter specification, leading to the target values $\{A_m, B_m, C_m, D_m, E_m\}$, and timekeeper execution, producing the intervals $\{A_m^*, B_m^*, C_m^*, D_m^*, E_m^*\}$, both reflect the hierarchical structure of the rhythm. This is expressed by the fact that both sets of variables refer to overlapping intervals, namely, the full, half, quarter cycle durations, etc. which characterize the rhythm. There are no timekeepers that produce the intercommand intervals $\{T_{1,m}^*, T_{2,m}^*, T_{3,m}^*, T_{4,m}^*\}$ directly; rather, these nonoverlapping 'serial' intervals are introduced for descriptive purposes only but have no representation in the rhythm program.

In the modified version of the rhythm program hypothesis, we still assume hierarchical parameter specification. Before the program is executed, nonoverlapping targets $\{T_{1,m}, T_{2,m}, T_{3,m}, T_{4,m}\}$ must first be constructed from the $\{A_m, B_m, C_m, D_m, E_m\}$ by serializing via:

$$T_{1,m} = C_m + D_m$$

$$T_{2,m} = B_m - C_m - D_m$$

$$T_{3,m} = E_m$$

$$T_{4,m} = A_m - B_m - E_m$$

This transformation yields the target values appropriate for the serial timekeeper structure. When the program is run, the intercommand intervals $\{T_{1,m}^*, T_{2,m}^*, T_{3,m}^*, T_{4,m}^*\}$ are produced by the timekeeper chain; corresponding to each intercommand interval there is now a timekeeper that controls the interval directly.

The effects of serializing the timekeeper targets are illustrated in Table 4.14 for the example above. The section labeled 'hierarchical–serial' displays the variance–covariance structure of the intercommand intervals as predicted from the error propagation and timekeeper execution parameters given above. Serialization has the desired effect on the variances of the intercommand intervals: as appropriate, piling up of the variance for the intervals late in the cycle is no longer predicted. Moreover, although the covariances have been changed (cf. the covariance matrix on the left), some of the intervals are still predicted to covary negatively with each other. Qualitatively, at least, the model is in agreement with the findings discussed above.

Note that the hierarchical as well as the serial component of the model is essential. Assuming that both parameter specification and timekeeper execution level are serially structured leads to the predictions labeled 'serial–serial' (Table 4.14). In a serial structure, target specification error (as distinct from timekeeper variability) produces positive dependence only. This may be appropriate as an account of the dependence structure for isochronous tapping but is contrary to the negative dependence found in rhythm production, as we discussed in Section 8.2.

These speculative arguments show that the rhythm program hypothesis may merit consideration. Parameter specification with error propagation in a hierarchical program, and serial timekeeping in the execution of the program, seem to be important ingredients for a theory of timing that has the potential of accounting for the findings above as well as other theoretical challenges that have not been addressed by quantitative models. One of them is *expressive* timing in music performance (Clarke, 1989; Shaffer and Todd, 1987). Distinguishing the processes whereby the parameters in an abstract representation of the rhythm program are specified from the program's execution, the model allows expressive modulation of performance in time by continuously changing the rate parameter, without destroying the temporal invariances that are essential for the rhythmic aspects of music. It remains to be seen whether speculations such as these will stand further analysis and experimental tests.

10 CONCLUSION

This chapter has been concerned with exploring mechanisms of human timing. It has focused on variation or, more precisely, covariation in the duration of intervals between events in a movement stream (responses). We have interpreted such statistical dependence in terms of a variety of linear models for the control of timing.

The simplest case that we considered involved tapping to reproduce a single target interval repeatedly. We reviewed evidence that indicates how observed intervals arise from the linear combination of intervals generated by a central timekeeper and more peripheral delays in motor execution processes associated with the pairs of movement events that define the boundaries of each interval. Although this model, proposed by Wing and Kristofferson (1973b) does not include feedback, it predicts commonly observed negative covariation between successive interresponse intervals. Dissociation of the estimates of the parameters of the model also constitutes evidence in support of the model.

We then showed how the basic model could be developed by including a simple feedback component (for synchronizing response with an external pacing stimulus). It was pointed out that the pattern of covariation in interresponse intervals obtained from such models reflects not only the two-level nature of timing but also the setting of the feedback correction term. The latter represents an additional complication in assessing the nature of timekeeping processes, and synchronization tasks are better avoided if the primary concern is with understanding timekeeping mechanisms.

The second half of the chapter was concerned with adding complexity to the timekeeper structure, based on a generalized version of the original two-level timing framework that does not restrict timekeeper intervals (or motor delays) to be independent. Various sources of dependence in timekeeper intervals were discussed. It was first shown that the rate-setting aspect of the motor program hypothesis could be treated within the two-level framework and predictions of serial versus parallel arrangements of timekeeper intervals were shown to be nearly indistinguishable. However, it was pointed out that there are interresponse interval covariance data from typing that provide evidence against appreciable variability of motor delays. This stands in contrast to tasks with explicit timing requirements such as music performance and indicates a possible limitation on the relevance of the two-level timing framework.

The remainder of the chapter was devoted to timing in rhythm production tasks. Models with hierarchically arranged timekeepers (which imply a grouping of intervals) were developed. While their predictions were shown to be in accord with some aspects of rhythmic tapping data, a limitation of simple hierarchies was identified in that they are unable to account for commonly observed positive covariation among interresponse intervals. This led to the exposition of a new hypothesis of rhythmic programming, which includes the concept of a multiplicative rate parameter. This acts to introduce positive correlations among intervals within a single hierarchical branch.

In conclusion, we have shown how psychologically interesting accounts of timing may be developed based on linear models that lead to testable predictions. We have attempted a tutorial approach, making clear our use of simple tools of probability, so that the reader may feel encouraged to go further in developing and applying these models in new fields. While there remain a number of issues in mapping theory onto data deserving of a more rigorous statistical analysis, we have tried to suggest practical solutions to some of these problems so that the psychologically interesting work may proceed.

ACKNOWLEDGEMENTS

This chapter has been long in the making. Over the years, we have had discussions with many persons who helped us to clarify our thoughts. We are grateful to Eric Clarke, Rolf Hambuch, Herbert Heuer, Steve Keele, Ron Knoll, Pim Levelt, Jiři Mates, Dirk-Jan Povel, Jeff Pressing, Hartmann Scheiblechner, Hans-Henning Schulze, András Semjen, Henry Shaffer, Saul Sternberg, Jeff Summers, Piet Vos, Ted Wright and Pienie Zwitserlood. Parts of this chapter were written during D.V.'s stays at the Max-Planck-Institut für Psycholinguistik, Nijmegen; we thank Pim Levelt for the hospitality. The help of Marianne Hempel in preparing the figures is greatly appreciated.

REFERENCES

Anderson, T. W. (1971). *The Statistical Analysis of Time Series*. New York: John Wiley.

Aschersleben, G. and Prinz, W. (1995). Synchronizing actions with events: The role of sensory information. *Perception and Psychophysics*, **57**, 305–317.

Bernstein, N. A. (1967). *The Coordination and Regulation of Movement*. London: Pergamon Press.

Box, G. E. P. and Jenkins, G. M. (1976). *Time Series Analysis: Forecasting and Control*, 2nd edn. San Francisco, CA: Holden Day.

Burgess-Limerick, R., Neal, R. J. and Abernethy, B. (1992). Against relative timing invariance in movement kinematics. *QJEP*, 44A, 705–722.

Clarke, E. (1989). The perception of timing in music. *Psychological Research*, **51**, 2–9.

Creelman, C. D. (1962). Human discrimination of auditory duration. *Journal of the Acoustical Society of America*, **34**, 582–593.

Dunlap, K. (1910). Reactions to rhythmic stimuli, with attempt to synchronize. *Psychological Review*, **17**, 399-416.

Fraisse, P. (1980). Les synchronizations sensori-motrices aux rhythmes. In J. Réquin (Ed.), *Anticipation et Comportement* (pp. 233–257). Paris: Editions du CNRS.

Gentner, D. R. (1982). Evidence against a central control model of timing in typing. *Journal of Experimental Psychology: Human Perception and Performance*, **8**, 793–810.

Gentner, D. R. (1987). Timing of skilled motor performance: Tests of the proportional duration model. *Psychological Review*, **94**, 255–276.

Gibbon, J., Church, R. M. and Meck, W. H. (1984). Scalar timing in memory. *Annals of the New York Academy of Sciences*, **423**, 52–77.

Goldberg, S. (1958). *Introduction to Difference Equations*. New York: John Wiley.

Hary, D. and Moore, G. P. (1987a). On the performance and stability of human metronome-synchronization strategies. *British Journal of Mathematical and Statistical Psychology*, **40**, 109–124.

Hary, D. and Moore, G. P. (1987b). Synchronizing human movement with an external clock source. *Biological Cybernetics*, **56**, 305–311.

Heuer, H. (1988). Testing the invariance of relative timing: Comment on Gentner (1987). *Psychological Review*, **95**, 552–557.

Huitema, B. E. and McKean, J. W. (1991). Autocorrelation estimation and inference with small samples. *Psychological Bulletin*, **110**, 291–304.

Ivry, R. B. and Keele, S. W. (1989). Timing functions of the cerebellum. *Journal of Cognitive Neuroscience*, **1**, 136–152.

Ivry, R. B., Keele, S. W. and Diener, H. C. (1988). Dissociation of the lateral and medial cerebellum in movement timing and movement execution. *Experimental Brain Research*, **73**, 167–180.

Jagacinski, R. J., Marshblum, E., Klapp, S. T. and Jones, M. R. (1988). Tests of parallel versus integrated structure in polyrhythmic tapping. *Journal of Motor Behavior*, **20**, 416–442.

Killeen, P. (1992). Counting the minutes. In F. Macar, V. Pouthas and W. J. Friedman (Eds), *Time, Action and Cognition*. Dordrecht: Kluwer.

Kristofferson, A. B. (1976). Low-variance stimulus–response latencies: Deterministic internal delays? *Perception and Psychophysics*, **20**, 89–100.

Koch, R. (1992). *Sensumotorische Synchronisation: Eine Kostenanalyse*, Paper 11/92. München: Max-Planck-Institut für Psychologische Forschung.

Lashley, K. S. (1951). The problem of serial order in behavior. In L. A. Jeffress (Ed.), *Cerebral Mechanisms in Behavior*. New York: John Wiley.

Löfquist, A. (1991). Proportional timing in speech motor control. *Journal of Phonetics*, **19**, 343–350.

Longuet-Higgins, C. (1987). *Mental Processes. Studies in Cognitive Science*. Cambridge, MA: MIT Press.

Martin, J. G. (1972). Rhythmic (hierarchical) versus serial structure in speech and other behavior. *Psychological Review*, **79**, 487–509.

McGill, W. A. (1962). Random fluctuations of response rate. *Psychometrika*, **27**, 3–17.

Michon, J. A. (1967). *Timing in Temporal Tracking*. Assen, Netherlands: Van Gorcum.

Ohala, J. J. (1975). The temporal regulation of speech. In G. Fant and M. A. A. Tatham (Eds), *Auditory Analysis and Perception of Speech* (pp. 431–453). London: Academic Press.

Ohala, J. J. and Lyberg, B. (1976). Comments on 'Temporal interactions within a phrase and sentence context'. *Journal of the Acoustical Society of America*, **59**, 990–992.

Povel, D. (1985). Time rhythms and tension: In search of the determinants of rhythmicity. In J. Michon and J. Jackson (Eds), *Time, Mind and Behavior*. Berlin: Springer.

Prinz, W. (1992). Why don't we perceive our brain states? *European Journal of Cognitive Psychology*, **4**, 1–20.

Restle, F. and Greeno, J. G. (1970). *Introduction to Mathematical Psychology*. Reading, MA: Addison-Wesley.

Rosenbaum, D. A. and Patashnik, O. (1980a). A mental clock setting process revealed by reaction times. In G. E. Stelmach and J. Réquin (Eds), *Tutorials in Motor Behavior* (pp. 487–499). Amsterdam: North-Holland.

Rosenbaum D. A. and Patashnik, O. (1980b). Time to time in the human motor system. In R. S. Nickerson (Ed.), *Attention and Performance*, vol. VIII. Hillsdale, NJ: Erlbaum.

Ross, S. (1983). *Stochastic Processes*. New York: John Wiley.

Ross, S. (1988). *A First Course in Probability*, 3rd edn. New York: Macmillan.

Schmidt, R. A. (1988). *Motor Control and Learning*, 2nd edn. Champaign, IL: Human Kinetics.

Schulze, H. H. (1992). The error correction model for the tracking of a random metronome: Statistical properties and an empirical test. In F. Macar, V. Pouthas and W. J. Friedman (Eds), *Time, Action and Cognition*. Dordrecht: Kluwer.

Schulze, H. H. and Vorberg, D. (19??)

Shaffer, H. and Todd, N. P. (1987). The interpretative component in musical performance. In A. Gabrielsson (Ed.), *Action and Perception in Rhythm and Music*. Stockholm: Royal Swedish Academy of Music.

Stevens, L. T. (1886). On the time sense. *Mind*, **11**, 393–404.

Townsend, J. T. and Ashby, F. G. (1983). *Stochastic Modeling of Elementary Psychological Processes*. Cambridge: Cambridge University Press.

Ulrich, R. and Stapf, K.-H. (1984). A double-response paradigm to study stimulus intensity effects upon the motor system in simple reaction time experiments. *Perception and Psychophysics*, **36**, 545–558.

Viviani, P. and Terzuolo, C. (1980). Space–time invariance in learned motor skills. In G. E. Stelmach. and J. Réquin (Eds), *Tutorials in Motor Behavior*. Amsterdam: North-Holland.

Viviani, P. and Terzuolo, C. (1982). On the relation between word-specific patterns and the central control model of typing: A reply to Gentner. *Journal of Experimental Psychology: Human Perception and Performance*, **8**, 811–813.

Voillaume, C. (1971). Modèles pour l'étude de la régulation de mouvements cadencés. *Anneès Psychologicques*, **71**, 347–358.

Vorberg, D. (1978). Problems in the study of response timing: Comments on Reece's (1976) 'A model of temporal tracking'. *Acta Psychologica*, **42**, 67–77.

Vorberg, D. (1992). Response timing and synchronization. In F. Macar, V. Pouthas and W. J. Friedman (Eds), *Time, Action and Cognition*. Dordrecht: Kluwer.

Vorberg, D. and Hambuch, R. (1978). On the temporal control of rhythmic performance. In J. Réquin (Ed.), *Attention and Performance*, vol. VII (pp. 535–555). Hillsdale NJ: Erlbaum.

Vorberg, D. and Hambuch, R. (1984). Timing of two-handed rhythmic performance. *Annals of the New York Academy of Sciences*, **423**, 390–406.

Vorberg, D. and Schulze, H. H. (submitted). Extending the two-level timing model to synchronization: Stochastic properties and parameter estimation.

Vorberg, D. and Ulrich, R. (1987). Random search with unequal search rates: Serial and parallel generalizations of McGill's model. *Journal of Mathematical Psychology*, **31**, 1–23.

Vos, P. and Helsper, E. L. (1992). Tracking simple rhythms: On-beat versus off-beat performance. In F. Macar, V. Pouthas and W. J. Friedman (Eds), *Time, Action and Cognition*. Dordrecht: Kluwer.

Vredenbregt, J. and Koster, W. G. (1971). Analysis and synthesis of handwriting. *Philips Technical Review*, **32**, 73–78.

Wann, J. P. and Nimmo-Smith, I. (1990). Evidence against the relative invariance of timing in handwriting. *Quarterly Journal of Experimental Psychology*, **42A**, 105–119.

Wing, A. M. (1980). The long and short of timing in response sequences. In G. E. Stelmach and J. Réquin (Eds), *Tutorials in Motor Behavior*. Amsterdam: North-Holland.

Wing, A. M. (1992). The uncertain motor system: Perspectives on variability in movement. In D. E. Meyer and S. Kornblum (Eds), *Attention and Performance*, vol. XIV: *Synergies in Experimental Psychology, Artificial Intelligence and Cognitive Neuroscience* (pp. 709–744). Cambridge, MA: MIT Press.

Wing, A. M., Church, R. M. and Gentner, D. R. (1987). Variability in the timing of responses during repetitive tapping with alternate hands. *Psychological Research*, **51**, 28–37.

Wing, A. M., Keele, S. W. and Margolin, D. I. (1984). Motor disorder and the timing of repetitive movements. *Annals of the New York Academy of Sciences*, **423**, 183–192.

Wing, A. M. and Kristofferson, A. B. (1973a). The timing of interresponse intervals. *Perception and Psychophysics*, **13**, 455-460.

Wing, A. and Kristofferson, A. B. (1973b). Response delays and the timing of discrete motor responses. *Perception and Psychophysics*, **14**, 5-12.

Woodrow, H. (1932). The effects of the rate of sequence upon the accuracy of synchronization. *Journal of Experimental Psychology*, **15**, 357–379.

Wright, T. W. (1974). Temporal interactions within a phrase and sentence context. *Journal of the Acoustical Society of America*, **56**, 1258–1265.

Chapter 5

Representational Issues in Motor Learning: Phenomena and Theory

Richard Ivry

University of California, Berkeley, USA

1 INTRODUCTION

After months of seemingly random flailing, the 6-month infant succeeds in grabbing an approaching toy. The 5-year-old begins to swim with her head below water, a feat that requires the coordination of upper and lower extremities as well as the muscles involved in breathing. The Olympic hopeful spends endless hours perfecting a 2-minute gymnastics routine. The 70-year-old relearns how to walk unassisted following the crippling effects of a stroke. As these examples demonstrate, learning is surely a continuous process across the life span, and this truism is especially apparent in terms of motor skills, the acquisition of coordinated behavior.

The goal of this chapter is to examine the processes required for motor learning. How can we account for the capabilities of the skilled performer in comparison with the novice? For example, how can a 60-kg person hoist a 180-kg weight over their head? The first intuition is to assume that there is something special about the physiology of the skilled athlete: perhaps a generous innate endowment of those muscle fibers needed for transient bursts of power or perhaps a more efficient use of calories. But such intuitive explanations do not seem sufficient to account for skills such as those that allow the professional baseball player to anticipate in less than 200 ms the location and arrival time of a 15-cm sphere traveling at almost 100 mph. Here intuitive physiological predictors of coordination are less obvious. Correspondingly, the study of individual differences over the past 50 years has revealed few physiological predictors of coordination (Fleishman, 1966) and even these account for little of the variance.

One inference to make from these observations is that an account of skilled performance must go beyond physiology and extend into psychology. The focus of this chapter will be on the psychological processes of motor learning. Central to this endeavor will be the notion of representation: the psychological structures and processes that allow us to utilize past experience in improving motor behavior.

The sections of the first half of this chapter will present related aspects of this problem. The first section on learning curves provides a macroscopic analysis of how performance changes with practice. The emphasis is on an examination of different theoretical accounts of how regularities in learning curves manifest changes in the representation of skill. A shared property of the most viable accounts of the learning curves is that the content of the skilled performer's memory is different from that of the novice, allowing for more efficient processing of information guiding performance.

The emergence of more efficient memory structures and processes is elaborated upon in the second section. Evidence for hierarchical control provides a more microscopic examination of an acquired, complex representation. Hierarchical representation not only allows for improved efficiency in control, but also introduces the notion that the skilled performer's domain of competence is enlarged. Constraints imposed by specific environmental contexts are reduced as the skilled performer's ability generalizes to novel situations. This issue is further developed in the third section on generalized motor programs. The focus of this section is on identifying those constraints that dominate once a skill has been acquired.

The last section of the first half of the chapter will address a different aspect of the constraints on skilled performance. Specifically, it is frequently stated that well-practiced skills are executed automatically. Conversely, there is the implication that unskilled performance requires greater involvement of attentional resources, or controlled processing. The implications of these inferences will be examined, focusing on what is meant by automaticity and the kinds of skill that can be acquired and executed without attention.

The second half of the chapter will present theories of motor learning. The selected theories are representative of current work in cognitive psychology, neuroscience and computational modeling. These theories will be assessed in terms of their ability to account for the psychological phenomena presented in the first half.

In choosing to emphasize the problem of representation, the chapter does not review a number of topics that have been central to other reviews of motor learning (e.g. Adams, 1987; Schmidt, 1988). The chapter does not provide a comprehensive review of the impressive literature on variables that affect motor learning such as the structure of practice trials and the availability of explicit feedback or knowledge of results. For both theoretical and applied reasons, issues such as these are clearly important in the study of motor learning (see Schmidt, 1988, for a comprehensive presentation). Nonetheless, for this review, these variables are examined only in terms of how they relate to the question of what is represented and how representations change with practice.

2 LEARNING FUNCTIONS

One formal technique for the quantitative study of motor learning involves the analysis of various summary performance measures as a function of trials or time. The general pattern of results can be summarized quite easily: not only does practice lead to improved performance, but the rate of improvement also changes over trials. During the early stages of learning, improvement is quite rapid, whereas later on improvement becomes much slower. The data points correspond to a linear function when plotted on log–log coordinates. This phenomenon has come to be referred to as the log–log linear learning law or the power law of practice (Newell

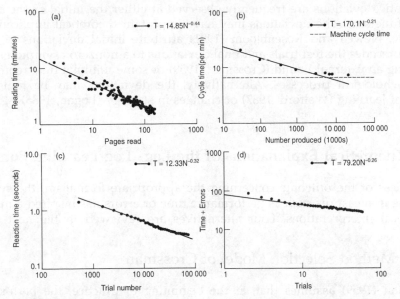

Figure 5.1. *Examples of log–log learning functions from four tasks. (a) Reading inverted text (Kolers, 1975); (b) cigar manufacturing (Crossman, 1959); (c) ten finger, 1023 choice reaction time (Siebel, 1963); (d) mirror tracing (Snoddy, 1926). [From Newell and Rosenbloom, 1981.]*

and Rosenbloom, 1981).[1] Newell and Rosenbloom (1981) provide many examples of this linear relationship (Figure 5.1), the generality of which led them to dub the relationship the 'ubiquitous law of practice' (p. 3).

Before examining the various theories offered to account for the power law of practice, a few caveats should be kept in mind. First, the phenomenon does not appear to be specific to perceptual motor learning. While most of the early examples focused on the acquisition of motor skills (Crossman, 1959; Siebel, 1963; Snoddy, 1926), similar functions have been observed in tasks in which the motoric demands are minimal (Logan, 1988; Newell and Rosenbloom, 1981; Neisser, Novick and Lazar, 1963). Thus, the scope of a unifying account of the power law must be quite broad.

Second, it cannot be unequivocally stated that practice curves are best described by a power function. Other functions such as hyperbolic (Newell and Rosenbloom, 1981) or square root (Welford, 1987) may also provide excellent fits. Third,

---

[1]A power function of learning takes the form:

$$p = a + b^x$$

where p is performance, x is the amount of practice, and a and b are constants. Taking the logarithm of both sides yields the linear equation:

$$\log (p - a) = x \log b.$$

Thus, a power function is linear when plotted on log–log coordinates.

systematic deviations are frequently observed at either the initial or the final tails of the functions. The deviations may have important theoretical implications. For example, Newell and Rosenbloom (1981) attribute initial deviations to learning which precedes the test trials and final deviations to a nonzero asymptote, perhaps reflecting an external bound (Crossman, 1959) or some minimal time requirements for psychological processes. Alternatively, the deviations may be indicative of stages of learning (Welford, 1987) or changes in strategy (Logan, 1988).

2.1 Theoretical Explanations of the Log–Log Learning Function

Regardless of the outcome concerning the appropriate formalism, the systematic decrease in measures such as performance time or errors has inspired a number of theoretical interpretations. Four alternatives are reviewed in the next sections.

2.1.1 Method Selection Model of Crossman

Crossman (1959) assumes that, at the beginning of practice, the performer has available a fixed repertoire of different methods, each associated with a specific execution time. Some of these methods will be well tailored for the task whereas others are poor alternatives. Crossman assumes that initially all of the methods have an equal probability of selection or what he terms 'habit strength'. Over repeated trials, a running average performance time is computed and the performance time on any specific trial can be compared with this cumulative average. When a given method is executed, its future probability of selection will be adjusted as a function of the difference between the time taken on average and the time taken by a particular method. What had initially been an equiprobable distribution will become, over time, highly skewed to favor the most efficient methods.

Crossman's (1959) model deserves a great deal of credit, not only because it was the first attempt to account for the power function, but also in that he provides an explicit learning mechanism. The theory, though, makes somewhat counterintuitive notions of what learning is all about. According to Crossman, learning is not a process of acquisition or restructuring. The optimal methods for performing a task are available at the beginning of training, but require experience in order to demonstrate their efficacy. This assumption, that all methods of performing a task are available initially, may be unlikely. However, the model does present a more fundamental and often overlooked insight: namely, that a complex task may be performed with different organizations of the component parts. The following models of log–log learning functions emphasize the organization of skill during learning; Crossman's emphasis on reorganization is worth retaining as well.

2.1.2 Chunking Model of Newell and Rosenbloom

The model of Newell and Rosenbloom (1981), steeped in the assumptions of cognitive psychology, was offered as an alternative. At the heart of their theory is the notion of a chunking process (Chase and Simon, 1973; Miller, 1956). Information capacity is increased by organizing input and output units into structured chunks.

There are perceptual chunks, motor chunks, internal-processing chunks, or chunks which link these three types of chunks. Not only can information be efficiently represented by chunking, but performance time also improves since the time to process a chunk is assumed to be less than the time to process all of the constituent chunks.

As an example of chunking, Newell and Rosenbloom (1981) examine the choice reaction time data of Siebel (1963). Siebel used a task in which there were ten lights situated over the subject's ten fingers. The subject was simultaneously to press the keys that corresponded to the illuminated lights. The number of lights illuminated on a trial could vary from 1 to 10. Given that there are 10 response effectors for which a binary decision must be made (respond or not respond), the task involves 1023 response alternatives ($2^{10} - 1$ since the zero light condition was not included). Newell and Rosenbloom (1981) propose that, at the beginning of practice, independent decisions must be made as to whether each finger should be part of the response. However, with experience, the subjects begin to treat the stimulus patterns as chunks. Stimulus–response groups which co-occur are coalesced into a single chunk. For example, at the lowest level of chunking, two adjacent lights will be treated as a unit. At the other extreme, a whole stimulus pattern may eventually be organized into a chunk. Since there are many more opportunities for any combination of two lights to be activated simultaneously than for a specific 10-element sequence, chunks of size two would be formed first. Initially, learning will progress rapidly as the frequently occurring low-level chunks are formed. Eventually, the rate of learning will slow down as the more complex and rarely occurring high-level chunks are slowly added to the subject's knowledge base.

According to this model, a single process – chunking – is proposed to account for performance gains. Given that the pool of potential chunks is limited, the opportunities for applying the chunking process become reduced over the course of learning. Newell and Rosenbloom (1981) assume that the rate of chunking is constant. Moreover, the time taken to process a single chunk is also assumed to be constant, regardless of complexity. These assumptions predict an exponential rate of learning. However, since the higher-level chunks are acquired relatively late and will be instantiated relatively infrequently, performance actually comes to resemble a power function (see Rosenbloom and Newell, 1987, for computer simulations of this phenomenon).

The most important contribution of the Newell and Rosenbloom model is that it specifies a learning process about how information is acquired and organized. The model is quite general: a chunking-based explanation has been successfully applied to account for learning in a variety of cognitive tasks (Anderson, 1983; Chase and Simon, 1973) and in a perceptual task involving basketball (Allard, Graham and Paarsalu, 1980). The model demonstrates how the structure of a skill can change with experience. Representations evolve from a collection of independent entities into a multistructured organization. Action can be guided by the different levels depending on the degree of experience.

2.1.3 Hierarchical Priming Model of MacKay

Before discussing MacKay's explanation of the log–log linear function, it is necessary to outline the fundamentals of his theory. Complex actions, according to

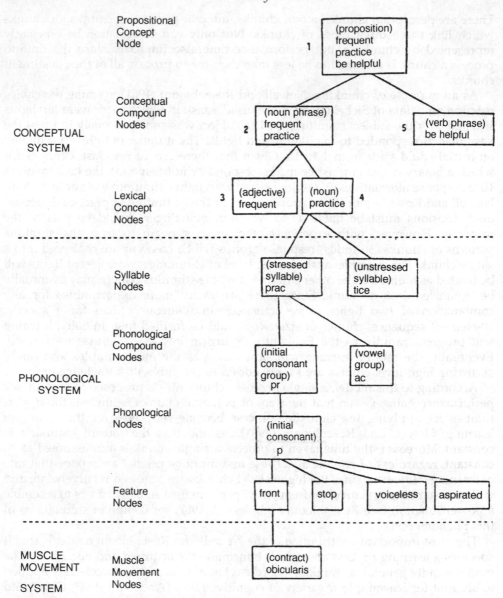

Figure 5.2. *Hierarchical model of sentence production.* [*From MacKay, 1982.*]

MacKay (1982), are organized hierarchically across a number of control systems (Figure 5.2). At the top of the hierarchy is the conceptual system in which the desired action is represented in an abstract form. In MacKay's example of sentence production, the conceptual system has nodes to represent the intended proposition as well as nodes to represent the decomposition of the proposition into constituent noun and verb phrases. At the bottom of the hierarchy is an implementation system. The nodes of this system represent concrete control structures, the selection of which determines the specific form of the output. Some nodes represent movements of speech articulators for spoken language, others represent hand movements for written language. In MacKay's complete example of speech production, a phonological system is inserted between the conceptual and muscle systems. This middle level of control is involved in the process of transforming the lexical concepts into a phonemic representation that triggers the final output.

Movement execution comes about in MacKay's (1982) model through the activation of output nodes beyond a triggering threshold. These nodes are activated, or primed, by all of the nodes to which they are connected. While activation involves a short-term, transient process, learning requires a more permanent mechanism. For this, MacKay (1982, p. 492) proposes that the rate of priming for every connection 'is an exponential function of the frequency with which that connection has been activated in the past'. Since the rate of priming increases as a function of frequency, connections that have been rehearsed will become activated more quickly than unused connections. This accounts for the basic improvement observed with practice. MacKay proposes that the specific shape of the priming function is exponential. This dictates that the form of the learning function is log–log linear. If a set of independent learning processes obeys an exponential learning function, the aggregate function will be linear in log–log coordinates.

In MacKay's model, the many connections that compose the hierarchy constitute the set of independent learning processes. Due to the exponential function, the relative strength of unpracticed nodes would be increased rapidly whereas additional practice would produce only small improvements in the strength of established connections. Since weak connections dominate during the early stages of learning, the overall learning rate should be fast. As strong connections become more prevalent, the learning rate will slow down.

Both MacKay (1982) and Newell and Rosenbloom (1981) postulate structural changes as a function of skill acquisition. Although superficially similar, the multilayered representation of Newell and Rosenbloom (1981) is not really a model of how action hierarchies emerge. Hierarchies are traditionally viewed as structures for distributed control (Keele, 1986; MacKay, 1982). The highest levels are concerned with the overall organization of the action whereas the lower levels are directly involved in specific implementations. Hierarchical control in this sense requires that all of the levels become involved in order for an action to be executed. The multilayered organization which emerges from chunking involves a shift in control. Higher levels come to supersede lower levels and are eventually able to bypass the lower levels by directly triggering the response. MacKay's (1982) hierarchical model does not involve a replacement process, but rather a mechanism for facilitation.

The two models also differ in terms of the foci of the structural changes. MacKay stresses the improved connections between the different nodes of a hierarchy. Newell and Rosenbloom, on the other hand, emphasize that processing demands are reduced as the units of information processing become larger with practice. MacKay accounts for the improved output behavior of a system while Newell and Rosenbloom focus on the improved efficacy of the input system in analyzing complex situations. The latter model has been criticized on the grounds that it may only be applicable to situations in which the stimuli are highly patterned, allowing for the formation of chunks at multiple levels (Logan, 1988; MacKay, 1982).

Nonetheless, in all of the tasks reported, it seems fairly straightforward to postulate reasonable chunking candidates. For example, in MacKay's sentence production task, the formation of phrases such as 'the three little pigs' is clearly less practiced at the beginning of training than the formation of the articulators for pronouncing the phoneme [pi]. It is not currently clear which model provides a more accurate account of the psychological process that underlies log–log learning functions.

2.1.4   Instance Model of Logan

Logan (1988) has offered another alternative which provides an interesting twist to the quantitative analysis of learning functions. According to him, performance on every trial can be accomplished through the use of one of two distinct memory retrieval processes. The first method is based on a general algorithm which is sufficient to perform the task. While Logan is vague as to what the algorithm consists of, the other theories discussed above make a similar assumption that the learner possesses, perhaps in a crude form, the prerequisite skills to accomplish the task. The second method involves a recall process in which task-specific solutions are retrieved from memory. The knowledge base is expanded with each trial even though there is no reorganization of the underlying structure such as the formation of chunks or strengthening of hierarchical connections. What is stored is simply a specific encounter with, and response to, a stimulus. Logan has dubbed his theory an 'instance theory of automatization'.

Performance on a given trial is determined by a race between the algorithm and the retrieval process. Both methods are instantiated and the one that finishes first controls the response. Moreover, within the retrieval process, there is a race between all of the stored processing episodes. The minimum of the overall race will guide performance. With practice, the memory process will come to dominate performance. This occurs because the algorithmic process is assumed to remain constant whereas the number of competing memory episodes will increase as a function of the number of practice trials.

Given these assumptions, log–log learning functions emerge. As the pool of specific instances increases, the likelihood of selecting an instance with a fast processing time also increases. This accounts for the general speed-up with practice. In contrast, the probability of obtaining an even faster processing time will decrease as the minimum is lowered, thus producing the negative acceleration of the learning rate. In his proof showing that the precise shape is a power function, Logan (1988) assumes a distribution of minima which is exponentially based.

The usefulness and generality of Logan's theory to motor learning remains to be seen. The two examples that Logan (1988) offers – lexical decision and alphabet arithmetic – make relatively minor demands on the motor system. Presumably Logan would argue that the same two processes operate when learning a skill such as hitting a golf ball. Whereas a person can invoke an algorithm to 'talk' their way through the task – keep the head down, arms straight, follow through over the shoulder – a memory of each swing is stored. Eventually performance is based on the retrieval of past experience rather than on the algorithm.

As with the theory of Newell and Rosenbloom (1981), the emphasis is on an expansion of the performer's knowledge base. However, Logan's model has little to say about what is actually stored. A specification of this structural change is lacking other than that each processing episode is stored. Indeed, some may see this as a strength of this approach: there is no need to postulate the construction of novel memorial structures such as chunks or hierarchies. However, if evidence points to the validity of such representational constructs, then it may not be advantageous to propose an alternative theory, even if the assumptions of the alternative are simpler.

2.2 Summary of Learning Functions

Schmidt (1988) has argued that the study of performance curves during skill acquisition are of little theoretical interest in the study of learning. The parameters of these functions will vary as a function of a number of variables related to the specifics of the training conditions. These idiosyncrasies will disappear under more rigorous tests of learning such as delayed recall or transfer to novel variations of the task. Given this, it is doubtful that strong inferences about mechanisms of learning can be derived from the exact shapes of the functions.

Nonetheless, this review of the theoretical accounts of the power law of practice was undertaken for three reasons. First, with few exceptions (see Welford, 1987), the data from a diverse set of tasks are well accounted for by a linear function in which the log transformation of a performance measure is plotted against the log transformation of the number of trials. Such quantitative results are rare in the area of motor learning and in psychology in general.

Second, although the log–log linear learning curves were originally derived to account for performance in perceptual motor tasks, they have come to be of equal utility in describing learning in many other cognitive tasks. Thus we have a clear instance in which motor learning appears to embody some of the same principles as learning in general. What should be inferred from this commonality across domains of learning? A skeptic may argue that this shows that gross performance measures such as reaction time or errors do not accurately reflect the contribution of the output system. Rather, they are more heavily weighted toward the input end such as the time to process a complex pattern or make some internal representational transformation. Alternatively, the parallel findings in motor and nonmotor tasks may help direct our attention to some fundamental principles that underlie all cognition and action (Newell and Rosenbloom, 1981).

Third, and most important, the theories reviewed all emphasize distinct processes, each of which is a central concept in the study of motor control and learning. A chunking process would be useful for the formation of motor programs, representational entities that extend beyond simple associations between individual events to encompass a patterned series of outputs (Keele, 1981). A motor program can thus be conceived of as a type of chunk. Priming ties in with the concept of levels of control. Although the idea of hierarchical representation has taken on many forms in motor control theory (Keele, 1986; Saltzman and Kelso, 1987), a constant supposition has been that this form of representation reduces the control demands on any single part of the system (Bernstein, 1967). MacKay's (1982) priming process offers one means for accounting for interactions across the levels of a hierarchy. Although not motivated by motor learning phenomena, Logan's instance theory emphasizes that action can be directly achieved without postulating complex, intermediary, representational structures (Lee, 1980; Warren and Whang, 1987). Learning centers on reducing the need for control structures as performance becomes more automated. These issues of motor programs, levels of representation, and automaticity are central to any discussion of motor learning. The next sections will continue this discussion drawing from forms of analysis other than the study of learning functions.

3   HIERARCHIES AND MOTOR PROGRAMS AS LEARNED, ABSTRACT REPRESENTATIONS OF MOVEMENT

The concepts of hierarchical representation and generalized motor programs can be seen as overlapping and complementary. The motor program is proposed as an abstract representation of an action (Keele, 1981). It exists independently of any specific effector system that may be used to implement the action. Similarly, hierarchical models such as MacKay's (1982, 1985) postulate that action can be represented in independent systems. While certain systems are specific to a given class of movements such as speech, the units in higher-level systems represent higher-level action concepts.

The following example may make this more concrete. Bernstein (1947, cited in Keele, Cohen and Ivry, 1990) presented a set of writing samples produced with a number of different movements (Figure 5.3). Samples 1 and 2 were produced with the subject's dominant right hand. For sample 3, the subject was required to move the hand as a unit. In samples 4 and 5, the pencil was attached to the arm, above the wrist and above the elbow, respectively, and in sample 6 to the shoulder. Samples 7 to 10 were produced by the right foot, teeth, left hand and left shoe. The similarities across the samples are quite striking: it seems quite reasonable to suppose that observers would recognize that the same writer has produced all of the samples. Nonetheless, the muscles actually used were vastly different. This would imply that the similarity results from a representation that is independent of a particular effector system, i.e. in a high-level, conceptual system such as postulated in hierarchical models.

Note that, despite the consistency across the writing samples, there are clearly differences in terms of legibility. The smooth, regular strokes of the hand-produced samples appear much more coordinated than the contours produced when the subject used his foot. If the same motor program (or high-level node in a hierarchical representation) is guiding the action in both situations, what accounts for the differences in performance? One answer is readily apparent: the subject has much more practice at writing with his hand than with his foot. Thus, at least some component of learning has occurred which is specific to the implementation system (see also, Wright, 1990).

MacKay's hierarchical theory (1981, 1985) is designed to account for these types of phenomenon. As discussed earlier, the theory assumes that an action can be conceptualized as a multilevel representation. There are at least two distinct reasons for postulating multiple layering. First, nodes in the various control systems represent different types of information. As seen in the example given in Figure 5.2,

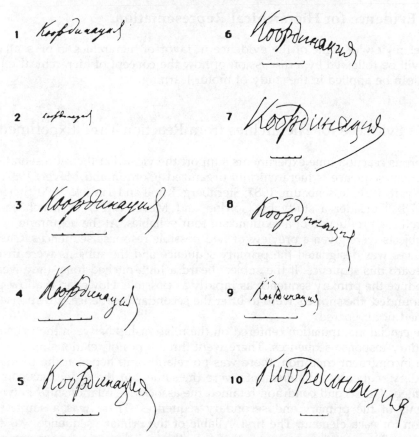

Figure 5.3. *Examples of handwriting with different effectors. See text for details. [From Keele, Cohen and Ivry, 1990.]*

MacKay assumes that three systems are involved in the production of a sentence. The nodes in the conceptual system represent concepts and propositions. The nodes in the phonological system provide a transformation of these concepts into units which are necessary for producing or perceiving speech. These nodes connect with the muscle movement system in which the nodes may represent activation of articulators. MacKay (1985) provides a more generalized version in which plan, movement concept and muscle movement systems are substituted for the sentential, phonological and muscle movement systems, respectively.

Second, the hierarchy involves multiple layering within a given system. For example, the propositional nodes are at the highest level in the conceptual system. Nested below these are compound nodes and further down are lexical nodes. All of these nodes share certain features characteristic of conceptual nodes. Most critical is that they are output-independent representations of concepts: the same nodes would become activated regardless of whether the concepts are spoken, written or heard (Caramazza, Miceli and Villa, 1986; Margolin, 1984). Nonetheless, there is a hierarchical arrangement in that the higher-level nodes represent more elaborate concepts.

3.1   Evidence for Hierarchical Representation

A brief review of some of the evidence in favor of hierarchies is presented next. This will be followed by a discussion of how the concept of hierarchical representation can be applied in the study of motor learning.

3.1.1   Evidence for Hierarchies from Reaction Time Experiments

Numerous reaction time experiments support the view that the representation of a movement sequence is hierarchically organized (Gordon and Meyer, 1987; Klapp and Wyatt, 1976; Rosenbaum, 1987; Sternberg, Knoll and Turock, 1990; Sternberg *et al.*, 1978). Consider a study by Gordon and Meyer (1987) in which each trial required the production of a sequence of four syllables. At the beginning of a trial, the subjects were given a preview of two possible response sequences. One of the sequences was designated the primary sequence and the subjects were instructed to prepare this sequence. If the subject heard a high-pitched tone, they were then to produce the primary sequence as rapidly as possible. However, if a low-pitched tone sounded, the subjects were to utter the secondary sequence, a response which they had not prepared.

The crucial manipulation centered on the relationship between the primary and secondary response sequences. There were three types of relationship (Table 5.1). In the incongruent condition, there was no relationship between the primary and secondary sequences. The elements were the same, but the order was completely reshuffled. The second condition retained the associative relationships between the elements of the primary and secondary sequences. There was a single shift in position for each element. The first syllable of the primary sequence was the last syllable of the secondary sequence and the other syllables moved up one position in order. Thus, the within-sequence order is identical for three of the members. The third condition involved a relationship that Gordon and Meyer (1987) labeled hierarchic. The secondary stimuli were constructed by reordering the stimuli as pairs. That is, the first and second elements of the primary sequence were the third and fourth elements of the secondary sequence and vice versa. Gordon and Meyer

Table 5.1. *Conditions and results of the Gordon and Meyer (1987) experiment. Results are the time to initiate the nonsense strings and error rates are the number of incorrect productions.* [From Gordon and Meyer, 1987]

Condition	Sequence type	Example	Reaction time (ms)	Errors (%)
Reshuffled	Primary	Bee-bay-bah-boo	291	5.7
	Secondary	Boo-bah-bay-bee	660	14.5
Associative	Primary	Bee-bay-bah-boo	298	4.5
	Secondary	Bay-bah-boo-bee	650	10.0
Hierarchic	Primary	Bee-bay-bah-boo	299	5.1
	Secondary	Bah-boo-bee-bay	640	7.5

(1987) assume that if the sequences are hierarchically represented, a reasonable parsing of a four-element sequence would be into chunks of two elements each (see Martin, 1972; Rosenbaum, Kenny and Derr, 1983, for evidence of binary parsing).

The reaction time and error data are given in the last two columns of Table 5.1. Primary sequence responses were more than 300 ms faster than secondary responses. Most interestingly, there are significant differences between the reaction times for the secondary conditions. Subjects were fastest in initiating a secondary response that retained a hierarchical relationship to the primary sequence in comparison with the two other conditions. This advantage is also evident in the error data. The results indicate that relationships between elements of a sequence are part of the representation of the sequence. Not only do the elements appear to be stored as linked items, but the evidence also indicates a preference for hierarchic organization. Note that there is no explicit, logical relationship for the pairwise representation. The sequences were composed of four unique, nonsense items, yet the subjects still utilized a hierarchic representation. Gordon and Meyer (1987) propose that this may either reflect the ubiquitous operation of a chunking mechanism or stem from rhythmic constraints which operate during speech.

3.1.2 Evidence for Hierarchies from the Analysis of Interresponse Intervals

A second source of evidence for hierarchical representation comes from studies which examine the temporal relationships between the elements of a movement sequence (Povel and Collard, 1982; Rosenbaum, Kenny and Derr, 1983). In Povel and Collard's (1982) study, subjects learned sequences composed of six key presses. The subjects used either three or four fingers for a given sequence. If the numbers 1, 2, 3 and 4 symbolize key presses with the index, middle, ring and little fingers, respectively, an example of a sequence involving three fingers would be (121323). At the beginning of a block of responses, the subjects would be presented with a numeric representation of a sequence to be learned. The subjects practiced the sequence cyclically until they had it memorized. That is, the sequences were produced continuously so that the first element followed the sixth. Then, for the experimental trial, the subjects were asked to produce the sequence six times in succession without pause. The data of interest were the interresponse interval (IRI) profiles for the last five cycles.

Povel and Collard (1982) applied a similar logic to Gordon and Meyer (1987) in the construction of their sequences. For example, one set of three stimuli included the sequences (123432), (234321) and (343212). Each of these sequences contains the same elements and, if viewed cyclically, the order is identical. The only difference is in the starting position. The second sequence (234321) is the same as the first sequence (123432) except that the initial element has been moved to the end. Similarly, the third sequence is identical except that the first two elements have been moved to the end. Povel and Collard (1982) consider two models which make distinct predictions of the IRI profiles. According to a linear association model, the IRI profiles should be similar when the sequences are aligned by finger transitions. This follows since the sequences are produced cyclically and all three sequences have the same associations. In this view, longer IRIs would reflect difficult finger transitions and short IRIs would imply easy transitions.

A hierarchic model, on the other hand, yields a very different prediction. Here, the main determinant of the IRI profiles is the hierarchic representation of the sequence. Although the hierarchic organization cannot be unambiguously stated *a priori*, Povel and Collard (1982) parse the sequences following some guidelines developed by Restle (1970). For example, the third sequence (343212) is predicted to be decomposed into two units of three elements (343) and (212). Each of these units can then be described as a higher-level unit: a trill. The model assumes that the transition time between elements of a sequence is determined by the number of hierarchical levels that need to be traversed (Restle, 1970; Rosenbaum, Kenny and Derr, 1983). Since relationships such as trills require a higher level in the hierarchy, the model predicts that the transitions between the trills will take the longest: a higher-level (trill) node must be activated before the next unit of three elements can be initiated. A different parsing is predicted for the other two sequences. The second may be parsed into two runs of (234) and (321) whereas a couple of alternative parsings are possible for the first sequence (123432), e.g. (1234) and (32), or (123) and (432).

The results for these three sequences are shown in Figure 5.4. Rather than show the actual reaction times, Povel and Collard (1982) employed an ordinal scale in which the transitions were ranked from one to six with lower numbers representing fast IRIs. The data shown are the mean ordinal rankings across 20 subjects. There is much greater correspondence across the three sequences when the IRIs are aligned by sequence position. The longest transitions tended to occur between the third and fourth elements and between the sixth and first elements. This indicates that the subjects have parsed each sequence into two three-element units. There is little correlation between the profiles when the sequences are aligned by finger transitions (Figure 5.4a). Thus, even though the three data points above a given finger number represent an identical finger transition, the IRIs are quite dissimilar. Clearly the three sequences have been coded differently, each with its unique hierarchic structure.

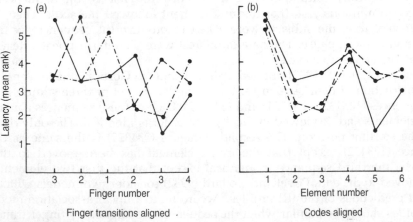

Figure 5.4. *Mean rank of response latencies for inter-tap intervals for the set of patterns (3-2-1-2-3-4), (2-1-2-3-4-3) and (1-2-3-4-3-2). Latencies arranged by: (a) finger, and (b) serial position. [From Povel and Collard, 1982.]*

3.2 Hierarchically Based Learning

How is improvement in speed with learning accounted for by hierarchical models? Previous discussion of the MacKay model has centered on the strengthening of connections between nodes. MacKay assumes that when any node in the hierarchy is activated, it sends activation to all of the nodes to which it is connected. This process not only produces short-term priming, but also strengthens the connection to yield long-term learning. Subsequent activation of the same node will produce even faster priming of its connecting nodes because of the increased strength (MacKay, 1982). This learning process would be expected to occur both within and across the different systems of the hierarchy.

A second mechanism of learning arises from the structuring within a system. The complexity of these subhierarchies will reflect the level of skill a person has at a given task (MacKay, 1985). In the model of Figure 5.2, propositional nodes may only retain some long-term permanence for well-practiced phrases such as 'whistle while you work'. Other, less practiced phrases such as 'the pelicans dove into the ocean' would presumably not be represented in long-term memory, but could be strung together through the activation of the constituent lexical concept nodes. Thus, one manifestation of learning will be that the complexity within a system increases.

The acquisition of morse code skills may provide an even better example of the two forms of learning (Bryan and Harter, 1899; McKay, 1985). To produce the letter 'v', the morse sender must make a series of three dots followed by a single dash. It is reasonable to assume that the conceptual node(s) for 'v' would be similar for the beginner and the expert. At this level, the output is independent of the form of implementation, namely morse code. Differences, however, would be expected at the other two levels as a function of skill. At the final output – the muscle movement level – the expert would be expected to be more consistent in the production of the individual dots and dashes. For example, the time for which the key is held to produce a dash might be less variable for the expert, thus minimizing any ambiguity between the two signals. This type of learning can be conceptualized as a strengthening of connections. In MacKay's (1985) model, there are nodes which represent 'key down', 'key hold' and 'key up'. The activation of these nodes is more regular due to increased strength of connections leading to them, i.e. there is an improved signal-to-noise ratio.

A different form of learning takes place within the movement concept system. Here MacKay (1985) postulates that the expert forms nodes that represent higher-order relationships. In the example of sending a 'v', a possible higher-order node is 'initial triple'. This node becomes activated, resulting in the dot signal being executed three times. In contrast, the beginner lacks this higher-order node and must iterate through the dot node three times. The beginner might then be expected to make an error such as sending 'u' instead of 'v' since 'u' is composed of two dots and a dash. The activation of the triple node would presumably prevent the expert from a similar error. In contrast, one might find that the expert mistakenly sends a 'j' for 'v' since this is composed of a dot followed by three dashes.

The hypothesis that expert performance involves the formation of higher-level nodes bears an obvious similarity to the chunking hypothesis (Newell and Rosenbloom, 1981) and many experiments have demonstrated this phenomenon (Allard, Graham and Paarsalu, 1980; Chase and Simon, 1973). However, the less intuitive prediction that the pattern of errors will change is more weakly supported. Analysis of errors in speech (Boomer and Laver, 1968; Foss and Hakes, 1978) or action (Norman, 1981; Reason, 1979) can be interpreted as evidence for higher-level nodes. For example, Boomer and Laver (1968) point out that Spoonerisms such as saying 'our queer old dean' when the intended sentence was 'our dear old queen' always involve swaps of phonemes from the same position. Thus, an initial position node is implicated. Reason (1979) cites analogous examples in movements. One subject reported unwrapping a piece of candy and putting the wrapper, rather than the candy, in her mouth. According to MacKay's model, this might be viewed as evidence that a higher-level node of 'place X in mouth' was activated and the wrong variable was inserted. Since these types of error occur most often in skilled action (Norman, 1981; Reason, 1979), the conjecture can be made that these types of node develop with practice.

3.3   Evidence for Hierarchies from Transfer Experiments

A striking example of how MacKay's hierarchic model can be useful for understanding learning comes from a couple of transfer experiments (MacKay, 1981; MacKay and Bowman, 1969; see also Cohen, Ivry and Keele, 1990; Keele, Cohen and Ivry, 1990). The subjects in both studies were bilinguals who were equally facile at German and English. In the study by MacKay and Bowman (1969), the subjects were presented with a string of words and asked to repeat them aloud 12 times in succession. The word strings were either grammatical sentences or scrambled versions of the grammatical stimuli. An example of the latter is 'morning in fourteen his I bed times rearranged one have' which is the scrambled version of 'I have rearranged his bed fourteen times this morning'. For a given sentence, the subjects practiced in either German or in English, but never both. The time to utter the sentences was measured and the subjects were instructed to speak as rapidly as possible.

The language of the transfer stimulus was always different from the preceding practice stimulus. The variable of interest was the relationship of the transfer stimulus to the practice stimulus. In one condition, the transfer sentence was a literal translation of the practice sentence in which word order as well as meaning was preserved. In another condition, the transfer sentence was similar in meaning but the word order was altered as in a passive to active transformation. In the third condition, the transfer sentence was unrelated to the practice sentence.

The data from MacKay and Bowman (1969) are presented in Table 5.2. There was considerable improvement in the production of both the normal and the scrambled sentences over the course of practice. Indeed, the learning curves from the 12 trials are linear when plotted on log–log coordinates. Most pertinent to the hierarchical model is the performance on the transfer sentences. The central finding is that there was no decrement in speaking rate when the translation preserved word order. Subjects were just as fast at speaking the sentence on the transfer trials as they had been on the last set of practice trials. This transfer occurred despite the fact that the test trials were spoken in a different language. Moreover, the benefits were specific

Table 5.2. *Mean time (seconds) to speak sentences early and late in practice and during transfer in MacKay and Bowman (1969). [From Keele, 1986]*

	Practice		Transfer		
	First four	Last four	Translation same order	Translation different order	New items
Normal sentences	2.33	2.03	2.03	2.24	2.44
Scrambled Sentences	2.90	2.38	2.83	—	2.79

to the practiced sentences. When the transfer sentences were related only in meaning but did not preserve word order or tense, subjects were significantly slower in their productions. Transfer to new sentences led to an even greater decrement. The production times on these stimuli were approximately equal to the time taken during the first set of practice trials.

These data strongly support the hypothesis of a multiple-system hierarchy. Prior experience with the subunits of the sentences exists for all of the subjects regardless of whether the sentences are spoken in German or in English. All of the sentences contain common words composed of sounds that the subjects have had extensive practice in producing. Thus, the lower parts of the hierarchy – the nodes and connections of the phonologic and muscle movement systems – are well established before the experiment begins. The benefits of learning accrued during the 12 practice trials would be expected to have negligible effect on these structures.

In contrast, it is unlikely that the conceptual nodes for the sentences as wholes existed at the beginning of the experiment. The subjects had probably never heard or spoken them, and it seems reasonable to assume that they had only modest experience with the constituent phrases. Therefore, the model assumes that the reduced response times observed during the practice phase reflect learning within the conceptual system. Conceptual-level nodes which represent the sentences are established during the practice trials. Since nodes at this level operate independently of the lower systems, any benefits of learning should persist even when the output system is changed. To restate this, the conceptual level is identical for the same sentence when spoken in either German or English. If learning is restricted to this level, transfer should be strong. Indeed, MacKay (1982) argues that the results provide the first demonstration of perfect transfer since the initial transfer response times are no slower than the last practice response times. However, given that the learning functions had not reached an asymptote, perfect transfer might require that the production times on the transfer trials be even faster than the production times of the last practice trials. Nonetheless, the results are impressive.

The data from the other conditions provide important controls for MacKay's interpretation. The finding that there was no transfer to novel sentences emphasizes that the benefits of practice cannot be attributed to general factors such as a warm-up effect, but rather are specific to the practiced material. It is interesting that there was a modest degree of transfer to the sentences that were related in meaning though different in word order. This would indicate that there are some shared nodes between the two forms of the sentences. This is in accord with many findings showing that memory is not restricted to the surface structure of a sentence, but may be based on more abstract representations (Sachs, 1967). Nonetheless, the transfer is only partial since the constituent phrases are different between the practice and transfer versions. It would seem that the transfer savings can be attributed to the highest levels of the hierarchy.

The results for the scrambled sentences are also accounted for by the model. Subjects improved during practice with these stimuli. However, response times following transfer to exact translation stimuli were no faster than transfer to stimuli composed of different words. MacKay (1982) argues that because of their nonsensicality, there is little conceptual-level representation of the scrambled sentences. It was the learning at this level of representation that had produced the transfer in the normal sentences. Since it is no longer relevant with the scrambled sentences, transfer is not observed.

Given this explanation, it is not clear why there was any improvement with practice on the scrambled sentences. If learning is occurring only at the highest levels, then there must be some conceptual-level learning going on during the practice trials. Yet this learning does not transfer. To account for this, MacKay proposes that this result may be an artifact of multitranslatability. A word that is ambiguous in meaning in one language may have multiple translations in another language, each of which is restricted in meaning. For example, the word 'right' in English has eleven different German forms such as 'recht', 'richtig' and 'ordnen'. Since there is no context provided by the scrambled sentences to restrict the meaning, the conceptual-level lexical nodes activated for a given word in practice may be different from those used following translation. This argument is required if MacKay is to argue that all of the benefits of practice are restricted to the higher levels – an argument that is a consequence of his belief that his results demonstrate perfect transfer. If, as pointed out above, the transfer is not truly perfect, then a simpler account can be offered for the practice functions: the learning reflects practice in the language-specific productions of the jumbled sentences.

Before leaving MacKay's model, one other clever manipulation should be noted. In addition to practice conditions in which the sentences are spoken aloud, MacKay has examined conditions in which the sentences were only practiced covertly (MacKay, 1981). Mental practice, by definition, should not involve the muscle movement system (Kohl and Roenker, 1980). However, since bilingual transfer is not the result of practice within this system, the model predicts that transfer should be just as great following mental practice as it is following overt practice. This novel prediction – that mental practice can be equally effective as actual practice – holds even when the transfer sentences must be spoken aloud. This result is exactly what was observed: MacKay (1981) observed a 200 ms advantage on transfer trials to literal translations compared with nontranslations following overt practice. The comparable figure on the transfer trials following mental practice was 230 ms.[2]

---

[2]MacKay did not observe perfect transfer in this experiment. There was an increase in response time between the training and transfer trials even when the subjects had overtly practiced the sentences. However, the transfer sentences in this experiment preserved meaning without retaining word order.

3.4 Parameters of Hierarchies and Generalized Motor Programs

In the preceding discussion, there has been little reference to possible constraints on the types of information that can be represented in the hierarchy. The section on chunking emphasized the ubiquitous nature of this mechanism: it was evident across a wide array of task domains. Does this mean that there are no constraints on chunking? Similarly, what determines the information represented by a node within a hierarchy? Are all aspects of a movement equally amenable to the node formation process or are some types of information more critical, perhaps given special status to ensure their long-term retention? The different levels discussed by MacKay offer only a weak constraint, namely, that there are different systems of nodes such as the conceptual and movement system. But this still leaves open the issue of whether certain types of information are more likely to be represented than other types of information.

3.4.1 Invariant Relative Timing

A number of researchers have argued that there is not a state of equipotentiality. In fact, one of the primary motivations for the notion of a generalized motor program is that there is some constraint on the type of information retained as a result of practice. It has been hypothesized that the essential information of the motor program is the relative timing between the different subcomponents of an action sequence (Armstrong, 1970; Carter and Shapiro, 1984; Shapiro *et al.*, 1981; Summers, 1975; Terzuolo and Viviani, 1980; Viviani and Terzuolo, 1980; Wulf and Schmidt, 1989; but see Gentner, 1987). According to this conceptualization, a generalized motor program may be instantiated in a single effector system or across effectors at different overall rates. However, once the output system and overall rate are selected, the timing within the action is determined. The relative timing remains invariant.

Consider an example from the literature on handwriting (Viviani and Terzuolo, 1980). In this experiment, people were asked to write letters of the alphabet at different speeds. The pen positions were recorded via a digitizing table and the velocity profiles could then be determined through differentiation. The subjects had no difficulty in producing a wide range of overall durations. For example, the time required to produce the letter 'a' varied from 245 to 680 ms for one subject. Despite this wide range, the temporal intervals between the velocity maxima and minima maintained a constant proportion of the overall duration. The parts of the letter that took the longest during the slow reproductions also took the relatively greatest amount of time during the fastest reproductions. This relative timing invariance is also evident in typing (Terzuolo and Viviani, 1980). The top panel in Figure 5.5a depicts the raw data from one subject typing the word 'ENCLOSED' 42 times. Each row represents a production of the complete word with the individual dots representing the times at which the individual letters were typed. The data are arranged according to overall duration for each production. In the bottom panel, the data are presented in terms of the proportion of time devoted to each interstroke interval relative to the total duration for that particular production. This transformation demonstrates the invariance of relative timing despite large fluctuations in the overall rate of performance. Terzuolo and Viviani (1980) interpret these results as

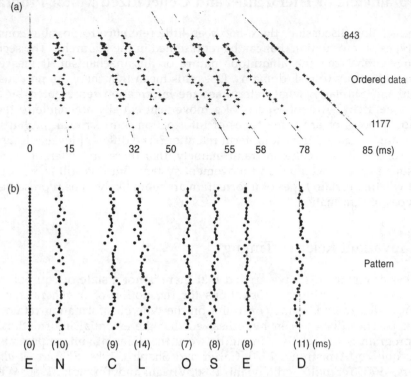

Figure 5.5. *Multiple productions for typing the word 'ENCLOSED'. (a) Depicts the raw trials arranged in order from fastest to slowest production. (b) Shows the inter-tap intervals when the data are normalized to equate the overall duration of each production. [From Terzuolo and Viviani, 1980.]*

indicating that a single rate parameter is being applied throughout the entire production.

If the relative timing hypothesis is a valid construct, then it could serve as a useful tool for examining the units of a motor program (Young and Schmidt, 1990). The hypothesis states that the invariance will apply across the segments of an action sequence. If two segments are from different motor programs, then the invariance is not expected to apply.

At a more atomic level, the hypothesis makes no explicit prediction concerning the parts of each segment. Consider a single button press within a sequence of key presses. There may be many parts to each button press: the time needed to depress the key, the time to release it and the lag time between presses. One can ask whether the proportional timing invariance is observed within the parts of a sequence element as well as across the different elements. This kind of reasoning has been applied in the literature of speech production (Kozhevnikov and Chistovich, 1965; Tuller, Kelso and Harris, 1982). Kozhevnikov and Chistovich (1965) asked subjects to vary the rate at which they repeated a set of phrases. The analyses examined the relative durations of the words, syllables, vowels and consonants. The results demonstrated that, whereas the relative durations of the words and syllables remained invariant across speaking rates, there was considerable variation in the relative durations of the vowels and consonants.

Similar results using electromyographic techniques have been reported by Tuller, Kelso and Harris (1982). Syllable lengths tended to be scaled proportionately, even when the muscular records of the articulators did not reveal any invariants. This last finding underscores three caveats for using relative timing as a means for identifying the units of a generalized motor program. First, the application of a single rate parameter may be restricted to higher-level representations of the action plan. Second, the motor program may not contain information about the lower, implementation levels of the action. Third, other sources of variability may dominate at the output level, obscuring invariant relationships (Wing and Kristofferson, 1973).

3.4.2   Additional Constraints on Motor Programs

It may be useful to reconsider the motivation for a hypothesis concerning invariant relative timing. For some researchers (i.e. Schmidt, 1975, 1988), invariant relative timing was one of the cornerstone pieces of evidence in support of the concept of abstract motor programs: the language of the memory was in terms of the relative temporal structuring of the components of the action. This sort of constraint is specific, or local, in nature. Any learned movement has certain relative temporal relationships and these are maintained across the various implementations of that specific action sequence. Moreover, invariant relative timing was a useful construct for reducing memory requirements. Only the relative timing profile needed to be stored rather than specific timing relationships. Thus, a number of different movements could be executed by changing single parameters of this representation.

However, there may be other, more global, factors which contribute to the appearance of an invariant. For example, Rumelhart and Norman (1982) present a model of typing in which certain temporal regularities arise because of peripheral constraints on interstroke intervals. A second example comes from the numerous studies showing that pointing and reaching movements are characterized by a bell-shaped velocity profile (Flash and Hogan, 1985; Kelso, Southard and Goodman, 1979; Soechting and Lacquaniti, 1981). While it may be tempting to argue that the scaling of this profile reflects some sort of invariant relationship between factors controlling the acceleration and deceleration phases of the movement, the result may be an indirect consequence of the operation of a different mechanism. For instance, Flash and Hogan (1985) argue that these profiles reflect a smoothness constraint: movements are made so as to minimize jerkiness. If a movement is made at a different speed, the same velocity profile will hold because the smoothness criterion will yield the same shaped velocity profile given any input. Thus, the presence of invariants need not be interpreted as demonstrating the existence of a stored parameter representing the relationship between segments of a learned motor program.

4.   ATTENTION, AUTOMATICITY AND LEARNING

An important theme in cognitive psychology over the past decade has been the comparison of controlled and automatic processes. The former mode of processing is characterized as slow, effortful and capacity limited such that concurrent demands will interfere with performance. In contrast, automatic processing is fast, parallel, basically effortless and may not be subject to interference from concurrent activities (Schneider and Shiffrin, 1977; Shiffrin and Schneider, 1977). This dichotomy has frequently been invoked as a useful concept to account for the acquisition of skilled performance. Early in practice, the performer must utilize controlled processes. Effort is directed at identifying the critical components of the task and developing effective strategies for accomplishing the desired action. With practice, the need for such control is diminished. The actions become freed from the conscious control of the performer and automatized in the sense that, once initiated, little mental effort is required for the control of the action.

The notion that skilled performance is performed automatically matches our intuition. We have great trouble describing to others how we perform many of our most skillful behaviors. Try, for example, to explain how to ride a bicycle or surfboard to someone who has never tried it. The shift in control away from a conscious or metacognitive level precludes the skilled performer from being able to describe how the task is executed. Thus, when asked what he thinks about during his performance, an Olympic gymnastics medalist responded, 'As I approach the apparatus... the only thing I am thinking about is... the first trick... I start the first trick, then my body takes over and hopefully everything becomes automatic...' (quoted in Schmidt, 1987, p. 85).

4.1 Dual-Task Methodology

The researcher must devise paradigms which can test these intuitions. One popular methodology has been the dual-task paradigm. The logic underlying this task runs as follows. In performing any given task, some attentional resources must be devoted to that task. If two tasks are performed simultaneously, then the performer must allocate resources to both tasks. Based on the assumption that there is some fixed limit to the amount of available resources, performance on two simultaneous tasks would be expected to be worse than performance on either task alone (Posner and Snyder, 1975). The allocation of resources will vary as a function of many factors such as the complexity of the task, the instructions given to the performer and the skill level of the performer. This last factor is most important for research on skill acquisition. If skilled behavior makes fewer demands on certain attentional resources, then a distractor task should produce less interference for a skilled performer than for an unskilled performer.

One of the most dramatic demonstrations of the ability to perform two tasks simultaneously comes from a study by Spelke, Hirst and Neisser (1976). Two subjects were tested over a 17-week period on their ability to write to dictation while reading short stories for comprehension. In the first weeks of the experiment, each subject's reading rate was markedly reduced when they concurrently wrote to dictation (Figure 5.6). However, when the subjects had simultaneously practiced the two tasks for over 25 hours, the reading rates were almost equal to that observed when the reading task was performed singly. Moreover, comprehension of the short stories was unaffected by the inclusion of the writing task. (However, these data may reflect a ceiling effect. Many of the comprehension tests were performed perfectly by each subject under both single- and dual-task conditions.) In latter

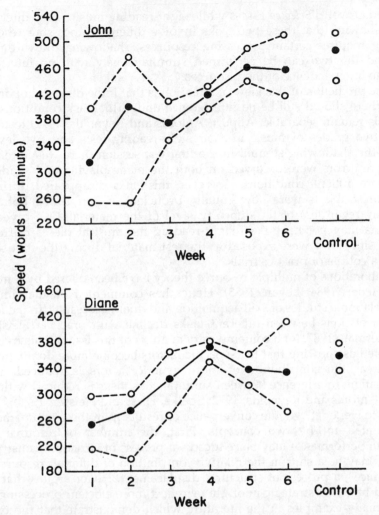

Figure 5.6. *Reading speed as a function of practice under dual-task conditions; weekly means and interquartile ranges. While reading for comprehension, the two subjects were required to write to dictation. The isolated points to the right of each function show reading speed without concurrent writing. [From Spelke, Hirst and Neisser, 1976.]*

phases of the experiment, the subjects were asked to monitor the dictation lists for semantic or phonological properties. Again, although reading speed originally decreased under these new task demands, the subjects were quickly able to achieve a rate comparable to the single-task results.

Demonstrations such as these have led to refined conceptions of what is meant by terms such as attentional resources and automatization (Allport, Antonis and Reynolds, 1972; McLeod and Posner, 1984; Shaffer, 1976; but see Navon, 1985). In particular, these studies have led to the notion of multiple resource pools: certain activities can be performed simultaneously when they tap separable resources or processing systems. Allport *et al.* found that skilled pianists are able to shadow passages from Orwell's *Selected Essays* while sight-reading music. They interpreted the data as showing that these two tasks involve different processing resources. Piano-playing requires certain processing resources, shadowing draws on other resources, and the two can be performed simultaneously with no interference because of the independence of the resources.

Indeed, one prediction of this view of attention is that if the difficulty of one task is increased there should still be no interference under dual-task conditions if the resource pools remain separable. Allport, Antonis and Reynolds (1972) tested this by utilizing two grades of music in their sight-reading tests and two levels of difficulty for the shadowing stimuli. In the first test session there was an effect of difficulty: more errors were observed on both the piano-playing and shadowing under the more difficult conditions. However, this effect disappeared during the second session. Subjects were now equally proficient at performing both tasks simultaneously regardless of the difficulty level of the material. One caveat: the skilled pianists may not have been sight-reading the musical pieces during the latter session since they were exposed to the test material during the first session as well as in a couple of practice trials.

Further elaborations of multiple resource theory have been offered by a number of authors (Heuer, 1984; Logan, 1985). Heuer has commented on the similarity between correlational studies of skill acquisition and dual-task results. In the former paradigm, correlations between different tasks decline with practice (Fleishman, 1966; see Ackerman, 1987, for a contemporary analysis of this issue). This trend has been interpreted as showing that task-specific factors become more dominant with practice whereas the contribution of more generic factors is reduced. In the dual-task situation, interference between simultaneous tasks is reduced with practice (Allport, Antonis and Reynolds, 1972; Spelke, Hirst and Neisser, 1976).

According to Heuer (1984), the convergence of results from these two paradigms can be accounted for by two concepts. First, the number of resource pools contributing to performance may be reduced – a process of structural constriction. Second, there may be a shift in the relative contribution of different resources for task performance – a process of structural displacement. Heuer argues that these changes could be either strategic in origin or reflect more efficient processing.

There are many examples in the literature which demonstrate that the type of information guiding performance may shift with practice. One example of a structural displacement may be seen in a typing study (West, 1967). Whereas visual feedback was found to be most important during the early stages of the skill acquisition process, kinesthetic feedback gradually assumed a pre-eminent role. A similar observation has been made by Fleishman and Rich (1963) in the learning of a bimanual task. The correlation between this task and a test of kinesthetic sensitivity increased with practice. Another example of structural displacement is seen in the work of Marteniuk and Romanow (1983). They found that subjects became sensitive to higher-order derivatives (e.g. target velocity rather than target position) with practice in a tracking task (see also Fuchs, 1962; Jagacinski and Hah, 1988).

In the preceding examples, constriction and displacement led to improvements in performance with practice. Less intuitive, these processes also predict that, under certain situations, two tasks may produce more interference following practice. Suppose two tasks, *A* and *B*, share a common resource pool, *R*. At the beginning of training, task *A* makes little use of *R* whereas task *B* is substantially dependent on

R. If, due to displacement, task *A* becomes more dependent on *R* with practice, there would be greater dual-task interference following practice than had initially existed. Examples supporting this prediction, however, are not readily evident in the literature, perhaps because we are biased to look for the benefits of practice.

An important point to be made from these reconceptualizations of attention and resource theory is that automaticity is a relative, rather than an absolute, concept. Qualification must be made of the assumption that, if there is no interference between two tasks, one of the tasks is performed automatically. Rather, little attention may be required for the performance of that task when paired with a particular secondary task. However, there may exist (and probably does exist) a different secondary task which would produce interference in the dual-task situation.

This point is clearly made by in a dual-task experiment by McLeod (1977). The primary task was to use a joystick to track a cursor that moved in a quasirandom fashion across a computer screen. For the secondary task, the subjects performed a tone discrimination task. When the responses to the tone task were made vocally, there was no significant reduction in tracking performance in comparison with when subjects only performed the tracking task. However, when the tone discrimination required a manual response with the nontracking hand, dual-task interference was extensive. Results such as these demonstrate that automaticity, at least as operationalized by dual tasks and other converging paradigms, becomes a fuzzy concept that can only be defined relative to the conditions under which it is observed.

4.2 Control and Awareness of Well-Developed Skills

When automatic processing and controlled processing are seen as a dichotomy, one inference, almost by definition, is that automatic processing involves less control on the part of the performer. In some theories, less control is explicitly equated with a reduction in conscious processing (Neumann, 1984; Schneider and Fisk, 1983). In other models the notion of 'less control' is more abstractly defined. Anderson (1987) argues that skilled activities can be implemented directly in a precompiled, or proceduralized, form once certain enabling conditions are met. An intermediate step between input and output can be bypassed as practice facilitates direct links between the input and output.

Skilled performers, when reflecting on their own performance, appear to share the belief that control processing is reduced during the execution of highly practiced movements. This was evident in the quote previously cited from the Olympic gymnast. Similarly, a common complaint of baseball professionals during hitting slumps is that they 'are thinking too much'. Nonetheless, evidence such as this is anecdotal.

More rigorous experimental study of this problem in the skills area has come from the study of error detection. Surprisingly, the evidence from movement studies is not supportive of the hypothesis that controlled processing is reduced in skilled performance. Rather, the studies tend to show that skilled performers are exquisitely sensitive to their actions. Rabbitt (1978) examined how quickly skilled typists were able to detect their own errors. He found that, when corrected, over 94% of the single keystroke errors were detected before the next keystroke had been executed. A second experiment demonstrated that this error detection process was active even before the erroneous keystroke was completed. By obtaining an indirect measure of the force of the keystrokes, Rabbitt (1978) was able to show that mistakes were more frequently executed with light keystrokes than were correct responses.

Logan (1982) has used a more direct method to study the ability of skilled typists to monitor their responses. While typing, the subjects were occasionally presented with a signal indicating that they should stop typing as quickly as possible. Logan (1982) reasoned that if skilled typists are executing their responses in chunks (i.e. whole words) more keystrokes should be produced when the stop signal occurs early in the trial than when it occurs late. The data did not support this prediction. In accord with Rabbitt (1978), Logan found that experienced typists are generally able to monitor each individual keystroke. The time to inhibit their responses was independent of the time of occurrence of the stop signal. The only exception was that subjects typically completed the word 'the' regardless of when the stop signal occurred.

One aspect of typing studies that has received little attention (Long, 1976; Rabbitt, 1978) is that many of the typing errors went undetected. The authors have focused on the rapid corrective ability of their subjects once they detect an error. It is unclear whether the skilled typists were worse than unskilled subjects at detecting errors – a prediction that would be made if automaticity and diminished control are equated. However, Schmidt and White (1972) have addressed this issue in a simple movement experiment. Subjects were trained to move a hand-held slide along a trackway with a goal movement time of 150 ms. After each trial, the subjects were asked to estimate their own errors. Subsequent to this, they were provided with their actual error. Schmidt and White (1972) calculated the correlation between the subjects' estimated error and actual error over the 2-day training period. If practice led to less control over performance, one would expect the correlation to decrease. In fact, the opposite occurred. The correlations rose from initial values of under 0.30 to values of about 0.90 during the last few blocks.

It should be noted that Schmidt and White did not use an online error detection task, but rather required an error estimate to be made after the end of the response. While the correspondence between these two measures of error sensitivity is unclear, the two measures provide converging evidence that skilled performance may involve an increase in the capability of controlled processing.

Schneider and Fisk (1983) offer a novel view of the role of controlled processes in skilled behavior, a role which is different from that needed during the acquisition process itself. Controlled processing is originally needed to establish automatic behaviors. Once established, controlled processing can be redirected to increasing the flexibility of the performer. For example, the skilled baseball batter is not only able to make contact with the ball regardless of where the pitch is thrown, but is also able to make adjustments in his/her swing so as to direct the ball to a desired location. According to Schneider and Fisk (1983), this adjustment in strategy is within the domain of controlled processes. However, once a given strategy is selected, the actual swing of the bat is automatically performed. At this level it seems doubtful that maintaining a distinction between controlled and automatic processes is more than a matter of semantics. The example does make a useful contribution, though, in showing that the use of controlled processing may be more specialized for skilled performers.

4.2.1 Automaticity as a Continuum of Skill Acquisition

The studies reviewed in the preceding paragraphs bode well with the conceptualization of automaticity as a relative process. The development of a skill is a continuous process. Skilled performers may learn to process information more efficiently (Allard, Graham and Paarsalu, 1980; Chase and Simon, 1973), use more appropriate forms of stimulus and feedback information (Fleishman and Rich, 1963; Marteniuk and Romanow, 1983; West, 1967), and develop better strategies (Schneider and Fisk, 1983). These abilities continue to be refined and improved upon at all levels of ability. Indeed, one of the most striking features of the learning curves reviewed previously is that, when plotted in log–log coordinates, there is no asymptote in performance other than might be imposed by external constraints (Crossman, 1959).

In an influential paper, Fitts (1964) has written of three phases in skill learning. The early phase, generally spanning only a short time, includes the period in which the performer comes to understand the instructions and establish the appropriate cognitive set for the task. During the second phase, the subject learns to associate certain responses with specific cues. The final phase is the period during which these associations are being refined and strengthened. Despite the use of the term 'phases', Fitts (1964) is quite adamant in stressing that skill acquisition is a continuous process. He writes,

'the fact that performance ever levels off at all appears to be due as much to the effects of physiological aging and/or motivation as to the reaching of a true learning asymptote or limit in capacity for further improvement.' (p. 268)

4.2.2 Is Attention Necessary for Learning to Occur?

Stating that automaticity is a relative concept does not contradict the hypothesis that there is a progression in skill acquisition from resource-limited performance to performance that places little demand on attention. The axiom that attention is required during the initial acquisition period is either explicitly stated or implicit in almost all papers on learning. This hypothesis has been the focus of a number of recent studies.

One set of studies has been conducted by Nissen and colleagues (Nissen and Bullemer, 1987; Nissen, Knopman and Schacter, 1987). In the basic experiment, four keys are paired with four stimulus locations. When a mark appears in one of the stimulus locations, the subject presses the corresponding key as quickly as possible. After 200 ms, the next stimulus appears, thus creating a sequential key-pressing task. Each block of trials was composed of a series of 100 presses. Nissen and Bullemer (1987) compared two methods of stimulus selection. In one method, each stimulus location was selected randomly. In the other method, the stimuli occurred in a fixed order. If the digits 1, 2, 3 and 4 are used to symbolize the stimulus locations from left to right, then the order used in the study was 4-2-3-1-3-2-4-3-2-1. This 10-element pattern recycled continuously 10 times over the course of a block of 100 presses. Sequence learning can be inferred if the response latencies are shorter on those blocks in which the stimuli appear in a fixed order in comparison with the blocks in which the stimuli are selected randomly.

For some conditions, subjects had to perform a secondary, distractor task while doing the key-pressing task. For the secondary task, a high- or low-pitched tone was played after each key press. The subjects were required silently to count the number of times the low tone occurred and report this number at the end of the block. This manipulation was adopted to distract attention, preventing the subject from observing the relationship between successive stimulus signals on the key-pressing task.

The primary findings showed that subjects could learn the sequence, but only when they did not have to perform the tone-counting task concurrently. In the single-task condition, mean response latencies in the ordered condition became much faster than in the random condition. However, under dual-task conditions, there were no significant differences in response times for the two groups. These results led Nissen and Bullemer (1987) to conclude that learning requires attention. In follow-up studies, however, they demonstrate that, whereas attention is necessary, awareness is not. Korsakoff patients (Nissen and Bullemer, 1987, experiment 4) and normal subjects with scopolamine-induced memory deficits (Nissen, Knopman and Schacter, 1987) demonstrate a performance advantage on the ordered trial blocks even when they are unaware that the stimuli and responses follow a fixed sequence.

These results are in accord with the hypothesis that skill acquisition is at least initially dependent on attention. However, we recently found that some forms of learning may have minimal requirements for attention during the initial acquisition phase (Cohen, Ivry and Keele, 1990; Keele, Cohen and Ivry, 1990; see also Pew, 1974). In our first experiment (Cohen, Ivry and Keele, 1990) we modified the procedure of Nissen and Bullemer by using only three stimulus locations. The stimuli appeared randomly or in sequences composed of five elements. An example of an ordered sequence is 1-3-2-3-2. Trial blocks were composed of 100 responses or 20 cycles of the sequence. The key-pressing task was performed concurrently with the tone-counting task. We included two levels of difficulty in the tone-counting task: on average, 37.5 target tones were presented during each block in the EASY conditions and 62.5 target tones occurred during each block of the HARD conditions. In sum, separate groups of subjects were tested on one of four conditions created by the factorial combination of two conditions: sequence (ORDERED or RANDOM) and tone difficulty (EASY or HARD).

The results for the four groups are shown in Figure 5.7. All of the groups became faster with practice. Presumably, the improvement for the random groups can be attributed to practice effects associated with general aspects of the task. More interestingly, both of the groups presented with the ordered sequence became faster than the groups in the random conditions. Thus, unlike the results of Nissen and Bullemer (1987), we found that subjects were able to learn a sequence under dual-task conditions. This learning occurred without any indication that the subjects were aware of the sequence. It is unlikely that the subjects were able to learn by switching attention between the two tasks. While reaction times were slower for the HARD conditions, the degree of learning was the same for the two groups of subjects in the ORDERED conditions. If subjects were switching attention between the key-pressing and the tone tasks, learning should have been reduced for the HARD group since their secondary task was more demanding.

We proposed that learning occurred in our experiment because of the presence of a unique association in the five-element sequences (Cohen, Ivry and Keele, 1990).

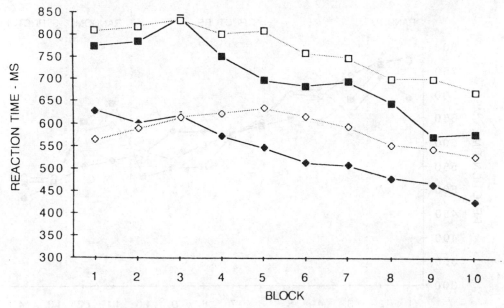

Figure 5.7. *Mean reaction time for each block of 100 responses. The stimuli followed a sequenced pattern for the groups represented by solid symbols and were* RANDOM *for the groups represented by open symbols. Squares refer to groups tested under easy secondary task conditions (average of 37 target tones). Diamonds refer to groups tested under difficult secondary task conditions (average of 62.5 target tones).*

For example, in the sequence 1-3-2-3-2 the stimulus location 1 occurs only once per cycle and is always followed by a stimulus in location 3. It is possible that this unique association provides a critical point for an associative learning mechanism. No comparable singularity was contained in the sequences of Nissen and Bullemer (1987).

To test this hypothesis, we compared performance on three different types of ordered sequences. AMBIGUOUS sequences involved three stimulus locations which were ordered into a series of six elements such as 1-3-2-3-1-2. In these sequences each stimulus position is presented twice within a single cycle and there are no unique pairwise associations. For example, stimulus 1 is followed by stimulus 3 at one point in the cycle and by stimulus 2 at another point. In contrast, UNIQUE sequences used five locations and responses, each of which occurred once within the sequence, creating five unique associations; an example is 1-3-2-5-4. HYBRID sequences were equated in length with the AMBIGUOUS sequence but had four stimulus locations. In these sequences two of the elements occurred twice and two occurred once: for example, 1-3-2-4-2-3. There are two unique associations in the HYBRID sequences (e.g. 1-3 and 4-2). In summary, unique associations exist in both the UNIQUE and the HYBRID sequences, but are not present in the AMBIGUOUS sequences.

Subjects were tested on a total of 14 blocks of 120 key presses each. For the first two blocks, the stimuli were selected randomly. Then, subjects completed eight blocks with their assigned ordered sequence. This was followed by two more

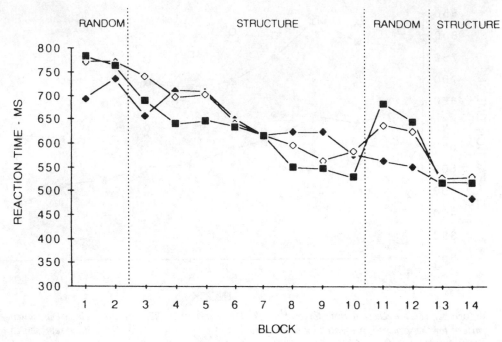

Figure 5.8. *Mean reaction time for each block of 120 responses for the three types of sequence. On blocks 11 and 12, the* ORDERED *sequences were replaced by* RANDOM *sequences. On blocks 13 and 14, the* ORDERED *sequences were resumed.* ◆—◆, AMBIGUOUS; ◇—◇, HYBRID; ■—■, UNIQUE. *[From Cohen, Ivry and Keele, 1990.]*

random blocks and two concluding ordered blocks. This method provides two tests of learning. First, if the sequence is learned, interference should be present following the switch from ordered to random conditions between blocks 10 and 11. Second, facilitation should be present following the return to ordered conditions between blocks 12 and 13. Subjects were tested under dual-task conditions.

Figure 5.8 presents the results. Only the UNIQUE and HYBRID groups show evidence of interference and facilitation as the stimuli switch from ORDERED to RANDOM and back. Although the response latencies decrease for subjects in the AMBIGUOUS group, there was no interference when following the switch to RANDOM sequences nor any significant facilitation following the return to the ORDERED sequences. The improvement for the AMBIGUOUS group appears to reflect non-specific benefits of practice.[3]

We believe that these results have important implications for the study of learning. First, the results indicate that learning does not always involve a simple progression in which the role of attention becomes diminished as learning progresses. Attentional manipulations had no effect on the rate of learning (Figure 5.7).

---

[3]Note that the subjects in the AMBIGUOUS condition are the fastest. This is presumably because their task is equivalent to a three-choice reaction time task whereas the HYBRID and UNIQUE groups face four- and five-choice reaction time tasks, respectively (Hick, 1952; Hyman, 1953).

Second, subtle changes in the task may produce large changes in the mechanisms needed for learning to occur. We have argued (Cohen, Ivry and Keele, 1990; Keele, Cohen and Ivry, 1990) that sequences which contain a unique association may be learned by an associative mechanism (Jordan, 1986). In contrast, sequences such as those used in our AMBIGUOUS conditions present ambiguities that are difficult for such a mechanism. To overcome these inherent ambiguities, an attention-demanding learning mechanism may be needed which can parse the sequence into subunits (see Jennings and Keele, 1990, for a simulation of these data). Differentiating between learning that requires attention and learning that does not require attention may prove fruitful in understanding the emergence of representational structures such as hierarchies. One hypothesis which remains to be fully explored is that hierarchical representation is not only useful as a way to represent complex actions, but may also provide a means for partitioning ambiguous subunits of an action. For example, in a hierarchical representation, the AMBIGUOUS sequence 1-3-2-3-1-2 could be broken into two chunks, 1-3-2 and 3-1-2, each containing unique associations.

4.2.3 Transfer Following Learning Without Awareness

As discussed previously, transfer experiments (MacKay, 1981; MacKay and Bowman, 1969) have shown that learning of an action sequence may occur independently of the output system with which the sequence is practiced. However, in previous studies, the subjects were aware of the learning task. Can transfer also occur following implicit learning?

To investigate this question, Cohen, Ivry and Keele (1990, experiment 2) had subjects perform the key-pressing task under dual-task conditions. Five element sequences that contained a unique association were used (e.g. 1-2-3-2-3). In the training phase, subjects responded by using three fingers, one for each stimulus location. For the transfer phase, subjects moved their arm back and forth so that all of the responses were made with the index finger. This mode of responding is akin to the 'hunt and peck' method of typing. During the transfer phase, the sequential stimulus pattern was continued for half of the subjects. For the other half of the subjects, the stimuli were randomly selected on the transfer blocks.

During the training phase, mean reaction time decreased by approximately 150 ms for both groups, replicating our finding of learning under dual-task conditions. Transfer produced a sharp dissociation between the two groups. The mean latencies for the group that shifted to the random stimuli increased dramatically. In contrast, there was little evidence of an increase in response time for the group that continued to respond to ordered sequences despite the change in response effectors. This result was replicated in a second transfer study (Keele, Cohen and Ivry, 1990) with an important control. Transfer performance across effectors was directly compared with conditions in which the subjects did not change effectors. There was no apparent advantage for the groups that used a single output system in comparison with the groups which switched effectors.

These transfer studies indicate that learning does not occur at a level of control linked to a specific output system. Instead, the sequence representation must be consolidated at an effector-independent level. Information at this level must either be in terms of where in the environment successive movements should be directed or where successive stimuli will occur. These representations can be acquired outside awareness.

5 THEORIES OF MOTOR LEARNING

The first half of this chapter has focused on some of the regularities and phenomena observed in the study of motor learning. Explanations of the log–log learning law were discussed in terms of possible mechanisms. However, mechanisms such as chunking, hierarchical construction and priming, and automaticity, have typically been discussed as generic processes. The content of the inputs and outputs for these processes is, at best, loosely described.

A true theory of motor learning requires greater specification. Consider a basketball player learning to shoot a jump shot. What are the essential sources of information for learning to occur? Does the player retain a record of the articulatory actions associated with each attempt and the context in which the shot was made? What about the importance of extrinsic, goal-based information? How does information about external events (i.e. whether the shot went in the basket or not) become merged with information intrinsic to the performer? What constitutes an error and how does the performer know when an error has occurred? How is an error signal used to produce improvements in future performance?

The issue of competence must also be considered. As defined by Chomsky (1965), a theory of competence can be distinguished from a theory of performance. Whereas the latter is restricted to observable behavior, the former aspires to account for the full extent of the performer's capability. For example, the basketball player will be required to make the jump shot from a near infinite number of positions and contexts in game situations. It is unlikely that every possible shot will be practiced, yet the skilled performer is still able to generate an appropriate action given the novel situation. Thus, a theory of motor learning requires some account of generalization. What is the extent of generalization? Is generalization incorporated into the representation of the skill or does it only become manifest during the execution of the skill?

The second half of this chapter will present a series of theories of motor learning. The theories were selected to span the disciplines of psychology, neuroscience and computer science, exemplifying the strengths and weaknesses of each. A cross-disciplinary review faces the obstacle that the theorists vary in terms of the types of movement and phenomena they seek to explain. Nonetheless, each theory presents an explicit statement of the mechanisms involved in learning.

5.1 Psychological Theories of Motor Learning

Two dominant theories of motor learning have emerged from psychology: Adams' (1971) closed-loop theory and Schmidt's (1975) schema theory. The theories share a common starting point in that they were developed to account for the large body of empiric data obtained in human performance laboratories. These movements primarily consist of relatively simple actions such as moving an object over a short distance in a specified time period. Performance measures will show rapid evidence of learning in such situations and, given that the subjects are humans, the experimenter can evaluate the performer's subjective experience as well as their overt actions. Despite these similarities, the two theories form a sharp dichotomy for contrasting basic principles of motor control and learning.

5.1.1 Adams' Closed-Loop Theory

As Adams notes in a retrospective (1987), the study of how motor skills are acquired was out of vogue through much of the 1940s, '50s and '60s. Adams attributes this to a number of factors. The decline of behaviorism had created a void for learning theory in general and, in particular, the early years of cognitive psychology were notable for their lack of interest in learning processes. Perhaps this latter trend can be attributed to the dominance of the computer metaphor for human cognition (Bower and Hilgard, 1981). Given that computers were not expected to learn (then), adherence to the metaphor discouraged the study of learning in animate organisms.

Nonetheless, research continued in other, more applied areas of study on the principles of learning. Physical education began to realize the benefits of becoming an experimental science (Adams, 1987). Engineers were exploring the capabilities of servomechanisms as cybernetic devices. Inspired by these two divergent realms of knowledge, Adams (1971) set forth one of the first comprehensive attempts to provide the field of motor control with a mechanistic theory of motor learning.

At the heart of Adams' theory is the idea that movement should be conceived of as a closed-loop process. Whereas behaviorist theories (Hull, 1943) tended to focus on the long-term role of feedback in strengthening habits, Adams emphasized that feedback is essential for the online production of skilled behavior. Indeed, every motor act is dependent on a matching process between the desired movement as stored in memory and the actual movement being produced. Thus, memory serves an active role, guiding the current movement by supplying the information which enables the performer to make the online adjustments necessary to achieve the desired action.

How is the memory established in order to provide this capability? It is one thing to postulate that movement is performed in a closed-loop manner, but it still remains to specify how the mechanisms of the closed-loop system acquire their knowledge of what constitutes a correct action and what constitutes an error. Adams (1971, 1976) provides explicit statements on these issues, focusing on two independent mechanisms.

The first is the notion of the perceptual trace. This is a reference mechanism, a representation of the feedback associated with each response. This representation is a composite of all of the sources of information produced by the action: the direct proprioceptive and tactile inputs that arise from the displacement of the limbs, as well as less direct visual and auditory stimuli that result from the movement. The perceptual trace accrues strength from each production of the movement. With practice, the perceptual trace comes to provide an accurate reflection of the skilled movement. This process is dependent on knowledge of results, informing the performer as to whether a particular production was accurate or not. When knowledge of results signals that a particular movement was in error, the difference between the feedback from that trial and the more stable perceptual trace can be used to modify the perceptual trace and therefore the next production. In this way, knowledge of results plays a vital role in the early stages of acquisition when the perceptual trace is relatively weak. Adams (1971) referred to this as the verbal-motor stage. However, as more correct movements are produced, the perceptual trace becomes solidified, providing a stable point of reference which can be used to null online errors. At this stage of learning, knowledge of results is no longer needed in order for skilled action to occur. The perceptual trace and response-produced feedback are sufficient for the subject to recognize accurate and erroneous responses. In Adams' (1971, 1976) terms, this corresponds to the motor stage of skill.

One of the predictions of the theory is that learning is still possible even when knowledge of results is eliminated. Adams refers to this process as subjective reinforcement. Indeed, at later stages of practice, the performer has little use of knowledge of results, relying entirely on the finely calibrated nulling process. This prediction may be difficult to test given that the small changes achievable at this stage may be obscured by measurement noise. However, the weaker form of this prediction is that performance will not deteriorate when knowledge of results is eliminated once the skill has achieved the motor stage.

This prediction has received support from a number of studies (Adams, Goetz and Marshall, 1972; Adams, Gopher and Lintern, 1977; Newell, 1974). Adams, Goetz and Marshall (1972) examined subjects' accuracy in moving a low-friction slide 10 inches. The amount of training with knowledge of results was varied, as was the type of online feedback provided to the subject. The results showed that, with extensive practice (150 trials) and augmented feedback, no decrement in performance was observed following the removal of knowledge of results. However, if the feedback was not augmented or if practice was minimal (15 trials), performance decrements were observed when knowledge of results was withdrawn. Presumably, the perceptual trace has not stabilized sufficiently under these conditions to guide performance solely.

One other aspect of the data should be noted. Except for the condition in which the removal of knowledge of results did not affect performance, the subjects' estimate of their error was considerably smaller than their actual produced error (Adams, Goetz and Marshall, 1972). Their overconfidence can be interpreted as further evidence that their variability in the task is not the result of performance deficiencies as much as it reflects a weak perceptual trace.

Adams (1971) argues that the perceptual trace by itself provides an insufficient account of how skilled movements are executed. As he writes:

'If the agent that fires the response also is the reference against which the response is tested for correctness, the response must necessarily be judged correct because it is compared against itself. Response activation and evaluation require independent mechanisms.' (pp. 125–126)

Moreover, since the perceptual trace becomes operative in the presence of feedback, it is unclear how movement would be initiated in the absence of feedback. For example: how would volitional movements begin? It can be argued that the logic underlying the first of these problems, the independence dilemma, is justified only if the execution process is assumed to be deterministic. As soon as the implementation of a command is assumed to be variable (Wing and Kristofferson, 1973),

Adams' dilemma disappears. However, the second problem – the need for feedback to render the memory trace operative – cannot be ignored.

The second mechanism of the closed-loop theory is proposed to account for the initiation of skilled actions (Adams, 1971). The memory trace is an independent entity, which serves to select and initiate the response. The memory trace is nonperceptual, requiring neither feedback nor a requisite context in order for its elicitation, although it is reasonable to suppose that these factors will contribute to the selection process. In this sense, the memory trace can be thought of as an abstract motor program (Adams, 1987). Selection of a memory trace will lead to the onset of an action, at which point the skilled execution of the movement will be carried out under the guidance of the error-sensing perceptual trace.

Newell and Chew (1974) tested the two-component aspect of Adams' (1971) theory by equating the perceptual and memory traces with recall and recognition memory processes, respectively. In support of the theory, Newell and Chew (1974) observed a dissociation between the two processes. When knowledge of results was withdrawn, performance (recall) did not deteriorate, but the subjects' estimates of their performance was more erroneous (recognition error). Newell and Chew (1974) view this dissociation as supportive of the hypothesis that the perceptual and memory traces are independent mechanisms.

The closed-loop theory has been criticized on a number of grounds. For instance, experiments have shown that, not only can performance be maintained when knowledge of results is eliminated, but also that subjects are able to show extensive motor learning when knowledge of results is not provided during the initial training period provided that subjects are supplied with an appropriate model of the task (Carroll and Bandura 1982; Newell, 1976). This would imply that significant learning can occur in the absence of movement itself. While the closed-loop theory does not provide a mechanism for this to occur, these results are not dissonant with any of the central tenets of the theory.

Other data, however, are at odds with the basic feature of Adams' theory. Most notable has been research demonstrating that animals and humans are able to produce skilled movements following either permanent or transient deafferentation. Under such conditions, feedback is no longer available for comparison with the perceptual trace and thus the theory would predict severe impairments for all movements, learned or novel. In a series of experiments, Taub and Berman (1968) found that monkeys were able to make unconstrained movements – locomotor, grasping and pointing – following bilateral dorsal root rhizotomy. In addition, the animals were able to learn novel, conditioned responses to avoid shock following deafferentation.

Similar evidence has been obtained with mice (Fentress, 1973), birds (Nottebohm, 1970), human patients (Rothwell *et al.*, 1982; Sanes *et al.*, 1985) and healthy human subjects (Kelso and Holt, 1980; Sanes *et al*, 1985). In the latter study, temporary deafferentation was achieved by reducing blood flow to the forelimb via a pressure cuff. Despite the failure to detect clinically signs of proprioceptive or cutaneous sensitivity, the subjects were able to perform a simple pointing task without a reduction in accuracy. These results mirror those obtained by Bizzi and his colleagues with primates who were surgically deprived of afferent information (Bizzi *et al.*, 1984; Polit and Bizzi 1979). It should be pointed out that the finding of relatively intact abilities following deafferentation is primarily observed with simple pointing tasks. When the movements become more complex or are repeated cyclically, performance tends to deteriorate (Rothwell *et al.*, 1982; Sanes *et al.*, 1985). On the other hand, the support for Adams' theory has been obtained almost entirely with movements as simple as those which are unimpaired following deafferentation. Moreover, the form of the deterioration in deafferented movements is instructive. The basic gestural sequence is maintained but the fine calibration is lost. For example, if trying to touch the thumb to each finger cyclically, the subject will move the effectors in the appropriate sequence but may have difficulty making contact at the distal tips. Adams' theory does not seem amenable to this partial form of deterioration. Rather, the model predicts that deafferentation should also produce a loss in the representation of the sequence.

Adams (1976) has countered that many of the deafferentation studies have involved the deprivation of proprioceptive, kinesthetic and cutaneous sources of feedback. Since the perceptual trace is a composite of all sources of feedback, the remaining inputs (i.e. vision or audition) may be sufficient to guide performance. Some of the more recent studies cited in the previous paragraph included controls in which these secondary sources of feedback were eliminated (Bizzi *et al.*, 1984). A problem which has received little experimental attention, however, is how much learning can occur in the absence of feedback. The study by Taub and Berman (reviewed in 1968) is a notable exception. (Adams (1976), however, points out that other exteroceptive sources of information may have been available to the monkeys.) The other studies with deafferented subjects have almost exclusively focused on whether performance deteriorates, not whether new movements can be learned.

To account for the competence of movements made in the absence of feedback, theorists have postulated open-loop models of motor control. Central to these schemes is the concept of the motor program. As defined by Keele (1981), the motor program is a central representation of an action that can lead to patterned movement in the absence of feedback. The emphasis in this definition should be on central representation, rather than the absence of feedback. Keele (1981) did not deny the importance of feedback in skilled action, arguing that an important component of the program may be in specifying how feedback should be incorporated into the ongoing action. Moreover, feedback is necessary for detecting errors should they occur. Without error detection, the program can continue but it cannot be corrected. Nonetheless, the essential idea of a motor program is that the action is instantiated in an open-loop manner rather than evolving from an interaction between the movement and feedback.

5.1.2 Schmidt's Schema Theory

How are motor programs learned? What do they specify and what is their content? Do they contain a specific description of the pattern of muscular activations needed to achieve an action? Or, perhaps more simply, does the program represent an abstract goal which is implemented via delegation through the various levels of the motor control system? A corollary of these questions concerns the storage and novelty problems which have faced all theories of memory and learning. Should individual motor programs be postulated for every movement within an organism's repertoire? And what of competency? We are capable of performing an infinite number of variations on an action, many instances of which are novel. Does each novel movement require the postulation of a new motor program?

Schmidt (1975, 1988) has put forth a comprehensive learning theory that embraces the notion of the motor program in a generalized form. To avoid the storage and novelty pitfalls that plagued earlier conceptualizations of the motor program, Schmidt (1975) proposed that the motor program did not contain instructions detailing the specifics of a movement, but rather generalized instructions for a given class of movement (see earlier discussion on generalized rate parameters). For example, one generalized motor program might cover how to shoot a jump shot in basketball. While the exact pattern of joint displacements and muscular activations will vary from shot to shot depending on factors such as distance, defense and fatigue, the same motor program will be called upon in each instance, with only certain parameters being free to vary.

Of course, the cost of replacing a single, movement-specific program with a generalized version is the loss of definitional precision. It now becomes incumbent for the theorist to provide a means for defining the extent and boundaries of a generalized motor program. While acknowledging this problem, Schmidt (1975) chooses to emphasize that the important point of the generalized motor program is that there is no longer a one-to-one match between motor programs and specific movements. It is this feature that provides for a natural link between a theory of movement execution and movement learning.

For the foundation of his learning theory, Schmidt (1975) has borrowed a concept that has proven useful to memory and perception researchers for over 50 years: the representational entity of the schema (Attneave, 1959; Bartlett, 1932; Posner and Keele, 1968). Like the generalized motor program, the schema is an abstract representational structure. In perceptual learning research (Posner and Keele, 1968), schemas refer to the composite memory that accrues following the presentation of a series of exemplars. The schema does not correspond to any specific exemplar but, rather, is a (weighted) composite in which the consistent and salient features have been abstracted. Storage demands are thus reduced since the specifics of a stimulus can be discarded once the essential features have been distilled and matched to stored schemata.

Schmidt (1975) brought the concept of the schema into the domain of movement. Rather than an abstraction over a set of stimuli, the motor response schema was postulated as an abstraction of the relationship between a set of stimuli and a corresponding set of actions. Moreover, the schema is not simply synonymous with the generalized motor program. Rather, it encompasses four sources of information:

(1) the initial conditions which serve to help select the appropriate action and are retained for movement evaluation;
(2) the specific response parameters generated to accomplish a given action;
(3) the sensory consequences associated with the response; and
(4) the response outcome, a cognitive source of feedback in which the response is evaluated in comparison with the desired action goal.

The schema is an abstraction of the functional relationship between these four sources of information, a way to link input conditions to an appropriate action. Thus, skill acquisition is the process in which experience allows the performer to form relationships between how muscles are activated and the end result of these activations (Schmidt, 1988). By relating the movement to the initial conditions, online feedback and knowledge of results, the schema is a malleable structure. The

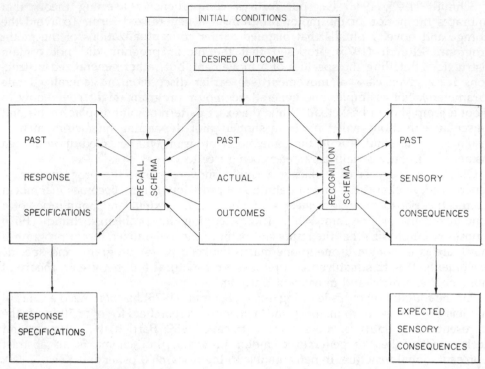

Figure 5.9. *Overview of schema theory of motor learning showing the component parts and sources of information. [From Schmidt, 1975.]*

basic notion of the generalized motor program did not contain a mechanism for learning (but see Keele and Summers, 1976).

Schmidt (1975) further partitions the schema into two subcomponents: the recall and the recognition schema (Figure 5.9). The recall schema is demanded for the selection of a specific response, not only from the repertoire of generalized motor programs (i.e. selection among schemata), but also for the programming of a specific response in a given situation (i.e. selection among the possible parameter-izations of a chosen generalized motor program). Two sources of information – the initial conditions and the desired goal – serve as input for the recall schema. When coupled with the person's memory of previous response specifications in similar situations, the movement is generated. In contrast, the recognition schema is important for the person to be able to evaluate the outcome of the movement. Here, the past sensory consequences and outcomes are coupled with the initial conditions to generate a representation of expected sensory consequences. This representation can then be compared with the inflow of sensory information both during and after the movement in order for the person to determine whether the response was successful or not. While the recognition schema bears a strong resemblance to the perceptual trace of Adams' theory (1971), its current usage is primarily for learning purposes rather than online control. The error signal is fed back into the schema, leading to modifications in the relationships between initial conditions and response specifications. Thus, sensory feedback is used analogously to knowledge of results (see Salmoni, Schmidt and Walter, 1984, for a review on the efficacy of knowledge of results). The learning process involves the continuous updating of the schema, a memory structure that initially emerged as a composite of numerous instances.

Schmidt (1975) argues that the strength of schema theory is its generality. The same model can be applied to fast and slow movements as well as to movements that occur in fixed contexts or those that take place in an unstable environment. For example, the same generalized motor program can be instantiated whenever a basketball player opts to shoot a jump shot, but the varying initial conditions, coupled with knowledge of the effects of these conditions on previous attempts, will lead to the appropriate response specification. Success in completing a novel shot such as a fade-away, arching shot over a seven-foot defender does not require a pre-existing perceptual trace of this movement. These initial conditions will yield a novel response. Note that the outcome may not be successful. The shot will most likely miss, perhaps because the schema does not have any stored information relating these conditions to successful response specifications. The important point here, however, is that novelty and versatility can be attributed to other (nonmotoric) components of the model rather than require an infinite number of motor programs or retained perceptual traces.

A strong prediction of schema theory is that variable practice will prove most effective in the long-term development of a stable schema. The basic paradigm used to test this prediction has been to train two sets of subjects. One group practices with a variable set of responses and the second group practices a constant response. Both groups are then transferred to a similar movement. Schema theory predicts that the variable practice group will be more competent on the novel task.

Hogan (1977) and McCracken and Stelmach (1977) utilized a linear movement task in which movement time was fixed and only the distance moved was varied. Both studies found that error was lower on a transfer task for subjects who were given variable practice. However, Zelaznik (1977) has argued that the design in these and many other similar studies confounds practice conditions with the degree of similarity between the transfer task and the practice tasks. Some of the movements in the variable practice conditions were more similar to the transfer task than the constant tasks. After controlling for this confound, Zelaznik found no difference in performance between variable and constant practice.

Developmental studies have also utilized this basic paradigm. Kelso and Norman (1978) tested three-year-olds on a task in which an object was propelled down a track with the goal being to have the object stop at a target location. When transferred to a novel distance, practice with a variable set of distances proved superior to practice with a single distance. This result was obtained regardless of whether the transfer distance was within the range of distances that the variable group had experienced or outside this range. Similarly, Kerr and Booth (1977) trained seven- and nine-year-olds to toss beanbags over either a variable distance or a single distance. When transferred to a new distance, the variable-practice group performed significantly better. More surprisingly, this same result was obtained even when the transfer distance was the same as that practiced by the constant-practice group (see also Carson and Wiegand, 1979; Kerr and Booth, 1977). This finding is in conflict with any prediction that would be formulated on the basis of Adams' closed-loop theory.

In a review paper, Shapiro and Schmidt (1982) concluded that, while the variable-practice prediction has received only mixed support in studies with adult subjects, experiments with children have consistently favored the prediction. Reconciling this inconsistency is problematic. One argument has been that the relatively small amount of variable practice given in the typical experiment pales in comparison with the variable practice that people experience in everyday life. Thus, adults benefit little from the artificial laboratory manipulation since their schemata are already well developed (Shapiro and Schmidt, 1982). Nonetheless, this argument fails to account for why learning does occur for both young and adult subjects in these experiments. In addition, in a meta-analysis, van Rossum (1990) questions the solidity of the conclusions regarding children.

In summary, Schmidt's (1975) schema theory has brought the area of motor control into the mainstream of cognitive psychology in terms of a conceptual explanation of learning. Learning is not viewed as a process in which every event or action is uniquely stored (as postulated in Logan's, 1988, theory). Instead, a generalized representation, the schema, provides the essential features, adding on the specific characteristics as a function of the context in which the action emerges. The model is quite broad, recognizing that a diverse set of information processing interactions takes place during the course of skilled action. Furthermore, unlike the closed-loop theory reviewed previously, the model seems sufficiently general that it can be applied beyond simple, discrete movements to complex skills which involve a series of movements.

However, perhaps because of its breadth, the theory lacks rigor and specificity. While some of the component parts may contain recognizable mechanisms such as the efference copy of the recognition schema, most of the theory is stated in terms well above a level that would lead to mechanistic explanations. For example, the manner in which the information from the different sources interact is unspecified. A similar reflection of the lack of concreteness is the fact that no formal version has been proposed for the theory in its entirety or for any of the component parts. The schema theory appears to capture the versatility of human motor competence in general terms. It remains unclear, however, how the outcome of schema processing, the response-specification process, leads to movement and how that movement is controlled.

In a series of recent studies, Koh and Meyer (1989, 1991) have attempted to develop a more rigorous analysis of the development of motor schema. They restate the problem as a case of inductive learning: the schema is a means to represent a functional relationship between a continuum of related stimulus conditions and the responses associated with these conditions. Since it is not possible to practice with all possible initial conditions, task competence requires the ability to generalize across the whole continuum. Thus, it is necessary to induce the functional relationship on the basis of limited experience.

Koh and Meyer (1989, 1991) use a simple paradigm to examine this induction problem. The stimulus continuum was defined as the horizontal distance between two vertical lines. The response continuum was defined as the duration between two key presses. Subjects were instructed that the target response duration was a function of the stimulus distance (e.g. length between the two lines) and their task was to learn the exact relationship. Although the movements are quite simple in this task, it is conceptually similar to much of the previous work on variable practice. For example, the beanbag-tossing task of Kerr and Booth (1977) also required that the subjects learn the relationship between a perceived distance and the action mapped to that distance.

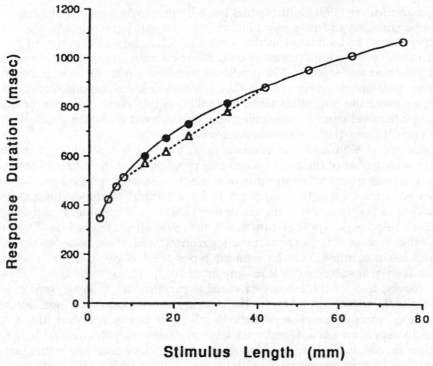

Figure 5.10. *Stimulus–response pairs for inductive learning experiment:* ○, *training pairs;* ●, *transfer pairs;* △, *predicted performance on the transfer trials if subjects use simple linear interpolation.* [*From Koh and Meyer, 1991.*]

In experiment 1 of Koh and Meyer (1991), the exact relationship was a power function: duration = 257.42 × length$^{0.33}$. The stimulus–response pairs are depicted in Figure 5.10. Subjects were initially trained with eight stimulus–response pairs, four from each end of the range. The critical question centered on their performance during transfer trials in which intermediate stimulus lengths were presented. Would the schema represent the exact relationship, the power function? Or would the schema involve a systematic distortion? Koh and Meyer formally derive a set of competing predictions based on different assumptions as to the constraints underlying schema formation. For example, simple linear interpolation between the stimulus–response pairs that border the transfer region would predict responses that fall on the dotted line of Figure 5.10.

The results were compeling. Subjects quickly learned the appropriate response durations during training. Moreover, performance was unimpaired on the transfer trials. Subjects were as accurate in responding to the novel stimulus lengths as they were in responding to the practiced lengths. There are at least two possible interpretations of these results. Subjects may have induced the power relationship, enabling them to perform accurately on the transfer trials. Alternatively, there may be a natural bias toward producing a power relationship and thus learning was facilitated because the experimenters used this function. In this case, the requirements for learning would be reduced to extracting the task-defined exponent for the power function.

Koh and Meyer (1991) address this issue by employing other functions relating the same stimulus and response dimensions. A logarithmic relationship was used in experiment 2 and a linear function with a positive slope in experiment 3. In both experiments, there were systematic distortions on both training and transfer trials during the first few sessions. The produced response durations were biased toward a power function. However, over the last few sessions, the response functions came to approximate the target functions. Note that, at this point, the transfer trials are no longer to novel stimuli. The subjects have completed numerous trials with these lengths on transfer trials in the earlier sessions.

The work of Koh and Meyer offers great promise for providing a means for making strong tests of the assumptions and predictions of the schema theory. Their study provides quantitative insights into the process of response specification. As shown with their task, there appears to be a natural tendency toward relating stimulus and response continua via power functions. Experiments utilizing other stimulus–response mappings can assess the generality of this bias. Despite this bias, subjects were able to abstract the logarithmic and linear relationships. Future research can determine constraints on the types of relationship that can be learned; it is unlikely that subjects can learn any arbitrary function.

Moreover, tests of the efficacy of variable practice can be reassessed given the analytic tools of Koh and Meyer. If the stimulus–response pairings selected for constant or variable practice conditions fall on a power function, there is little reason to expect an advantage for variable practice given the natural bias for this function. Indeed, typical studies of variable practice have used linear functions with an intercept of zero – a special case of a power function where the exponent equals one. However, if the stimulus–response pairings are defined by a different function, then variable practice appears to be essential for successful transfer. Constant practice may not provide sufficient stimulus–response pairings for the subjects to induce the relationship, whereas variable practice could. However, the advantage of variable practice would not become evident until sufficient trials had been completed for the subjects to abstract this relationship and overcome the bias toward a power function. The finding that the advantage of variable practice is most evident in research with children may reflect the fact that biases are not well established in these subjects.

5.2   Neural Models of Motor Learning

Eccles (1986) argues that the study of motor learning encompasses three distinct classes of phenomena. The first class includes the learning of automatic movements such as those involved in eye movements or conditioned reflexes. The second and third classes include all other motor skills and are arbitrarily distinguished by those that can be learned by animals (the second class) and those that are only observed in human behavior (the third class). In Eccles' scheme, a continuum is formed in terms of the degree of consciousness required for the learning of the movements within a class. Eccles (1986) points out that very little is known about the neural basis of the highest class of motor learning. He assumes that the neural basis for learning advanced skills is not discontinuous from the processes involved in the learning of simple movements. Rather, increased neocortical participation supplements those subcortical structures that dominate the learning of more primitive skills. Nonetheless, a comprehensive neural theory of advanced skill learning is lacking (but see Goldberg, 1985, for a model based primarily on neuroanatomic considerations). Thus, the focus of this section will be on neural models of simple motor learning.

The cerebellum has long been known to play an essential role in the execution of coordinated movements (Holmes, 1939). Lesions in the cerebellum cause disturbances in both postural and volitional movements. The latter are characterized by intentional tremor, dysmetria (inability to match movement end-point to target location) and dysadiochokinesia – the inability to produce rapid alternating movements. Interestingly, cerebellar lesions have not been associated with apraxia. The patients appear to know what the proper movement is for a given situation and are able to activate the appropriate muscles. However, the metrics are askew. This perhaps could be a cardinal sign of a deficit in pure 'motor learning'. The cognitive intent for movement and the overall structure is intact, but the patient is unable to accurately implement a plan of action.

5.2.1 Marr–Albus Model of Cerebellar Learning

Marr (1969; Bloomfield and Marr, 1970) and Albus (1971) independently developed theories of cerebellar motor learning, drawing their initial inspiration from anatomy. While densely packed with approximately 50% of all the neurons in the central nervous system, the organization of the cerebellar cortex is homogeneous and simple. The Purkinje cells are the only output cells of the cerebellar cortex. There are two major input sources to the Purkinje cells: the parallel and the climbing fibers, originating in the pontine (via mossy fibers) and olivary nuclei, respectively. Whereas each Purkinje cell may have dendritic synapses with up to 200 000 parallel fibers, only a single climbing fiber will terminate in the dendritic tree of a Purkinje cell. The parallel and climbing fibers also differ in terms of their respective physiological effects. Parallel fibers produce small, local increases in the membrane potential of the Purkinje cell – a response that is called the simple spike. In contrast, activation of a climbing fiber produces a complex spike, a strong response which leads to an action potential in the Purkinje cell.

The Marr–Albus model assumes that most of the normal output from the Purkinje cells is the result of summated parallel fiber input. The array of parallel fibers arriving on a Purkinje cell are hypothesized to convey a multimodal representation of the current state of the organism as well as information from premotor association areas (Ito, 1984). This input leads the animal to select the appropriate parameters for action.

The central tenet of the Marr–Albus learning hypothesis is that synapses between the parallel fibers and the Purkinje cells are modified under the guidance of the climbing fiber system. The two models differ in the specific role they place on the climbing fiber system. Marr (1969; Bloomfield and Marr, 1970) argues for a facilitatory role. As a movement is rehearsed, complex spikes will strengthen currently active parallel fiber–Purkinje cell synapses. The mechanism proposed by Albus (1971) has the opposite effect. The complex spikes provide an error signal leading to a process that reduces the strength of recently active parallel fiber–Purkinje cell synapses. For example, olivary cells in the cat produce complex spikes when an unexpected obstacle is encountered during the course of voluntary movement, but remain silent if the same stimulus is expected (Gelman, Houk and Gibson, 1985; Schwartz, Ebner and Bloedel, 1987). This complex spike is postulated to inhibit the mossy fiber pattern from producing the erroneous response in the future.

Despite the difference in the predicted direction of synaptic modifiability, Marr and Albus are in agreement on the basic features of their learning theories. The cerebellum is essentially viewed as a pattern recognition device and the essential motor learning takes place in the cerebellar cortex. The patterns are transmitted via the mossy fiber system and are matched to appropriate actions through the interaction of the parallel fibers and Purkinje cells. The climbing fibers play a feedback role. The massive number of parallel fiber–Purkinje cell synapses enables this structure to learn the near-infinite number of contexts that will be encountered over the course of an animal's life. The appropriate response can thus be tailored to match a specific context. Marr (1969) calculated that a single Purkinje cell should be able to learn up to 200 different mossy fiber input patterns without appreciable confusion. Combining this figure with the density of Purkinje cells, Albus (1971) estimates the pattern-expansion capacity of a square millimeter of cerebellar cortex to be in the order of $50^{50\,000}$. The computational and memorial ability of such a system would be immense, even if only a small fraction of the capacity were tapped. Albus (1971) argues that a similar capability is not found in the cerebral cortex, perhaps because the computational goals of this structure are quite distinct.

Experimental tests of the Marr–Albus hypothesis of motor learning have presented technological and logical challenges to cerebellar researchers. Twenty years after the original conjectures, the hypothesis remains controversial. Two aspects of the hypothesis can be tested. First, the neurophysiologist can investigate the degree of plasticity of the cerebellar cortex. Second, the behavioral neuroscientist can determine the importance of the cerebellum in motor learning vis à vis other neural structures in the motor pathways.

5.2.2   Modification of the Vestibular–Ocular Reflex

One behavior that has received extensive study is the vestibular–ocular reflex (VOR). The VOR effectively maintains visual image stability by producing eye movements that counteract head movements. For example, when the head rotates to the left, the eyes must move toward the right in order to maintain fixation of an object. Ito (1984) has proposed that the cerebellum is essential in long-term calibration of the gain and phase of the VOR. In other words, Ito argues that the cerebellum ensures that the metrics of the reflexive eye movements will succeed in maintaining fixation across the range of possible stimuli.

The VOR has been a favorite tool for studying motor learning because of its adaptability. A striking demonstration of this was performed by Gonshor and Melville-Jones (1976; see also Ito *et al.*, 1974). These researchers had human subjects wear prism glasses which produced a left–right reversal of the visual world. When tested in the dark, the gain of the VOR of these subjects rapidly adapted. Whereas the normal gain values hover around 0.90, the reversible glasses led to a rapid decrease in the gain and gradual phase shifts. The effect of these two changes was functionally adaptive: in tracking a visible object, the new values would be relatively effective at maintaining image stability whereas an unadapted VOR under reversing conditions would cause the image to move at nearly twice the speed in the opposite direction of a head movement.

Ito (1984) reviews lesion and physiological evidence in support of the hypothesis that the flocculus, a posterior lobe of the cerebellum, is essential for VOR plasticity (see Lisberger and Pavelko, 1988, for an alternative view of VOR adaptation). Large lesions which include the flocculus prevent modification of the VOR (Ito *et al.*, 1974) as do focal lesions produced by application of kainic acid (cited in Ito, 1984). Moreover, recordings from flocculus Purkinje cells during VOR adaptation show large phase shifts in simple spike activity (Watanabe, 1984). Thus, in agreement with the Marr–Albus hypothesis, the learned response was correlated with simple spike activity. That this change in responsiveness is brought about by climbing fiber activity is less clear and currently rests on indirect evidence. Similar recordings of complex spikes have shown that this activity is modulated in opposite phase of simple spike activity. While causality could logically proceed in either direction, Ito (1984) assumes that climbing fiber activity produces the shift in simple spike activity.

5.2.3 Other Evidence for a Cerebellar Role in Motor Learning

In addition to the work on adaptation of the VOR, a second paradigm has focused on the role of the cerebellum in learning associated with reflexive behavior. Laboratories headed by Thompson (reviewed in Thompson *et al.*, 1984; see also Thompson, 1986) and Yeo (Yeo, Hardiman and Glickstein, 1985) have studied classic conditioning of the nictitating membrane response (NMR) in the rabbit. For example, McCormick and Thompson (1984) trained rabbits to retract the nictitating membrane following the presentation of a tone (the conditioned stimulus, CS) to avoid an aversive puff of air (the unconditioned stimulus, US). Initially, the CS was uninformative to the animal and thus the animal made an NMR only after the US. With repeated pairing, however, the rabbits learned to make a conditioned response (CR) prior to the onset of the US in order to avoid the aversive puff of air. The unconditioned response (UR) would still occur, but it was now manifest on top of the CR.

The advantage of this paradigm in comparison with the VOR adaptation work is that there are two independent responses. The UR is assumed to depend on a simple reflex arc whereas the learned CR involves other networks that are subject to modification. Thus, it is possible that a dissociation can be made between the neural systems necessary for performance and those necessary for learning. A lesion which impairs only the learning and/or memory processes would be expected to have an effect only on the CR.

The work of these two research teams has emphasized that cerebellar lesions produce a selective effect on the learned response (but see Welsh and Harvey, 1989). Whereas the UR is relatively unaffected, cerebellar lesions can lead to complete and permanent abolition of the CR (Figure 5.11). Effective lesions can be restricted to

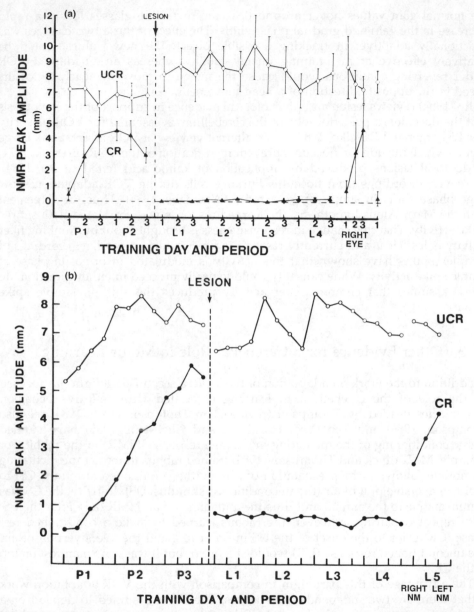

Figure 5.11. *Effects of cerebellar lesions on conditioned and unconditioned responses of the nictitating membrane reflex with the left eye. (a) Effects of lesions of the cerebellar cortex; (b) effects of lesions of the cerebellar nuclei. Note that learning occurs when training commences with the right eye. [From Thompson* et al., *1984.]*

either the cerebellar nuclei (McCormick and Thompson, 1984) or the cortex (Yeo, Hardiman and Glickstein, 1985). Thompson and colleagues (Thompson, 1986; Thompson *et al.*, 1984) have worked through a series of experiments to delineate the memory trace circuits involved in the learned NMR. Both Purkinje and nuclear cells undergo response modification which mirrors the learned response. These cells are initially activated just prior to the onset of the UR. After learning, the activation precedes the CR.

Stimulation experiments have supported the hypothesis that the mossy and climbing fibers convey the CS (Lavond *et al.*, 1987) and US (Mauk, Steinmetz and Thompson, 1986) information, respectively. Furthermore, extinction has been reported following lesions of the olive (McCormick, Steinmetz and Thompson, 1985). Thus, the essential ingredients for classic conditioning are apparent in the two major afferent systems that feed into the cerebellum. Since their first point of convergence is in the cerebellar cortex, it seems most parsimonious that this would be the source of learning.

The VOR adaptation and NMR conditioning research offer excellent paradigms for the study of the neural basis of motor learning. The experiments reviewed above are in accord with theoretical views of how motor learning could occur. The evidence and theory emphasize the role of the cerebellum as an adaptive device for long-term learning (but see Lisberger and Pavelko, 1988).

These preparations fall within the first class of motor learning in Eccles' (1986) scheme: the learning of automatic or conditioned reflexes. It remains to be seen whether the neural basis for more complex motor learning is built upon the same mechanisms or whether distinct processes are involved. Two primate studies involving the learning of arm movements have reported results demonstrating plasticity in the cerebellar pathways during the learning of voluntary arm movements. Gilbert and Thach (1977) recorded from Purkinje cells while animals learned a one-dimensional forearm movement task. As predicted by Albus (1971), a depression in simple spike activity was observed following learning. More recently, Ebner (1989) has utilized a two-dimensional movement task in which the input–output gain relationship can be changed. His preliminary results show that climbing fiber activity is high during the period of recalibration, thus supporting the hypothesis that this information serves as an error signal for learning.

The role of the cerebellum in human learning of complex skills has received scant attention. Certainly cerebellar lesions in humans can lead to severe coordination problems. However, the critical research with patients has not yet been done which dissociates performance from learning deficits.

5.2.4 Timing in Motor Learning

The Marr–Albus hypothesis centers on two critical features. First, the pattern of divergence and convergence within the cerebellar cortex is amenable for learning large numbers of input patterns. Second, the distinct climbing and mossy fiber inputs are suitable for a learning process, perhaps based on error detection and correction (Albus, 1971). A third feature of at least some, if not all, types of motor learning is not explicitly captured by the model. Many adaptive responses have precise temporal requirements. For example, the rabbit learns to make an avoidance response, the NMR, following the presentation of a CS. However, the CR is not time-locked to the CS, but rather to the US. In the Thompson paradigm, the CS–US interval is 550 ms. In the Yeo paradigm, the CS–US interval is 250 ms. In either situation, the conditioned NMR is most adaptive if the response approaches peak amplitude just prior to the presentation of the US in order to minimize the aversive effects of the airpuff. This is exactly what happens. Thus, even if the CR is triggered by the CS, the animal must have the flexibility in terms of timing the CS–CR interval.[4]

Keele and Ivry (1991) have argued that the cerebellum can be characterized as an internal timing mechanism (see also Braitenberg, 1967). They hypothesize that, at least for movements that are temporally constrained, the cerebellum provides the necessary timing computations. Moreover, the timing capabilities of the cerebellum extend beyond the motor domain. Perceptual tasks that require timing also utilize the cerebellar timing system. Patients with cerebellar lesions were found to be impaired in comparing the durations of two successive intervals (Ivry and Keele, 1989) and in judging the velocity of a moving stimulus, even when fixation was maintained (summarized in Keele and Ivry, 1991). While a timing deficit is sufficient to account for many of the motor problems seen in cerebellar disorders, alternative explanations are possible. However, evidence that these lesions also impair perceptual processes that require accurate timing makes the timing hypothesis most parsimonious.

Keele and Ivry (1991) postulate that the timing capabilities of the cerebellum are another unique feature of this neural structure which makes it essential for learning. In its current form, the Marr–Albus hypothesis serves as a useful model for associating input and output patterns (see also Pellionisz and Llinas, 1982). Skilled action, however, is not a matter of simply chaining together inputs and outputs. Temporal requirements and constraints, such as those seen in classic conditioning of the NMR, must also be captured by the learning mechanism. The evidence (Ivry and Keele, 1989) suggests that the cerebellum is capable of providing the necessary computations. Combining a timing function with pattern recognition and error detection/correction mechanisms would make the cerebellum a powerful tool for motor learning.

However, the kind of information represented by the cerebellum and the putative computations performed by this system probably limits the types of learning that it encompasses. The VOR and NMR are highly context dependent. When calibrated correctly, the VOR is perfectly coupled to the stimulus. Similarly, as argued above, the NMR is only adaptive if timed precisely to anticipate the aversive stimulus. Motor learning in these cases is of concrete actions. The loss of coordination following cerebellar lesions in humans can similarly be characterized as a breakdown in the coupling of the various components of an action sequence. The person is able to activate the appropriate muscles to reach for a glass of water, but is unable smoothly to coordinate the grasping actions of the hand with the extensions of the arm.

In contrast, there is no evidence that the cerebellum is involved in the establishment of abstract, hierarchical structures of action sequences of the sort emphasized in the first half of this review. It is reasonable to suppose that other neural systems are essential for the more abstract aspects of motor learning. Precise timing capabilities would probably not be an essential feature of these systems since the

---

[4]While the change in gain during VOR adaptation has received the most attention, a phase shift is also observed. It is unclear, however, whether the temporal properties of this latter process need be explicitly represented in an analogous manner to the NMR. There are at least two ways in which a phase shift could be implemented. One method would be to remap input–output relationships – there need be no explicit timing computation if the delay between inputs and outputs remains constant. The second method would be to retain old mappings but vary the delay between inputs and outputs. This method would require some sort of explicit timing mechanism.

representation is independent of any specific implementation. Similarly, systems that learn abstract relationships may not need access to a precise representation of the stimulus and context associated with an action. Systems lower down in the hierarchy, including the cerebellum, could implement the abstract plan into a specific action.

5.3   Computational Models of Motor Learning

A third theoretical approach to the study of motor learning has emerged from research in the field of artificial intelligence (AI), or specifically, robotics. Dexterous machines have been developed which can accomplish everything from mundane, assembly-line tasks to much more complex actions such as navigating through a room littered with objects. The emphasis in this work has been on developing efficient control algorithms. What variable(s) need be computed in order to plan an action? Are separate controllers needed for each effector or action? Should sensory information be used in providing online control? The issue of learning was even less evident in computer science during the 1970s and early '80s than in experimental psychology. Intuitively, it appeared that learning was one area in which the machine would be hard pressed to lend insight into biological capabilities.

Recent computational work has begun to question the wisdom of this belief. A number of computer models of learning have been presented. The motivation for this work is twofold. First, many AI researchers utilize computer models as a way of studying biological information processing. Since adaptability is a central feature of living organisms, the processes that underlie learning cannot be ignored by any model which hopes to capture the breadth of biological competence. Second, a robotics model that does not encompass learning will always require a human programmer for building in the movement plans that make up the robot's repertoire. A dynamic area of AI research centers on how robot programming can be incrementally automated. Thus, the issue of learning can no longer be ignored.

5.3.1   Atkeson's Adaptive Model of the Effector System

Atkeson (1987, 1989) has presented a theory of robotic motor learning. Following the wisdom of Marr (1982), Atkeson has carefully developed the model on three fronts. First, he considers the computational goals of a learning theory. Second, he explores possible algorithms for achieving those goals. Only then does he consider how these algorithms might be implemented: the current research focuses on machine implementations, but Atkeson (1989) acknowledges the need for biological testing.

Atkeson (1987; see also Hollerbach, 1990) starts by partitioning the motor control problem into two components. One component involves planning – the process of specifying an action in a task coordinate space. Planning can be described in macroscopic terms (e.g. ride a bicycle) or at a more microlevel of description (e.g. the trajectory needed to move my arm from point A to point B). The second component is movement execution. The plan needs to be converted from task to effector coordinates and there needs to be a method for generating the commands required to propel the effector. This method may involve feedback, feedforward or hybrid strategies (Hollerbach, 1990).

The effects of learning can similarly be partitioned. The planning component can obviously be improved by the use of better plans. Atkeson (1987) does not address this issue other than to point out that these learning mechanisms can be assumed to be independent of mechanisms contributing to movement execution learning. This latter form of learning can be effected in a number of ways. For example, the internal model of the context in which an action occurs can be improved by enriching the representation. Feedback can be made more efficacious by using an adaptive feedback controller which incorporates the effects of previous corrections (see Astrom, 1983).

The focus of Atkeson's current model (1987, 1989) is on how improvements can be built into a third subcomponent of the execution system: the feedforward controller. Motor learning can be used in two distinct ways. First, movements (and postural sensing) can be used to build and refine internal models of the motor apparatus. Second, these internal models can be used to transform performance errors into command corrections.

The ideal feedforward controller requires a model of the systems dynamics, or more precisely, a model of the inverse of the system (Atkeson, 1987). This dynamical model is essential for transforming information about kinematics (i.e. trajectories) into mechanically useful information regarding the required forces and torques (Hollerbach, 1990). An inverse dynamic transformation could produce a set of joint forces which in turn produce a linear displacement of a distal effector from one position to another. These transformations are limited by the accuracy of the internal model. If the model is poor or unstable, the subsequent transformations will mirror these inaccuracies.

Control schemes that require accurate internal models have generally been criticized in the AI literature as implausible in that the input requirements for building the models are too extensive. Atkeson (1987), however, observes that the prerequisites for developing a stable model of effector dynamics are not extensive. Data obtained from exploratory movements and postures can provide all of the necessary information for estimating the relatively small set of inertial parameters that describe the dynamics. The computations are further simplified by the fact that the parameters appear linear in the dynamical equations. These inertial parameters (i.e. mass, center of mass, moments of inertia) can be estimated given a system capable of sensing peripheral forces and torques as well as information concerning position, velocity and acceleration during movement. All of these inputs seem biologically plausible.

Atkeson's (1987) current implementation involves a threefold process. First, the algorithm is applied to estimate the inertial parameters associated with any load the system may encounter. Thus, the computations center on the most distal aspect of the effector system. A basketball-playing robot, for example, might manipulate a basketball to determine the characteristics of the robot hand. Then, the same process is applied to estimate the inertial parameters associated with each of the proximal segments of the effector system such as the upper 'limbs'. The only additional computational problem here is that the effects from distal segments need to be summed and transmitted to the more proximal segments. The third process is a filtering method for improving the parameter estimation processes. Certain inputs such as velocity and acceleration tend to be noisy and would thus lead to parameter estimation errors. Optimal, nonlinear filtering is one technique for reducing the effects of this obstacle.

An internal model of the system dynamics is global in the sense that it allows for powerful generalization (Atkeson, 1987, 1989). As long as the structure of the internal model matches the actual motor system, the same model can be used for all types of movement. If the load is changed, the internal model can be rapidly updated since only a few parameters need to be re-estimated. Once re-estimated, the new parameters will apply to all movements made with that load. Such generalization is not possible with robotic schemes of motor learning based on a table look-up strategy (Albus, 1971; Pellionisz and Llinas, 1982; Raibert, 1978). In these implementations, the system stores a set of input–output mappings. Generalization to a novel movement is only achieved by interpolating between movements that are retained in memory. Thus, these types of models only allow for generalization between similar movements (Atkeson, 1987). Load changes require storage of a completely different set of input–output mappings. A global, internal model is much more flexible. The model can be built up through one set of movements and then be tested with a dissimilar set of movements.

The drawback to global modeling is that any error is maintained throughout the domain of the model. To overcome this problem, Atkeson (1987) proposes a second, local level of modeling. This local model is nested within the global model. Error information from a movement can be used to tune the global model, at least in a way which will improve performance on subsequent executions of that particular movement.

The algorithm for correcting specific trajectories is based on three processes. First, the feedforward controller issues a set of commands in order to execute a movement. As with all movements, the commands are originally in kinematic form of a trajectory. Second, the movement is executed after the trajectory commands are translated through inverse dynamics into actuator commands. Third, the feedforward controller is modified on the basis of the outcome of the movement. Atkeson (1987) assumes the existence of a correct actuator command history, that is, a representation of an error-free set of commands. However, the internal model is not error-free and thus the movement will not be perfectly accurate. An error signal could be obtained either by comparing the current commands to the correct commands or, if the global model is assumed to be linear, by directly comparing the actual trajectory to the correct commands. The latter method is favored by Atkeson (1987) since the computations are based directly on the actual feedback signal. The difference between the actual trajectory and the correct commands then constitutes an error signal which can be used to update the current model. The error will be smaller on subsequent trials since the current model is always modified so as to reduce the difference between the two signals.

Atkeson (1987, 1989) emphasizes the strengths of this approach. First, the inverse dynamical model is specified as the only learning operator. It is developed globally and then applied and tuned locally. The trajectory learning algorithm converges rapidly regardless of whether the error is the result of an imperfect model, external disturbances or noisy information processing. The local process makes explicit use of feedback information but does not require a specific feedback operator. Any operator will work since only the output is required for the comparison process.

The algorithm, however, depends on two strong assumptions. First, the error is assumed to be solely the result of a faulty model. While Atkeson (1987) acknowledges that there are other potential sources of error, he assumes that the modeling errors outweigh sensing errors or disturbance errors. Evidence for this assumption is not provided and may not be possible given differences in units between model error and other types of error. Second, the algorithm requires that the actor has knowledge of the correct actuator commands. Thus, there must be at least two independent representations: knowledge of what the system needs to do and knowledge of what the system can do as encompassed in the current dynamical model.

More recently, Atkeson (1989) has modified the process so that the error signal is derived by comparing the final position achieved with the desired position and then working back to a kinematic description of the joint angles that would correspond to these positions (see Bullock and Grossberg, 1988, for a similar scheme in which error is only computed at the end of a movement). Here, the correct commands would only have to correspond to the accurate perception of the desired position. This modification, however, produces two new difficulties. First, the information used to modify trajectories would no longer be in kinematic form. Second, transforming the information into kinematic form would require an inverse kinematic model (Hollerbach, 1990). Atkeson (1989) has pointed out that such models present difficult calibration problems, especially for biological systems.

5.3.2   Jordan's Connectionist Model of Sequence Learning

Atkeson has focused on modeling single movements between a starting position and a final position. The model is not intended to simulate a sequence of actions between a series of target positions. Presumably, this process would entail computing independent trajectories for each of the segments of the sequence. In contrast, Jordan (1986, 1990; Jordan and Rosenbaum, 1989) has started with the goal of modeling sequential behavior. In order to do this, he has adopted a different computational architecture which encompasses the processes and constraints necessary to achieve this goal.

The architecture is a variant of a connectionist model. As in the Atkeson and Marr–Albus model, a set of input units is linked to output units. The inputs may correspond to sensory patterns (Albus, 1971) or task goals (Atkeson, 1989) and the learning process involves learning the mapping between the inputs and outputs. As with most connectionist models, Jordan includes an additional level of units – the hidden layer–that acts as an intermediary between the inputs and outputs. All of the input units are connected to each hidden unit and every hidden unit is connected to each output unit. The strengths of these connections are adjustable. Learning involves modifying these connections on the basis of an error signal that is generated following each cycle of the model. One way of thinking about the representation embodied in the hidden units is as representing combinations of inputs. The inclusion of an intermediate level is what gives a connectionist system its power as a learning system. The hidden layer transforms the system from that of a linear associator to a system that is capable of learning nonlinear associations (Rumelhart, Hinton and McClelland, 1986).

The sequence learning model proposed by Jordan (1990) is shown in Figure 5.12. This model contains a number of features which differ from the basic connectionist scheme. Jordan's model contains two distinct types of input units. One set of inputs is labeled the plan units. The vector of activation across these units represents the plan for a given sequence of actions. For example, there would be one pattern of

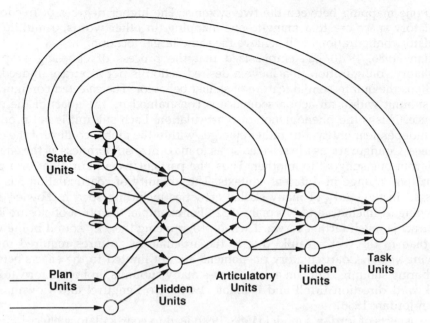

Figure 5.12. *Overview of a connectionist model for learning sequential movements. Nodes represent the units of the network and arrows indicate the connections. [From Jordan, 1990.]*

activity in the plan units representing an action sequence that travels from point 1 to point 2 to point 3. A second pattern would represent the reverse path; a third the path from point 2 to point 1 to point 3. The plan units are activated at the beginning of the execution of the sequence and are fixed. They do not change their output while the sequence is being executed. The state units reflect the changing context of the action. The connections from the target units allow the state units to be continually updated as the action unfolds. Thus, each part of the sequence occurs within a specific context. Moreover, as shown in Figure 5.12, each state unit contains autoconnections and is linked with the other state units. These features build a continuity property into the system (Jordan, 1990). This ensures that the output from the state units will not change radically from one cycle to the next.

A second unique feature of Jordan's connectionist model (1990) is the upper layer of connectivity between the articulatory units and the target units. This feature is necessary because of the problem domain modeled by Jordan. As seen in the discussion of Atkeson's model, motor control is complicated by the fact that different coordinate spaces are required for the enunciation of movement goals and the actions which achieve those goals. The plan and state units issue signals coded in terms of task space. In Jordan's simulations (1990) these correspond to points in a two-dimensional Cartesian coordinate space. These task-space coordinates are represented by the two target units. The actions, though, are executed by a multijoint manipulandum which has six degrees of freedom. Each degree of freedom is represented by one of the articulatory units. As seen in the work of Atkeson (1987), a translation is needed between these different coordinate systems. Moreover, this translation is made more complicated by the fact that there is not a one-to-one mapping between the two systems. The higher degrees of freedom in articulatory space create a many-to-one mapping. In other words, a multitude of articulator configurations will achieve the same target location.

Jordan (1986, 1990) has emphasized that the process of choosing a specific articulatory configuration to achieve a desired action is not arbitrary. Indeed, this is perhaps the quintessential feature of skilled behavior. The selected configuration for a subunit within an action sequence is constrained by the goals of the entire sequence. This is the phenomenon of coarticulation. Each subunit is not produced as an independent entity, but rather emerges within the global context of the entire sequence. Configurations are selected so as to maximize smoothness as the effectors move from one subgoal to another. Thus, the particular configuration for a given subgoal will change in different contexts. The ubiquity of coarticulation has been discussed in the study of many skilled activities including speech (Fowler, 1980) and typing (Rumelhart and Norman, 1982). For example, the point of closure in the vocal tract is much farther forward when pronouncing the /k/ sound in the word 'key' than in the word 'caulk' due to the articulatory gestures required for the following vowel. Coarticulatory phenomena are not limited to the effects between neighboring subunits, but can extend across many subunits, in both a forward and a backward direction (Moll and Daniloff, 1971; also Bengurel and Cowan, 1974, cited in Jordan, 1986).

Two aspects of Jordan's model (1986, 1990) lead to coarticulatory effects. First, as discussed previously, the structure of connectivity is designed so that each subunit of the sequence takes place within a specific context. This is achieved by having the state units receive input from the output units, other state units, and via the recurrent connections. These time-varying units are thus provided with a continuous record of the current context. This process is not really a learning process since the inputs are unaffected by whether the action is correct or not. However, the second feature contributing to coarticulation can involve an error signal. For this, Jordan (1990) exploits the fact that output (either articulatory or target) units do not always need to be specified or, at least, completely specified for each subunit of the sequence. By associating not only the articulatory actions needed to achieve a subgoal, but also the context, these units can take on values that minimize subsequent transitions. For example, when typing the word 'example', the right hand does not strike a key until the fourth letter, the 'm'. Thus, its position need not be specified during the production of the first three letters, 'exa'. However, the skilled typist will begin to configure the right hand for typing 'm' during the production of the preceding letters (Rumelhart and Norman, 1982).

Jordan (1990) uses the metaphor of coupled springs to capture the effects of these processes. Springs are attached to the articulatory outputs for each subunit of the sequence. The stiffness of each spring is an inverse function of the distance in time between each pair of subunits. The springs bias the values that the articulatory units adopt so as to minimize the transition between the subunits.

This associative process is nested within a more general learning scheme. As with Atkeson (1987), Jordan (1990) postulates a two-stage learning model. The first stage involves only the upper level of the network: the mappings from the articulatory units to target units must be learned. For example, the typist must learn the mapping between the fingers and keyboard. Or, in speech, the mapping would be between movements of the articulators and the sounds produced by these actions. Rather than apply an inverse mapping solution as Atkeson (1987) has done, Jordan favors forward modeling (1990; Jordan and Rosenbaum, 1989; note that Atkeson modeled inverse dynamics, not inverse kinematics). The process is quite simple and the requirements are minimal. Each learning trial only requires that a set of articulatory units be activated which are associated with an intended target. Since the initial weights between the units in the network are randomly set, the action that is produced will be quite different from the intended goal. An error signal is generated by comparing the output that would correspond to the intended target with the actual output. This error signal is then used to modify the weights so as to reduce the difference.

The algorithm implemented by Jordan uses the error signal not only to modify the weights between the target units and the hidden units, but is also propagated back through the system to modify the weights between the hidden units and the articulatory units (see Rumelhart, Hinton and Williams, 1986). After many such trials, the weights become configured so as to reflect the nonlinear mapping between the articulatory units and the target units. Indeed, the learning capability of connectionist systems is primarily derived from the fact that the inclusion of a hidden layer allows the system to learn nonlinear mappings.

Jordan (1990) refers to this first stage of learning as the 'babbling stage'. The system characteristics become known as a consequence of seemingly random events in a manner similar to how an infant appears to learn to speak. The cooing sounds of the six-month-old bear little resemblance to adult speech sounds. However, the infant could use the output to facilitate learning of the linkage between a specific articulatory pattern and sound. The difference between the infant's expectation of what sound will be produced (i.e. target unit activity) and the actual sound produced (output unit activity) can serve as an error signal. Note that, unlike Atkeson's model (1987), the capability of the system will be constrained by the range of data sampled during the learning phase. The controller will probably fail if asked to execute movements which are outside the domain of the training movements.

The upper level of the network, the output controller, thus learns a forward model of the input–output relationships for single actions. After this is achieved, Jordan (1990) fixes the connection weights for this part of the network, no longer allowing them to be modified from further experience. Now the second stage of learning commences in which the same basic scheme is applied to the lower level of the network in order to learn sequential behavior (Jordan, 1986). A pattern of activity is activated across the plan units. This plan vector corresponds to a given sequence of actions. Combined with the inputs from the state units, this vector produces a series of articulatory outputs over time which lead to a series of target actions. Note that, unlike the first stage, the plan/target no longer corresponds to isolated movements, but rather sequences of actions. For example, rather than attempting to produce the sound 'da', the target may be a whole word such as 'daddy'. Of course, the output early on will not correspond to the target sequence and an error signal will be generated from the mismatch.

Unlike standard, single-level, connectionist models, the error signal is generated quite distal from the input: the target unit output is compared with the intended plan. This error signal, reflecting the difference in these two vectors, is then propagated back through the upper level (without modifying any weights) and then through the lower level. The weights in the lower level are adjusted so as to reduce the error. When the weights achieve a stable state, learning can be observed in two ways. First, a given plan vector will produce the desired target output. Second, the trajectory across the subunits will be smooth, reflecting the coarticulatory capabilities of the model.

Jordan (1990) has implemented this model on the network shown in Figure 5.12. It is difficult to evaluate the effects of these simulations. What are the biological counterparts to the components of the model? What is the equivalent of a simulation training epoch? Nonetheless, the simulation can perhaps be best evaluated as an existence proof. Jordan (1990) reports that after approximately 2000 trials the upper level of the network has achieved a stable forward model of the input–output relationships. Following this, sequence learning is quite rapid due to the error minimization algorithm.

Of greater interest are certain phenomena that are not obvious consequences of the learning algorithm. The model exhibits both generalization and interference (Jordan, 1990). Simulations were run in which the general relationship between the successive target positions was retained, but the exact positions were shifted. If the shift was below a certain distance, positive transfer was evidenced by the few trials required to learn the new sequence. When the shift was increased, learning took even longer than a control condition in which learning of the initial sequence was not simulated. The model shows an additional form of generalization. The speed with which a learned sequence is executed can be adjusted by solely varying the weights between the state units. Thus, the model would appear to have the capability of producing flexible sequential actions which obey an invariant timing principle.

5.3.3   Comparison of the Two Computational Models

Many of the similarities between the models proposed by Atkeson (1987) and Jordan (1986, 1990) have been discussed previously. Both models require a two-step learning process. First, a model of the feedforward controller must be learned so that movements can be generated which do not require feedback guidance. Atkeson models this as an inverse process whereas Jordan chooses a forward model. Once the controller characteristics are mastered, specific trajectories (Atkeson, 1987) or sequences of trajectories (Jordan, 1986) can be acquired and fine-tuned. The two models are quite different in both architecture and algorithm. Atkeson represents the various components as symbolic entities, each assigned an identifiable process. In contrast, Jordan uses a distributed representation where the summed activity across many processing units accomplishes the comparable process. The respective learning algorithms reflect these architectural constraints.

Jordan (1990; Jordan and Rosenbaum, 1989) argues that there are a number of advantages to forward modeling. The modeling process is simplified: the only requirements are pairs of inputs and intended targets. Whatever is produced as the actual output can be used to derive an error signal to correct the system. Inverse modeling requires that a series of dynamical equations be known. Jordan (1990) has also simulated the effects of noise in a forward model. The results show that, while the rate of learning is slower and the trajectories lose their smoothness, the model is still able to complete the sequence accurately. All of the targets are achieved in the correct order. As discussed earlier, inaccuracies in an inverse model are globally perpetuated producing a constant error in the final output.

Two other advantages of forward modeling are also useful for learning (Jordan and Rosenbaum, 1989). Forward modeling is naturally goal-directed since the error signal is formulated in the coordinates of target space. Moreover, a forward model is efficient for predicting the expected outcome of an input. Predictive information would be useful for two purposes. First, predictive information could be used as efference copy. The actor would be provided with a copy of the expected feedback and could monitor incoming afferent signals for mismatches signaling errors. Second, predictive information could allow for practice in the absence of movement (i.e. mental practice) by generating an error signal necessary to modify the action.

The minimal constraints required for learning by a connectionist model, however, have been viewed by some as a major weakness (see Pinker and Prince, 1988). The learning theory of Atkeson (1987, 1989) takes advantage of constraints imposed by the fact that we move in an environment with stable characteristics. Presumably, action systems have evolved to exploit, or at least operate within the bounds of, these constraints. Given that gravitational forces are fixed, the equations needed to describe the dynamics of a known rigid system do not entail complex computations. The model that will result is perfectly suited to perform within this context. Moreover, this model will encompass the full competence of the system within this context and can be easily modified if the system properties are changed, such as when a load is applied.

Connectionist learning schemes do not exploit these constraints. As seen in Jordan's model, the connections between the different layers are initialized randomly, with an organized structure emerging during the course of learning. Thus, Jordan (1990) is able to use a 'babbling' method to train his network: he randomly pairs vectors of activation across the articulatory units with target goals. It is unclear what constrains this powerful learning capability. However, it may be that the constraints underlying motor behavior are not imposed by learning processes, but rather by other aspects of motor performance (Gentner, 1987; Kay *et al.*, 1987; Kugler, Kelso and Turvey, 1980).

6 INTEGRATING THEORY AND PHENOMENA

In evaluating the disparate theories of motor learning presented above, it is useful to identify the scope of the theories. What types of movement and learning phenomenon are encompassed by the theory? Is the generalizability of a theory inherently limited to only those aspects of motor learning considered in its original formulation? Once these issues have been addressed, it is then possible to evaluate how well the theories account for the phenomena and regularities discussed in the first half of this chapter.

A central concept that emerged in both the study of learning functions and motor programs was the idea that complex movements entailed a hierarchical representation. The lower levels of the hierarchy correspond to the interface of a movement plan with the effector system chosen to implement the plan. At higher levels in the hierarchy, however, the representation becomes more abstract. It is this abstract representation that allows a movement representation to be effector independent or retain certain invariant characteristics (i.e. relative timing) across different implementations. Which of the existent theories of motor learning are amenable to hierarchical representation?

The psychological theory of Adams (1971) and the Marr–Albus neural theory do not appear suited for this form of generalization. Both models are based on mapping inputs to outputs. In Adams' (1971) theory, the inputs are sensory consequences from an ongoing movement. This work was antecedent to much of the work on abstract motor programs, although recent evaluations of the model (Adams, 1987) have not addressed this issue. In the Marr–Albus theory, the inputs could arise either from sensory inputs or from an efference copy signal. Each of these requirements directly links the learning process to a specific effector system. Learning centers around associating the desired response to a specific pattern of inputs. Indeed, the question of effector independence does not seem appropriate for the movements studied within the context of the Marr–Albus theory of cerebellar learning. Maintaining fixation of a stationary object during head rotation requires a nulling eye movement and an eyeblink is the only adaptive response available to the rabbit in the classic conditioning paradigm.

Little research has been devoted to neural models of more abstract learning processes. One provocative result from the nictitating membrane research has been the finding that cells in the hippocampus are modified in a manner similar to the cerebellar cells (Thompson et al., 1984). These cells do not appear to be essential for the animal to acquire or retain the conditioned response since hippocampal ablation does not impair performance. Nonetheless, the response profile of hippocampus cells is modified over the course of learning so that they come to mirror the learned response. It has been argued that the hippocampus plays a role in a higher-level memory system (Mishkin, Malamut and Bachevalier, 1984; Nissen, Knopman and Schacter, 1987; Squire, 1987; Thompson, 1986). The exact role of this system is unspecified but seems to be for meta-memory functions such as awareness, memory of factual information and abstract learning. This declarative memory system is contrasted with performance-based memory systems such as the system which includes the cerebellum. Abstract, hierarchical representations may thus require models that replicate information in forms that are progressively detached from the implementation system.

This separation of the representation from a specific implementation is, of course, at the heart of the concept of generalized motor programs. Schmidt (1975) proposes that these representations are composed into perceptual-motor schema as a function of learning. There is a parallel between the schema idea as proposed by Schmidt and the computational models of Atkeson and Jordan. Motor schemas can be viewed as representing a functional relationship between an input and an output. Indeed, the recent work of Koh and Meyer (1989, 1991) has shown that subjects can inductively derive fairly complex relationships, and that, once derived, the schema is as competent in producing novel movements as it is with practiced movements. The computational models also emphasize that learning involves a process of abstracting the relationships between states rather than the learning of specific instances. While Atkeson does have to assume the existence of a fixed, internal model during the initial stages of learning, the system can generalize quite easily once the relationship between inputs and outputs becomes known, even if the model is changed.

What about other aspects of higher-level learning? In addition to the schema abstraction process, the concept of generalized motor programs has been developed into a theoretical framework in which control is hierarchically represented. This representation can provide a parsimonious account of the differential effects of learning across the continuum of skill acquisition. MacKay (1982) has described conditions where learning may be restricted to the conceptual levels of the hierarchy. Similarly, Atkeson and Jordan have both adopted a two-stage approach to learning. Analogous to the lower level of MacKay's hierarchy (Figure 5.2), both computational models postulate an early stage of learning during which the output nodes are mastered. Learning of more complex sequences involves modifications at a different level – a process clearly seen in Jordan's model.

Nonetheless, it is important to consider how well the computational models can account for other aspects of hierarchic representation. Jordan (1986) has argued that a multiple-level model can be implemented to capture the features of hierarchic representation. Output units from higher levels would serve as the plan units for lower levels, and backward connections would be needed from the state units of one layer to the state units of a preceding layer to capture context constraints. By this method, a sequence of plans can be learned in the same way that a sequence of actions is currently learned from a single plan.

This model can be expected to mimic the latency data reviewed previously. For example, the time to initiate a response becomes longer as the response becomes more complex (Klapp and Wyatt, 1976; Sternberg *et al.*, 1978). In an elaborated version of Jordan's model, movement would occur after the higher-level plan units activate lower-level plan units, which in turn activate output units. This process would be expected to take more time as more levels are traversed. Similarly, the profiles of interresponse intervals should be successfully simulated since the model would need to return to higher levels in the hierarchy only when a new plan was activated. Chunking would correspond to the unification of previously separate plan units and automaticity would arise when an action sequence had been coalesced into a single plan.

Despite the fact that Jordan's theory can be adapted to capture hierarchical representation, movements would still be bound to particular effector systems. That is, the model is not able to account for the positive transfer that occurs when a learned movement is implemented in a novel manner (Keele, Cohen and Ivry, 1990; MacKay, 1981). The output units in the adapted model are driven by a particular effector system. Sequence learning involves transmitting an error obtained by comparing this output with a desired output and propagating the signal back through the network. Thus, the error is dependent on a specific output system. This problem could be overcome either by postulating that independent error signals are generated for different levels of the network or by conceiving of the output units as at a different level than the effector system (Keele, Cohen and Ivry, 1990).

These solutions are possible given that Jordan (1986) uses information coded in target coordinates to generate the actual outcome. Presumably the plan units at all levels would represent information in similar goal-oriented coordinate space. However, such a solution would seem to eliminate or minimize the role of the state units, thus stripping Jordan's theory of one of its critical features. State units, by definition, automatically introduce constraints in an effector system.

An alternative is presented by Atkeson's (1989) model. His scheme is amenable to global generalization. The model requires that the structure of the system be known. Given this, the inverse kinematics mapping any desired output onto articulatory space can be solved. Thus, the model is capable of producing an action with an unlimited number of output systems as long as the structure of each of the systems is known. It is reasonable to suppose that the parameters describing each effector system could be determined through the sampling algorithm proposed by Atkeson (1987). Whether this algorithm is biologically feasible remains to be tested. In addition, Atkeson's learning process for refining single trajectories is clearly tied to specific effectors.

Keele, Cohen and Ivry (1990) discuss one other approach to reconciling the theoretical problems posed when the phenomena of coarticulation and abstract representation are jointly considered. Effector independence may only be present for simple, well-practiced skills. Each of the movement components in the bilingual transfer experiments of MacKay (1981) and the button-pressing experiment of Keele and associates (Cohen, Ivry and Keele, 1990; Keele, Cohen and Ivry, 1990) are well practiced. During the early stages of acquisition, sequence performance may be dominated by the near-automatic execution of these components. This would appear as effector independence since, for example, individual button presses can be rapidly executed by either finger or arm movements. The effects of sequential interactions, an effector-specific event, would only become apparent following extensive practice (Grudin and Larochelle, 1982). Empirical data in support of this hypothesis are lacking. Experiments showing extensive positive transfer have focused on movements that involve simple actions. It would be useful to employ transfer paradigms with more complex skills. It is easy to demonstrate that skills such as shooting a basketball cannot be readily performed with the nondominant hand. The failure of learning to generalize in such situations should be informative in the study of skill acquisition.

The issues discussed in this section point out some difficult problems that need to be addressed by a theory of motor learning. Nonetheless, this is a time for optimism among students of motor learning. Learning has resurfaced at the forefront of research in psychology, neuroscience and computation. As exemplified by the neural and computer modeling work, current theoretical conjectures contain a much finer degree of specificity and rigor than previous psychological theories. It should be expected that initial efforts would focus on the acquisition of relatively simple and restricted actions. The coming years should bode well for the study of the acquisition of complex skills and the generalizability of these skills.

ACKNOWLEDGEMENTS

The author was supported by an Office of Naval Research Contract (N00014-87-K-0279) and a fellowship from the Sloan Foundation. Critical readings of this manuscript were provided by Richard Schmidt, Don MacKay and especially the editors, Steven W. Keele and Herbert Heuer.

REFERENCES

Ackerman, P. L. (1987). Individual differences in skill learning: An integration of psychometric and information processing perspectives. *Psychological Bulletin*, **102**, 3–27.

Adams, J. A. (1971). A closed-loop theory of motor learning. *Journal of Motor Behavior*, **3**, 111–150.

Adams, J. A. (1976). Issues for a closed-loop theory of motor learning. In G. E. Stelmach (Ed.), *Motor Control: Issues and Trends* (pp. 87–107). New York: Academic Press.

Adams, J. A. (1987). Historical review and appraisal of research on the learning, retention, and transfer of human motor skills. *Psychological Bulletin*, **101**, 41–74.

Adams, J. A., Goetz, E.T. and Marshall, P.H. (1972). Response feedback and motor learning. *Journal of Experimental Psychology*, **92**, 391–397.

Adams, J. A., Gopher, D. and Lintern, G. (1977). Effects of visual and proprioceptive feedback on motor learning. *Journal of Motor Behavior*, **9**, 11–22.

Albus, J. S. (1971). A theory of cerebellar function. *Mathematical Biosciences*, **20**, 25–61.

Allard, F., Graham, S. and Paarsalu, M.E. (1980). Perception in sport: Basketball. *Journal of Sport Psychology*, **2**, 14–21.

Allport, D. A., Antonis, B. and Reynolds, P. (1972). On the division of attention: A disproof of the single channel hypothesis. *Quarterly Journal of Experimental Psychology*, **24**, 225–235.

Anderson, J. R. (1983). *The Architecture of Cognition*. Cambridge, MA: Harvard University Press.

Anderson, J. R. (1987). Skill acquistion: Compilation of weak-method problem solutions. *Psychological Review*, **94**, 192–210.

Armstrong, T. R. (1970). *Training for the Production of Memorized Movement Patterns*, Tech. Report No. 26. Ann Arbor: University of Michigan, Human Performance Center.

Astrom, K. J. (1983). Theory and applications of adaptive control – a survey. *Automatica*, **19**, 471–486.

Atkeson, C. G. (1987). *Roles of Knowledge in Motor Learning*, Tech. Report No. AI-TR-942. Cambridge, MA: Massachusetts Institute of Technology, Department of Brain and Cognitive Sciences.

Atkeson, C. G. (1989). Learning arm kinematics and dynamics. *Annual Review of Neuroscience*, **12**, 157–183.

Attneave, F. (1959). *Applications of Information Theory to Psychology*. New York: Holt.

Bartlett, F. C. (1932). *Remembering: A Study in Experimental and Social Psychology*. Cambridge: Cambridge University Press.

Bernstein, N. (1967). *The Coordination and Regulation of Movement*. New York: Pergamon Press.

Bizzi, E., Accornero, N., Chapple, W. and Hogan, N. (1984). Posture control and trajectory formation during arm movement. *Journal of Neuroscience*, **4**, 2738–2744.

Bloomfield, S. and Marr, D. (1970). How the cerebellum may be used. *Nature*, **227**, 1224–1228.

Boomer, D. S. and Laver, J. D. M. (1968). Slips of the tongue. *British Journal of Disorders of Communication*, **3**, 1–12.

Bower, G. H. and Hilgard, E. R. (1981). *Theories of Learning*, 5th edn. Englewood Cliffs, NJ: Prentice-Hall.

Braitenberg, V. (1967). Is the cerebellar cortex a biological clock in the millisecond range? *Progress in Brain Research*, **25**, 334–346.

Bryan, W. L. and Harter, N. (1899). Studies on the telegraphic language. The acquisition of a hierarchy of habits. *Psychological Review*, **6**, 345–375.

Bullock, D. and Grossberg, S. (1988). Neural dynamics of planned arm movements: Emergent invariants and speed–accuracy properties during trajectory formation. *Psychological Review*, **95**, 49–90.

Caramazza, A., Miceli, G. and Villa, G. (1986). The role of the (output) phonological buffer in reading, writing, and repetititon. *Cognitive Neuropsychology*, **3**, 37–76.

Carroll, W. R. and Bandura, A. (1982). The role of visual monitoring in observational learning of action patterns: Making the unobservable observable. *Journal of Motor Behavior*, **14**, 153–167.

Carson, L. and Wiegand, R. L. (1979). Motor schema formation and retention in young children: A test of Schmidt's schema theory. *Journal of Motor Behavior*, **11**, 247–251.

Carter, M. C. and Shapiro, D. C. (1984). Control of sequential movements: Evidence for generalized motor programs. *Journal of Neurophysiology*, **52**, 787–796.

Chase, W.G. and Simon, H.A. (1973). The mind's eye in chess. In W.G. Chase (Ed.), *Visual Information Processing*. New York: Academic Press.

Chomsky, N. (1965). *Aspects of the Theory of Syntax*. Cambridge, MA: MIT Press.

Cohen, A., Ivry, R. I. and Keele, S.W. (1990). Attention and structure in sequence learning. *Journal of Experimental Psychology: Learning, Memory, and Cognition*, **16**, 17–30.

Crossman, E. R. F. W. (1959). A theory of the acquisition of speed-skill. *Ergonomics*, **2**, 153–166.

Ebner, T. (1989). Cerebellar involvement in motor learning. Presented at *Symposium of Current Controversies in Cerebellar Theory*, Tuebingen, West Germany, July 1989.

Eccles, J. C. (1986). Learning in the motor system. *Progress in Brain Research*, **64**, 3–18.

Fentress, J. C. (1973). Development of grooming in mice with amputated forelimbs. *Science*, **179**, 704–705.

Fitts, P. M. (1964). Perceptual-motor skill learning. In A. W. Melton (Ed.), *Categories of Human Learning* (pp. 243–285). New York: Academic Press.

Flash, T. and Hogan, N. (1985). The coordination of arm movements: An experimentally confirmed mathematical model. *Journal of Neuroscience*, **5**, 1688–1703.

Fleishman, E. A. (1966). Human abilities and the acquisition of skill. In E. A. Bilodeau (Ed.), *Acquisition of Skill*. New York: Academic Press.

Fleishman, E. A. and Rich, S. (1963). Role of kinesthetic and spatial–visual abilities in perceptual motor learning. *Journal of Experimental Psychology*, **66**, 6–11.

Foss, J. P. and Hakes, D. T. (1978). *Psycholinguistics, An Introduction to the Psychology of Language*. Englewood Cliffs, NJ: Prentice-Hall.

Fowler, C. A. (1980). Coarticulation and theories of extrinsic timing. *Journal of Phonetics*, **8**, 113–133.

Fuchs, A.H. (1962). The progression–regression hypothesis in perceptual-motor skill learning. *Journal of Experimental Psychology*, **63**, 177–182.

Gelman, R., Houk, J. C. and Gibson, A. R. (1985). Inferior olivary neurons in the awake cat: Detection of contact and passive body displacement. *Journal of Neurophysiology*, **54**, 40–60.

Gentner, D.R. (1987). Timing of skilled motor performance: Tests of the proportional duration model. *Psychological Review*, **94**, 255–276.

Gilbert, P. F. C. and Thach, W. T. (1977). Purkinje cell activity during motor learning. *Brain Research*, **128**, 309–328.

Goldberg, G. (1985). Supplementary motor area structure and function: Review and hypotheses. *Behavioral and Brain Sciences*, **8**, 567–616.

Gonshor, A. and Melville-Jones, G. M. (1976). Extreme vestibulo-ocular adaptation induced by prolonged optical reversal of vision. *Journal of Physiology*, **256**, 381–414.

Gordon, P. C. and Meyer, D. E. (1987). Control of serial order in rapidly spoken syllable sequences. *Journal of Memory and Language*, **26**, 300–321.

Grudin, J. T. and Larochelle, S. (1982). *Digraph Frequency Effects in Skilled Typing*, CHIP Report No. 110. La Jolla, CA: University of California, San Diego, Center for Human Information Processing.

Heuer, H. (1984). Motor learning as a process of structural constriction and displacement. *Cognition and Motor Processes*, **18**, 297–305.

Hick, W. E. (1952). On the rate of gain of information. *Quarterly Journal of Experimental Psychology*, **4**, 11–26.

Hogan, J. C. (1977). The effect of varied practice on the accuracy of ballistic movement error in ballistic skill acquisition. *Journal of Motor Behavior*, **10**, 133–138.

Hollerbach, J. M. (1990). Planning of arm movements. In D. N. Osherson, S. M. Kosslyn and J. M. Hollerbach (Eds), *Visual Cognition and Action: An Invitation to Cognitive Science*, vol. 2 (pp. 183–212). Cambridge, MA: MIT Press.

Holmes, G. (1939). The cerebellum of man. *Brain*, **62**, 1–30.

Hull, C. L. (1943). *Principles of Behavior*. New York: Appleton-Century.

Hyman, R. (1953). Stimulus information as a determinant of reaction time. *Journal of Experimental Psychology*, **45**, 188–196.

Ito, M. (1984). *The Cerebellum and Neural Control*. New York: Raven Press.

Ito, M., Shiida, N., Yagi, N. and Yamamoto, M. (1974). The cerebellar modification of rabbit's horizontal vestibulo-ocular reflex induced by sustained head rotation combined with visual stimulation. *Proceedings of the Japanese Academy*, **50**, 85–89.

Ivry, R. I. and Keele, S. W. (1989). Timing functions of the cerebellum. *Cognitive Neuroscience*, **1**, 136–152.

Ivry, R. I., Keele, S. W. and Diener, H. C. (1988). Dissociation of the lateral and medial cerebellum in movement timing and movement execution. *Experimental Brain Research*, **73**, 167–180.

Jagacinski, R. J. and Hah, S. (1988). Progression–regression effects in tracking repeated patterns. *Journal of Experimental Psychology: Human Perception and Performance*, **14**, 77–88.

Jennings, P. J. and Keele, S. W. (1990). *A Computational Model of Attentional Requirements in Sequence Learning*. Tech. Report No. 90-5. Institute of Cognitive and Decision Sciences, University of Oregon, Eugene.

Jordan, M. I. (1986). *Serial Order: A Parallel Distributed Processing Approach*, ICS Report No. 8604. Institute for Cognitive Science, University of California, San Diego.

Jordan, M. I. (1990). Motor learning and the degrees of freedom problem. In M. Jeannerod (Ed.), *Attention and Performance*, vol. XIII: *Motor Representation and Control* (pp. 796–836). Hillsdale, NJ: Erlbaum.

Jordan, M. I. and Rosenbaum, D. A. (1989). Action. In M. I. Posener (Ed.), *Foundations of Cognitive Science* (pp. 727–768). Cambridge, MA: MIT Press.

Kay, B. A., Kelso, J. A. S., Saltzman, E. L. and Schoener, G. (1987). Space–time behavior of single and bimanual rhythmical movements: Data and limit cycle model. *Journal of Experimental Psychology: Human Perception and Performance*, **13**, 178–192.

Keele, S. W. (1981). Behavioral analysis of motor control. In V. Brooks (Ed.), *Handbook of Physiology*, vol. 2: *Motor Control* (pp. 1391–1414). Bethesda, MD: American Physiological Society.

Keele, S. W. (1986). Motor control. In L. Kaufman, J. Thomas and K. Boff (Eds), *Handbook of Perception and Performance*. New York: John Wiley.

Keele, S. W. and Summers, V. (1976). The structure of motor programs. In G. Stelmach (Ed.), *Motor Control: Issues and Trends* (pp. 109–142). New York: Academic Press.

Keele, S. W., Cohen, A. and Ivry, R. (1990). Motor programs. In M. Jeannerod (Ed.), *Attention and Performance*, vol. XIII: *Motor Representation and Control* (pp. 77–110). Hillsdale, NJ: Erlbaum.

Keele, S. W. and Ivry, R. (1991). Does the cerebellum provide a common computation for diverse tasks: A timing hypothesis. *Annals of the New York Academy of Sciences*, **608**, 179–211.

Kelso, J. A. S. and Holt, K. G. (1980). Exploring a vibratory systems analysis of human movement production. *Journal of Neurophysiology*, **43**, 1183–1196.

Kelso, J. A. S. and Norman, P.E. (1978). Motor schema formation in children. *Developmental Psychology*, **14**, 153–156.

Kelso, J. A. S., Southard, D. L. and Goodman, D. (1979). On the coordination of two-handed movements. *Journal of Experimental Psychology: Human Perception and Performance*, **104**, 147–153.

Kerr, R. and Booth, B. (1977). Specific and varied practice of motor skill. *Perceptual and Motor Skills*, **46**, 395–401.

Klapp, S. T. and Wyatt, E. P. (1976). Motor programming within a sequence of responses. *Journal of Motor Behavior*, **8**, 19–26.

Koh, K. and Meyer, D.E. (1989). Induction of continuous stimulus–response relations. In G. M. Olson and E. E. Smith (Eds), *Proceedings of the 11th Annual Conference of the Cognitive Science Society* (pp. 333–340). Hillsdale, NJ: Erlbaum.

Koh, K. and Meyer, D. E. (1991). Function learning: Induction of continuous stimulus–response relations. *Journal of Experimental Psychology: Learning, Memory, and Cognition* **17**, 811–836.

Kohl, R. M. and Roenker, D. L. (1980). Bilateral transfer as a function of mental imagery. *Journal of Motor Behavior*, **12**, 197–206.

Kolers, P. A. (1975). Memorial consequences of automatized encoding. *Journal of Experimental Psychology: Human Learning and Memory*, **1**, 689–701.

Kozhevnikov, V. A. and Chistovich, L. A. (1965). *Speech Articulation and Perception*. (U.S. Department of Commerce, Transactions.) Clearinghouse for Federal, Scientific and Technical Information, Washington, DC.

Kugler, P. N., Kelso, J. A. S. and Turvey, M. T. (1980). On the concept of coordinative structures as dissipative structures: I. Theoretical line. In G.E. Stelmach and J. Requin (Eds), *Tutorials in Motor Behavior* (pp. 3–37). Amsterdam: North-Holland.

Lavond, D. G., Knowlton, B. J., Steinmetz, J. E. and Thompson, R. F. (1987). Classical conditioning of the rabbit eyelid response with a mossy-fiber stimulation CS: II lateral reticular nucleus stimulation. *Behavioral Neuroscience*, **101**, 676–682.

Lee, D. N. (1980). Visuo-motor coordination in space–time. In G. E. Stelmach and J. Requin (Eds.), *Tutorials in Motor Behavior* (pp. 281–285). Amsterdam: North-Holland.

Lisberger, S. G. and Pavelko, T. A. (1988). Brain stem neurons in modified pathways for motor learning in the primate vestibulo-ocular reflex. *Science*, **242**, 771–773.

Logan, G. D. (1982). On the ability to inhibit complex movements: a stop-signal study of typewriting. *Human Perception and Performance*, **3**, 778–792.

Logan, G. D. (1985). Skill and automaticity: Relations, implications, and future directions. *Canadian Journal of Psychology*, **39**, 367–386.

Logan, G. D. (1988). Toward an instance theory of automatization. *Psychological Review*, **95**, 492–527.

Long, J. (1976). Effects of delayed irregular feedback on unskilled and skilled keying performance. *Ergonomics*, **19**, 183–202.

MacKay, D. G. (1981). The problem of mental practice. *Journal of Motor Behavior*, **13**, 274–285.

MacKay, D. G. (1982). The problem of flexibility and fluency in skilled behavior. *Psychological Review*, **89**, 483–506.

MacKay, D. G. (1985). A theory of representation, organization, and timing of action with implications for sequencing disorder. In E. Roy (Ed.), *Advances in Psychology*, vol. 23: *Neuropsychological Studies of Apraxia and Related Disorders*. New York: Academic Press.

MacKay, D. G. and Bowman, R. W., Jr. (1969). On producing the meaning in sentences. *American Journal of Psychology*, **82**, 23–39.

Margolin, D. I. (1984). The neuropsychology of writing and spelling: Semantic, phonological, motor, and perceptual processes. *Quarterly Journal of Experimental Psychology*, **36A**, 459–489.

Marr, D. (1969). A theory of cerebellar cortex. *Journal of Physiology*, **202**, 437–470.

Marr, D. (1982). *Vision*. San Francisco, CA: W. H. Freeman.

Marteniuk, R. G. and Romanow, S. K. E. (1983). Human movement organization and learning as revealed by variability in movement, use of kinematic information, and Fourier analysis. In R. A. Magill (Ed.), *Memory and Control of Action* (pp. 167–198). Amsterdam: North-Holland.

Martin, J. G. (1972). Rhythmic (hierarchical) versus serial structure in speech and other behavior. *Psychological Review*, **79**, 487–509.

Mauk, M. D., Steinmetz, J. E. and Thompson, R. F. (1986). Classical conditioning using stimulation of the inferior olive as the unconditioned stimulus. *Proceedings of the National Academy of Sciences*, **83**, 5349–5353.

McCormick, D. A., Steinmetz, J. E. and Thompson, R. F. (1985). Lesions of the inferior olivary complex cause extinction of the classically conditioned eyeblink response. *Brain Research*, **359**, 120–130.

McCormick, D. A. and Thompson, R. F. (1984). Neuronal responses of the rabbit cerebellum during acquistion and performance of a classically conditioned nictitating membrane– eyelid response. *Journal of Neuroscience*, **4**, 2811–2822.

McCracken, H. D. and Stelmach, G. E. (1977). A test of the schema theory of discrete motor learning. *Journal of Motor Behavior*, **9**, 193–201.

McLeod, P. (1977). A dual task response modality effect: Support for multiprocessor models of attention. *Quarterly Journal of Experimental Psychology*, **29**, 651–667.

McLeod, P. A. and Posner, M. I. (1984). Priviledged loops from percept to act. In H. Bouma and B. Bowhuis (Eds), *Attention and Performance*. Hillsdale, NJ: Erlbaum.

Miller, G. A. (1956). The magical number seven, plus or minus two: Some limits on our capacity for processing information. *Psychological Review*, **63**, 81–97.

Mishkin, M., Malamut, B. and Bachevalier, J. (1984). Memories and habits: Two neural systems. In J. L. McGaugh, G. Lynch and N. M. Weinberger (Eds), *Neurobiology of Learning and Memory*. New York: Guilford Press.

Moll, K. L. and Daniloff, R. G. (1971). Investigation of the timing of velar movements during speech. *Journal of the Acoustical Society of America*, **50**, 678–684.

Navon, D. (1985). Attention division or attention sharing? In M. I. Posner and O. S. Marin (Eds), *Attention and Performance*, vol. XI (pp. 133–146). Hillsdale, NJ: Erlbaum.

Neisser, U., Novick, R. and Lazar, R. (1963). Searching for ten targets simultaneously. *Perceptual and Motor Skills*, **17**, 427–432.

Neumann, O. (1984). Automatic processing: A review of recent findings and a plea for an old theory. In W. Prinz and A. F. Sanders (Eds), *Cognition and Motor Processes*. Berlin: Springer.

Newell, A. and Rosenbloom. P. S. (1981). Mechanisms of skill acquisition and the law of practice. In J. R. Anderson (Ed.), *Cognitive Skills and their Acquisition* (pp. 1–55). Hillsdale, NJ: Erlbaum.

Newell, K. M. (1974). Knowledge of results and motor learning. *Journal of Motor Behavior*, **6**, 235–244.

Newell, K. M. (1976). Motor learning without knowledge of results through the development of a response recognition mechanism. *Journal of Motor Behavior*, **8**, 209–217.

Newell, K. M. and Chew, R. A. (1974). Recall and recognition in motor learning. *Journal of Motor Behavior*, **6**, 245–253.

Nissen, M. J. and Bullemer, P. (1987). Attentional requirements of learning: Evidence from performance measures. *Cognitive Psychology*, **19**, 1–32.

Nissen, M. J., Knopman, D. S. and Schacter, D. L. (1987). Neurochemical dissociation of memory systems. *Neurology*, **37**, 789–794.

Norman, D. A. (1981). Categorization of action slips. *Psychological Review*, **88**, 1–7.

Nottebohm, F. (1970). Ontogeny of bird song. *Science*, **167**, 950–956.

Pellionisz, A. and Llinas, R. (1982). Space–time representation in the brain. The cerebellum as a predictive space–time metric tensor. *Neuroscience*, **7**, 2949–2970.

Pew, R. W. (1974). Human perceptual-motor performance. In B. H. Kantowitz (Ed.), *Human Information Processing: Tutorials in Performance and Cognition*. Hillsdale, NJ: Erlbaum.

Pinker, S. and Prince, A. (1988). On language and connectionism: Analysis of a parallel distributed processing model of language acquisition. *Cognition*, **28**, 73–193.

Polit, A. and Bizzi, E. (1979). Characteristics of motor programs underlying arm movements in monkeys. *Journal of Neurophysiology*, **42**, 183–194.

Posner, M. I. and Keele, S. W. (1968). On the genesis of abstract ideas. *Journal of Experimental Psychology*, **77**, 353–363.

Posner, M. I. and Snyder, C. R. (1975). Attention and cognitive control. In R. I. Solso (Ed.), *Information Processing and Cognition*. Hillsdale, NJ: Erlbaum.

Povel, D.-J. and Collard, R. (1982). Structural factors in patterned finger tapping. *Acta Psychologica*, **52**, 107–123.

Rabbitt, P. (1978). Detection of errors by skilled typists. *Ergonomics*, **21**, 945–958.

Raibert, M. H. (1978). A model for sensorimotor control and learning. *Biological Cybernetics*, **29**, 29–36.

Reason, J. (1979). Actions not as planned: The price of automatization. In G. Underwood and R. Stevens (Eds), *Aspects of Consciousness*. London: Academic Press.

Restle, F. (1970). Theory of serial pattern learning: Structural trees. *Psychological Review*, **77**, 481–495.

Rosebaum, D. A. (1987). Hierarchical organization of motor programs. In S. Wise (Ed.), *Higher Brain Functions: Recent Explorations of the Brain Emergent Properties* (pp. 45–66). New York: John Wiley.

Rosenbaum, D. A., Kenny, S. B. and Derr, M. A. (1983). Hierarchical control of rapid movement sequences. *Journal of Experimental Psychology: Human Perception and Performance*, **9**, 86–102.

Rosenbloom, P. S. and Newell, A. (1987). An integrated computational model of stimulus–response compatibility and practice. In G. H. Bower (Ed.), *The Psychology of Learning and Motivation, Advances in Research and Theory*, vol. 21: (pp. 3–49). London: Academic Press.

Rothwell, J. C., Traub, M. M., Day, B. L., Obeso, J. A. and Marsden, C. D. (1982). Manual motor performance in a deafferented man. *Brain*, **105**, 515–542.

Rumelhart, D. E., Hinton, G. E. and McClelland, J. L. (1986). A general framework for parallel distributed processing. In D. E. Rumelhart, J. L. McClelland and The PDP Research Group (Eds), *Parallel Distributed Processing: Explorations in the Microstructure of Cognition*, vol. 1: *Foundations* (pp. 45–76). Cambridge, MA: MIT Press.

Rumelhart, D. E., Hinton, G. E. and Williams, R. J. (1986). Learning and relearning in Boltzmann machines. In D. E. Rumelhart, J. L. McClelland and The PDP Research Group (Eds), *Parallel Distributed Processing: Explorations in the Microstructure of Cognition*, vol. 1: *Foundations* (pp 318–362). Cambridge, MA: MIT Press.

Rumelhart, D. E. and Norman, D. A. (1982). Simulating a skilled typist: A study of skilled cognitive-motor performance. *Cognitive Science*, **6**, 1–6.

Sachs, J. S. (1967). Recognition memory for syntactic and semantic aspects of connected discourse. *Perception and Psychophysics*, **2**, 437–442.

Salmoni, A. W., Schmidt, R. A. and Walter, C. B. (1984). Knowledge of results and motor learning: A review and critical reappraisal. *Psychological Bulletin*, **95**, 355–386.

Saltzman, E. and Kelso, J. A. S. (1987). Skilled actions: A task dynamic approach. *Psychological Review*, **94**, 84–106.

Sanes, J. N., Mauritz, K. H., Dalakas, M. C. and Evarts, E. V. (1985). Motor control in humans with large-fiber sensory neuropathy. *Human Neurobiology*, **4**, 101–114.

Schmidt, R. A. (1975). A schema theory of discrete motor skill learning. *Psychological Review*, **82**, 225–260.

Schmidt, R. A. (1987). The acquisition of skill: Some modifications to the perception–action relationship through practice. In H. Heuer and A. F. Sanders (Eds), *Perspectives on Perception and Action* (pp. 77–103). Hillsdale, NJ: Erlbaum.

Schmidt, R. A. (1988). *Motor Control and Learning: A Behavioral Emphasis*. Champaign, IL: Human Kinetics.

Schmidt, R. A. and White, J. L. (1972). Evidence for an error detection mechanism in motor skills: A test of Adams' closed-loop theory. *Journal of Motor Behavior*, **4**, 143–253.

Schmidt, R. A. and Young, D. E. (1987). Transfer of movement control in motor skill learning. In S. M. Cormier and J. D. Hagman (Eds), *Transfer of Learning* (pp. 47–79). New York: Academic Press.

Schneider, W. and Fisk, A. D. (1983). Attention theory and mechanisms for skilled performance. In R. A. Magill (Ed.), *Memory and Control of Action*. Amsterdam: North-Holland.

Schneider, W. and Shiffrin, R. M. (1977). Controlled and automatic human information processing: I. Detection, search, and attention. *Psychological Review*, **84**, 1–66.

Schwartz, A. B., Ebner, T. J. and Bloedel, J. R. (1987). Responses of interposed and dentate neurons to perturbations of the locomotor cycle. *Experimental Brain Research*, **67**, 323–338.

Shaffer, L. H. (1976). Intention and performance. *Psychological Review*, **83**, 375–393.

Shapiro, D. C. and Schmidt. R. A. (1982). The schema theory: Recent evidence and developmental implications. In J. A. S. Kelso and J. E. Clark (Eds), *The Development of Movement and Control and Coordination* (pp. 113–173). New York: John Wiley.

Shapiro, D. C., Zernicke, R. F., Gregor, R. J. and Diestel, J. D. (1981). Evidence for generalized motor programs using gait pattern analysis. *Journal of Motor Behavior*, **13**, 33–47.

Shiffrin, R. M. and Schneider, W. (1977). Controlled and automatic human information processing: II. Perceptual learning, automatic attending, and a general theory. *Psychological Review*, **84**, 127–190.

Siebel, R. (1963). Discrimination reaction time for a 1023-alternative task. *Journal of Experimental Psychology*, **66**, 215–226.

Snoddy, G. S. (1926). Learning a stability. *Journal of Applied Psychology*, **10**, 1–36.

Soechting, J. F. and Lacquaniti, F. (1981). Invariant characteristics of a pointing movement in man. *Journal of Neuroscience*, **1**, 710–720.

Spelke, H., Hirst, W. and Neisser, U. (1976). Skills of divided attention. *Cognition*, **4**, 215–230.

Squire, L. R. (1987). *Memory and Brain*. New York: Oxford University Press.

Sternberg, S., Knoll, R. L. and Turock, D. L. (1990). Hierarchical control in the execution of action sequences: Tests of two invariance properties. In M. Jeannerod (Ed.) *Attention and Performance*, vol. XIII: *Motor Representation and Control* (pp. 1–56). Hillsdale, NJ: Erlbaum.

Sternberg, S., Monsell, S., Knoll, R. L. and Wright, C. E. (1978). The latency and duration of rapid movement sequences: Comparisons of speech and typewriting. In G.E. Stelmach (Ed.), *Information Processing in Motor Control and Learning*. New York: Academic Press.

Summers, J. J. (1975). The role of timing in motor program representation. *Journal of Motor Behavior*, **7**, 229–241.

Taub, E. and Berman, A. J. (1968). Movement and learning in the absence of sensory feedback. In S. J. Freedman (Ed.), *The Neuropsychology of Spatially Oriented Behavior*. Homewood, IL: Dorsey Press.

Terzuolo, C.A. and Viviani, P. (1980). Determinants and characteristics of motor patterns used for typing. *Neuroscience*, **5**, 1085–1103.

Thompson, R. F. (1986). The neurobiology of learning and memory. *Science*, **233**, 941–947.

Thompson, R., Clark, G., Donegan, N., Lavond, D., Madden, J., Mamounas, L., Mauk, M. and McCormick, D. (1984). Neuronal substrates of basic associative learning. In L. Squire and N. Butters (Eds), *Neuropsychology of Memory*. New York: Guilford Press.

Tuller, B., Kelso, J. A. S. and Harris, K. S. (1982). Interarticulator phasing as an index of temporal regularity in speech. *Journal of Experimental Psychology: Human Perception and Performance*, **8**, 460–472.

van Rossum, J. H. A. (1990). Schmidt's schema theory: the empirical base of the variability of practice hypothesis. *Human Movement Science*, **9**, 387–435.

Viviani, P. & Terzuolo, C. (1980). Space–time invarience in learned motor skills. In G. E. Stelmach and J. Requin (Eds), *Tutorials in Motor Behavior*. Amsterdam: North-Holland.

Warren, W. H. and Whang, S. (1987). Visual guidance of walking through apertures: Body–scaled information for affordances. *Journal of Experimental Psychology*, **13**, 371–383.

Watanabe, E. (1984). Neuronal events correlated with long-term adaptation of the horizontal vestibulo-ocular reflex in the primate flocculus. *Brain Research*, **297**, 169–174.

Welford, A. T. (1987). On rates of improvement with practice. *Journal of Motor Behavior*, **19**, 401–415.

Welsh, J. P. and Harvey, J. A. (1989). Cerebellar lesions and the nictitating membrane reflex: Performance deficits of the conditioned and unconditioned response. *Journal of Neuroscience*, **9**, 299–311.

West, L. J. (1967). Vision and kinesthesis in the acquisition of typewriting skill. *Journal of Applied Psychology*, **51**, 161–166.

Wing. A. and Kristofferson, A. (1973). Response delays and the timing of discrete motor responses. *Perception and Psychophysics*, **14**, 5–12.

Wright, C. E. (1990). Generalized motor programs: Reevaluating claims of effector independence. In M. Jeannerod (Ed.), *Attention and Performance*, vol. XIII: Motor Representation and Control (pp. 294–320). Hillsdale, NJ: Erlbaum.

Wulf, G. and Schmidt, R. A. (1989). The learning of generalized motor programs: Reducing relative frequency of knowledge of results enhances memory. *Journal of Experimental Psychology: Learning, Memory, and Cognition*, **15**, 748–757.

Yeo, C., Hardiman, M. and Glickstein, M. (1985). Classical conditioning of the nictitating membrane response of the rabbit. II. Lesions of cerebellar cortex. *Experimental Brain Research*, **60**, 99–113.

Young, E. G. and Schmidt, R. A. (1990). Units of motor behavior: Modifications with practice and feedback. In M. Jeannerod (Ed.), *Attention and Performance*, vol. XIII: Motor Representation and Control (pp. 763–795). Hillsdale, NJ: Erlbaum.

Zelaznik, H. N. (1977). Transfer in rapid timing tasks: An examination of the role of variability in practice. In R. W. Christiana and D. M. Landers (Eds), *Psychology of Motor Behavior and Sport – 1976*. vol. 1: *Motor Behavior* (pp. 36–43). Champaign, IL: Human Kinetics.

Part II

Particular Skills

Chapter 6

Posture and Locomotion

Marjorie Hines Woollacott and Jody L. Jensen

*Institute of Neuroscience and Department of Exercise and Movement
Science, University of Oregon, USA*

1 INTRODUCTION

Studies on the control of posture and locomotion over the past century have taken
a variety of experimental perspectives, including neurophysiological, biomechanical and, more recently, a dynamical systems perspective. In the following pages we
will review the theoretical underpinnings of each perspective and their evolution
over time. We will then summarize the research from each of these areas which has
contributed to our current understanding of the control of posture and locomotion.

1.1 The Neurophysiological Perspective

Sherrington was one of the first neurophysiologists to study posture and locomotion. Through experiments in which he stimulated restricted sensory inputs, he was
able to map out and classify a variety of reflexes and to describe the contributions
of these reflexes to the control of posture and locomotion (Sherrington, 1906, 1910).
For example, he noted that stepping movements can be elicited by a number of
stimuli, including hip extension, and rubbing, squeezing or pinching the skin in a
number of places, including the foot, the back or the tail.

This research contributed significantly to our understanding of the way sensory
inputs modulate posture or locomotor control. However, this approach involved
stimulating an inactive organism, and measuring the reactions of individual body
segments to discrete stimuli – an approach that was later called the 'stimulus–
response approach' to understanding motor control. Sherrington's conclusions
concerning nervous system organization reflect this restricted stimulus–response
approach. In his book, *Integrative Action of the Nervous System*, Sherrington comments that, with the whole nervous system intact, the simple reflexes are combined
into actions, which in their continuity may be termed the 'behavior' of the
individual.

Sherrington only examined reflexes, and only asked questions about the nervous
system related to reflexes. He modeled the function of the nervous system and of
postural and locomotor control in a manner that was skewed toward reflex control.

Handbook of Perception and Action, Volume 2
ISBN 0-12-516162-X

Thus, even today, some classic texts view posture control as being made up of vestibular reflexes, spinal stretch reflexes and visually elicited reflexes.

Explanations for the sequencing and timing of motor behaviors were part of the appeal of a reflex-based strategy for motor control. In this view, sequencing and timing were the indirect result of a series of stimulus–response pairs. This reflex-chaining hypothesis subsequently fell into disfavor in large part with the demonstration that stereotypic sequences of movements continued to exist when the system was deafferented (sensory inputs removed). With the removal of sensory inputs, triggers for successive reflexes were no longer available–yet purposive behavior continued to be manifest (for a review, see Taub, 1976).

The results from deafferentation studies could not be accounted for by a reflex-chaining hypothesis, but such results were not antithetical to the construct of a central pattern generator for the control of rhythmical locomotor movements or a function generator for control of nonrhythmical movements, like posture control. If input from the periphery was not necessary to drive the behavior, then a representation of the behavior had to exist within the motor system. A logical supposition was that some central mechanism was the source. From this perspective, central pattern or function generators prescribe the sequencing and timing of the motor act and impose this structure on the periphery (Delcomyn, 1980). Experimental evidence grew to support the concept of the central pattern generator controlling locomotor output in a wide variety of lower vertebrates and mammals (for reviews, see Edgerton *et al.*, 1976; Grillner, 1981). In decorticate and deafferented preparations, pattern generation persisted.

It was also becoming clear, however, that patterns generated under impoverished neural conditions (e.g. deafferentation) were not identical to the patterns created by the intact animal. Further, sensory inputs appeared to play an important role in adapting the pattern to the context. Just as Sherrington's conclusions were limited by his *a priori* expectations about reflex control, a conclusion about the importance of the central pattern generator, independent of peripheral and higher central inputs, also has become a limited view of the process of pattern generation (see the critique by Pearson, 1987).

The arguments that combined to weaken the concept of a central pattern generator (and function generator) as the exclusive explanatory construct for the sequencing and timing of patterned motor behavior included: (1) the recognition that isolated neural preparations often produced behavior quite different from that seen in the intact animal; and (2) the demonstration of the modulating influence of sensory inputs. This evidence does not argue against the existence of central pattern generators but denies their sole prescriptive control over the observable behavior. One could thus argue that certain aspects of the behavior are prescribed (with specific details influenced by sensory feedback) and the 'prescription' is filtered through a mechanical system that influences form.

1.2 The Biomechanical Perspective

The biomechanical perspective has a history in classic mechanics and Newton's laws of motion wherein the machine metaphor plays a dominant role in questions that drive the research. Muscles are equated with torque motors and limbs with levers, and the mathematical techniques of trigonometry and calculus make the function of muscle accessible in a way not revealed by investigations of muscle physiology. The perspective is captured by Elftman's (1941) description of muscle function:

'Muscles are useful in the body primarily because they are able to exert tension between their points of attachment. Their ultimate effect must therefore be mechanical in nature, such as the production of movement, the stopping of movement, or the maintenance of equilibrium by opposing other forces which are present.' (p. 191)

In the mechanics of rigid body motion, forces create rotation of a segment by acting at some distance from the axis of rotation. The effectiveness of any force to produce rotation is a product of the force magnitude and the perpendicular distance from the line of action of the force to the axis of rotation. This product is referred to as 'torque' (see Elftman, 1941, for a very readable tutorial on muscle force and resultant torque). The sum of the torques causing limb segment rotations is explicitly known from Newtonian equations of motion – in essence, the sum of the torques is a product of the segment's moment of inertia (a measure of segmental mass and its distribution) and the segmental angular acceleration. The torques contributed by external forces such as gravity and the reactive torques due to the mechanical interaction of adjacent segments are also explicitly known from the kinematics of the motion, i.e. the spatial trajectories of movement as a function of time (for recent formulations of equations of motion see Dillman, 1971; Hoy and Zernicke, 1986; Miller and Nelson, 1973). By subtracting all known torques from the sum, the muscle torque (the only torque not directly measured) may be estimated. Knowledge of the anthropometric characteristics of the body and the kinematics of motion (i.e. position–time histories of joints and segments from which velocities and accelerations may be derived) allows the kinetic (force) characteristics of motion to be determined. This procedure has become a standard biomechanical practice known as *inverse dynamics* – from knowledge of the kinematics of motion we estimate the forces that are responsible.

Elftman (1939, 1941) was among the pioneers in estimating the contribution of muscle to the sum of the forces that produce human locomotion (see also Braune and Fischer, 1895; and Bernstein, 1935, in Whiting, 1984). These techniques continue to play an important role in our investigation of locomotor performances (Pedotti, 1977; Phillips, Roberts and Huang, 1983; Winter and Robertson, 1978). From the perspective of biomechanics we have gained insight to the function of muscles in the generation and control of movement. Passive forces due to gravity, inertia and the mechanical interaction of limb segments also contribute to movement. A central insight of the biomechanical approach is that movement is a product not only of muscle forces as prescribed by the nervous system, but of these other factors as well. It is in this sense that the nervous system cannot directly prescribe movement without an account of the entire complex of factors.

A weakness of past research from the biomechanical perspective is that the nervous system has often been ignored. The literature contains numerous descriptions of the muscular and nonmuscular forces that combine to produce motor behavior, and the complementarity of these forces has always been recognized (Elftman, 1940). It was Bernstein (1967; Whiting, 1984), however, who expressed this complementarity of forces as a control problem for the nervous system. How does the nervous system deal with the mechanical constraints of the neuromotor system and the impingements of the external environment?

1.3   Dynamical Systems Perspective

A new perspective on the control and coordination of motor behavior has evolved with the rediscovery of the works of N.A. Bernstein (1967; Whiting, 1984) and the application of the principles of pattern generation in physical systems (Haken, 1983) to human movement (e.g. speech: Kelso and Tuller, 1984a; hand movements: Haken, Kelso and Bunz, 1985; infant limb movements: Thelen, Skala and Kelso, 1987). Rather than neural pattern generation, this new perspective may be considered in terms of dynamic pattern generation (Schöner and Kelso, 1988a, b). Central to this perspective is that patterned behavior grows out of an interaction among central and peripheral inputs, as well as the dynamics of the context where the spatiotemporal details of the movement cannot be anticipated, and *planned* for, in advance. As Kugler, Kelso and Turvey (1980) write:

> '... it is the tendencies in dynamics – the free interplay of forces and mutual influences among components tending toward equilibrium or steady states – that are primarily responsible for the order of biological processes.' (p. 6)

Bernstein reminded us of an obvious but sometimes forgotten condition for human movement: the motor system never operates independently of the physical environment, and muscles never act in an isolated context. Given this interdependence, however, we are left with the question of coordination. As Bernstein asked: how are the very many degrees of freedom that constitute the human motor system and relevant context marshaled toward a task-specific end? Those who focus on the neural control of pattern generation (what we will refer to as the neurophysiological perspective) have sought answers to this question in the descriptions of the circuitry and sensory feedback that supports each behavioral form. For example, it has been suggested that by functionally linking groups of muscles together, the degrees of freedom requiring control will be reduced and postural or locomotor control becomes simplified. The name postural 'synergies' has been used to describe these linkages (Gelfand *et al.*, 1971; Nashner and Woollacott, 1979). Temporal patterning of muscle activation becomes a critical representation of the circuitry, the mechanism that produces the pattern.

The alternative perspective, dynamic pattern generation (for the purposes of this paper referred to as the dynamical perspective) seeks to understand the compression of the degrees of freedom not in the form of hard-wired neural circuitry, but rather as a function of the natural tendency of physical systems to seek stability, or move toward steady states. This 'natural tendency' is driven by the laws of thermodynamics and applies to all physical systems. Temporal patterning from the dynamical perspective is representative of the solution not the prescription.

As we proceed in our review, we will return frequently to the neurophysiological and dynamical perspectives, asking how each perspective would interpret the data. From behavior alone, one cannot distinguish between the neural and dynamical aspects of pattern generation. From each theory, however, we can make predictions about what the system will do under conditions of perturbation. Perturbation is the scientist's way of asking questions of nature.

The exploration of neural pattern generation has focused on the mechanisms, the physical instantiation of the 'plan'. New behavioral forms are examined for changes in the circuitry, but *how* transitions occur and the emergence of new forms has not been a critical question from this perspective.

The emergence of new behaviors is a fundamental issue from the dynamical perspective. Understanding dynamic pattern generation precipitates the search for the organizational principles behind the coordination of elements and subsystems and the impetus that leads to instability and the emergence of new stable forms (Kelso and Schöner, 1988).

In summary, understanding the generation of coordinated behavior as a function of the interactions between central and peripheral sources of information and the external environment continues to be the fundamental challenge facing movement scientists. This chapter will explore how our understanding of posture control and locomotion is enhanced by each perspective.

2 POSTURE

In the following section we will give an overview of previous and current neurophysiological, biomechanical and dynamical systems research on the control of balance in normal adults, as well as its developmental changes across the life span. In addition, we will discuss the changes in balance control and balance development that result from pathology.

2.1 The Concept of Synergies

Biological systems are composed of a great many elements, each of which is potentially free to vary independently. Yet patterned behavior, not randomness, is the hallmark of biologic systems. What is the source of this organization and pattern? The term 'synergies', or coordinative structures, refers to the functional coupling of groups of muscles such that they are constrained to act as a unit, and has been proposed by many as the functional unit of the nervous system (Bernstein, 1967; Gelfand *et al.*, 1971; Kugler, Kelso and Turvey, 1980; Turvey, Shaw and Mace, 1978). The presence of synergies would greatly compress the degrees of freedom of the motor system and simplifies the problem of control. Further, the constraining of muscles into functional units implies the production of a stable pattern each time the synergies are invoked.

Behavioral patterning may be accounted for by synergies in both neural and dynamical perspectives, but the source of synergies or the constraints that lead to the packaging of muscle action is unclear. For Sherrington, reflexes were the source of the synergies. The reflex-based perspective is no longer held tenable as the primary account of motor control. In its place is the perspective that there is neural encoding or a central prescription of muscle action plans, which is modulated by sensory input. As the next section reveals, neurophysiologists have focused on the search for the discrete muscle synergies that reveal the central plan and the sensory inputs that modulate their output.

Synergies are also an important concept for dynamic pattern generation. From this perspective, however, synergies are 'softly assembled cooperative states, not hard-wired mechanisms' (Kelso and Schöner, 1988; see also Kugler and Turvey, 1987). First consider pattern formation in physical systems. Haken (1983) describes numerous systems (e.g. lasers, cloud formations, fluid dynamics) in which order emerges from disorder. Manipulating the energy in the system leads to abrupt phase transitions from one level of order to another. The energy, or scaled parameter, is a nonspecific input. That is, it contains no information that specifies or *prescribes* the emergent order or pattern. In terms of dynamical systems, these ordered and stable behaviors are *attractor states*. Changing some variable to which the system is sensitive leads to transitions from one stable attractor to another. These system-sensitive parameters are termed *control parameters*.

What biological systems share with the physical systems in Haken's examples is the very many degrees of freedom at the microscopic level that self-organize into coherent and well-defined macroscopic behaviors. In this view, synergies in biological systems are not constructed from some central representation or neural code. Rather, the patterned behavior emerges as the result of a stable interaction among the actor (or motor system – in which the neural substrate is a substantive contributor), environment and task constraints.

2.2   The Search for Muscle Synergies

In order to determine the extent to which the human nervous system uses synergies in the control of posture, a number of investigators have studied the characteristics of muscle responses activated when a subject is quietly standing or exposed to external threats to balance. Many of these experiments have manipulated the sensory information available to the subject in order to determine the extent to which visual, vestibular and somatosensory information contribute to balance control.

Gurfinkel and his colleagues (Elner, Popov and Gurfinkel, 1972; Gurfinkel and Shik, 1973; Gurfinkel *et al.*, 1976) performed the first extensive experiments on the contributions of peripheral and central neural control mechanisms to posture during quiet stance. Elner *et al.* (1976) and Gurfinkel, Lipshits and Popov (1979) showed that the state of excitability of the monosynaptic stretch reflex decreases during stance (compared with lying down, sitting or standing with support). They hypothesized that this is due to the wider range of adaptability of longer latency responses (latencies from 70 to 125 ms, which may be spinally or supraspinally mediated) which would be more useful in postural control. They also suggest that this reorganization in neural output, reflected in the change in reflex sensitivity when going from sitting to standing, is a manifestation of the functioning of central programs that coordinate the activity of different muscle groups during postural control.

More recent work by Nashner (1977) and Nashner and Woollacott (1979) asked the question: are the neuromuscular responses activated in muscles of the leg and trunk in response to external threats to balance the result of: (1) a neurally programmed response (i.e. a synergy), or (2) an independent stretch of the individual muscles due to a mechanical coupling of the ankle and hip motions. In order to test these alternate hypotheses they asked subjects to stand on a platform programmed to move unexpectedly. The platform could move each foot independently either horizontally, rotationally or vertically (Figure 6.1). Each of the platform motions was designed to destabilize the posture in a unique way, requiring the activation of different muscle groups in order to regain balance. The presence of muscle response synergies was determined by recording the surface

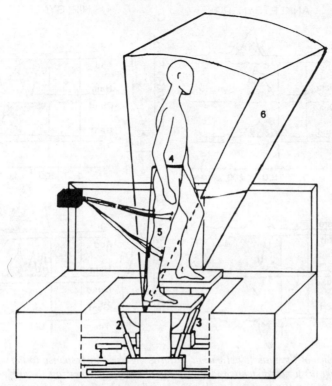

Figure 6.1. *Diagram of the experimental set-up. The hydraulically activated platform may be: (a) translated in the anteroposterior (AP) direction (hydraulic cylinder 1 is moved); (b) rotated about an axis colinear with the ankle joints (cylinders 2/3 moved reciprocally); or (c) moved vertically (cylinders 2/3 moved symmetrically). A belt (4) attached to the hips measures AP sway. Electromyograms record from the muscles of the leg (5). A visual enclosure (6) may be used to eliminate sway-related visual cues, by rotating the enclosure with body sway. [From Woollacott, Shumway-Cook and Nashner, 1986. © Baywood Publishing Co., Inc.. Reproduced with kind permission.]*

electromyographic (EMG) responses from the gastrocnemius (G), tibialis anterior (TA), hamstrings (H) and quadriceps (Q) muscles which contribute to the control of the movements of the ankle, knee and hip.

In response to platform translations inducing anterior sway, gastrocnemius, the stretched ankle muscle was activated at approximately 90 ms after platform movement onset, followed 20 ms later by the hamstrings muscle. Note that this response is about 50 ms later than a monosynaptic stretch reflex, suggesting that the postural response involves more complex neural circuitry. Anterior translations caused activation of the stretched tibialis anterior muscle, followed by the quadriceps (Figure 6.2). The authors hypothesized that the synergy was neurally preprogrammed by the system and not the result of independent stretch of the individual muscles due to a mechanical coupling of the ankle and hip motions because platform rotations, which directly rotated the ankles without causing movements at the other joints, caused activation of the same complementary pairs of leg muscles. This evidence supported the hypothesis of a neurally programmed synergy.

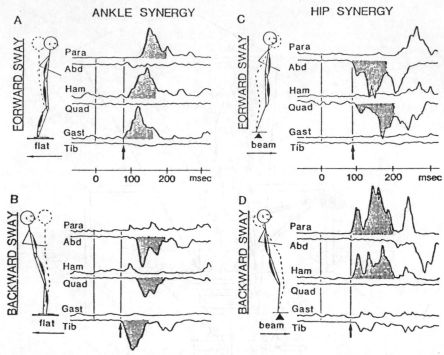

Figure 6.2. *Examples of the muscle activation patterns observed in response to horizontal platform translations causing: (a) forward sway, and (b) backward sway, and eliciting the ankle synergy. Note that the responses start in the stretched ankle muscle, followed by the leg and trunk muscles. (c), (d) Patterns observed when subjects balanced on a 9-cm long support surface (restraining the use of ankle torque) while the platform moved to cause: (c) forward sway, or (d) backward sway, and elicited the hip synergy. [From Horak and Nashner, 1986. Adapted with kind permission.]*

In order to determine whether ankle joint rotation was necessary to elicit the response, the platform was moved forward, and during the movement was rotated to keep the ankle joints at a constant 90 degrees, thus eliminating ankle rotation. In this case, the postural responses were delayed. Since the response was delayed when ankle rotation was eliminated, the authors concluded that the early response was activated primarily by ankle joint inputs, and that a later response, possibly activated by vestibular inputs, served to stabilize balance. Since the coupling of ankle and hip extensor muscles served a sway-stabilizing function, the response was termed the 'sway synergy'.

In response to moving one platform surface upward and one downward, flexing one leg and extending the other, the opposite relationships between proximal and distal leg muscles were observed. Muscles that extend and flex the ankle and knee together (G-Q or T-A-H) contracted in a fixed pattern. To determine whether this pattern was also preprogrammed, and was not caused by independent stretch of the proximal and distal muscles, one of the platform bases was rotated during a vertical movement so that the ankle motion was unexpectedly dissociated from that of the knees and hips. The response was unaltered by this ankle rotational input. They thus concluded that this synergy is activated whenever the predominant somatosensory input is knee rotation. Since this synergy helped to stabilize the body vertically, it was called the 'suspensory synergy'.

Later, Horak and Nashner (1986) showed that, in response to conditions which restrained the use of ankle torque (subjects balanced on a 9-cm long support surface, which was significantly shorter than the foot), subjects had to rely on shear forces to return balance to normal. In this case subjects responded to forward and backward platform displacements by first contracting the thigh and trunk muscles on the unstretched aspect of the leg (Horak and Nashner, 1986) (see Figure 6.2c, d). This pattern generated both hip and ankle motions, the hip motion as a direct result of the contractions, and the ankle motion indirectly through inertia (McCollum, Horak and Nashner, 1985). Since the synergy served to aid balance through hip movement rather than ankle movement, it was called the 'hip synergy'.

The above experiments suggest that the synergies are discrete entities. An understanding of the effect of these synergies, if not their formation, may be enhanced by consideration of the biomechanics of the postural system. Nashner and McCollum (1985) devised a scheme for understanding the organization of human postural adjustments. Equating limbs to rigid bodies and muscles to force vectors, they made principled predictions about the behavior of this mechanical system in a gravitational environment. Two additional limiting assumptions were made: (1) a minimum number of muscles will be used, and (2) frequently used movements will be organized to require minimal decision making. Out of this biomechanical and neural scheme, Nashner and McCollum propose that a limited number of combinations of muscle contractions and movement trajectories can be used for performing postural adjustments. These combinations are those of the ankle, hip and suspensory strategies described above.

According to Nashner and McCollum (1985), the system determines the region into which it has been moved by postural perturbations and then selects a control strategy which functions within that region (Figure 6.3). For example, Figure 6.3a shows a contractile muscle pattern that, according to the mechanical model, shifts

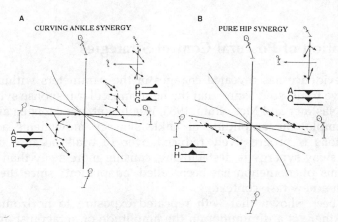

Figure 6.3. *Possible control strategies for trajectories in the ankle–hip plane. (a) Predicted EMG patterns (P, H, G or A, Q, T) to move the body toward the origin in a clockwise curved trajectory, by swaying about the ankle (ankle synergy). (b) EMG patterns (A, Q or P, H) for moving the body to hip-flexed and hip-extended positions (balancing in a nonerect position) by using the hip strategy. P, paraspinals; H, hamstrings; G, gastrocnemius; A, abdominals; Q, quadriceps; TA, tibialis anterior. [From Nashner and McCollum, 1985. © Cambridge University Press. Reprinted with kind permission.]*

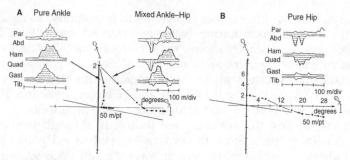

Figure 6.4. *(a) Examples of EMG and sway trajectories of a subject in response to backward platform movements causing forward sway. The points in position space are taken from motion analysis of the body positions at successive 50-ms intervals. The muscle responses on the left were produced on a regular flat support surface; the patterns on the right were observed immediately after switching from a beam to the normal surface. (b) Patterns produced when perturbed after adapting to standing on a short beam. [From Nashner and McCollum, 1985. © Cambridge University Press. Reprinted with kind permission.]*

the center of mass relative to the center of foot support by rotating the body about the ankle joint. In Figure 6.3b a contractile pattern appropriate to the hip synergy moves the body toward a position of balance with respect to gravity but not to a position of erect stance. Figure 6.4 shows actual muscle contraction patterns elicited within regions of pure ankle, pure hip and boundary regions between the two predicted strategies. Where the synergy-specific regions meet and overlap, an interaction between hip and sway synergies occurs. Nashner and McCollum noted that in the 5–10 trials after a transition, subjects mixed ankle and hip synergies, using a limited range of possible combinations. They suggest that the limited use of possible mixtures supports the concept of discrete synergies controlling posture.

2.3 Modulation of Postural Control Strategies

Experimental evidence has revealed changes in the parameters within a synergy across successive trials, suggesting that the neuromuscular response synergies may be fine-tuned (Nashner and McCollum, 1985; Woollacott, von Hofsten and Rosblad, 1988). For example, the amplitude of ankle synergy movements activated by platform rotations is progressively reduced over 10 trials because under these conditions the sway synergy is destabilizing, causing more sway than the perturbation itself. This phenomenon has been called 'adaptation', since the synergy is fine-tuned to fit a new task context.

It has also been shown that with repeated exposure to horizontal platform displacements, there is a diminution in the amplitude of antagonist ankle muscle responses. This also corresponded with smaller displacements of the body (Woollacott, von Hofsten and Rosblad, 1988), as if the subjects were changing their postural set during the course of the experiment.

As mentioned above, Nashner and McCollum (1985) also hypothesize that more complex patterns of muscle activation are formed by combining several synergies, during points in time when subjects are adapting responses to changing support surface conditions. These responses have been termed 'mixtures', and have been proposed to be combinations of more than one elemental synergy.

2.4 Variance and Invariance in Muscle Synergies

Although it had previously been shown that humans always respond to an unexpected perturbation in the anterior or posterior direction with appropriate combinations of output patterns to compensate for the task, these studies only examined responses to perturbations in the sagittal plane. It might be asked whether giving several different angles of platform motion would cause subjects to: (1) use different combinations of a few distinct synergies; or (2) show continuous variation in response patterns. Moore *et al.* (1988) performed this experiment by perturbing subjects as they stood on a platform in a variety of positions. They were asked to pivot at 15-degree increments between blocks of 10 trials (5 forward and 5 backward trials randomly presented for each of 8–12 orientations about the vertical axis).

Moore *et al.* (1988) noted that EMG activity and, in some cases, onset latency of individual muscle responses varied continuously as a function of perturbation direction. Continuous variation of response organization with perturbation direction does not, however, support or refute the hypothesis that automatic postural responses are simple mixtures of a few synergies. As discussed by Moore *et al.*, the data show that the postural response organization is determined by sensory cues which include directionality. Response organization in directions near the cardinal sagittal plane (300–15 degrees) showed a relatively constant onset latency relationship between muscles, with responses in the gastrocnemius, hamstrings and trunk extensors, as predicted, along with an early response in the abdominals (probably because of the high velocity of perturbation: $25\,\mathrm{cm\,s^{-1}}$ versus $13\,\mathrm{cm\,s^{-1}}$ used in earlier experiments). Similar relationships were seen for tibialis anterior, quadriceps and abdominals (with an early trunk extensor response) for directions of 165–225 degrees. However, in other directions latency relationships varied continuously. While the latency relationships may provide some evidence for discreteness in the postural responses, sharp transitions in latency and/or amplitude were not seen. An acknowledged limitation of the study was that EMG recordings were taken primarily from muscles involved in flexion and extension, and not those that would be responsive to perturbations in the lateral direction, so they could not describe a 'lateral synergy'.

Similar experiments have been performed using cat postural control as the model system (MacPherson, 1988; Rushmer *et al.*, 1988), recording ground reaction forces and postural muscle responses in the cat in response to horizontal platform perturbations in 16 different directions. MacPherson (1988) noted that the biomechanical strategy used by the cat involved primarily the hindlimbs and showed invariance in the direction of the vector of force they generated. For any of the 16 perturbation directions, the system made a simple two-choice response for vector direction: either backward/outward or forward. She states that this behavioral strategy may simplify the control process, since the animal can make a simple choice between two vector directions rather than computing a new direction of force to be exerted by each hindlimb for every direction of perturbation. Thus, once the direction is established, only the amplitude needs to be adjusted.

In contrast, the muscle response data did not support the concept that the simplification of the control process is achieved by constraining all the muscles in the response to act as a single unit. Although some of the muscles were comodulated, and could have been activated by a central command, others were controlled independently. The muscles that were comodulated included most of the hip muscles and distal muscles, such as the gastrocnemius. Other muscles (e.g. gracilis) were controlled independently.

MacPherson (1988) thus concluded that invariances were observed in: (1) the direction of horizontal plane force generation by the two hindlimbs; and (2) the spatial grouping of certain hindlimb muscles. But other muscles were clearly controlled independently and possibly used to 'tune' the synergy in order to produce the biomechanical goal of the production of specific ground reaction forces.

2.5   Alternative Approaches to the Definition of Functional Synergies

The search for neuromuscular strategies based on the monitoring of selected muscle groups is subject to criticism based on the inherently limiting nature of the methodology (see discussion of Moore *et al.*, 1988, above). The need to select muscle groups for monitoring necessarily excludes other muscles that may be participating. Thus, the full nature of the neuromotor cooperativity may not be revealed. Further, without independent measures of performance, we face the difficulty of assessing the suitability of the expressed synergy and subsequent changes. This issue is particularly relevant for investigating developmental changes in synergies. For example, do age-related changes in the neuromuscular synergies of the older adult reflect a decrement in performance, or an appropriate functional adaptation to compensate for accumulating deficiencies in the neuromotor system?

In an attempt to address these issues Yang, Winter and Wells (1990a, b) have taken an alternative approach to the determination of balance strategies. Based on model and experimental data, Yang *et al.* suggest that a fixed relationship among the joint torques about the hip, knee and ankle may be the more appropriate control variable for the motor system rather than a centrally driven pattern of muscle activation. Here, the joint torque is defined as the torque due to the active contraction of muscle and the viscoelastic properties of the musculotendinous unit.

The suitability of this approach may be argued from two major points. First, there is no one-to-one mapping between muscle activation and joint trajectories. Change in the limb segment behaviors that contribute to joint motion is the result of both active (muscle) and passive forces (gravity and the forces due to the mechanical interaction among segments). Gravity and motion-dependent forces are dependent upon context. Thus identical joint trajectories under different circumstances (e.g. the body in motion versus the body in a static posture) would require different muscle involvement. Further, the joint torques reflect the *net* effect of muscle activation for all muscles crossing the joint. As a simple example, a net joint torque of zero may be obtained at any number of gain settings in which antagonist muscles are coactive and lead to equivalent but opposite torques.

A relevant example of the mutable relationship between muscle activation (thus joint torque) and joint trajectory comes from Winter's (1980) work in which he describes the extensor, or 'support', moment for the stance limb during locomotion. Winter's data show that it is possible to have a functionally appropriate net extensor moment for the limb with an extensor *or* flexor joint torque at the knee. In the case of a flexor torque, compensation occurs in the torque magnitudes at the hip and ankle to prevent collapse of the limb. Thus, function may be maintained despite modulation or fluctuations in the pattern of muscle contribution.

The second point to be made is that the analysis of the joint torques may reveal a stability of pattern not observed at finer levels of analysis. Citing Nashner's (1976) experience of finding nearly 50% of the subjects who failed to exhibit the muscle synergies of the proposed models, Yang, Winter and Wells (1990a) suggest such individual differences may be functionally insignificant. Other measures, perhaps joint torque relationships, may be better representative of synergistic response to task demands.[1]

In support of their arguments, Yang *et al.* compared model and experimental results from perturbations to stance. The mathematical model consisted of a three-link system (the lower legs, the thighs and the trunk) with appropriate inertial characteristics. Perturbations could be applied to the model as disturbance forces acting at the model hip, knee or shoulder and as a horizontal acceleration at the ground contact point (a simulation of the platform translation paradigm) and the model response was created by idealized torque generators at the ankles, knees and hips. The simulation was designed to determine the set of joint torque combinations that would restore balance given a specific disturbance. In the experimental paradigm a mechanical perturbation was applied to the subject while in a static symmetrical stance. Joint torques were estimated from recorded kinematic and ground force reaction data using the standard techniques of inverse dynamics.

Model and experimental results were in good agreement. The model results revealed multiple mechanical solutions for the same initial conditions and disturbance force. Figure 6.5a shows a set of results obtained from the model when a disturbance of 160 N was applied for 80 ms. The shaded areas represent combinations of hip, knee and ankle torques that led to successful returns to balance.

The experimental results revealed individual strategies in the muscle response patterns and joint torques. Despite the range of responses, the average joint torque for each subject fell within the predicted solution space generated from the model (Figure 6.5b). The density of the solution set for physiologically appropriate responses is low because of the small subject pool ($n = 5$). Nevertheless, these initial results suggest an appropriate match between model assumptions and physiological reality.

The model results further predict that postural control may be obtained through a fixed relationship between the joint torques: a 1.5 ratio of hip to knee and a 2.0 ratio between ankle and knee torques. An invariant relationship among joint torques could be an effective control strategy in reducing the complexity of the multidimensional system at the muscle level and is consistent with the assumptions of dynamic pattern generation and the accommodation of task demands.

---

[1]Nashner's results were subsequently demonstrated to be a function of the perturbation velocity, the velocity being at or near the threshold velocity necessary to elicit the synergistic response. Nevertheless, Nashner published results in 1977 which supported the contention of individual differences, even with perturbation velocities well above threshold.

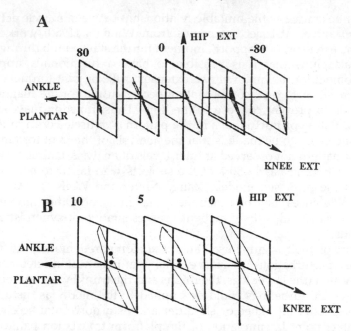

Figure 6.5. *(a) Solution space for conditions of a disturbance force of 160 N applied for 80 ms. Model configuration was erect stance with the disturbance applied as a forward force at the level of the knee. Movement along the horizontal axis reflects changes in the torque about the ankle. The plantarflexor torque increases with movement to the left. Hip torque is represented along the vertical axis, and knee torque along the third orthogonal axis (moving into and out of the plane of the page). (b) Comparison of model and experimental results. The model results are generated from conditions equivalent to (a) and are indicated by the outlined area. Average joint torque values for five experimental subjects are marked with dots. The scale in (b) has been expanded to yield greater resolution of the graph. [Adapted from Yang, Winter and Wells, 1990.]*

The results of Yang, Winter and Wells (1990a,b) are intriguing and lead to interesting questions. As heuristic devices, models such as these may help us to explore the region of overlapping solution sets that represent mechanical possibility and physiological reality – not unlike the approach taken by Nashner and McCollum (1985). But models are limited by simplifying assumptions. Of particular relevance here is that in the model developed by Yang *et al.*, the joint torques at hip, knee and ankle were simultaneously initiated – unlike physiological data that show a sequencing of muscle activation. Questions regarding the effect of shifts in the temporal patterning of muscle activation are left unexplored. Thus the model does not provide a critical test of neural versus dynamic pattern generation. The results of this study, however, add to the growing body of literature that hints at an organizational scheme for motor control that is broader in dimension and more context sensitive than discrete neural codes – even with modulating sensory inputs – can explain.

What we are seeking is a principled account of patterned behavior and the immediate compensatory actions that are observed in response to perturbation. The foundation of the neural perspective is that discrete muscle synergies exist *a priori* and are elicited under selected proprioceptive conditions. Adaptation of the synergies occurs over trials as a result of supraspinal influences using knowledge of results and assimilating relevant sensory information.

Alternatively, Saltzman and Kelso (1985, 1987) argue that postural control is not rooted in preprogrammed discrete muscle synergies, but in the formation of control laws that are task specific, but muscle independent. In the dynamical perspective, it is the function or the task that drives the organization. For example, perturbation to the jaw during vocalization of certain syllables alters the trajectory of some of the physical components of the motor system. Function is maintained by immediate, and first trial, compensatory trajectory changes in the movement of the lips (Kelso and Tuller, 1984b). The response appears reflexive, but not in a hard-wired, preplanned manner. That is to say, information from some source is modifying subsequent behavior in a task-relevant way, and in a manner that appears to avoid the replanning of the movement and the invoking of a new plan.

Both neural and dynamical perspectives acknowledge that parsimonious control is served by constraining the free variables and reducing the degrees of freedom, and minimizing executive function (Kugler, Kelso and Turvey, 1980; Nashner and McCollum, 1985). It is in the source of the synergies that the perspectives diverge. From a dynamical perspective, Saltzman and Kelso (1985, 1987) offer a reinterpretation of existing data on postural control and the compensatory responses seen after perturbation. Their position offers a counterpoint to the neural perspective that hypothesizes postural control as a function of modular synergies triggered by sensory inputs. The EMG patterns reflect a functional synergy that exists *a priori* and is elicited under selected proprioceptive conditions.

Alternatively, motor control begins with a control law based on the task: e.g. maintain upright stable balance. This control law specifies the corrective joint torques that maintain function. The joint torques subsequently specify the muscle involvement that leads to appropriate corrective torques. The result is that the task demands lead to the EMG burst patterns appropriate to generating the proper torques (Saltzman and Kelso, 1985). This position finds additional support in the work of MacPherson (1988) and Yang, Winter and Wells (1990a, b).

Evidence for one or the other perspective may be observed at the boundary regions where proposed functional synergies should be competing and/or overlapping (see article by Nashner and McCollum, 1985, with commentary by Saltzman and Kelso, 1985). Are the mixed synergies observed at the boundaries a reflection of competing neural synergies or a reflection of the instabilities and bifurcations of a multicomponent system seeking a new stable mode? These questions await further exploration.

2.6 Hypothetical Experiment–From the Dynamical Perspective

Beyond the Saltzman and Kelso (1985, 1987) reconceptualization of existing postural data, little research has been initiated on postural control that begins with an explicit expression of hypotheses rooted in the dynamical perspective. Here we present the outlines of an experiment designed to expand our knowledge of postural control, particularly during strategy transitions.

In the terminology of the dynamical perspective, the ankle and hip synergies are independently stable attractors – preferred but not mandatory behavioral patterns. Following the theoretical propositions of Schöner and Kelso (1988a) for dynamic pattern generation, the stability of the attractor is characteristically described by low variability about the mean behavior, resistance of the pattern to perturbation, and quick return of the system to a stable posture after perturbation. To monitor the behavior of the system and the transition between synergies we need to define a *collective variable* – a variable that reflects essential characteristics of the movement patterns and whose behavior reflects the attractor states. What we are looking for is a representative variable that captures the qualitative change in the pattern. Thus, when the behavioral pattern is stable, the values of the collective variables should also remain stable. When the pattern changes, the value of the collective variable should reflect that change (Scholz, 1990). For example, the *ratio* of hip to ankle joint movement may be a better expression of the selected synergy, than some singular kinematic descriptor (e.g. linear translation of the hip joint center). A low ratio would be obtained when the ankle strategy was used and a high ratio value would occur if the hip strategy was used, but translation of the hip joint center might be equivalent in both patterns. Further, we need to define one or more *control parameters* – variables that when scaled up or down move the system through its attractor states. Perturbation velocity and length of the support surface (as it affects the ability to produce torque about the ankle) are both potential control parameters. For simplicity in the discussion that follows, we will use perturbation velocity as the control parameter.

By scaling up and down on perturbation velocity, we expect to push the system into and out of attractor states. At low velocities we expect consistent use of the ankle synergy. At high velocities we would predict predominant use of the hip synergy.[2] Over multiple trials, we predict the transition periods to be observable in increased variability about the collective variable mean (Figure 6.6a), increased sensitivity to perturbation during the transition, and slower returns to stable posture after the perturbation.

Once stable and unstable response regions have been found, we can look at the strength of the attractor state. Testing the strength of the attractor requires us to 'poke' the system during a response to a platform perturbation – that is, a secondary perturbation. This 'poke' might take the form of an added mass to the trunk, or conflicting optic flow information. From the theory, we would predict that, at low velocities when the ankle synergy was stable, the second perturbation would have no effect. The same result would occur at high velocities after the switch to the more stable hip synergy. However, during intermediate velocity trials, when the ankle synergy still predominated, but with greater variability, the addition of the secondary perturbation would push the system into the hip synergy.

Support for dynamic pattern generation would be further enhanced if we could demonstrate hysteresis in the response pattern between scaling up and scaling down on the control parameter. In this example, this scaling corresponds to increasing or decreasing velocity of the platform perturbation. Hysteresis exists if the trajectory of the x-y plot as the control parameter is scaled down does not follow

---

[2]Diener, Horak and Nashner (1988) attempted this velocity scale perturbation but did not seek the switch from ankle to hip strategy. It is conceivable that the tested velocities were of insufficient magnitude to elicit the switch.

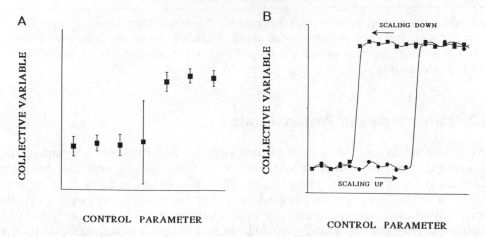

Figure 6.6. (*a*) *Hypothetical means (SD) resulting from manipulation of the control parameter. Mean behavior remains constant and standard deviations are small for selected values of the control parameter. The transition from one stable behavior to another is marked by increased variability about the mean. (b) Predicted hysteresis: the transition from one stable behavior to another occurs at different values of the control parameter when scaling up versus scaling down.*

the same trajectory formed during scaling up (Figure 6.6b). From the neural perspective, muscle synergies are modulated by sensory inputs. Qualitative changes in behavior may be elicited as sensory inputs change through the scaling of the control parameter. Under identical conditions, however, the same behavior should occur. If hysteresis is present, then the transition between stable states is not a simple function of additive stimulus inputs. Rather, the hysteresis reveals a classic property of dynamical systems – namely, that at the same value of a control parameter, two or more stable states may exist. Further, the stable state attained by the system depends on the history of the system (Prigogine and Stengers, 1984).

Could such data be accounted for by both perspectives? Neural pattern generation has been the dominant explanation for synergic responses, and could explain much of the predicted results from our hypothetical experiment. From this neural perspective, however, there is no easy account of transition instability or the presence of multiple stable behavioral states at constant values of a control parameter. The dynamical systems perspective offers a complementary view. At another level of analysis, specific predictions regarding the behavior of the collective variables and their reflection of the variability of behavioral systems in transition may be derived from the propositions of dynamical systems theory. Dynamic pattern generation as an explanatory construct may add to our knowledge of postural control by accounting for a different part of the data set: the transition periods to new states.

Each perspective, then, contributes to our understanding of the behaviors observed in this hypothetical experiment and to understanding postural control in general. The contrast between neural and dynamic pattern generation as explanatory constructs may arise, in part, from the discontinuity in the levels of analysis to which the perspectives typically have been applied. The strength of the dynamical systems perspective is, however, that its propositions for pattern formation are level independent. That is, organization at the neuronal level is governed by the same pattern formation processes that operate at the behavioral level. A merging of perspectives may come when we can reconcile 'hard-wired' synergies with strong attractors, and synergy elicitation as a function of scaling on system-sensitive control parameters.

2.7   Other Issues in Posture Control

We have tried to contrast theories of motor control and show the relevance of the dynamical perspective to understanding posture control – an area that has been dominated by the neural perspectives. The task of re-examining all existing literature from the dynamical perspective is prohibitive. What we hope is that the above discussion will encourage others to examine the literature from multiple theoretical perspectives. Thus, what follows is a simple description of additional research relevant to our understanding of postural control.

2.7.1   How Modifiable are Synergies?

The theory of dynamic pattern generation is not restricted only to events at the behavioral level. Animal studies have shown that the motor cortex is organized spatially not only in a task-dependent manner, but that it is also continuously modulated by immediate past experience, i.e. it appears dynamically organized. Humphrey and his colleagues (Humphrey, 1986; Humphrey and Reed, 1983) have performed experiments which suggest that there is a spatial organization within the primate motor cortex that would allow spatially simple afferent inputs to evoke muscle synergies that are necessary for a variety of simple movements. Although his work focuses on muscles of the arm and hand, it will be reported here since it relates to the question of the organization of muscle response synergies. His mapping experiments were carried out on adult rhesus monkeys equipped with chronically implanted recording and stimulation chambers. He showed that a single muscle could be represented at more than one focus within the motor cortex, and that such a focus could activate several other muscles when higher, but still moderate, stimulation intensities were used. In addition, the evoked muscle synergies were functionally useful: they were exactly those required for the production of a specific movement, along with postural or stabilizing responses required at adjacent joints.

Thus, postural responses associated with balance control could be activated in a similar manner, with a simple set of sensory inputs activating: (1) primary postural muscles at the joint that is focal for restabilizing the center of mass; and (2) additional muscles at adjacent or nearby joints which contribute to stabilization.

More recent work by Humphrey et al. (1990) indicates that the motor cortical representation can be shaped by sensory experience. They found consistent expansion of the forelimb zone of the rat motor cortex after passive movements of the elbow over a period of 90–120 minutes, with no increase in this zone under other movement conditions. (Shrinkage occurred after vibrissae movements, as a resuslt of expansion of the adjacent vibrissae zone.) They interpret this movement-induced expansion to be caused by changes in the synaptic strengths of afferent pathways converging onto the forelimb motor control cells at the periphery of the zone. This suggests that the amount of cortex controlling a given set of muscles is regulated by competitive dynamic processes.

2.7.2   Are Muscles Other than Leg and Trunk Muscles Involved in the Synergies?

Two studies (Keshner, Woollacott and Debu, 1988; Woollacott, von Hofsten and Rosblad, 1988) examined the body movement kinematics and the responses of leg, trunk and neck muscles of subjects who were given support surface translations in order to determine whether responses radiating upward from the ankle joint represented part of a large ascending synergy encompassing axial muscles along the entire length of the body, or whether muscles of the neck and possibly the trunk could be independently activated by vestibular, visual or other proprioceptive inputs. The results support the hypothesis of multiple control of upper body muscles. Posterior platform translations, causing anterior sway, elicited an ascending pattern of response in the extensor muscles of the body, radiating upward from gastrocnemius, to hamstrings, trunk extensor and neck extensor muscles. In addition to this pattern ascending from the stretched ankle muscles, there were very short latency responses in the neck flexor and abdominal muscles.

In order to determine whether these neck muscle responses were activated by vestibular or neck proprioceptive inputs, Woollacott, von Hofsten and Rosblad (1988) examined head and trunk movement kinematics in response to platform translations. They noted small vertical movements of the head and shoulder as early as 40 ms after platform movement onset, which could be responsible for activating the early neck muscle responses. In order to differentiate between vestibular and neck proprioceptive contributions to neck muscle response activation, they repeated the experiment on one of their subjects with a neck stabilization device, to restrict neck movement and stretch of the neck muscles. In this condition, they found normal neck muscle responses, supporting the hypothesis that these responses are mainly activated by the vestibular system, with possible contributions by the ankle proprioceptors.

2.7.3   Latencies of Postural Responses

The responses described above are elicited by support surface displacements at latencies of 80–110 ms, and are usually referred to as medium latency responses or automatic postural adjustments, since they are too short to have a voluntary component. In addition to these responses, shorter monosynaptic latency responses can occasionally be elicited in normal standing adults.

Some laboratories (Diener and Dichgans, 1986; Diener *et al.*, 1984) have performed postural experiments using platform rotations rather than translations to destabilize subjects. They have described postural responses in the ankle muscles to ankle-dorsiflexing (toes-up) platform rotations as M1, M2 or M3 depending on their latencies. Thus M1 (55–65 ms) is a monosynaptic reflex, observed in the stretched gastrocnemius muscle, M2 (108–123 ms) is the medium latency response in the gastrocnemius, and M3 is a longer latency response, seen in the antagonist tibialis anterior musculature (130–145 ms). They state that the first two responses, M1 and M2, activated by stretch of the ankle muscles, are destabilizing in this condition, since they enforce the induced backward displacement, but the third response, M3, activated in the antagonist muscle and involving more complex pathways (possibly vestibular), is used to return the center of mass to its original position. They noted that the area under the rectified EMG curve was linearly related to the amplitude of platform rotation, and that the slope of this function (gain) was smaller for the destabilizing M1 and M2 responses than for the stabilizing M3 response in the antagonist, thus showing a functionally adaptive modulation of gain. The M2 response is equivalent to that described above for platform translations.

2.7.4   Sensory Inputs Contributing to Postural Control

Three sensory systems contribute to the maintenance of upright stance: the visual, vestibular and somatosensory systems. A number of research labs have performed experiments to determine the relative contributions of these inputs to postural control under normal and restricted sensory conditions. It has been shown that if there is a deficit in sensory information from two of these systems it may cause severe impairment of posture control. For example Paulus, Straube and Brandt (1987) analyzed postural control in a patient with severe deficits of vestibular function and the somatosensory system (as a result of sensory poly-neuropathy). This patient was able to stand and to walk slowly with eyes open. However, with eyes closed, with low visual acuity or with stroboscopic illumination he lost balance within seconds.

It was originally suggested that, within the neural pathways for postural stabilization, each of these three systems had a separate frequency range for optimal function, with some overlap between ranges. For example, Nashner (1970) suggested that the normal subject uses a combination of high-frequency (semicircular canal and ankle joint somatosensory receptors, responding in the range of 90–100 ms) and low-frequency (otolith and vision, responding in the range of 180 ms) systems for stabilization. However, more recent work suggests that otoliths and the visual system have high-frequency components as well. Allum and Pfaltz (1985) have shown that EMG responses are evoked in ankle muscles within 80 ms after head acceleration onset, when a subject is perturbed by ankle rotational perturbations. In addition, Nashner and Berthoz (1978) have shown that visuomotor reaction time to platform perturbations can be as early as 100 ms.

Visual Contributions to Posture

In the 1970s, Lishman and Lee (1973) performed an experiment to show that motion in the visual field by itself can induce the sensation of postural sway and an accompanying compensatory response. The experiment involved using a room with a stable floor, but with walls and ceiling which moved forward or backward. When the room moved forward, the subjects perceived they had swayed backward and compensated by swaying in the direction of the room's movement. When the room oscillated, adults showed postural sway oscillations at the same frequency as the room's movements. In addition, adults could be made to rely more heavily on the visual information if they stood cross-wise on a beam, reducing their support surface information coming from the feet. Thus it was shown that visual movement by itself could give the perception of body sway and cause postural compensations, even when somatosensory and vestibular information did not signal sway.

The above research suggests that there are two possible perceptual interpretations of visual movement: either self motion or object motion. In the case of the moving room experiments, the subject mistakenly assumes object motion is self motion. Brandt (1988) states that the relative retinal shift of a viewed scene is greater the nearer the objects are to the eyes, and thus when a person is close to stationary objects, balance improves. This also explains height vertigo, which is experienced when the distance between the observer's eye and the nearest non-moving object becomes critically large (Brandt).

Although it has been shown that visually guided behaviors such as locomotion and postural stabilization depend on visual information mediated by peripheral visual inputs, recent research suggests that central areas of the visual field play a dominant role in fine-tuning of postural control (Amblard and Carblanc, 1980; Brandt, 1988; Leibowitz, Rodemer and Dichgans, 1979). Brandt (1988) notes that foveal stabilization becomes important for correction of small lateral body sway relative to structures in grasping space.

Somatosensation

Research has shown that adults, under normal circumstances, are more reliant on somatosensation than visual inputs in correcting for body sway (Nashner and Berthoz, 1978; Roos, Bles and Bos, 1988). Thus, for example, when a normal adult is asked to stand on a platform in a room that is dynamically tilting, they almost always perceive the room as tilting and the platform as stable (Roos, Bles and Bos, 1988).

It has also been shown that vibratory stimuli to postural muscles induce kinesthetic illusions and associated motor responses (Eklund, 1972). Work by Roll and Vedel (1982) has shown that the afferent information underlying kinesthetic sensation is almost entirely of muscle spindle origin. They have shown, through recording from sensory nerves coming from the vibrated muscle, that a vibratory stimulus preferentially activates the Ia afferents of muscles. Roll and Roll (1988) have further explored the relative contributions of proprioceptive inputs from ankle, neck and eye musculature in regulating body sway, through this same method of muscle vibration. To vibrate eye muscles, they created minivibrators which were attached to a helmet and aligned so that the superior recti, inferior recti, or medial or lateral recti muscles could be vibrated. They showed that application of vibration to the eye muscles of a standing subject with eyes closed elicited, within 1–2 seconds, whole body postural shifts, whose direction depended on the muscle vibrated. Similar effects of backward body displacement were elicited when either the inferior rectus muscles of the eye, the sternocleidomastoid muscles of the neck or the soleus muscles of the leg were stimulated. Stimulation of the superior recti, splenii or tibialis anterior muscles causes forward body displacement. In addition, when costimulation of muscles of these three areas was performed, the effects were additive, with no clear domination of one proprioceptive influence over another. This thus suggests that extraocular proprioception as well as neck and ankle proprioception plays an important role in the organization of whole body posture.

Vestibular System

In order to explore the contributions of the vestibular system to posture control, experiments have been performed on patients with vestibular deficits to determine any differences in their postural responses compared with normal subjects. Under normal support surface conditions, with eyes open, patients with vestibular deficits show normal muscle response synergies to horizontal perturbations (Nashner, Black and Wall, 1982; Shupert *et al.*, 1988). This would be expected, since it has previously been shown that the ankle synergy is mediated primarily by support surface inputs (Nashner, 1977).

However, patients with vestibular deficits have more difficulty balancing when subjected to platform rotations, especially with eyes closed. As was mentioned earlier, ankle dorsiflexing platform rotations cause stretch-induced responses in the gastrocnemius/soleus ankle joint muscles, which are destabilizing, and adapt to low levels within a few trials, but at slightly longer latencies responses are also activated in the tibialis anterior muscle, which counteracts the body sway. By recording responses of vestibular patients to platform rotations, it was shown that approximately 80% of the earliest tibialis anterior (TA) activity (occurring at 80 ms after platform movement onset) is due to stabilizing reactions originating in the vertical semicircular canal system when vision is not available (Allum and Pfaltz, 1985) (Figure 6.7). Comparison of results for eyes open versus closed conditions indicates that an interaction between the visual and vestibulospinal systems occurs

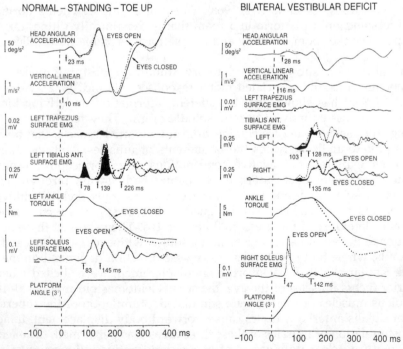

Figure 6.7. *Responses of a normal subject and a patient with bilateral deficit to toe-up platform rotations with eyes open versus closed. Note that the early tibialis anterior response in the normal subject is almost absent in the vestibular patient. [From Allum and Pfaltz, 1985. Reproduced with kind permission.]*

in the TA responses. It has been hypothesized that the vestibulospinal reflexes may also be influenced by visual inputs, or alternatively that the visual system may act directly on TA motor neurons via tectospinal tracts (Allum and Pfaltz, 1985).

2.7.5   Controlling Posture Under Changing Sensory Conditions

It has been hypothesized that within the postural control system, the vestibular system is an inertial–gravitational orientation system and is thus a reference against which support surface and visual inputs are compared and quickly inhibited if they conflict with this vestibular reference (Nashner, Black and Wall, 1982). This hypothesis is based upon the fact that patients with vestibular deficits cannot cope with disturbances in support surface and visual inputs (Begbie, 1967), and that the vestibular system is an accurate inertial–gravitational sensory system for normal movement speeds. In order to test this hypothesis the equilibrium strategies of normal and vestibular system-impaired subjects were compared as they balanced within changing support surface and visual environments. Experiments required the subjects to: (1) balance on the platform when ankle joint somatosensory inputs and/or visual inputs were made incongruent with postural sway, by rotating the platform and/or a visual box surrounding the subject in direct correlation with body sway. This kept the ankle joint at a constant 90 degrees and/or the visual world stationary with relation to the body; or (2) balance under similar ankle joint conditions, but with vision absent.

It was shown that patients with mild vestibular impairment balanced in the absence of useful support surface and visual inputs, yet could not balance when exposed to conflicting support surface and visual stimuli. Normal subjects balanced well under all conditions. Nashner, Black and Wall (1982) thus propose that in normal adults the major determinant of the short-term weighting of support surface and visual inputs during stance is their congruence with the inertial–gravitational reference provided by the vestibular system. Their experiments indicate that in normal adults conflicting orientation inputs from the visual or somatosensory systems are suppressed quickly in favor of those that are congruent with the vestibular system. However, in patients with vestibular deficits there is no internal mechanism for selecting the correct sensory reference when incongruence occurs between visual and somatosensory inputs.

2.7.6   Postural Preparatory Processes Before Voluntary Movements

Although postural adjustments can regulate body sway during quiet stance, they are also activated in advance of voluntary movements to maintain equilibrium during the movement. Studies in both humans (Belen'kii, Gurfinkel and Pal'tsev, 1967; Cordo and Nashner, 1982; Lee, 1980; Massion, 1984) and cats (Massion, 1979) have shown that the execution of potentially destabilizing movements is preceded by activation of postural muscles. These postural adjustments act to oppose the forces created by the voluntary movement and thus compensate in advance for changes in equilibrium caused by the movement.

Belen'kii, Gurfinkel and Pal'tsev (1967) showed that for rapid arm-raising movements these postural responses were of short latency (80–100 ms after a response signal for biceps femoris) compared with those for voluntary reaction times (150–200 ms) and preceded the onset of the primary mover muscle response by 40–50 ms. More recently, other researchers (Cordo and Nashner, 1982; Hugon, Massion and Wiesendarger, 1982) have shown that anticipatory postural adjustments are specific to other voluntary movements as well, including arm flexion/extension movements, active unloading of the arm and pointing. It has also been shown that the same muscle response organization used in stabilizing posture after an external threat to balance (G-H-TE) is used to stabilize posture before activation of the prime mover muscle (biceps) in an arm flexion task (Cordo and Nashner, 1982).

To study animal models of the coordination of posture and voluntary movement, Massion and his colleagues (Massion, 1984) have studied the activation of postural muscles in the standing quadruped when one of the legs is lifted from the support base, either in response to a cue or in response to stimulation of the motor cortex. Massion noted that the activation of the prime mover and that of the postural muscles were fairly synchronous, and hypothesized that the movement control pathway delivered postural signals through a command mediated by internal collaterals of the pathway. To test this hypothesis, they stimulated the motor cortex in the area required for activation of the prime mover muscle. They observed that both the contralateral prime mover and the appropriate postural support activity were elicited by activation of this area. Thus the activation of prime mover muscles and their associated postural support synergies appears to be tightly coupled in the motor cortex.

2.7.7   The Development of Balance Control

The maturation of a variety of nervous system and musculoskeletal components contributes to development of balance control in infants. Thus one could view the onset of independent stability as an emergent behavior, depending on the maturation of certain rate-limiting components which can be identified as those that push the system to a new level of postural control when they have matured. The following variables could be rate-limiting: (1) the development of the muscle response synergies used in maintaining balance; (2) the development of somatosensory, visual or vestibular systems; (3) the development of adaptive mechanisms to allow the child to change the weighting of different sensory inputs used in posture control; (4) development of muscle strength or change in the relative mass of different body segments. The following sections will discuss the progressive stages in the cephalocaudal development of balance control in children, and within each section will include the available research on the relative contributions of the above variables to balance.

Posture Control in the Neonate

Jouen (1984, 1988) has studied the development of visual postural reactions in the neonate. To determine whether the visual system could activate postural responses he used a sequentially activated pattern of lights to create the illusion of forward or backward sway, and measured subsequent head postural compensation by the infant who was supported in an infant seat. He noted head postural reactions to optical flow in the 3-day-old infant, which suggests that vision may exert a proprioceptive function in the control of posture from birth.

Posture Control in the Newly Sitting Child

The effect of visual flow fields on posture control in infants able to sit independently has also been tested, by using the moving room described above (see 'Visual contributions to posture'). Pope (1984) showed that at the onset of crawling, at about 6 months, there was a decline in the susceptibility to the effects of visual feedback from the moving room. However, the susceptibility occurred again when the infant gained control over the trunk. In more recent experiments the extent to which peripheral versus central visual cues are instrumental in activating the infant's response to optical flow was explored (Bertenthal and Bai, 1988; Stoffregen, Schmuckler and Gibson, 1987). It was shown that global flow is not necessary for inducing postural sway in infants, and that flow along the edges of the visual field induces greater responsiveness than flow in the center of the field.

The role of other sensory inputs such as proprioception on posture control, and the time course of the emergence of postural synergies, has also been studied in the infant from 4 to 14 months of age, by using support surface displacements to activate postural responses (Woollacott, Debu and Mowatt, 1987). Infants were placed in an infant seat if they were unable to sit independently. Responses of the flexors and extensors of the neck and trunk were recorded. Infants of 5–6 months of age, who could not yet sit independently, showed responses only in the muscles of the neck. When vision was occluded, the combined proprioceptive and vestibular systems were mature enough to give directionally specific responses in all of the trials. Postural response synergies of independently sitting infants aged 8–14 months included muscles of both the neck and trunk, and were directionally specific to compensate for the platform-induced sway: thus when the platform was moved backward, causing forward sway, the trunk extensor and neck extensor muscles were activated. These experiments show a gradual development of posture control moving in the cephalocaudal direction, with postural responses first appearing in the neck and then the trunk, as children develop from birth to 8 months of age.

Postural Development in the Standing Child

Research on posture control in the newly standing child (Forssberg and Nashner, 1982; Shumway-Cook and Woollacott, 1985; Woollacott, Debu and Mowatt, 1987; Woollacott and Sveistrup, 1992) has used the platform paradigm described above to investigate the organization of postural muscle responses during this transition period. It has previously been hypothesized that animals go through specific phases in the development of behavior where movements initially show excessive degrees of freedom, then are simplified as the new skill level is mastered, and are finally re-elaborated as the young animal learns to reach the same end-point through variable means (Bernstein, 1967; Fentress, 1989). In order to determine whether this hypothesis is true for the developmental stages seen in children's balance control, the transition to independent stance was studied in infants from 9 to 14 months of age in both cross-sectional and longitudinal studies (Woollacott, Debu and Mowatt, 1987; Woollacott and Sveistrup, 1992).

Figure 6.8a shows examples of the longitudinal changes in the muscle response onset latencies of one infant to backward platform perturbations, causing forward sway, between the period of 9 and 14 months of age. With the initial emergence of 'pull to stand' behavior (9 months) postural responses were disorganized, with delayed and highly variable onset latencies. Responses were also infrequently activated in response to support surface perturbations (Figure 6.8b). This behavior began to improve with experience in dependent stance (10 months). However, at

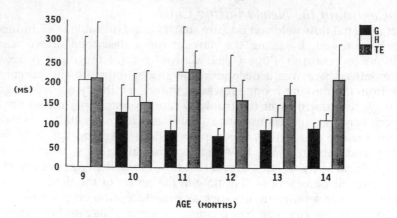

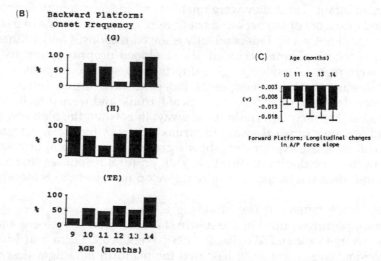

Figure 6.8. (a) Means and standard deviations of onset latencies of G (gastrocnemius), H (hamstrings) and TE (trunk extensor) muscles activated in response to backward platform translations causing forward sway, for ages 9–14 months. (b) Frequency (percentage of total trials) with which a response was observed in individual muscles for ages 9–14 months. (c) Changes in the slope of the anterior–posterior force curve of the infant (ages 10–14 months) for the first 50 ms after the platform starts to move. This would indicate background stiffness characteristics of the system, before active muscle contraction has been elicited. [From Woollacott and Sveistrup (1992). © Elsevier. Reproduced with kind permission.]

the onset of independent stance, the muscle response patterns show a regression, toward longer onset latencies and higher variability (11 months). With improved ability at independent stance and the onset of independent walking the postural response organization became consistent and latencies were shortened to more mature levels (Figure 6.8a, b; 13–14 months). Variability of response onsets was also reduced and responses were activated whenever the child's balance was disturbed.

In analyzing the movement of the children's hip, knee and ankle joints when quietly standing on the platform, we noted that there was a large amount of background 'wobble' or movement of the joints over the first few months of dependent stance, which disappeared when the children began independent stance. This could be due either to: (1) a low level of muscle stiffness at early ages, which was correlated with an inability to stand independently; or (2) the infant exploring postural space, in order to calibrate a 'sensorimotor map', to be used at the onset of independent stance. In the second case one would not expect a low level of background stiffness in the muscles during this period, since the wobble would be due to an active exploration of space.

In order to explore these two hypotheses the slope of the torque trace (time rate of change of the locus of the anterior–posterior (AP) force) was measured during the initial 50 ms of the platform perturbation, before the onset of any active muscular compensation, to determine whether there were changes in these slopes with development. Figure 6.8c shows that the slopes of the torque trace (for forward platform movements, causing backward body sway) almost doubled between 10 and 12 months of age. This corresponds to a drop in muscle stiffness, as the child learned to stand independently. Thus this does not support the first hypothesis, which predicts that the background movement was wobble due to lack of muscle stiffness, and gives some support for the second hypothesis, that the background movement was a form of exploration of the postural sensorimotor space. In addition, it suggests that with experience in balance control the background muscle stiffness levels drop–a characteristic change that is found in the learning of other motor tasks as well.

Forssberg and Nashner (1982) also noted that postural muscle responses of children first learning to stand showed more antagonist coactivation, and were also more variable and slower than those of adults. They noted that sway excursions were larger and more oscillatory than in older children, because of slower EMG responses and faster rates of sway acceleration. Responses in the 15–31-month-old age range were also consistently larger in amplitude and longer in duration than those of adults (Shumway-Cook and Woollacott, 1985). Figure 6.9 shows examples of responses to three successive platform perturbations in infants from three age groups (15–31 months, 4–6 years, 7–10 years), compared with adults to show these changes in response characteristics.

The changes seen during the transition to independent stance appear to mirror those seen during the development of intersensory integration abilities in posture control in the 4–6-year-old child. In this transition, postural response onsets show a delay and a high degree of variability at the onset of the new phase; then, as the children gradually master the ability to reweight sensory inputs under different sensory conditions, there is a return of short muscle response latencies and reduced variability (Shumway-Cook and Woollacott, 1985).

Haas and Diener (1988) have also performed studies on the development of posture control in children aged 6 months and older, using the platform rotation paradigm described earlier, causing toes-up rotations. Haas and Diener state that all the children they tested showed an M3 (long latency, stabilizing response) in the tibialis anterior muscle in response to rotations. However, in children younger than 1 year the response was neither sufficiently large nor fast enough to compensate for the induced sway, and the children lost balance. The response onset latencies,

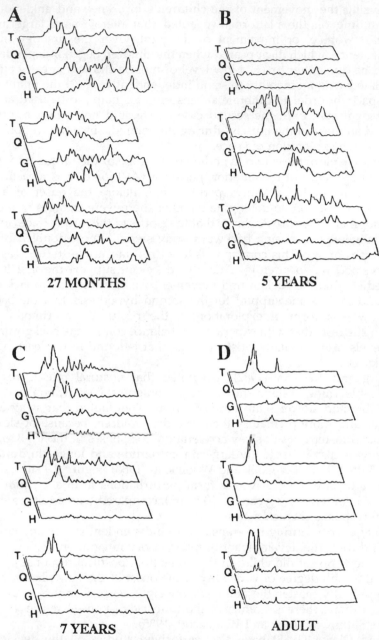

A

27 MONTHS

B

5 YEARS

C

7 YEARS

D

ADULT

Figure 6.9. *Examples of muscle response patterns to three platform translations in the forward direction, causing backward sway from children in three age groups and an adult: (a) 27 months old; (b) 5 years old; (c) 7 years old; (d) adult. Note the coactivation of antagonist muscles in the 27-month-old. The 5-year-old also shows increased variability compared with the other age groups (see section 2.7.7.). [From Shumway-Cook and Woollacott, 1985. Reprinted with permission of the Helen Dwight Reid Educational Foundation. © Heldref Publications, 4000 Albemarle St. NW, Washington, DC 20016, USA.]*

normalized to 1 meter body height, were 650 ms in the 6-month-old, 350 ms in the 9-month-old and 80 ms in the adult. It is not clear whether the 650 ms response in a 6-month-old could truly be in the same functional category as either a 350 or 80 ms response found in the adult. However, if this response is equivalent in the different ages, and is of vestibulospinal origin as suggested by Allum and Pfaltz (1985), it implies that vestibulospinal control may be present, though not functional, as early as 6–9 months of age.

The strong effect that visual flow fields have on postural control in the newly standing child was first shown by Lee and Aronson (1974). They used the visual room described earlier to show that these children would fall, stagger or sway in the direction of the room movement, compensating for their perceived but nonexistent sway. This effect gradually diminished over the first year of experience in standing. It is possible that this high susceptibility to incongruent visual information is due to the infant having poorer information from the ankles and feet than the adult. Lee and Young (1986) note that adults can be made to rely on visual information if they are asked to stand cross-wise on a beam, thus reducing their support surface information.

Balance Control in the Older Adult

Among the theories that attempt to explain the decline in nervous system function seen in the elderly, one hypothesizes a decline in nervous system function over time, with various abnormalities in motor function appearing as neuron numbers in specific brain areas decrease below a threshold for normal function. A second is that with normal ageing the nervous system continues to function at a high level until death, unless a specific pathological condition causes dysfunction in a specific neural subsystem. In research on posture control certain studies, using no selection criteria beyond age range, show significant deterioration in postural and locomotor function (Gabell and Nayak, 1984; Imms and Edholm, 1981). Other studies, using an older population selected to have no pathology, show no change in function of the postural systems with age, supporting the second model. The literature review on postural changes in the elderly will examine the extent to which the subject populations included older adults with nervous system changes indicative of pathology.

Early studies on postural sway in the elderly through 80 years of age (Sheldon, 1963) indicated significant increases in postural sway during quiet stance when compared with younger adults. These studies included a random sample of older adults, in which pathological conditions were not specifically excluded. In order to determine whether there was a relationship between the frequency of falls in older adults and the extent of their postural sway during quiet stance, Fernie, Gryfe and Holliday (1982) studied 205 institutionalized elderly with an average age of 82 years. Their results indicated that the elderly who had fallen one or more times in the previous year showed significant increases in the average speed of sway, compared with the other older adults. However, they noted that the mean sway of even the nonfallers was greater than had been earlier reported for non-institutionalized elderly. Given the institutionalized status of subjects in this study, it is possible that pathology and not age *per se* is the cause of increased sway and falling.

Research by Woollacott et al. (1982, 1986, 1988) has examined the neuromuscular synergies of older adults which are activated in response to external perturbations of balance. They compared the muscle response characteristics of 12 older (61–78 years) and younger (19–38 years) adults, using the platform translations and rotations as described above. They noted that the automatic postural responses of older adults showed the following changes in both timing and amplitude characteristics compared with the young adults: (1) increases in the absolute latency of distal muscle responses, specifically the tibialis anterior muscle, in response to platform translations causing posterior sway; (2) intermittent reversals in the normal distal to proximal sequence of leg muscle contractions so that quadriceps was activated before the tibialis anterior; (3) a larger incidence of short latency spinal monosynaptic reflexes, when subjected to platform rotations; (4) a second study (Manchester et al., 1989) also indicated that older adults coactivated antagonist muscles significantly more than young adults when responding to platform translations.

The older adults were also less efficient in balancing under conditions of reduced or conflicting sensory information. When first asked to balance under conditions of incongruent somatosensory and visual inputs, half of the older adults lost balance and needed the aid of an assistant, while none of the young adults lost balance. However, in most instances the older adults were able to balance when given repeated exposures to the condition.

Since subclinical manifestations of pathology could contribute to these changes in balance control, Manchester et al. (1989) performed a neurological examination on the older adults in their study. Although none of the older adults had any history of neurological dysfunction, one half of the group had an indication of borderline peripheral or central nervous system pathology (e.g. mild peripheral neuropathy, diminished ankle reflexes, distal muscle weakness, slight dyspraxia or slight left hemisphere deficits). Losses of balance in sensory conditions in which ankle joint proprioception and peripheral vision were minimized occurred in those subjects whose diagnosis revealed borderline pathology. Moreover, 52% of the losses of balance were from the data of two of the older adults. These two subjects were diagnosed as borderline abnormal with pathology of central nervous system origin.

In addition, there was a relationship between response sequencing and balance loss. For 6 of the 10 older adults who lost balance, falls occurred for trials in which the muscle sequencing was different from their predominant response strategy. Also for 7 of the 10 adults who lost balance, loss occurred when the sequencing was not the normal distal–proximal ankle strategy. In summary, losses of balance occurred when the muscle sequencing was unusual, with respect to either the subject's habitual sequencing or the most efficient strategy used by young adults.

2.8 Posture Summary

Sherrington was one of the first researchers to study the neural mechanisms that underlie posture control, classifying a variety of reflexes and describing the contributions of these reflexes to posture. Although his research contributed significantly to our understanding of reflex function, it dealt with a narrow aspect of neural function and did not take into account interactions between different neural systems in posture control.

Bernstein and his colleagues approached posture control from a broader perspective, examining the contributions of neural, musculoskeletal and environmental factors to posture, and hypothesizing the presence of synergies of muscles or segments acting as a unit to compress the degrees of freedom of the motor system and simplify the problem of posture control.

More recently, researchers have attempted to define the degree to which the posture control process is simplified by constraining muscles to act as a unit. Studies using a movable platform to destabilize balance in the anterior or posterior direction have suggested that there are discrete postural synergies used in balance control and that specific sensory inputs are used in their activation. Responses have been classified as ankle, hip or suspensory (flexion at the ankle, knee and hip) synergies in accordance with the joint(s) that showed the predominant movements in postural compensation.

Experimental evidence has revealed changes in the parameters of the synergies across successive trials, suggesting that they may be fine-tuned to the task and context. When cats were perturbed at different angles about the sagittal plane the biomechanical strategy showed invariance in the direction of the vector of force generated, but muscle responses were not invariant. Although some muscles were comodulated, and could have been activated by a central command, others were controlled independently and possibly used to tune the synergy. A recent model of balance control suggests that a fixed relationship among joint torques may be a more appropriate control variable for the motor system rather than simply centrally driven muscle activation patterns.

Research from a variety of laboratories has attempted to determine the relative contributions of visual, vestibular and somatosensory inputs to posture control under different task contexts, and it has been shown that deficits in any two of these systems may cause severe impairment in balance function.

There are certain similarities between the postural responses of the child and the older adult, including more coactivation of antagonist muscles. However, these may simply imply the use of a strategy of agonist–antagonist coactivation to stiffen the ankle joint and thus limit the degrees of freedom that they need to control.

3 LOCOMOTION

Since the time of Borelli (1685), scientists have been fascinated by the complexities of animal locomotion. In the following sections we provide an overview of past and current research on animal and human locomotion, with particular focus on walking. As we did with the previous section on posture, this review reflects the neurophysiological, biomechanical and dynamical perspectives. We begin with a description of the walking gait. This is followed by a section on the initiation of gait and the transition from static balance to steady-state progression velocity. The final section addresses the control of locomotion and issues of neural versus dynamic pattern generation. Where pertinent, we will raise issues relative to age-related changes in the acquisition of locomotor skill, for the developmental perspective has provided an important window on the mechanisms and processes of control and coordination in locomotion.

3.1 Descriptors of the Gait Cycle

We begin with a description of mature gait–its spatiotemporal features and the muscle activation patterns that underlie the observable behavior. The description is expanded to the joint kinetics that drive the behaviors. Subsequently, we take up issues of change: how selected gait parameters change with the speed of progression, and changes in gait that accompany skill acquisition and the decline associated with ageing.

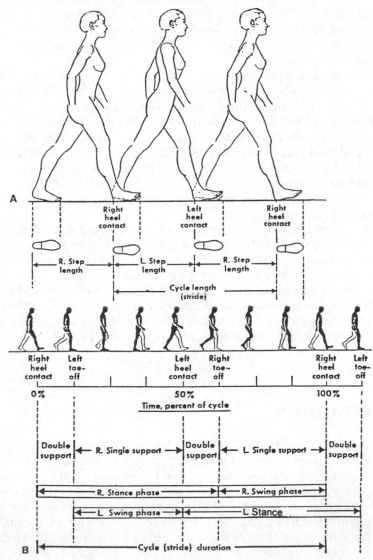

Figure 6.10. *Temporal and distance dimensions of the gait cycle. (A) Distance dimensons of the gait cycle. (B) Temporal characteristics of the gait cycle. [From Inman, Ralston and Todd, 1981. ©Williams and Wilkins. Reprinted with kind permission.]*

3.1.1   Temporal Features of Human Locomotion

Upright bipedal locomotion is an alternating, or symmetric, gait in which the relationship between the two limbs is described by a phase lag of 0.5 (Grillner, 1981). A phase lag of 0.5 means that one limb initiates its step cycle as the opposite limb reaches the midpoint of its own cycle (Figure 6.10). For example, if the cycle duration is defined as the time between ipsilateral footstrikes (right heel contact to right heel contact, Figure 6.10a), then the contralateral limb begins its cycle midway through the ipsilateral stride cycle.

The symmetric, or alternating, gait is the first pattern to appear in the independent locomotor repertoire of the developing motor system. Raibert (1986) suggests that the functional significance of the symmetric gait may lie in the fact that symmetry provides for the greatest dynamic stability for bipedal gait while minimizing regulatory demands.

The single limb cycle is also a common descriptor of the gait cycle and is frequently defined in terms of relative time spent in stance and swing (Figure 6.10b). At freely chosen walking speeds, adults typically spend approximately 60% of the cycle duration in stance, and 40% in swing (Murray *et al.*, 1984; Rosenrot, Wall and Charteris, 1980).

3.1.2   Description of Joint Action

Simply, locomotion is the translation of the body from one location to another. Yet, while we think of this translation as the linear path between starting and ending locations, the construction of the human body necessitates that this translation be produced out of a complex series of limb segment rotations about joints. The result is that the center of mass (CM), as a marker of the body's location, moves not in a straight line, but in a series of subtle undulations.

Saunders, Inman and Eberhart (1953) described six characteristics of normal gait (see also Inman, Ralston and Todd, 1981; McMahon, 1984). First, the 'compass gait' results when the only motion allowed is *flexion and extension at the hip* (stiff knee). Within the single-limb step cycle, the hip joint goes through a single flexion–extension wave (Figure 6.11). Limiting joint action in walking to 'compass gait' characteristics leads to a sinusoidal path of the CM in the sagittal (anterior–posterior) plane. Adding *pelvic rotation* about the vertical axis contributes to an increase in stride length and flattens the amplitude of the sinusoidal oscillations of the CM. The path of the CM becomes smoother and the transition from step to step a little less abrupt.

With the addition of the *pelvic tilt* (rotation of the pelvis about an anterior–posterior axis), the path of the CM flattens further. The pelvic tilt occurs as the swing-side hip lowers as the swing limb is unweighted in preparation for toe-off. A concomitant to pelvic tilt is knee flexion in the swing limb to prevent the swinging foot from contacting the ground prematurely.

Two characteristics of the walking gait are particularly related to the stance limb: *knee flexion during stance* and *plantar flexion at the ankle* (Figure 6.11). The effect of knee flexion during stance is further to flatten the vertical excursions of the CM.

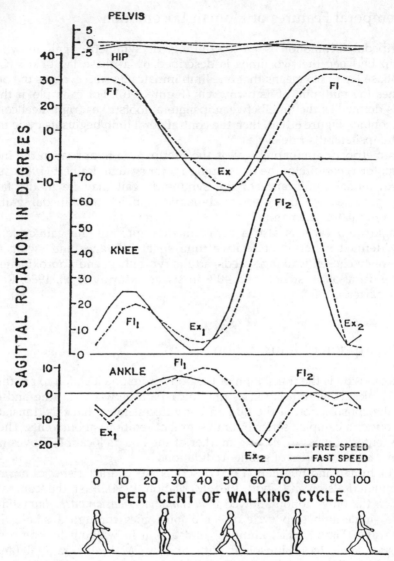

Figure 6.11. *Joint angle rotations associated with the adult step cycle. [From Murray et al., 1966.* © *Williams and Wilkins. Reprinted with kind permission.]*

Plantar flexion of the stance ankle contributes to a smooth transition from step to step and establishes the initial velocity conditions for the swing limb.

Finally, normal gait is characterized by a *lateral shift in the pelvis* that occurs as stance is alternately shifted from limb to limb. The width of the step determines the magnitudes of the shift of the CM in a transverse (horizontal) plane.

In summary, the step cycle is a complex series of joint rotations. Taken independently, the rotations create an undulating path of the CM in the sagittal and transverse planes. Taken together, the undulations are minimized in what appears to be a strategy to reduce the energy cost of walking (Eberhart, 1976; Saunders, Inman and Eberhart, 1953).

3.1.3 Muscle Activation Patterns During the Step Cycle

The muscle activation patterns that accompany the gait cycle have been of interest to numerous investigators (e.g. Basmajian, 1979; Battye and Joseph, 1966; Brandell, 1973; Dubo *et al.*, 1976; Eberhart, Inman and Bresler, 1954; MacConaill and Basmajian, 1977; Milner, Basmajian and Quanbury, 1971; Van der Straaten, Lohman and Van Linge 1975), and the following discussion summarizes the major points from these works. Despite subject- and condition-specific differences in the EMG patterns, some consistencies have been identified. In general, muscles in the stance limb first act to stabilize and then propel the body. Muscle activity in the swing limb is largely confined to the beginning and end of the swing phase, while the leg swings much like a jointed pendulum under the influence of gravity (McMahon, 1984). Typical EMG patterns during a series of steps are shown in Figure 6.12.

The task demands of the stance phase include stabilization of the stance limb against the impact force of footstrike and subsequent force generation to propel the body forward into the next step. Two behavioral patterns are particularly related to force absorption: a knee flexion wave at the initiation of stance and the distribution of the footstrike impact from heel contact to the foot-flat stance. Thus at the initiation of stance we typically see activity in the knee extensors (rectus femoris and vasti muscles – the quadriceps) and the ankle dorsiflexors (pretibial muscles). Both muscle groups initially act to oppose the direction of motion. The quadriceps control the small knee flexion wave that is used to absorb the impact of footstrike. The anterior tibial muscles decelerate the foot upon touchdown, opposing and slowing the plantar flexion that results from heelstrike. Muscles that

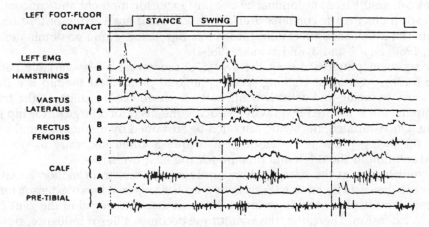

Figure 6.12. *Electromyographic patterns associated with the adult step cycle. [From Murray et al., 1984. Reprinted with kind permission.]*

contribute to trunk extension, thus controlling forward sway of the trunk, and tilt of the pelvis on the femur are also active during the early force-absorbing phase of stance.

By midstance, the quadriceps is predominantly inactive as are the pretibial muscles. The propulsive force is generated by activity in the ankle plantar flexors (gastrocnemius and soleus) after the CM has passed the vertical and the stance heel has lost contact with the floor. The hip and knee extensors (hamstrings and quadriceps, respectively) may exhibit a burst of activity late in stance as a contribution to propulsion, although this activity typically is of lesser magnitude than that observed during the force-absorption phase.

The early swing phase is often characterized by a burst of activity from the quadriceps to generate the forward acceleration of the thigh. By midswing, however, the quadriceps is virtually inactive. The hamstrings become active at the end of swing to slow the forward rotation of the thigh in preparation for footstrike. Knee extension occurs not as the result of muscle activity, but is the passive result of nonmuscular forces (Winter and Robertson, 1978). The pretibial group is also active late in swing to ensure toe clearance during swing and preparation of the foot for the next footfall.

3.1.4   Joint Kinetics

The kinetic parameters associated with the normal gait pattern are less stereotyped than the kinematic descriptors. The joint moments (active and passive muscle forces) that generate a stereotyped behavior are themselves quite variable. During stance the algebraic sum of the joint moments at the hip, knee and ankle, the 'support moment' (Winter, 1980), is an extensor torque (Figure 6.13b). The net extensor torque is necessary to keep the limb from collapsing while bearing weight. However, this net extensor resultant may be achieved in a variety of ways. Individual subject data have demonstrated that the functional extensor support moment can result from a dominance of a hip extensor moment and concomitant knee flexor moment. The converse is also true: knee and ankle extensor torques can maintain the extensor support moment while a hip flexor torque predominates (see Winter, 1980, Figs 2 and 3, and Winter, 1983a).

Joint moment patterns during the swing phase reveal a less variable pattern (Figure 6.13b). At normal walking speeds, the joint moment at the hip is a flexor torque early in swing and actively contributes to flexion of the thigh on the trunk. Early hip flexion is assisted by gravity, reducing the need for a large flexor hip joint moment. Once initiated, the swing can often be sustained by momentum and at the end of the swing phase an extensor joint torque is often necessary to slow the forward rotation of the thigh and prepare for the next heelstrike.

The joint torque at the knee predominantly acts to constrain motion about the knee, not to generate its motion. Early swing is characterized by an extensor torque that slows joint flexion early in swing and contributes to reversal of the joint from flexion to extension. Thereafter, the joint torque becomes a flexor influence, slowing extension at the knee in preparation for the next football (Cavanagh and Gregor, 1975; Winter, 1983a; Winter and Robertson, 1978).

At the initiation of stance, a small dorsiflexor torque is generated at the ankle to control the force plantarflexion brought about by heelstrike. Thereafter, a plantar-

(a)

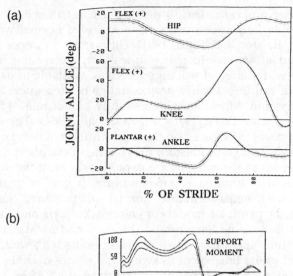

(b)

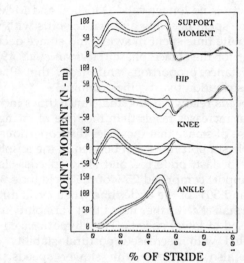

Figure 6.13. *(a) Averaged (n = 9) joint angle time histories, and (b) joint torque patterns associated with the adult step cycle. Stance: 0–60% of the stride; swing: 60–100% of the stride. Positive joint moments contribute to joint extension (plantar flexion at the ankle). [From Winter, 1984. Adapted with kind permission.]*

flexor joint torque builds to a peak at approximately 50% of the stride. This peak occurs after knee flexion has begun and just as the ankle begins to plantarflex (Figure 6.13). The largest joint torque occurs at the ankle and is largely responsible for accelerating the limb into the next swing phase.

3.1.5 Changes in Gait Characteristics Associated with Changes in Velocity

The speed of walking is a function of stride length and stride frequency. Increases in walking speed are typically generated by changes on both dimensions: the stride lengthens and the pace quickens. Thus a direct linear relationship exists between stride length and stride frequency over a wide range of normal walking speeds (Grieve, 1968; Inman, Ralston and Todd, 1981). Ultimately, an upper limit to stride length is achieved and subsequent increases in walking speed come from increases in step rate. While a wide range of walking speeds is available to us, the majority of self-selected speeds fall into a fairly narrow range of step rates. Preferred step rates average 110 steps min^{-1} for men with a slightly higher rate ($+5$ steps min^{-1}) for women (see Finley and Cody, 1970; Murray *et al.*, 1984). The selection of a preferred step rate appears to be based on the minimization of energy requirements (Ralston, 1976; Zarrugh, Todd and Ralston, 1974). When pendular properties of the leg and elastic properties of the muscles are exploited, at least the swing phase of locomotion can occur with little energy expenditure. It may be that seeking this energy minimum is what helps to define 'normal' or 'preferred' gait speeds. At slower or higher speeds, pendular models of gait break down, and the assumption of minimal muscle activity is no longer valid (Mochon and McMahon, 1980).

The proportion of time spent in swing and stance shifts with walking speed. As speed increases the absolute time spent in swing and stance declines, although the rate of decline is greater for the stance phase (Herman *et al.*, 1976; Murray, 1967). Ultimately, the swing/stance proportions shift from the 40/60 distribution of walking to the 60/40 distribution that typifies running.

At slower walking speeds relative swing and stance times increase and, again, it is the time of stance that increases faster than the time of swing. In addition, it is the double support phase of stance that increases disproportionately. A disproportionate increase in double support times can be seen in the absolute times reported by Murray *et al.* (1984) for fast, preferred and slow speeds. Herman *et al.* (1976) observed that double support comprised 25% of the cycle time with step durations of approximately 1.1 s, and 50% of the cycle time when cycle duration increased to approximately 2.5 s. Herman *et al.* further noted that variability in cycle time, swing and stance times increased at lower speeds. They hypothesized that the increased variability was associated with decreased postural stability during the single support period, which also lengthens with slower speeds. Alternatively, the variability in temporal parameters may be related to the dynamics of the motion and variability in force modulation at uncommon speeds.

Joint angle patterns are quite stereotyped across a range of speeds (Murray *et al.*, 1966, 1984; Winter, 1983a). Winter's analysis of normal gait revealed the stability of joint angle patterns across the gait cycle of self-selected slow, natural and fast cadences. Differences as speed increased appeared limited to changes in amplitude, not to changes in timing.[3] Higher impact forces occur at faster cadences (Soames and Richardson, 1985), thus the increased knee flexion observed in the early part of stance may be attributed to the absorption of this larger force. The slight increase in hip variability was attributed to changes in trunk posture across the speeds, not to a change in behavior of the lower extremity.

---

[3]The joint angle time histories in Murray's work (Murray *et al.*, 1966, 1984 e.g. Fig. 3) suggest shifts in timing as well as amplitude across changes in speed. Both Murray and Winter (1983a) have reported the data on a normalized time axis (cycle duration = 100%), thus it is not possible to determine the exact magnitude of the temporal shift. However, part of the difference may be the result of differences in sampling rate. Murray's data were collected at a sampling rate of 20 Hz. Winter did not report a sampling rate in the 1983a paper, but typically uses 50 Hz (Winter, 1980, 1983b). Murray's slow sampling rate potentially attenuates curve peaks and may misrepresent the timing of those peaks.

Winter (1983a) also observed stability in the EMG patterns of lower extremity muscles across changes in speed. Changes in ensemble averages of the EMG linear envelope appeared temporally stable, but the 'gain', or amplitude, decreased with slower speeds. The gains were not, however, increased or decreased linearly across the cycle duration. Greatest gain changes were observed in the rectus femoris and the vastus medialis and associated with early stance (force absorption) and the push-off into swing. The biceps femoris showed uneven gain changes across the cycle with the greatest differences associated with early stance (control of hip at touchdown) and late swing (slowing the thigh and knee in preparation for touchdown).

While stability was the hallmark of joint angle and EMG patterns, joint torque patterns appear more variable. Joint moments show similar 'gain' changes as cadence goes up or down. With increased cadence, joint moment magnitudes increase (Cavanagh and Gregor, 1975; Winter, 1989; Zernicke, Schneider and Buford, 1991). Large variability, however, characterizes ensemble averages of joint moments. Winter (1983a) reported average coefficients of variation of 45, 150 and 144% for joint moments of force at the ankle, knee and hip, respectively, during a natural cadence. The coefficients of variation decreased at fast speeds and increased at slow speeds (see also Winter, 1984).

3.1.6 The Development of Mature Gait

Anyone who has watched the hesitant and sometimes careening first steps of an independently walking child will recognize, as Statham and Murray (1971) expressed, 'that a child is not an adult in miniature' (p. 19). While certain qualitative and functional characteristics of a 1-year-old's first steps bear similarity to the mature adult pattern, quantitative analyses reveal the disparities and help us track the development of the mature pattern. Depending on the variable of interest, infants, toddlers and children approximate the adult pattern as early as 3 months of independent walking experience, to as late as 7–9 years of age.

An infant's first independent steps are characterized by excessive flexion at the hip, knee and ankle (Statham and Murray, 1971). Stance begins with a flexion bias in the lower extremities and the subsequent joint excursions during extension are limited relative to the adult pattern. Swing, too, is marked by excessive flexion primarily at the hip and leads to the characteristic high stepping (McGraw, 1963). Statham and Murray also observed greater hip flexion in infant steps over that observed in adults, but suggest the high stepping may be more an impression than fact, contributed to by the forward lean of the trunk. This claim is supported by their failure to find excessive foot-floor clearance during the swing phase.

The flexion bias of the support limb is seen also in the EMG recordings of trunk and lower extremity muscles. Cocontraction of antagonist muscle pairs typifies the stance phase in the new walker (Okamoto and Goto, 1985). The gastrocnemius and tibialis anterior are coactive in the newly walking infant and reciprocal in the adult. For the infants, the early activation in stance of the gastrocnemius corresponds to the flat-foot touchdown and the early acceptance of a large proportion of body weight. This is unlike the adult heel-to-toe footstrike pattern that distributes the weight onto the foot over time. Knee flexor and hip extensors are also coactive in the stance phase of new walkers, with the vastus medialis, rectus femoris and biceps femoris active through much of the stance phase (Okamoto and Goto, 1985).

The new independent walker progresses forward lacking the smooth transitions that characterize the mature walk. The new walker displays a stereotypic joint reversal pattern of knee, then hip, and finally ankle, in the transition from stance to swing. This is the same pattern used by adults. Unlike the adult, though, activation of the rectus femoris and the vastus medialis during the swing phase suggests the infant actively lifts and extends the knee. Knee extension occurs passively in the swing phase of the adult gait.

The transition from swing to stance is more troublesome. At the initiation of stance, the adult first yields at the knee and then extends. The yield absorbs the impact of the footstrike. The adult also achieves distribution of the impact force across the foot by rolling the foot from heel to toe. Neither of these mechanisms is employed by the new walker. The infant begins in a flexed knee posture during swing and extends upon a flat-foot touchdown.

Infants in the first week of independent walking show a strong discharge pattern in the rectus abdominis (Kazai, Okamoto and Kumamoto, 1976; Okamoto and Goto, 1985). During the first week, the trunk appears held in a more erect posture when compared with the slight forward lean typical of later walking, and the rectus abdominis assists in posture control, pulling the trunk forward over the lower extremities. With experience in the order of 1 to 2 weeks, activation of the rectus femoris is observed less often as the trunk assumes a slightly forward-inclined posture. Cocontraction of the tibialis anterior and gastrocnemius also subside, with tibialis activity decreasing after the initial impact of the footstrike, and the gastrocnemius activation weakening at the initiation of stance. The changes in the tibialis anterior and gastrocnemius muscle reflect a change toward the adult pattern.

Walking proficiency is gained quickly. The gait pattern of new walkers is characterized by imprecision and the cocontraction of antagonist muscles. With relatively little experience, cocontraction begins to decline and reciprocal muscle activation patterns appear. By 3 months of walking experience, infants have achieved the stable pattern of muscle activations that will be maintained until about 3 years of age (Okamoto and Goto, 1985).

The interlimb coordination of the lower extremities also becomes adult-like in consistency after approximately 3 months of walking experience. Studying the walking patters of infants with 0, 0.5, 1 and 6 months of walking experience as well as the patterns of adults, Clark, Whitall and Phillips (1988) documented the experience-related changes in selected temporal and distance phasing measures of the stepping pattern.

In a symmetric gait such as walking, the step cycle actions of one limb are 50% out of phase with the other limb (a phase lag of 0.5). Consistent with accepted convention, Clark, Whitall and Phillips (1988) use temporal phasing to refer to the proportion of time during the ipsilateral limb's cycle when the contralateral limb begins its own cycle. In a symmetric gait, temporal phasing is expected to be 50%. Clark *et al.* define distance phasing as the proportional distance contributed by one step to the total stride (refer again to Figure 6.10). In a symmetric gait, the distance phasing also is expected to be 50%. Further, in the mature gait pattern, variability in the phasing measures would be expected to be small.

Clark, Whitall and Phillips (1988) found no differences in mean temporal phasing across all groups studied. That is, new walkers (those capable of walking three steps before falling) were as accomplished as adults in achieving a mean temporal phasing of 50%. However, statistically significant differences were found in the variability of the temporal phasing exhibited by the walking groups. In essence, those with walking experience of 0.5 and 1 month were more variable than those with 3 months or more walking experience. Variability in the temporal phasing decreased with experience across all groups, but after as little as 3 months the variability no longer differed from that of those with more experience – including adults. The distance phasing results were quite similar. By 3 months' walking age, the variability in the distance phasing was similar to that of the 6-month walkers and the adults.

Soon after the onset of independent walking the 40/60 swing/stance ratio of the adult appears to stabilize in the child. The very first steps of new walkers may be characterized by a disproportionate amount of the time spent in stance (e.g. as high as 80%; Phillips and Clark, 1987). Nevertheless, Statham and Murray (1971) reported average stance phase proportions of 62% in new independent walking although the values ranged from 50 to 71%. Others have reported similar values, although the age range was more broadly defined to include subjects between the ages of 12 and 24 months (e.g. Beck *et al.*, 1981: swing/stance = 39/61; Sutherland *et al.*, 1980: swing phase = 32%). Despite variability, the patterns seem relatively stable across the moderate range of speeds that the young child is capable of generating (Bril and Breniere, 1989; Clark and Phillips, 1987, Fig. 5).

By 18 months of age, a reciprocal armswing and heelstrike are present (Sutherland *et al.*, 1980). Sutherland *et al.* also reported that the mature gait, as assessed by measures of single-limb stance duration, step length, ratio of pelvic width to step width during double support, cadence and progression velocity, is well established by 3 years of age. This is also the age at which Okamoto and Goto (1985) reported the next significant change in muscle activation patterns.

From the data of Sutherland *et al.* (1980) we see that walking velocity increases with age while cadence declines. Thus, longer strides are being taken during the step. This suggests that single-limb support times should increase concomitantly with these changes, and they do. At the same time, the stride width is becoming narrower. While these parameters continue to change to 7 years or later, the greatest rates of change are observed between the onset of independent walking and 3–3.5 years of age.

The additional changes observed around 3 years of age by Okamoto and Goto (1985) include the preheelstrike EMG activity from the tibialis anterior signaling the preparation of heelstrike and the eccentric control of the initial plantarflexion of the foot. The child also assumes a more erect posture, and activity in the biceps femoris and gluteus maximus decreases or disappears after the initial shock absorption. By 7 years of age, the adult muscle activation pattern is complete. Sutherland (1984) also reported that the adult EMG pattern was the appropriate comparator for children aged 7 years and older.

In summary, the acquisition of mature gait characteristics takes place most rapidly between the onset of independent walking and 3–3.5 years of age. Thereafter, changes in gait kinematics and muscle activation patterns continue to be refined to approximately 7–8 years of age. By this time the mature gait pattern is in place, although some have reported minor changes to the gait pattern continuing until 16 years of age (Norlin, Odenrick and Sandlund, 1981).

3.1.7 Gait Characteristics of the Older Adult

A number of laboratories have studied changes in locomotor patterns from prenatal development through old age in order to determine the relative contributions of different neural and musculoskeletal subcomponents to the emergence and deterioration in this behavior across the life span. This section deals with the gait characteristics of the older adult.

Spielburg (1940) was one of the first investigators to systematically observe age-related changes in gait. He described three age-related stages in the decline of walking performance. For stage 1 (60–72 years) he observed a slower walking velocity, shortened steps, a lower cadence, less vertical excursion of the center of gravity and disturbed coordination between the upper and lower extremities. Stage 2 (72–86 years) was typified by a loss of the normal arm–leg synergy, an overproduction of 'unwanted' movements and a diminished flexion in the swing phase. During stage 3 (86–104 years) there was rapid disintegration of the gait pattern, arrhythmia in step rate and absence of any arm swing movement.

Craik (1989), in reviewing Spielburg's (1940) observations, concludes that the gait disorders described by Spielburg are due to more than the effects of age alone. She notes the lack of any health screening for Spielburg's subjects. When Spielburg made his observations, the effect of clinical disorders like multi-infarct dementia, normal pressure hydrocephalus and Parkinson's disease on gait were not clearly identified. Thus it is possible that these walking disorders include a combination of disease and age-related changes. In fact, Spielburg's descriptions of stages 2 and 3 are more similar to those for clinical walking disorders, than the walk of healthy older adults which have been described more recently.

As Craik (1989) notes, the consensus is that older adults walk more slowly, but she questions whether the changes in other gait variables simply reflect the reduced walking velocity, or whether they also reflect age-related deterioration. Craik demonstrated that younger adults also show similar changes in gait variables when they walk more slowly, including a shortened step length, diminished single support time, and the foot coming into ground contact with a more plantarflexed position. In addition there is a decreased amplitude of hip and shoulder rotation, a change in the pattern of interlimb coordination (shoulders flex with the hip cycle for both lower extremities) and a decreased amplitude of EMG activity.

Gabell and Nayak (1984) studied age-related changes in locomotion in order to determine the relative contributions of deterioration in automatic stepping mechanisms versus balance mechanisms in locomotor pattern deterioration. They hypothesized that increased variability in stride width and double support time would be caused by decreased balance control, while increased variability in stride timing and step length would be attributable to deterioration of gait patterning mechanisms. In order to obtain subjects who were free from pathology, they selected only 32 older adults from an initial population of 1187 persons over 64 years of age, due to exclusion criteria including disorders of the musculoskeletal, neurological or cardiovascular systems, or any previous history of falls. In comparing their elite older adults to young adults, they found no differences in variability for any of the parameters measured, and concluded that any age-related increases in variability of gait parameters must be the result of pathology.

Murray, Kory and Clarkson (1969) examined walking patterns of 64 men aged 20–87 years. Each subject had normal strength, range of motion and was asymptomatic. Subjects over 65 years of age were given physical examinations to rule out neurological deficits. They compared 'normal' and fast walking across ages. Men in the three oldest age groups (between 67 and 87 years) showed significantly slower walking speeds: 150 cm s^{-1} for young versus 118–123 cm s^{-1} for the older groups. Stride length was also significantly shorter especially for fast walking, and stride width was wider for men over 74, but not significantly. Toeing out was greater for men over 80. It was also noted that beyond the age of 65 the subjects spent a longer time in stance phase and a shorter time in swing phase. Hip, knee and ankle flexion were less than in younger adults, the vertical excursion of the head was smaller and the lateral excursion was larger. In addition, the arms extended further backward, and did not flex as far forward, showing less elbow rotation.

Murray, Kory and Clarkson (1969) further noted that the men in this study did not have a gait that appeared pathological. Although it was not vigorous, it was also not labored. Instead, it appeared to be guarded or restrained as if in an attempt to obtain maximum stability, and resembled that of someone walking on a slippery surface or someone walking in darkness. This description thus appears to be that of someone with a postural problem, with possible reduction in sensory inputs controlling posture, rather than that of a simple locomotor problem.

In comparing the locomotor pattern characteristics in the young child and the older adult one sees both similarities and differences. Similarities include shorter relative step length, slower velocity, and more coactivation of antagonist muscles during the gait cycle than seen in young adults. However, many if not all of these changes could be due to problems with balance control, causing the young child and the older adult to walk more slowly, while keeping the center of mass nearer to the base of support, and continuing to make balancing adjustments in both agonist and antagonist muscles during the step cycle. Further, like the studies on age-related changes in posture control, these studies on locomotor abilities in elite older adults also tend to support the hypothesis that the nervous system continues to function at a relatively high level until death, unless there is a specific catastrophe or disease that causes a rapid decline in function of a specific brain area.

3.2 The Initiation of Gait

How does one move from static to dynamic balance? In the following sections we review this transition first in adults exhibiting a mature gait, and then in infants and children with immature patterns.

3.2.1 The Transition from Stance to Progression

The transition from standing to walking has the simple appearance of falling and regaining one's balance by stepping forward. The initiation of gait from a static, symmetric stance begins with the relaxation of selected postural muscles (Carlsöo, 1966; Herman *et al.*, 1973). In quiet stance, a dorsiflexor torque about the ankle occurs if the vertical projection of the body's center of mass (CM) moves forward of the ankle joint. This motion is inhibited by a plantarflexor torque generated by muscle activation of soleus and gastrocnemius muscles. The transition from balance to imbalance is characterized first by a reduction in the activation of these postural muscles followed by activation of the tibialis anterior which assists dorsiflexion and moves the CM forward in preparation for toe-off. Static balance can be regained if posterior leg and trunk muscles are activated before the horizontal position of the CM moves forward of the toes. Nevertheless, once the vertical projection of the CM moves forward of the base of support, balance can be regained only by stepping forward.

Falling seems, if somewhat inelegant, a simple and effective means of setting the body in motion and making the transition between static and dynamic behavior. Indeed, toddlers just learning to walk show all the characteristics of falling into their first steps (Breniere, Bril and Fontaine, 1989). Continued analyses of adult gait, however, have revealed a complexity in gait initiation previously unobserved, which suggests that there is more to the initiation of gait than a simple fall.

Mann *et al.* (1979) traced the center of pressure during the initiation of gait by normal adults. The center of pressure is positioned just posterior to the ankle and midway between both feet prior to any movement (Figure 6.14). As subjects begin to move, the center of pressure first moves posteriorly and laterally toward the *swing* limb before shifting toward the stance limb and forward (these results have also been observed by Breniere, Do and Bouisset, 1987; Cook and Cozzens, 1976; Yamashita and Katoh, 1976). Movement of the center of pressure toward the swing limb occurs simultaneously with hip and knee flexion and ankle dorsiflexion as the swing limb prepares for toe-off. Subsequently, the center of pressure shifts rapidly toward the stance limb and toe-off of the swing limb occurs as the center of pressure shifts from lateral movement to forward progression over the stance foot. The purpose of the initial shift in the center of pressure toward the swing limb is not clear, but Mann *et al.* (1979) hypothesized that this is a strategy for setting the CM in motion, perhaps using the momentum of the CM to assist in creating the loss of balance that leads to the first step.

The complexity of the center of pressure trajectory is supported by a sophisticated neuromuscular response in the lower extremities (Herman *et al.*, 1973; Mann *et al.*, 1979). As the center of pressure moves posteriorly and toward the swing limb, the stance limb is stabilized against backward sway by activation of anterior leg

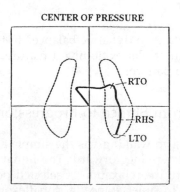

Figure 6.14. *Trajectory of the center of pressure during the initiation of gait from a balanced, symmetric stance. Prior to movement, the center of pressure is located midway between the feet. RTO, right toe off; RHS, right heel strike; LTO, left toe off. [From Mann et al., 1979. The initiation of gait.* Journal of Bone and Joint Surgery, **61A**, 232–239. *Reprinted with kind permission.]*

and thigh muscles. The tibialis anterior subsequently causes dorsiflexion in the stance ankle, pulling the lower leg over the foot. Anterior thigh muscles activate to oppose the knee flexion so that the leg as a unit rotates forward over the foot. Hip abductors are active to prevent lateral tilt of the pelvis toward the swing limb side as the swing limb is unloaded and the stability of the stance ankle is enhanced by the peroneals. Once toe-off occurs the muscles in the stance leg contribute less to stability and more to propulsion – the primary active muscles being gastrocnemius and hamstrings.

3.2.2   Transition to Steady-State Progression Velocity

The achievement of a steady-state progression velocity marks the end of the transitory gait initiation phase. Still unresolved is the question of how long it takes to achieve steady state in adult gait. The consensus view is that steady state may be achieved in the range of one step (Breniere and Do, 1986) to three steps (Cook and Cozzens, 1976; Mann *et al.*, 1979). Although still awaiting the explicit test, the final answer seems likely to be dependent on the magnitude of the steady-state progression velocity. Breniere, Do and Bouisset (1987) looked at time to peak progression velocity across speeds, but the speeds were relative rates of slow, normal and fast as self-selected by their subjects. Thus the systematic manipulation of speed, either absolute or relative to stature, has yet to be done.

At least at slow to moderate speeds, the duration of the initiation phase appears invariant and independent of the target progression velocity (Breniere and Do, 1986). Peak progression velocity is achieved at the end of the first step with time to peak velocity independent of the velocity. Time to peak velocity appeared to be a function of individual anthropometric parameters: mass, moment of inertia and location of the body's CM. Breniere and Do modeled the body as an inverted pendulum and calculated the time to peak velocity. Their calculated times were comparable to their experimental results.

The model results of Breniere and Do (1986) are consistent with conceptualizing the initiation of gait as a fall. The same model, however, specifies the limits of applicability where the target velocity exceeds the velocity that can be passively generated by gravity (see also Alexander, 1984). Slow speeds also present a problem. If the peak velocity of the first step is a function of unmodulated mechanics then only a small range of velocities would be available at the end of step 1, and subsequent steps would be needed to speed up the body or to slow it down.

Alternatively, Cook and Cozzens (1976) suggest that with knowledge of the task (or target velocity) subjects make adjustments in the central programming of the motor outcome, regulating muscle activation levels (see also Breniere, Do and Bouisset, 1987). Muscle function is regulated to delay or exacerbate the loss of balance. Maintaining tone in the posterior postural muscle would delay gait initiation whereas activation of the tibialis anterior would precipitate the fall. Subsequent modulation of muscle activity determines the joint torques that contribute to propulsion should the target velocity exceed what gravity alone could generate. The experimental results of Cook and Cozzens support this regulation hypothesis. Linear relationships were shown to exist between target velocity and the instantaneous velocity of the CM at selected times (e.g. at the time of swing-side toe-off, swing-side heelstrike, stance-side toe-off) – as if the system was proportionally scaling the propulsive impulses across a multistep gait initiation process.

3.2.3 Developmental Trends in the Initiation of Gait and Transition to Steady-State Velocity

Breniere, Bril and Fontaine (1989) investigated the initiation of gait and the transition to steady-state velocity in children who had been walking independently for between 90 and 200 days. While children with 3 months' walking experience display in their gait many adult-like features (Clark, Whitall and Phillips, 1988), they lack fine-tuning. These young subjects demonstrated the 'fall' strategy in the initiation of the step cycle. Like adults under certain conditions (see Breniere and Do, 1986, above), the time to peak progression velocity in the first step of the children's gait was independent of their steady-state velocity. Adults may exploit this mechanical falling strategy to initiate gait, but the evidence is also clear that adults support that strategy with a context- and task-dependent muscle activation pattern. Breniere *et al.* did not record the muscle activation patterns of the children but their results support the conclusion that these children lack the stability and functionality of the center of pressure pattern typical of adult gait initiation. Further, these children require 2–3 steps to achieve steady-state progression velocity.

3.3 Control Issues in Locomotion

The apparent simplicity of rhythmic, alternating bipedal gait belies the complexity of bringing all the components and subsystems together for coordinated action. The act of locomotion is in fact a complex pattern of limb segment rotations that produce a balanced combination of force generation and force absorption such that forward progression and dynamic balance are maintained. How is this coordination achieved?

The historical perspective has been to assign proximate cause for the appearance of new behaviors to cortical maturation or the development of complex neural structures (Forssberg, 1985; McGraw, 1940). The focus of neurophysiological research has been on the neural structures and mechanisms that generate the locomotor pattern in much of its detail. In this, the animal research has presented compeling evidence for neural pattern generation.

The dynamical perspective offers the alternative view. As in posture control, it is not the neural substrate that supports the behavior that is denied, but rather the prescriptive control over pattern formation. From both perspectives, the search for synergies is as important in locomotion as it is in posture control. It is the organizational principles behind the synergy formations that are at issue. From the dynamical perspective, the oscillatory behavior of the legs in locomotion displays features of organization consonant with the periodic attractors that describe patterned behavior in physical systems (Haken, Kelso and Bunz, 1985). These attractor states are softly-assembled from the elements of the motor system, the environment, the task and all attendant constraints.

In the sections that follow, we review the literature from the neural perspective on pattern formation in locomotion. This work comes predominantly from animal research. Following that, we review the biomechanics of pattern generation in cat locomotion. Finally, we address pattern generation in human locomotion. Unlike posture control research, there is a growing body of research on the coordination of limbs in oscillatory movements that begins from the tenets of dynamical systems theory. Thus in the following sections we discuss what each perspective brings to our understanding of the control of human bipedal gait.

3.3.1 Pattern Generation in Locomotion – the Neurophysiological Perspective

During the past 20 years there has been a dramatic increase in the research related to the nervous system control of the basic rhythmic movements underlying locomotion. Results of these studies have indicated that central pattern generators play an important role in the production of these movements (Grillner, 1973; Smith, 1980). In the late 1800s, Sherrington and Mott (Mott and Sherrington, 1895; Sherrington, 1898) performed experiments which showed that the hind limbs continued to exhibit alternating movements after the spinal cord had been severed and thus the influence of higher brain centers had been eliminated. In addition, in monkeys, they unilaterally sectioned the dorsal roots of the spinal cord which innervated the fore and hind limbs, thus eliminating the influence of sensory feedback on locomotion on one side of the body. They noticed that the monkeys would not use the deafferented limbs during walking and thus concluded that sensory feedback was necessary for locomotion. As a result they modeled locomotion as being controlled by a set of reflex chains, with the output from one phase of the step cycle acting to stimulate the next phase in a reflexive manner.

However, within a little more than a decade Brown (1911) showed that, in animals with bilateral dorsal root lesions, severing the spinal cord caused rhythmic walking movements which lasted for more than a minute following the section. The difference in the results of the two labs appears to lie in the fact that Sherrington only severed the dorsal roots on one side of the spinal cord. Taub and Berman (1968) have more recently shown that animals who would not use a limb when the dorsal roots were sectioned unilaterally would regain use of the limb with a bilateral section of the dorsal roots.

Although it has been shown that locomotor movements persist without peripheral feedback, the difference in movement characteristics in deafferented preparations compared with controls has been widely discussed, with some laboratories indicating 'reasonably normal' electromyograms in these preparations (Grillner and Zangger, 1979) and others indicating greater differences (Smith, 1980). The characteristics of central pattern generators have also been more extensively investigated, with research indicating that the spinal cord, when deprived of all supraspinal influence and peripheral input, can continuously generate rhythmic alternating contractions in muscles of all joints, with a structure similar to that of the step cycle (Grillner and Zangger, 1979).

Smith (1980) and others (Grillner, 1973) have indicated that there are limitations in the capacity of the lumbosacral spinal cord to produce locomotor patterns, with age of transection and exercise being critical in contributing to its manifestation. Spinal cord transection must be made in kittens under 3 months of age and coupled with daily treadmill exercise of the affected limbs for optimal treadmill performance. Grillner showed that the locomotor abilities of spinalized kittens were such that they could generate enough muscle force to support the weight of hindquarters, and could vary the speed of the step cycle with that of the treadmill, from speeds of 0.1 to 1 m s^{-1}. He noted that the stance phase was reduced from 600 to 200 ms during this increase in speed, while the swing phase remained at about 300 ms.

Electromyographic activity in spinalized cats was also similar to that seen in normal cats walking on a treadmill (Forssberg, Grillner and Rossignol, 1977). Forssberg *et al.* showed that the extensor muscles of the knee and ankle were activated prior to paw contact and were terminated prior to lift off. This indicates that extension is not simply a reflex in response to contact, but is predetermined. Flexor muscles were activated at the beginning of the swing phase. Smith, Smith and Dahms (1979) also showed that spinal cats were capable of fully recruiting motor units within the spinal cord when progressing from a walk to a gallop.

Chronic spinal cats are also capable of adapting responses to perturbations of the limbs during ongoing locomotor activity (Forssberg, Grillner and Rossignol, 1977). Forssberg *et al.* applied mechanical tactile stimuli (a plexiglass rod) to the dorsum of the paw during various phases of the step cycle, and showed that stimulation during the swing phase activated a flexion response in the stimulated leg with concomitant extension of the contralateral leg. However, stimulation during stance caused an increased ipsilateral extension. Thus the same stimulus activated functionally separate sets of muscles depending on the phase of the step cycle. The spinally mediated responses to perturbations would thus be functional in normal locomotor conditions in compensating for an obstacle impeding the movement of the paw.

As mentioned above, it appears that the basic neuronal circuitry for generating the patterned locomotor output is present within the spinal cord of the cat and does not depend on feedback from the periphery to produce the pattern. Grillner and Zangger (1979) showed that cyclical stepping movements could be produced in a chronic spinal cat which had undergone a transection of the dorsal roots L3 to S4, in order to deafferent the hind limbs. Although the pattern was not spontaneously generated, it could be elicited by either an injection of the noradrenergic precursor 3,4-dihydroxyphenylalanine (DOPA) or by continuous electrical stimulation of either the dorsal column or the dorsal roots of the spinal cord. They also curarized the preparations to be sure that no movement-related information was activating the neural pattern generator and studied 'fictive locomotion', that is, the output of the muscle nerves, in the spinalized and deafferented preparation. A most common type of interlimb coordination was an alternating activity of the muscles of the two legs. They also noted that when the stimulation strength was increased the pattern changed from the alternation which would be used in a walk to a gallop pattern, with a phase difference between legs of 0.2. This shift in pattern usually came on as a sudden transition in activity.

Although these characteristics of normal locomotion were present, there were also differences in these spinalized and deafferented animals. For example, the duration of the step cycle, measured as the time between the midpoint of two repetitions of a muscle burst, was significantly longer than those seen in a chronic spinal cat without deafferentation. It is thus possible that sensory information from the limb contributes to appropriate stepping frequency.

It has been suggested that joint receptors may play a critical role in normal locomotion, with the position of the ipsilateral hip joint being an important contributor to the initiation of swing phase (Grillner and Rossignol, 1978; Smith,

1980). In addition, it has been shown that cutaneous information from the paw of the chronic spinal cat can have a powerful influence on the spinal pattern generator, as was discussed above (Forssberg, Grillner and Rossignol, 1977).

Descending influences from higher brain centers are also important for modulating locomotor activity. Decerebrate cats will walk normally on a treadmill when tonic electrical stimulation is applied to a particular region of the brainstem known as the mesencephalic locomotor region (Shik, Severin and Orlovsky, 1966). Grillner and Zangger (1979) noted that the effects of electrically stimulating the mesencephalic locomotor region can be duplicated by injections of L-DOPA. It is hypothesized that the L-DOPA increases the amount of norepinephrine released from the terminals from descending pathways. Grillner and Zangger also noted that when spinal pattern-generating circuits are stimulated by tonic activation, they produce, at best, a bad caricature of walking. They say this is due to the lack of important modulating influences from brainstem and cerebellum. For example, it has been shown that in each step cycle discharges from the vestibulospinal, rubrospinal and reticulospinal pathways act directly on motoneurons to fine-tune the movements according to the needs of the task (Grillner and Zangger, 1979).

In addition, Arshavsky and colleagues (1972a, b) have shown that the cerebellum has a special role in fine-tuning locomotor movements. They recorded from the dorsal and ventral spinocerebellar tracts during locomotion and showed that they were phasically active. The dorsal spinocerebellar tract neurons, receiving synaptic inputs from muscle afferents, were no longer phasically active with locomotion after deafferentation. Thus they appeared to function to send the cerebellum information about sensory feedback during locomotion. However, the ventral tracts still showed phase-dependent modulation. They thus hypothesized that the ventral neurons functioned in part to send a copy of the central pattern generator output for locomotion to the cerebellum.

It is also possible that the cerebellum has a different function in the modulation of the locomotor pattern. Keele and Ivry (1991) hypothesize that the cerebellum may also allow modulation not to correct error but to alter stepping patterns. For example, as an animal crosses uneven terrain, the legs must be lifted higher or lower depending on the obstacles. The locomotor pattern may be modulated through the following steps. First, the locomotor rhythm is conveyed to the cerebellum. The cerebellum extrapolates forward in time to specify when the next flexion is to occur. The cerebellum then facilitates descending commands that originate with vision to alter the flexion phase at precisely the correct time.

In sum, these results suggest that natural locomotor behavior emerges through a continuous interaction between the central pattern generators, descending corrections and peripheral feedback. Higher centers may also contribute to locomotion through feedforward modulation of patterns in response to environmental demands.

3.3.2   The Biomechanics of Pattern Generation

The importance of the interactions between central and peripheral sources of information is further demonstrated by recent analyses of the limb dynamics of the cat hind limb motion during the paw shake response and swing phase of locomotion (Hoy and Zernicke, 1985, 1986; Hoy, Zernicke and Smith, 1985; Smith and Zernicke, 1987; Wisleder, Zernicke and Smith, 1990). Using methods of inverse dynamics, it is possible to determine the joint moments of force (torque) responsible for the observed behavior. Knowledge of the limb trajectory and an appropriate anthropometric model make possible the calculation of the net torque acting on each segment and the subsequent partitioning of the net torque into components due to gravity, the mechanical interaction among segments (motion-dependent torques), and a generalized muscle torque. Thus, what this type of analysis allows us to do is assess the roles of muscular and nonmuscular forces in the generation of the behavior.

It is intuitively obvious that nonmuscular forces, such as gravity, play a role in the construction of all movement. What is revealed by analysis of the limb dynamics, however, is the relative importance of the muscular and nonmuscular contributions. For example, Hoy, Zernicke and Smith (1985) examined the paw shake response in adult spinal cats. The paw shake response is a series of rapid oscillations at the hip, knee and ankle as the animal attempts to remove some irritant on the paw. Their analyses revealed that the muscular torque at the ankle was the dominant contributor to the net torque. That is, a plot of the time series of the muscle and net torque components revealed the two curves to be nearly identical. The passive forces were relatively unimportant in determining motion of the paw. In contrast, the muscle and net torque curves at the knee were not parallel. Large muscle torques at the knee were required to counterbalance the large inertial torque, particularly due to paw angular acceleration. Thus, at the ankle, the muscles contributed to the control of the paw angular acceleration, whereas at the knee the muscles acted to control the motion-dependent torques arising from the mechanical interactions of adjacent segments.

The different roles played by muscles about the ankle and knee lead to questions of control. What features of the paw shake response are preplanned? The limited influence of motion-dependent terms on the net torque about the ankle suggest a limited need to consider the intersegmental dynamics at the ankle. However, the compensatory muscle response at the knee suggests that an important role is, in fact, played by motion-dependent feedback. As Hoy, Zernicke and Smith (1985) ask: is it possible that neural circuitry responsible for generating activity in the ankle musculature waits on motion-dependent feedback to produce the compensatory effects at the knee?

Perturbing the paw shake response by the application of a cast to the limb (Sabin and Smith, 1984) or weights to the paw (Hart et al., 1986) led to disruption of the activation patterns of the knee muscles but not the activity of the ankle flexors and extensors. These results appear to confirm the immutability of the neural pattern generator for ankle muscle activity and a context sensitivity to intersegmental dynamics and subsequent knee muscle recruitment. Such a dialog between the neural pattern generator and the periphery appears quite useful in that the use of motion-dependent feedback would allow neural adaptation to the ongoing or emerging limb dynamics (Smith and Zernicke, 1987).

Sensitivity to context appears all the more important in locomotion. Each segment of the cat hind limb is subject to a complex set of muscular and nonmuscular forces. Changes in speed lead to changes in the interactive patterns among the torque components (Hoy and Zernicke, 1985; Wisleder, Zernicke and Smith, 1990). In exemplar trials, Hoy and Zernicke report that the muscle torque at the knee was predominantly flexor early in the swing of the walking gait, becoming extensor just prior to knee reversal to extension. Subsequently, the knee muscle torque turned flexor again, controlling the extension of the joint while a large extensor torque due to leg angular acceleration sustained the extensor motion. In contrast, the gallop required an extensor knee muscle torque early in the swing phase to counterbalance the flexor influence of leg angular acceleration. Knee extension was also sustained by a passive extensor torque, counterbalanced by a flexor muscle torque. At higher speeds, the muscle torque was used more often to counterbalance the motion-dependent torques, not explicitly to drive the behavior. Similar results have been observed at the hip joint (Wisleder, Zernicke and Smith, 1990).

How the dialog between the periphery and the neural pattern generating circuits occurs is still unclear, although both the discharge from muscle spindles and the mechanical advantages of biarticular muscle undoubtedly play a role (Hoy, Zernicke and Smith, 1985; Wisleder, Zernicke and Smith, 1990). What is revealed in the dynamic analysis of limb movements is the intricacies of the interaction among active and passive forces. How is movement preplanned in its entirety in the face of reactive phenomena?

3.3.3 Pattern Generation in the Leg Movements of Humans

We begin with a discussion of swing-limb dynamics and the contribution of nonmuscular forces to the behavior. Subsequent sections focus on infant stepping and pattern generation from both neural and dynamical perspectives. Much of the research on locomotor pattern generation in humans comes from infant studies. Infants provide a unique window to pattern generation because they represent the naive motor system and the spontaneous leg movements of infants reveal an intrinsic organization. First in supported stepping movements and later in locomotion, we address the issues of pattern formation. In the final section we discuss dynamic pattern generation in other gait forms such as running and galloping.

Swing-Limb Dynamics in Adult Locomotion
For biomechanists, locomotion has provided fertile ground for the kinetic analysis of the mechanical interaction among segments of the lower extremity. The methods of inverse dynamics go beyond descriptions of limb trajectories and yield the causative factors behind the observed behavior. The simplifying model assumptions appropriate to the swing phase (e.g. planar motion, free-acting distal segment) have made this part of the gait cycle particularly attractive for investigation. The questions typically are concerned with how much of the limb behavior can be explained by the mechanical interaction among the limb segments, or to what extent does muscle drive the behavior versus controlling mechanical and/or gravitational effects?

Nonmuscular forces play a substantial role in the trajectory formation of the swing phase of gait. Winter and Robertson (1978) determined that 80% of the torque necessary to accelerate the shank forward during the swing phase was produced by nonmuscular forces (inertia of the limb, linear acceleration of the knee joint and gravity). In fact, during most of the swing phase, the muscle torque at the knee opposes the direction of motion (Winter and Robertson, 1978; see also Figs 4 and 5 in Zernicke, Schneider and Buford, 1991). Phillips, Roberts and Huang (1983), using a direct dynamics approach, further demonstrated the importance of nonmuscular forces in trajectory formation in the swing phase of running.

The direct dynamics approach involves the use of joint moments of force as inputs to the model with subsequent prediction of the model kinematics. This approach contrasts the methods of inverse dynamics in which the joint moments of force are predicted from the kinematics. An advantage of the direct dynamics approach is the potential for exploring perturbations to systems that cannot easily be accomplished experimentally. For example, Phillips, Roberts and Huang (1983) modeled the lower extremity as a two-segment link model–the thigh and a combined shank–foot segment. Inputs to the model were experimentally determined and included the linear kinematics of the hip joint, the muscle torque at the hip and the initial angular kinematics for the two segments. The model manipulation was to 'set' the muscle torque about the knee to zero at selected points in the swing phase to assess the role of other contributing torques.

Phillips, Roberts and Huang (1983) found that the removal of the muscle torque at the knee early in the swing phase led to continued knee flexion. The attendant motion-dependent torques were insufficient to produce knee joint reversal. If the influence of the knee muscle torque was removed later in the swing, just before the thigh reached maximum flexion velocity, then joint reversal occurred but its occurrence was delayed and the peak joint extension velocity was of lower magnitude than that observed in normal running. In a final manipulation, the knee joint muscle torque was set to zero 60% into the swing. At this time, knee reversal from flexion to extension had already occurred, and the rate of thigh flexion was slowing in preparation for the next heelstrike. In this case, the simulated motion closely approximated the experimentally obtained data until 65 ms before heelstrike. As the thigh ultimately slowed and reversed direction of rotation, the simulated shank motion increased in forward rotational velocity and the model exhibited hyperextension at the knee well beyond anatomic limits.

The work of Phillips, Roberts and Huang (1983) provides continuing support–in a more dramatic context (running versus walking)–for the importance of nonmuscular forces in trajectory formation. Further, the role of muscle in the swing phase of locomotion appears complementary, rather than antagonistic, to the nonmuscular forces. For example, Zernicke *et al.* (1991) have shown that counterbalancing effects from leg angular acceleration (tending to flex the knee) and the combined effect of thigh angular velocity and hip linear acceleration (tending to extend the knee) permit the muscle torque to remain small at the time of knee joint reversal (independent EMG analyses confirm minimal muscle activation at this time). Thus, while reversal could be generated solely by passive force, albeit delayed (Phillips *et al.*), the complementarity of muscular and nonmuscular forces combine for task-appropriate behavior.

At different speeds, slower walking or sprinting, the precise combination of muscular and nonmuscular forces may be quite different. For example, Mena, Mansour and Simon (1981) and Mochon and McMahon (1980) achieved reasonable success with direct dynamic models of the swing phase of walking driven predominantly by gravity. Mochon and McMahon developed a simple model of walking in which the stance limb had the characteristics of an inverted pendulum and the swing limb a passive compound pendulum. For normal speeds, model assumptions of a compound pendulum swinging under the influence of gravity led to approximately correct kinematics and ground reaction forces. Muscle forces were hypothesized to be used only to create the initial conditions prior to toe-off, and at high speeds, to brake the motion prior to heelstrike. Pendular models have met with some success, but it is also agreed that they are limited in application within a small range of speeds (Elftman, 1939; Grieve and Gear, 1966; Mochon and McMahon, 1980).

From models such as those described above, we see that the relative importance of muscular and nonmuscular forces is highly context dependent. The production of purposeful movements necessitates an ongoing interaction between neural pattern generators and the peripheral dynamics. There is a confluence of behavioral, electromyographic and kinetic data supporting the cooperativity between neural pattern generation and the advantageous exploitation of peripheral dynamics.

Infant Stepping and the Development of Locomotion – the Neural Perspective

When newborn infants are held under their arms in an upright position, tilted slightly forward, with the soles of their feet touching a surface, they often perform coordinated movements that look much like erect locomotion (Andre-Thomas and Autgarden, 1966). This behavior is much more difficult to elicit after the first few weeks, and by 2 months of age the behavior is seldom seen. The nature of this stepping behavior, the underlying neural mechanisms and the cause of its disappearance in the majority of children have been the focus of numerous investigations (Forssberg, 1985; Okamoto and Goto, 1985; Sutherland *et al.*, 1980; Thelen and Cooke, 1987; Thelen, Fisher and Ridley-Johnson, 1984).

Using a longitudinal design, Forssberg (1985) studied stepping during the newborn period, during supported locomotion just prior to the onset of independent locomotion and during early independent locomotion, in order to determine what changes occurred in the kinematics of the movement and in the neural patterning as the child developed independent mobility. Forssberg analyzed the behavior of 156 infants tested at 1, 3, 4, 5 and 10 months, in addition to 24 neonates, 5–6 days old. The infants were gently pulled over a flat surface while EMGs were recorded from the gastrocnemius, tibialis anterior, hamstrings and quadriceps. All 24 newborns could perform at least one step, with 7 able to execute a series of regular steps. Of the 156 infants tested longitudinally, 94 made one or more steps at 1 month, 18 stepped at 3 months, and 2 stepped at 4 and 5 months. Thus there was a significant decline in stepping frequency with an increase in age up to 5 months. At 10 months, however, stepping reappeared with all 156 stepping with support and 18 stepping without support.

Thelen and colleagues obtained similar results. In a study of 65 neonates (mean age 43.2 ± 17.1 hours), all infants performed at least one step, with a mean of 7.75 steps for the right leg (range 0–20) and 7.93 for the left (range 1–17) (Thelen, Fisher *er al.*, 1982). Between 2 and 6 weeks of age, a significant decline in steps was also observed (Thelen, Fisher and Ridley-Johnson, 1984).

The stepping patterns of infants are quite variable both within and between subjects, but general characteristics prevail. Young infants exhibit a dominant flexor bias at both the hip and the knee. The motor response patterns are characterized by a high degree of synchronized activity and coactivation of antagonistic muscles. Joint behaviors at the hip, knee and ankle are also tightly coupled (Forssberg, 1985; Thelen and Cooke, 1987).

In most infants, the stepping behavior declines significantly with increasing age. Forssberg (1985) noted an inactive period in 152 of 156 infants that occurred just after 2 months of age (4–8 months' duration), during which spontaneous stepping did not occur. The infants resumed locomotion first as crawling, then supported locomotion. At 10 months of age, all 156 children were stepping with support and 18 were stepping independently.

With the reappearance of the stepping behavior during supported locomotion, Forssberg observed greater regularity in the step frequency, reduction in the hyperflexion of the knee, as well as a reduction in the synchrony of joint action. The EMG patterns of the 10-month-olds during supported locomotion were similar to the patterns of the newborn, although some increase in regularity of muscle firing and increased activation amplitudes was observed. The heel and toe were still lowered to the ground together, and while all children could produce vertical forces exceeding their own body weight and could produce forward and backward thrusts, there was no double peak in vertical force, as is seen in adult locomotion. The valley between the vertical force peaks is a dynamic response to the swing limb, and the lack of such a valley suggests the push-off into the swing phase is still weak.

The onset of independent locomotion is the next step in the gradual transformation of the locomotor movements during the first year of life. The trend is toward a dissolution of the uniform pattern of joint movements to a more dissociated pattern in the adult. Forssberg (1985) tested four children 1–2 weeks after they began to walk without support. While they had achieved independence in gait, Forssberg concluded that their movement and EMG patterns were not significantly different from those seen during supported locomotion.

Forssberg (1985) argues that infant locomotion is like that of digitigrade quadrupeds: they show high knee/hip flexion and do not have heelstrike stepping. The transformation to adult-like gait happens during the later part of the second year (heelstrike in front of body, reversed ankle coordination, asynchronous EMG pattern), and not upon the appearance of independent locomotion. Based on this developmental pattern and the observation that anencephalic infants can perform a similar pattern of infant stepping (Peiper, 1961), Forssberg concludes that the locomotor network must be organized at or below the brainstem. The neural pattern generator appears to be innate and not reflexively activated by ankle muscle stretch, since extensor activity is activated prior to foot touchdown. Learning to walk, then, has nothing to do with a change in rhythm generation, but appears to result from maturation of the equilibrium system.

In sum, Forssberg (1985) contends that human locomotion is controlled by a hierarchical system. In support of this position he notes that children with cerebral palsy, children with mental disabilities and habitual toe-walkers do not develop a plantigrade gait. Further, adults may revert to immature locomotion through hemiplegia or Parkinson's disease. From this view, the gradual transformation in gait over the second year could be the result of: (1) new rhythm generating circuits gradually taking over or a rewiring of the original circuit; (2) changed peripheral feedback, from the distal leg, modifying the output; or (3) a new central system could influence the original network and modify it.

Forssberg, then, is a proponent of the neurophysiological perspective. The locomotor pattern is organized and controlled by a system in which an innate pattern generator creates the basic rhythm. Descending driving systems would establish control in the first year to give the child the ability to control the activity but adaptive systems for equilibrium control develop over a longer period and subsequently modify the central pattern generator.

There are those, however, who argue that rhythmic behavioral patterns, including locomotor patterns, derive from dynamical interaction among systems in which descending driving influences are de-emphasized (Kugler, Kelso and Turvey, 1982; Turvey, Shaw and Mace, 1978). In the sections that follow we review the application of this perspective to investigations of locomotor pattern generation in developmental and real time.

Infant Stepping and the Development of Locomotor Patterns – the Dynamical Perspective

For some years now, Thelen has been a major voice in the promotion of a dynamical systems approach to the study and explanation of developmental processes (Thelen, 1986a, 1988, 1989b; Thelen, Kelso and Fogel, 1987). From this perspective, Thelen offers explanations for the disappearance of the stepping pattern early in the first year of life, and the emergence of patterned leg movements from birth through the achievement of independent locomotion.

In dynamical systems, patterned behaviors form spontaneously from the unique interactions of all the component parts. The phrases 'self-organization', 'self-assembly' and 'soft-assembly' refer to this spontaneous pattern formation. In this view, the trajectory of an infant's kicks or steps is not coded anywhere in the nervous system. Rather, it is a behavior that emerges from the soft-assembly of many elements, including the neural circuitry, anatomical linkages, body composition, arousal level and gravitational conditions (Thelen, Ulrich and Jensen, 1989b). No single element holds the 'plan', and no single element is sufficient to specify the behavior. Thus, the movement behavior at any moment is a product of all the functionally related elements acting cooperatively, in context, and not simply the result of the activation of a neural pattern generator.

The contextual dependence and self-organization of infant leg behaviors is supported by the mutability of the leg pattern under a variety of conditions (Thelen, 1988; Thelen, Ulrich and Jensen, 1989a). The 5-month-old who performs few if any steps when held upright will perform well-coordinated steps when placed on a motorized treadmill (Thelen and Ulrich, 1991). The treadmill steps of a 7-month-old are coordinated and demonstrate a dissociated hip/knee pattern that approximates more mature forms of locomotion. Yet when the 7-month-old steps without the context of the treadmill, the hip and knee revert to the more immature patterns of synchronous joint flexions and extensions (Thelen, 1986b). Perhaps one of the most dramatic behavioral demonstrations of the soft-assembly of the elements that support the coordinated alternating stepping patterns of infants comes from the split-belt paradigm studies by Thelen, Ulrich and Niles (1987). When placed on a split-belt treadmill where each leg moved backward at a different rate, these 7-month-old infants adjusted the stepping pattern of each leg to maintain the 0.5 phase lag that typifies alternating gait. In fact, between 1 and 10 months, when treadmill steps can be elicited, infants demonstrate an ability (which improves as the alternating step pattern becomes dominant) to accommodate changes in bilateral belt speed as well as split-belt speed differences (Thelen and Ulrich, 1991).

From the earliest ages there is a strong tendency to produce coordinated, alternate leg movements. These behaviors are observed in a variety of postures and environmental contexts. Ulrich, Jensen and Thelen (1991) argue that such evidence supports the contention that the pattern generation for alternate stepping (or kicking) is not the product of highly specific muscle synergies, but a general ensemble characteristic of the neuromotor system that provides for the continuity of the alternate pattern and the flexibility to adapt to changing conditions.

Dynamical systems are complex cooperative systems composed of many elements. An assumption of the dynamical systems approach to developing phenomena is that these elements develop asynchronously and in a nonlinear fashion (Thelen, Ulrich and Jensen, 1989b). Different components develop at different rates, and the slower developing components become the rate-limiters. The emergence of a new behavior awaits the availability of all relevant components. Thus, while certain components may be available well in advance of the onset of the behavior, their expression must await the further development of the slower developing or rate-limiting elements. For example, in this section we discuss the shifting of locomotor patterns to higher levels of maturity by providing the missing component (posture control) or artificially enhancing what otherwise would be a rate-limiting element. It was from this perspective, also, that Thelen approached the questions surrounding the disappearance of the stepping reflex.

In a programmatic series of studies, Thelen and colleagues have made a cogent argument for the appearance and disappearance of the infant stepping behavior as a function of the asynchronous development and contextually dependent interaction of subsystems. First, kinematic (Thelen, Bradshaw and Ward, 1981) and electromyographic (Thelen and Fisher, 1982) similarities were demonstrated between the supine kicks and upright steps of infants. From this evidence, Thelen and Fisher argued that both behaviors were generated from the same neural circuitry. They hypothesized that the disappearance of the stepping pattern at 2 months of age was due to an increase in adipose tissue in the body, decreasing the strength-to-weight ratio – the leg becomes too heavy to lift. Supine kicking might remain if strength deficits in the upright posture could be compensated by mechanical and gravitational advantages in the supine posture. Given the present inability precisely to measure muscle moment arm lengths and experimentally to determine the force–length relationship of muscles in infants, it seems that the next best test of Thelen's hypothesis is an experimental manipulation of kinetic context. If the stepping behavior is susceptible to contextual influence such as manipulation of the mechanical load, then easing the load should facilitate the behavior, as increasing the load should inhibit it. Thelen, Fisher and Ridley-Johnson (1984) altered the mechanical load for 4-week-old infants first by adding weights to the legs, and then submerging the (unweighted) legs in water. As predicted, weighting the legs led to a reduction in steps and stepping increased dramatically in both rate and amplitude when the infants were submerged up to the trunk in water.

Finally, we consider the emergence of new behaviors. From the dynamical systems perspective, discontinuity often characterizes the shift between one behavioral mode (or attractor state) and another. What makes the discontinuity noteworthy is that the shift occurs as the system inputs are scaled up continuously. In the abstract, as the energy inputs into the system increase, the system moves through different stable behavioral modes associated with selected energy ranges. (In the terminology of dynamical systems, the stable behavioral modes are the attractor states and energy is the control parameter that moves the system from one stable attractor to another.) We addressed this issue explicitly in the hypothetical experiment discussed in Section 2.6. As the velocity of the platform perturbation was increased on a continuous scale, we predicted qualitatively different, but stable, behavioral responses – first the ankle synergy at low velocities, then the hip synergy at high velocities. The transition from walk to trot to gallop in animal locomotion with scalar changes in speed is another example. Thelen (1984) hypothesized that the emergence of independent locomotion awaits critical levels of strength and balance. The emergence of later appearing locomotor patterns may also be influenced by achieving critical values in subsystems. Control parameters that shift the system from a walk to a run may be force production and posture control, and the transition from running to the asymmetry of galloping may be a function of critical levels of force differentiation between the legs as well as other equilibratory responses to the force asymmetries (Clark and Whitall, 1989).

Dynamic Pattern Generation in Real Time – Comparing Supported and Independent Locomotion

Manipulations of task and context can be used to explore the developmental status of pattern generation and its rigidity/plasticity in response to perturbations. The contrast between supported and independent locomotion is one of the contextual manipulations that has been used to explore pattern generation in the developing human motor system (Clark, Whitall and Phillips, 1988; Forssberg, 1985; Kazai, Okamoto and Kumamoto, 1976; Okamoto and Goto, 1985).

The basic neural and behavioral patterns characteristic of upright bipedal locomotion are in place long before the infant is capable of independent walking. At 6 months of age the infant propels herself when supported by an infant walker (Kauffman and Ridenour, 1977; Okamoto and Goto, 1985). From that age forward, infants held upright will take steps forward with greater or lesser degrees of skillfulness. As the child matures and gains experience, cocontraction of the antagonist musculature begins to give way to reciprocal patterns of activation, the dominant flexor bias of the lower extremity relaxes, and the hip, knee and ankle joints begin to flex and extend independently of one another.

A critical test of the plasticity of the neuromotor system, however, is the comparison of behavioral and neural patterns from supported and independent locomotion within the same subject and at the same developmental age. For example, Kazai, Okamoto and Kumamoto (1976) compared EMG patterns during supported and independent walking from the same subject on the first and sixth day of independent walking and again at the end of the first month. On the first day, independent steps were characterized by cocontraction of antagonist muscles. With support, activation levels of the lower extremity and trunk muscles were reduced and evidence of a reciprocal pattern between the biceps femoris and rectus femoris was observed. Cocontraction of antagonist muscles continued to dominate the pattern on the sixth day of independent locomotion, but a reduction in the activation levels of the rectus abdominis could already be seen. Once again, when given support, an overall reduction in activation was observed. In addition, there was a decrease in the discharge of the tibialis anterior during stance and a reciprocal pattern between the tibialis anterior and the gastrocnemius appeared. Activity in the gastrocnemius and soleus during the swing of supported walking also appeared.

Okamoto and Goto (1985) observed a similar reduction in antagonistic coactivation and the shift toward more reciprocal patterns in selected muscle pairs in a 9-month-old preindependent walker. Their comparison was between supported walking in an unstable posture (erect trunk and full weight bearing) and supported walking in a stable posture (slight forward inclination of the trunk and reduction of the load on the legs). In the stable, supported walk there was a reduction in the activation of the rectus femoris and vastus medialis during the swing phase. This implies a lesser tendency to lift and extend the knee actively during swing. A reciprocal pattern between the tibialis anterior and gastrocnemius during stance could also be seen. Okamoto and Goto concluded that the provision of posture control and reduced mechanical load could shift the EMG patterns to those observed in stable independent walking.

Clark, Whitall and Phillips (1988) also compared independent and supported walking within the same experimental test session. Their subjects were new walkers who were filmed within 2 days of generating their first three independent steps. No difference was observed between supported and independent conditions for mean temporal phasing; however, the supported condition led to a significant reduction in the temporal phasing variability (see Section 3.1.6 for a more complete description of the Clark *et al.* study and the definition of the dependent measures). In fact, new supported walkers were similar in temporal phasing variability to those with 3 months of walking experience. Supporting the new walker did lead to significant differences in distance phasing, an effect the authors attribute to the facilitating effect of the postural support. Like temporal phasing variability, supporting the new walker led to a reduction of the distance phasing variability such that they were not significantly different from infants with 0.5 or 1 month of walking experience.

The contrast of supported and independent locomotion within the same test session has revealed a plasticity in the neuromotor system that is difficult to observe in cross-sectional or even longitudinal studies. Forssberg (1985) had concluded that neither movement nor EMG patterns differed substantially between the time a child could walk with support and some later time when the child could walk independently. On some relative scale, this conclusion is warranted by the evidence. Yet, the within-session comparisons demonstrate a shift toward mature gait patterns both at the neural level (Kazai, Okamoto and Kumamoto, 1976; Okamoto and Goto, 1985) and in the kinematics (Clark, Whitall and Phillips, 1988) when support is present. These results suggest that, while the appearance of mature gait patterns is influenced by the evolution of central structures, it is also quite susceptible to the precise integration of all contributing systems whether they be neuromuscular, equilibratory, perceptual, etc.

Dynamic Pattern Generation – Locomotion as the Coupling of Nonlinear Limit Cycle Oscillators

Previously we described walking as an alternating gait described by a phase lag of 0.5. The ubiquity of this interlimb pattern – evident in treadmill stepping, at the onset of independent locomotion, and in the mature adult gait – prompts the question of how *interlimb* coordination is achieved. Appealing again to theories of pattern formation in physical systems, the interlimb coordination achieved in locomotion (or between two or more limbs) has been modeled as the coupling of nonlinear limit cycle oscillators (Kelso, Putnam, and Goodman, 1983; Kelso *et al.*, 1981, 1987). Here, a brief divergence into some definitions is warranted.

An oscillator is a device that exhibits repetitive motion. A pendulum swings, or oscillates, back and forth. An ideal pendulum, or frictionless device, would continue to oscillate indefinitely. But real systems are dissipative structures – that is, they dissipate energy and ultimately the oscillation is damped out. To sustain motion, energy is added to the system periodically and in an amount that, on average, equals the energy dissipated during the cycle. Over many repetitions the system settles into a 'near-isochronous motion of fixed amplitude independent of sporadic disturbances and initial conditions' (Kelso and Tuller, 1984a).

If the oscillatory pattern is perturbed by a push that increases the amplitude of the oscillation, then more energy will be dissipated in the cycle than can be provided by the forcing function, and the amplitude of the cycle will decline until energy dissipation and the forcing function become balanced. Likewise, for any perturbation that leads to a reduced amplitude, the energy imbalance will be in favor of the forcing function and the cycle will grow until a balanced state is achieved. It is the quality of nonlinearity that allows the system to return to the same stable pattern – the limit cycle – regardless of whether the perturbation pushes the systems 'in' or 'out'. Linear systems do not return to a preferred trajectory when perturbed, but assume new states.

Nonlinear limit cycle oscillators display three fundamental properties (Kelso *et al.*, 1981). First, they tend to maintain a stable trajectory (in amplitude and frequency) despite perturbation. This property is referred to as 'structural stability'. A second important property of such oscillatory systems is their tendency to interact. This interaction is observed in the entrainment of one oscillator to another. That is, two oscillators with different initial frequencies will become matched (identical frequencies) or one oscillator will assume a frequency that is an integer multiple of the other (subharmonic entrainment). A third related property of coupled nonlinear limit cycle oscillators is that they tend to be stable only in limited phase relationships (Kelso *et al.*, 1987). For example, in the flexion/extension cyclic movement of two hands a stable phasing relationship is observed only when the two hands are cycling in phase with each other (0 or 360 degrees) or out of phase (180 degrees). These two phase relationships are stable, attractor states. The in-phase relationship is stable in all ranges of oscillation frequencies; the 180 degrees phasing is stable only at low frequencies (Kelso, 1984).

Interlimb coordination in upper extremity motion has been explored in some detail, but little work has been done explicitly to test the properties of nonlinear limit cycle oscillators as they might apply to locomotion. An exception is the work by Whitall (1989) which explored interlimb coordination in running and galloping.[4] Four children's groups, 2.5–3.5, 3.5–4.5, 6–7 and 9–10 years of age, and an adult group were included for study. The phase mode specific to each gait was assessed by measures of mean temporal and amplitude phasing. Entrainment was revealed

---

[4]The gallop is a gait pattern in which the lead limb performs a walking step and the rear limb performs a running step. The rear limb never moves ahead of the lead limb.

by the variability in the temporal and amplitude phasing, and structural stability was tested by adding weight to one limb.

Distinct phase-locked modes were identified in both the run and the gallop, and these phasing relationships were consistent across all ages. For the run, a 50/50% mean phasing relationship (1:1 ratio) was found in both temporal and amplitude phasing. This is the expected relationship in a mature symmetric gait and concurs with the earlier reported 50 phasing relationships in new walkers (Clark, Whitall and Phillips, 1988). The gallop was also characterized by stable temporal phase-locked modes, but there appeared to be individual differences with 2:1 and 3:1 ratios being the most attractive across all age groups. A mean amplitude phasing of 40/60% for the rear/front limbs was stable across all age groups. Amplitude phasing was more variable than temporal phasing, but this appeared to be because of the disparity in length of the initial step compared with subsequent steps (subjects started from rest).

The addition of a weight (4% of body weight) to one limb did not alter the temporal or amplitude phasing relationship between the limbs in the run. This resistance to perturbation argues in favor of structural stability although a more robust test would be to test the system response to a range of weights and/or to perturb the legs in the midst of the cyclic behavior.

The addition of weight did affect the temporal phasing of the gallop, causing a shift to a different phase mode without subsequent re-entrainment. Amplitude phasing was also affected by the weight, but re-entrainment occurred within one step cycle. Whitall (1989) hypothesized that the differential regulation of the force between the limbs is a system-sensitive parameter and the intentional modification of the forces to accommodate the weight pushes the system into a new phasing relationship. The amplitude phasing re-entrains – perhaps for balance consider-ations – while the temporal phasing is the result of limb dynamics.

The results of this study generally concur with predictions based on properties of nonlinear limit cycle oscillators, and developmental differences were generally confined to differences between the youngest age group and the others.

In summary, the limbs participate in stable repetitive processes during locomo-tion in which each gait is described by a fixed-phase relationship between or among the limbs. The gait of prewalking infants, new walkers and new gait forms are all characterized by well-coordinated patterns of movement at the start. The modeling of gait as ensembles of nonlinear limit cycle oscillators may provide a theory-driven account of this apparently intrinsic interlimb coordination and the abrupt phase transitions that occur as speed increases.

3.4   Locomotion Summary

The human upright bipedal gait is a symmetric gait characterized by largely stereotypic yet functionally adaptive behaviors at all levels of analysis (neural through kinematic outcomes). Mature gait has a developmental history that begins (postnatally) with the earliest steps of the newborn and exhibits the most dramatic changes in the first 3 years of life. Mean temporal and distance step cycle characteristics are remarkably adult-like at the onset of independent locomotion, although the variability is quite high. Posture control appears to be an important modifier. Providing the new walker with postural support shifts the behavioral pattern to more mature levels of performance. At the other end of the age continuum, the decrements apparent in the gait of the elderly also appear to be, in part, a function of changes in posture control.

The evidence from deafferented and spinal-transected animal preparations lends support to hypotheses of neural origins for locomotor pattern generation. Modification of these neural patterns arise from biomechanical constraints and context-sensitive reflex responses. Reactive mechanical forces appear accommodated while the precise mechanisms for such contextually sensitive control remains unclear.

Recent theoretical perspectives on pattern generation in locomotion have de-emphasized prescriptive neural plans in favor of pattern formation as the emergent and softly-assembled result of multiple subsystem contributions. This dynamical systems perspective draws upon the analogy between biological systems and other complex physical systems where spontaneous pattern formation has been demonstrated to result from manipulating the energy inputs to the system or scaling on some system-sensitive parameter. Support for the dynamical systems perspective comes from demonstrations of the sensitivity of the stepping or locomotor pattern to tasks and contextual manipulations, the biomechanical contributions to pattern formation, and the success of physical system models in approximating pattern formation in biological systems. Such results do not exclude the neurophysiological perspective as a potent explanatory perspective. Descending neural commands themselves may follow dynamic processes, being altered in specific ways as a function of scaling on some system-sensitive parameter. Moreover, return afference, from a dynamic viewpoint, may directly interact with neural circuitry, altering its behavior in ways consistent with dynamic principles – that is, the same neural circuitry may behave differently depending on the nature of afferent feedback. A mark of a dynamic systems perspective, in contrast to earlier neural perspective views is, therefore, to emphasize interaction of feedback with existing circuitry.

4 FINAL COMMENTS

The purpose of this paper was to review the extant literature on posture and locomotion. We organized this review around the historical and contemporary theoretical perspectives that have driven the research on these topics. This review is not all-inclusive, but we believe it is sufficiently thorough to demonstrate how each perspective has informed and shaped our attitudes and expectations about pattern generation and motor control with particular regard to posture and locomotion.

Research grounded in the neurophysiological perspective has supplied us with information of increasing detail regarding the specific elements of the neuromotor system that participate in synergistic ways in pattern formation and perturbation responses. Yet the increasing detail about *which* elements are involved in each behavior does not answer questions about *how* these elements are coordinated. Past theories based primarily on models of neuronal central pattern generators whose output is modulated by relevant sensory information are being altered by dynamical models in which systems are softly-assembled and self-organizing. This paradigmatic shift is not a denunciation of the past, but rather an acknowledgement that the present knowledge base requires a broader theoretical perspective. Our descriptions of the neural, kinematic and kinetic events that surround postural tasks and locomotion are quite robust. We hope that future research will turn increasingly toward the rigors of hypothesis testing and theory development.

ACKNOWLEDGEMENT

This study was supported by NIA Grant R23 AG05317.

REFERENCES

Alexander, R. McN. (1984). Walking and running. *American Scientist*, **72**, 348–354.

Allum, J. H. J. and Pfaltz, C.R. (1985). Visual and vestibular contributions to pitch sway stabilization in the ankle muscles of normals and patients with bilateral peripheral vestibular deficits. *Experimental Brain Research*, **58**, 82–94.

Amblard, B. and Carblanc, A. (1980). Role of foveal and peripheral visual information in maintenance of postural equilibrium in man. *Perception and Motor Skills*, **51**, 903–912.

Andre-Thomas, and Autgarden, S. (1966). *Locomotion from Pre- to Postnatal Life*. Lavenham, Suffolk: Spastics Society.

Arshavsky, Yu. I., Berkinblit, M. B., Fukson, O. I., Gelfand, I. M. and Orlovsky, G. N. (1972a). Recordings of neurones of the dorsal spinocerebellar tract during evoked locomotion. *Brain Research*, **43**, 272–275.

Arshavsky, Yu. I., Berkinblit, M. B., Gelfand, I.M., Orlovsky, G. N. and Fukson, O. I. (1972b). Activity of the neurones of the ventral spino-cerebellar tract during locomotion. *Biophysics*, **17**, 926–935.

Basmajian, J. V. (1979). *Muscles Alive*, 4th edn. Baltimore, MD: Williams and Wilkins.

Battye, C. K. and Joseph, J. (1966). An investigation by telemetering of the activity of some muscles in walking. *Medical and Biological Engineering*, **4**, 125–135.

Beck, R. J., Andriacchi, T. P., Kuo, K. N., Fermier, R. W. and Galante, J.O. (1981). Changes in the gait patterns of growing children. *Journal of Bone and Joint Surgery*, **63A**, 1452–1456.

Begbie, G. H. (1967). Some problems of postural sway. In A. V. S. de Reuck and J. Knight (Eds), *Myotatic, Kinesthetic and Vestibular Mechanisms* (pp. 80–92). London: Churchill.

Belen'kii, V. Y., Gurfinkel, V. S. and Pal'tsev Y. I. (1967). Elements of control of voluntary movements. *Biofizika*, **12**, 135–141.

Bernstein, N. (1967). *Co-ordination and Regulation of Movements*. New York: Pergamon Press.

Bertenthal, B. I. and Bai, D. L. (1988). Infants' sensitivity to optical flow for controlling posture. In C. Butler and K. Jaffe (Eds), *Visual-Vestibular Integration in Early Development*: *Technical and Clinical Perspectives* (pp. 43–61). Washington, DC: RESNA.

Borelli, G. A. (1685). *De Motu Animalium*. Rome.

Brandell, B. R. (1973). An analysis of muscle coordination in walking and running gaits. *Medicine and Sport*, vol. 8: *Biomechanics III* (pp. 278–287). Basel: Karger.

Brandt, T. (1988). Sensory function and posture. In: B. Amblard, A. Berthoz and F. Clarac (Eds), *Posture and Gait: Development, Adaptation and Modulation* (pp. 127–136). Amsterdam: Elsevier.

Braune, W. and Fischer, O. (1895). *Der Gang des Menschen*. Leipzig: Hirzel.

Breniere, Y., Bril, B. and Fontaine, R. (1989). Analysis of the transition from upright stance to steady state locomotion in children with under 200 days of autonomous walking. *Journal of Motor Behavior*, **21**, 20–37.

Breniere, Y. and Do, M. C. (1986). When and how does steady state gait movement induced from upright posture begin? *Journal of Biomechanics*, **19**, 1035–1040.

Breniere, Y., Do, M. C. and Bouisset, S. (1987). Are dynamic phenomena prior to stepping essential to walking? *Journal of Motor Behavior*, **19**, 62–76.

Bril, B. and Breniere, Y. (1989). Steady-state velocity and temporal structure of gait during the first six months of autonomous walking. *Human Movement Science*, **8**, 99–122.

Brown, T. G. (1911). The intrinsic factors in the act of progression in the mammal. *Proceedings of the Royal Society of London*, **84**, 308–319.

Carlsöo, A. (1966). The initiation of walking. *Acta Anatomica*, **65**, 1–9.

Cavanagh, P. R. and Gregor, R. J. (1975). Knee joint torques during the swing phase of normal treadmill walking. *Journal of Biomechanics*, **8**, 337–344.

Clark, J. E. and Phillips, S. J. (1987). The step cycle organization of infant walkers. *Journal of Motor Behavior*, **19**, 421–433.

Clark, J. E. and Whitall, J. (1989). Changing patterns of locomotion: From walking to skipping. In M. Woollacott and A. Shumway-Cook (Eds), *The Development of Posture and Gait Across the Lifespan* (pp. 128–151). Columbia: USC Press.

Clark, J. E., Whitall, J. and Phillips, S. J. (1988). Human interlimb coordination: The first 6 months of independent walking. *Developmental Psychobiology*, **21**, 445–456.

Cook, T. and Cozzens, B. (1976). Human solutions for locomotion: III. The initiation of gait. In R. M. Herman, S. Grillner, P. S. G. Stein and D. G. Stuart (Eds), *Neural Control of Locomotion* (pp. 65–76). New York: Plenum.

Cordo, P. and Nashner, L. (1982). Properties of postural adjustments associated with rapid arm movements. *Journal of Neurophysiology*, **47**, 287–302.

Craik, R. (1989). Changes in locomotion in the aging adult. In M. Woollacott and A. Shumway-Cook (Eds), *The Development of Posture and Gait Across the Lifespan* (pp. 176–201). Columbia: USC Press.

Delcomyn, F. (1980). Neural basis of rhythmic behavior in animals. *Science*, **210**, 492–498.

Diener, H. C. and Dichgans, J. (1986). Long loop reflexes and posture. In W. Bles and T. Brandt (Eds), *Disorders of Posture and Gait* (pp. 41–51). Amsterdam: Elsevier.

Diener, H. C., Dichgans, J., Bootz, F. and Bacher, M. (1984). Early stabilization of human posture after a sudden disturbance: Influence of rate and amplitude of displacement. *Experimental Brain Research*, **56**, 126–134.

Diener, H. C., Horak, F. B. and Nashner, L. M. (1988). Influence of stimulus parameters on human postural responses. *Journal of Neurophysiology*, **59**, 1888–1905.

Dillman, C. J. (1971). A kinetic analysis of the recovery leg during sprint running. In J. Cooper (Ed.), *Selected Topics on Biomechanics: Proceedings of the CIC Symposium on Biomechanics* (pp. 137–165). Chicago, IL: The Athletic Institute.

Dubo, H. I. C., Peat, M., Winter, D. A., Quanbury, A. O., Hobson, D. A., Steinke, T. and Reimer, G. (1976). Electromyographic temporal analysis of gait: Normal human locomotion. *Archives of Physical Medicine and Rehabilitation*, **57**, 415–420.

Eberhart, H. D. (1976). Physical principles of locomotion. In R. M. Herman, S. Grillner, P. S. G. Stein and D.G. Stuart (Eds), *Neural Control of Locomotion* (pp. 1–11). New York: Plenum.

Eberhart, H. D., Inman, V. T. and Bresler, B. (1954). The principle elements in human locomotion. In P. E. Klopsteg and P. D. Wilson (Eds), *Human Limbs and their Substitutes* (pp. 437–471). New York: McGraw-Hill.

Edgerton, V. R., Grillner, S., Sjostrom, A. and Zangger, P. (1976). Central generation of locomotion in vertebrates. In R. M. Herman, S. Grillner, P. S. G. Stein and D. G. Stuart (Eds), *Neural Control of Locomotion* (pp. 439–464). New York: Plenum.

Eklund, G. (1972). Position sense and state of contraction: the effect of vibration. *Journal of Neurology, Neurosurgery and Psychiatry*, **35**, 606–611.

Elftman, H. (1939). Forces and energy changes in the leg during walking. *American Journal of Physiology*, **125**, 339–356.

Elftman, H. (1940). The work done by muscles in running. *American Journal of Physiology*, **129**, 672–684.

Elftman, H. (1941). The action of muscles in the body. *Biologica Symposia*, **3**, 191–209.

Elner, A. M., Gurfinkel, V. S., Lipshits, M. I., Mamasakhlisov, G. V. and Popov, K.E. (1976). Facilitation of stretch reflex by additional support during quiet stance. *Agressologie*, **17**, 15–20.

Elner, A. M., Popov, K. E. and Gurfinkel, V. S. (1972). Changes in stretch-reflex system concerned with the control of postural activity of human muscles. *Agressologie*, **13**, 19–24.

Fentress, J. C. (1989). Developmental roots of behavioral order: Systemic approaches to the examination of core developmental issues. In M. R. Gunnar and E. Thelen (Eds), *Systems in Development: The Minnesota Symposia in Child Psychology*, vol. 22 (pp. 35–76). Hillsdale, NJ: Erlbaum.

Fernie, G. R., Gryfe, C. I. and Holliday, P. J. (1982). The relationship of postural sway in standing to the incidence of falls in geriatric subjects. *Age and Ageing*, **11**, 11–16.

Finley, F. R. and Cody, K. A. (1970). Locomotive characteristics of urban pedestrians. *Archives of Physical Medicine and Rehabilitation*, **51**, 423–426.

Forssberg, H. (1985). Ontogeny of human locomotor control I. Infant stepping, supported locomotion and transition to independent locomotion. *Experimental Brain Research*, **57**, 480–493.

Forssberg, H., Grillner, S. and Rossignol, S. (1977). Phase dependent reflex reversal during walking in chronic spinal cats. *Brain Research*, **85**, 121–139.

Forssberg, H. and Nashner, L. (1982). Ontogenetic development of postural control in man: Adaptation to altered support and visual conditions during stance. *Journal of Neuroscience*, **2**, 545–552.

Gabell, A. and Nayak, U. S. L. (1984). The effect of age on variability in gait. *Journal of Gerontology*, **39**, 662–666.

Gelfand, I. M., Gurfinkel, V. S., Tsetlin, M. L. and Shik, M. L. (1971). Problems in the analysis of movements. In V. S. Gurfinkel, S. V. Fomin and M. L. Tsetlin (Eds), *Models of the Structural–Functional Organization of Certain Biological Systems* (pp. 329–345). Cambridge, MA: MIT Press.

Grieve, D. W. (1968). Gait patterns and the speed of walking. *Biomedical Engineering*, **3**, 119–122.

Grieve, D. W. and Gear, R. J. (1966). The relationship between length of stride, step frequency, time of swing and speed of walking for children and adults. *Ergonomics*, **9**, 379–399.

Grillner, S. (1973). Locomotion in the spinal cat. In R. B. Stein, K. G. Pearson, R. S. Smith and J. B. Redford (Eds), *Control of Posture and Locomotion* (pp. 515–535). New York: Plenum.

Grillner, S. (1981). Control of locomotion in bipeds, tetrapods, and fish. In V. B. Brooks (Ed.), *Handbook of Physiology – The Nervous System*, vol. II: *Motor Control* (pp. 1179–1236). Baltimore, MD: Williams and Wilkins.

Grillner, S. and Rossignol, S. (1978). On the initiation of the swing phase of locomotion in chronic spinal cats. *Brain Research*, **146**, 269–277.

Grillner, S. and Zangger, P. (1979). On the central generation of locomotion in the low spinal cat. *Experimental Brain Research*, **34**, 241–261.

Gurfinkel, V. S., Lipshits, M. I., Mori, S. and Popov, K. E. (1976). The state of stretch reflex during quiet standing in man. *Progress in Brain Research*, **44**, 473–486.

Gurfinkel, V. S., Lipshits, M. I. and Popov, K. E. (1979). Kinesthetic thresholds in the orthograde posture. *Agressologie*, **20**, 133–134.

Gurfinkel, V. S. and Shik, M. L. (1973). The control of posture and locomotion. In A. A. Gydikov, N. T. Tankov and D. S. Losarov (Eds), *Motor Control* (pp. 217–234). New York: Plenum.

Haas, G. and Diener, H. C. (1988). Development of stance control in children. In B. Amblard, A. Berthoz and F. Clarac (Eds), *Posture and Gait: Development, Adaptation and Modulation* (pp. 49–58). Amsterdam: Elsevier.

Haken, H. (1983). *Synergetics: An Introduction*. Heidelberg: Springer.

Haken, H., Kelso, J. A. S. and Bunz, H. (1985). A theoretical model of phase transitions in human hand movements. *Biological Cybernetics*, **51**, 347–356.

Hart, T. J., Cox, E. M., Hoy, M. G., Smith, J. L. and Zernicke, R. F. (1986). Intralimb kinetics of perturbed paw-shake response. *Biomechanics*, **X–A**, 471–477.

Herman, R., Cook, T., Cozzens, B. and Freedman, W. (1973). In R. B. Stein, K. G. Pearson, R. S. Smith and J. B. Redford (Eds), *Control of Posture and Locomotion* (pp. 363–388). New York: Plenum.

Herman, R., Wirta, R., Bampton, S. and Finley, F. R. (1976). Human solutions for locomotion I. Single limb analysis. In: R. U. Herman, S. Grillner, P. Stein and D. G. Stuart (Eds), *Neural Control of Locomotion* (pp. 13–49). New York: Plenum.

Horak, F. and Nashner, L. (1986). Central programming of postural movements: Adaptation to altered support surface configurations. *Journal of Neurophysiology*, **55**, 1369–1381.

Hoy, M. G. and Zernicke, R. F. (1985). Modulation of limb dynamics in the swing phase of locomotion. *Journal of Biomechanics*, **18**, 49–60.

Hoy, M. G. and Zernicke, R. F. (1986). The role of intersegmental dynamics during rapid limb oscillations. *Journal of Biomechanics*, **19**, 867–877.

Hoy, M. G., Zernicke, R. F. and Smith, J. L. (1985). Contrasting roles of inertial and muscle moments at knee and ankle during paw-shake response. *Journal of Neurophysiology*, **54**, 1282–1294.

Hugon, M., Massion, J. and Wiesendanger, M. (1982). Anticipatory postural changes induced by active unloading and comparison with passive unloading in man. *Pflugers Archiv*, **393**, 292–296.

Humphrey, D. R. (1986). Representation of movements and muscles within the primate precentral motor cortex: Historical and current perspectives. *Federation Proceedings*, **45**, 2687–2699.

Humphrey, D. R. and Reed, D. J. (1983). Separate cortical systems for the control of joint movement and joint stiffness: Reciprocal activation and coactivation of antagonist muscles. *Advances in Neurology*, **39**, 347–372.

Humphrey, D. R., Qiu, X. Q., Clavel, P. and O'Donoghue, D. L. (1990). Changes in forelimb motor representation in rodent cortex induced by passive movements. *Neuroscience Abstracts*, **16**, 422.

Imms F. J. and Edholm, O. G. (1981). Studies of gait and mobility in the elderly. *Age and Ageing*, **10**, 147–156.

Inman, V. T., Ralston, H. and Todd, F. (1981). *Human Walking*. Baltimore, MD: Williams and Wilkins.

Jouen, F. (1984). Visual–vestibular interactions in infancy. *Infant Behavior and Development*, **7**, 135–145.

Jouen, F. (1988). Visual–proprioceptive control of posture in newborn infants. In B. Amblard, A. Berthoz and F. Clarac (Eds), *Posture and Gait: Development, Adaptation and Modulation* (pp. 13–22). Amsterdam: Elsevier.

Kauffman, I. B. and Ridenour, M. (1977). Influence of an infant walker on onset and quality of walking pattern of locomotion: An electromyographic investigation. *Perceptual and Motor Skills*, **45**, 1323–1329.

Kazai, N., Okamoto, T. and Kumamoto, M. (1976). Electromyographic study of supported walking of infants in the initial period of learning to walk. *Biomechanics*, **V**, 311–318.

Keele, S. and Ivry, R. (1991). Does the cerebellum provide a common computation for diverse tasks? A timing hypothesis. In A. Diamond (Ed.), *Developmental and Neural Bases of Higher Cognitive Function*, pp. 179–211. New York: New York Academy of Sciences.

Kelso, J. A. S. (1984). Phase transitions and critical behavior in human bimanual coordination. *American Journal of Physiology: Regulatory Integrative Comparative Physiology*, **240**, R1000–R1004.

Kelso, J. A. S., Holt, K. G., Rubin, P. and Kugler, P. N. (1981). Patterns of human interlimb coordination emerge from the properties of non-linear, limit cycle oscillatory processes: Theory and data. *Journal of Motor Behavior, 13,* 226–261.

Kelso, J. A. S., Putnam, C. A. and Goodman, D. (1983). On the space–time structure of human interlimb coordination. *Quarterly Journal of Experimental Psychology, 35A,* 347–375.

Kelso, J. A. S. and Schöner, G. (1988). Selforganization of coordinative movement patterns. *Human Movement Science, 7,* 27–46.

Kelso, J. A. S., Schöner, G., Scholz, J. P. and Haken, H. (1987). Phase-locked modes, phase transitions and component oscillators in biological motion. *Physica Scripta, 35,* 79–87.

Kelso, J. A. S. and Tuller, B. (1984a). A dynamical basis for action systems. In M. S. Gazzaniga (Ed.), *Handbook of Cognitive Neuroscience* (pp. 321–356). New York: Plenum.

Kelso, J. A. S. and Tuller, B. (1984b). Converging evidence in support of common dynamical principles for speech and movement coordination. *American Journal of Physiology: Regulatory, Integrative and Comparative Physiology, 246,* R928–R935.

Keshner, E., Woollacott, M. and Debu, B. (1988). Neck, trunk and limb muscle responses during postural perturbations in humans. *Experimental Brain Research, 71,* 455–466.

Kugler, P. N., Kelso, J. A. S. and Turvey, M. T. (1980). On the concept of coordinative structures as dissipative structures: I. Theoretical lines of convergence. In G.E. Stelmach and J. Requin (Eds), *Tutorials in Motor Behavior* (pp. 3–47). New York: North-Holland.

Kugler, P. N., Kelso, J. A. S. and Turvey, M. T. (1982). On the control and co-ordination of naturally developing systems. In J. A. S. Kelso and J. E. Clark (Eds), *The Development of Movement Control and Co-ordination* (pp. 5–78). New York: John Wiley.

Kugler, P. N. and Turvey, M. T. (1987). *Information, Natural Law, and the Self-Assembly of Rhythmic Movement.* Hillsdale, NJ: Erlbaum.

Lee, D. N. and Aronson, E. (1974). Visual proprioceptive control of standing in human infants. *Perception and Psychophysics, 15,* 529–532.

Lee, D. N. and Young, D. S. (1986). Gearing action to the environment. *Experimental Brain Research Series 15* (pp. 217–230). Berlin: Springer.

Lee, W. (1980). Anticipatory control of postural and task muscles during rapid arm flexion. *Journal of Motor Behavior, 12,* 185–196.

Leibowitz, H. W., Rodemer, C. S. and Dichgans, J. (1979). The independence of dynamic spatial orientation from luminance and refractive error. *Perception and Psychophysics, 25,* 75–79.

Lishman, J. R. and Lee, D. N. (1973). The autonomy of visual kinaesthesis. *Perception, 2,* 287–294.

MacConaill, M. A. and Basmajian, J. V. (1977). *Muscles and Movements.* New York: R. E. Krieger.

MacPherson, J. M. (1988). The neural organization of postural control–do muscle synergies exist? In B. Amblard, A. Berthoz and F. Clarac (Eds), *Posture and Gait: Development, Adaptation and Modulation* (pp. 381–390). Amsterdam: Elsevier.

Manchester, D., Woollacott, M., Zederbauer-Hylton, N. and Marin, O. (1989). Visual, vestibular and somatosensory contributions to balance control in the older adult. *Journal of Gerontology, 44,* M118–127.

Mann, R. A., Hagy, J. L., White, V. and Liddell, D. (1979). The initiation of gait. *Journal of Bone and Joint Surgery, 61-A,* 232–239.

Massion, J. (1979). Role of motor cortex in postural adjustments associated with movement. In H. Asanuma and V. J. Wilson (Eds), *Integration in the Nervous System* (pp. 239–260). Tokyo: Igaku-Shoin.

Massion, J. (1984). Postural changes accompanying voluntary movements. Normal and pathological aspects. *Human Neurobiology, 2,* 261–267.

McCollum, G., Horak, F. B. and Nashner, L. M. (1985). Parsimony in neural calculations of postural movements. In J. Bloedel, J. Dichgans and W. Precht (Eds), *Cerebellar Functions* (pp. 52–66). Heidelberg: Springer.

McGraw, M. B. (1940). Neuromuscular development of the human infant as exemplified in the achievement of erect locomotion. *Journal of Pediatrics*, **17**, 747–771.

McGraw, M. B. (1963). *The Neuromuscular Maturation of the Human Infant*. New York: Hafner.

McMahon, T. A. (1984). *Muscles, Reflexes and Locomotion*. Princeton, NJ: Princeton University Press.

Mena, D., Mansour, J. M. and Simon, S. R. (1981). Analysis and synthesis of human swing leg motion during gait and its clinical applications. *Journal of Biomechanics*, **14**, 823–832.

Miller, D. I. and Nelson, R. C. (1973). *Biomechanics of Sport*. Philadelphia, PA: Lea and Febiger.

Milner, M., Basmajian, J. V. and Quanbury, A. O. (1971). Multifactorial analysis of walking by electromyography and computer. *American Journal of Physical Medicine*, **50**, 235–258.

Mochon, S. and McMahon, T. A. (1980). Ballistic walking. *Journal of Biomechanics*, **13**, 49–57.

Moore, S. P., Rushmer, D. S., Windus, S. L. and Nashner, L. M. (1988). Human automatic postural responses: Responses to horizontal perturbations of stance in multiple directions. *Experimental Brain Research*, **73**, 648–658.

Mott, F. W. and Sherrington, C. S. (1895). Experiments upon the influence of sensory nerves upon movement and nutrition of the limbs. Preliminary communication. *Proceedings of the Royal Society of London*, **57**, 481–488.

Murray, M. P. (1967). Gait as a total pattern of movement. *American Journal of Physical Medicine*, **46**, 290–333.

Murray, M. P., Kory, R. C. and Clarkson, B. H. (1969). Walking patterns in healthy old men. *Journal of Gerontology*, **24**, 169–178.

Murray, M. P., Kory, R. C., Clarkson, B. H. and Sepic, S. B. (1966). Comparison of free and fast speed walking patterns of normal men. *American Journal of Physical Medicine*, **45**, 8–24.

Murray, M. P., Mollinger, L. A., Gardner, G. M. and Sepic, S. B. (1984). Kinematic and EMG patterns during slow, free, and fast walking. *Journal of Orthopaedic Research*, **2**, 272–280.

Nashner, L. M. (1970). *Sensory Feedback in Human Posture Control*. Massachusetts Institute of Technology Report MVT–70-3.

Nashner, L. M. (1976). Adapting reflexes controlling the human posture. *Experimental Brain Research*, **26**, 59–72.

Nashner, L. M. (1977). Fixed patterns of rapid postural responses among leg muscles during stance. *Experimental Brain Research*, **30**, 13–24.

Nashner, L. and Berthoz, A. (1978). Visual contribution to rapid motor responses during postural control. *Brain Research*, **150**, 403–407.

Nashner, L., Black, F.O. and Wall, C. (1982). Adaptation to altered support and visual conditions during stance: Patients with vestibular deficits. *Journal of Neuroscience*, **2**, 536–544.

Nashner, L. M. and McCollum, G. (1985). The organization of human postural movements: A formal basis and experimental synthesis. *Behavioral and Brain Sciences*, **8**, 135–172.

Nashner L. M. and Woollacott, M. H. (1979). The organization of rapid postural adjustments of standing humans: An experimental–conceptual model. In R. E. Talbot and D. R. Humphrey (Eds), *Posture and Movement* (pp. 243–257). New York: Raven Press.

Norlin, R., Odenrich, P. and Sandlund, B. (1981). Development of gait in the normal child. *Journal of Pediatric Orthopedics*, **1**, 261–266.

Okamoto, T. and Goto, Y. (1985). Human infant pre-independent and independent walking. In S. Kondo (Ed.), *Primate Morphophysiology: Locomotor Analyses and Human Bipedalism* (pp. 25–45). Tokyo: University of Tokyo Press.

Paulus, W., Straube, A. and Brandt, Th. (1987). Visual postural performance after loss of somatosensory and vestibular function. *Journal of Neurology, Neurosurgery and Psychiatry*, **50**, 1542–1545.

Pearson, K. G. (1987). Central pattern generation: A concept under scrutiny. In H. McLennan, J. R. Ledsome, C. H. S. McIntosh and D. R. Jones (Eds), *Advances in Physiological Research* (pp. 167–185). New York: Plenum.

Pedotti, A. (1977). A study of motor coordination and neuromuscular activities in human locomotion. *Biological Cybernetics*, **26**, 53–62.

Peiper, A. (1961). *Cerebral Functions in Infancy and Childhood*. New York: Consultants Bureau.

Phillips, S. J. and Clark, J. E. (1987). Infants' first unassisted walking steps: Relationships to speed. *Biomechanics*, **X-A**, 425–428.

Phillips, S. J., Roberts, E. M. and Huang, T. C. (1983). Quantification of intersegmental reactions during rapid swing motion. *Journal of Biomechanics*, **16**, 411–417.

Pope, M. J. (1984). *Visual Proprioception in Infant Postural Development*. Unpublished PhD thesis, University of Southampton.

Prigogine, I. and Stengers, I. (1984). *Order out of Chaos*. New York: Bantam.

Raibert, M. (1986). Symmetry in running. *Science*, **231**, 1292–1294.

Ralston, H. J. (1976). Energetics of human walking. In R. M. Herman, S. Grillner, P. S. G. Stein and D. G. Stuart (Eds), *Neural Control of Locomotion* (pp. 77–98). New York: Plenum.

Roll, J. P. and Roll, R. (1988). From eye to foot: A proprioceptive chain involved in postural control. In B. Amblard, A. Berthoz and F. Clarac (Eds), *Posture and Gait: Development, Adaptation and Modulation* (pp. 155–164). Amsterdam: Elsevier.

Roll, J. P. and Vedel, J. P. (1982). *Experimental Brain Research*, **47**, 177–190.

Roos, J. W. P., Bles, W. and Bos, J. E. (1988). Postural control after repeated exposure to a tilting room. In B. Amblard, A. Berthoz and F. Clarac (Eds), *Posture and Gait: Development, Adaptation and Modulation* (pp. 137–144). Amsterdam: Elsevier.

Rosenrot, P., Wall, J. C. and Charteris, J. (1980). The relationship between velocity, stride time, support time and swing time during normal walking. *Journal of Human Movement Studies*, **6**, 323–335.

Rushmer, D. S., Moore, S. P., Windus, S. L. and Russell, C. J. (1988). Automatic postural responses in the cat: Responses of hindlimb muscles to horizontal perturbations of stance in multiple directions. *Experimental Brain Research*, **71**, 93–102.

Sabin, C. and Smith, J. L. (1984). Recovery and perturbation of the pawshake response in spinal cats. *Journal of Neurophysiology* **51**, 680–688.

Saltzman, E. and Kelso, J. A. S. (1985). Synergies: Stabilities, instabilities, and modes. *Behavioral and Brain Sciences*, **8**, 161–163.

Saltzman, E. and Kelso, J. A. S. (1987). Skilled actions: A task-dynamic approach. *Psychological Review*, **94**, 84–106.

Saunders, J. B. de C. M., Inman, V. T. and Eberhart, H. D. (1953). The major determinants in normal and pathological gait. *Journal of Bone and Joint Surgery*, **35-A**, 543–558.

Scholz, J. P. (1990). Dynamic pattern theory – Some implications for therapeutics. *Physical Therapy*, **70**, 827–843.

Schöner, G. and Kelso, J. A. S. (1988a). Dynamic pattern generation in behavioral and neural systems. *Science*, **209**, 1513–1520.

Schöner, G. and Kelso, J. A. S. (1988b). Dynamic patterns of biological coordination: Theoretic strategy and new results. In J. A. S. Kelso, A. J. Mandell and M. F. Schlesinger (Eds), *Dynamic Patterns in Complex Systems* (pp. 77–102). Singapore: World Scientific Publishers.

Sheldon, J. H. (1963). The effect of age on the control of sway. *Gerontologia Clinica*, **5**, 129–138.

Sherrington, C. S. (1898). Decerebrate rigidity, and reflex coordination of movements. *Journal of Physiology (London)*, **22**, 319–332.

Sherrington, C. S. (1906). *Integrative Action of the Nervous System*. New York: Scribner.

Sherrington, C. S. (1910). Flexion-reflex of the limb, crossed extension reflex, and reflex stepping and standing. *Journal of Physiology (London)*, **40**, 28–121.

Shik, M. L., Severin, F. V. and Orlovsky, G. N. (1966). Control of walking and running by means of electrical stimulation of the mid-brain. *Biophysics*, **11**, 756–765.

Shumway-Cook, A. and Woollacott, M. (1985). The growth of stability: Postural control from a developmental perspective. *Journal of Motor Behavior*, **17**, 131–147.

Shupert, C. L., Black, F. O., Horak, F. B. and Nashner, L. M. (1988). Coordination of the head and body in response to support surface translations in normals and patients with bilaterally reduced vestibular function. In B. Amblard, A. Berthoz and F. Clarac (Eds), *Posture and Gait: Development, Adaptation and Modulation* (pp. 281–289). Amsterdam: Elsevier.

Smith, J. L. (1980). Programming of stereotyped limb movements by spinal generators. In G. E. Stelmach and J. Requin (Eds), *Tutorials in Motor Behavior* (pp. 95–115). Amsterdam: North-Holland.

Smith, J. L., Smith, L. A. and Dahms, K. L. (1979). Motor capacities of the chronic spinal cat: Recruitment of slow and fast extensors of the ankle. *Neuroscience Abstracts*, **5**, 387.

Smith, J. L. and Zernicke, R. F. (1987). Predictions for neural control based on limb dynamics. *Trends in Neuroscience*, **10**, 123–128.

Soames, R. W. and Richardson, R. P. S. (1985). Stride length and cadence: Their influence on ground reaction forces during gait. *Biomechanics*, **IX-A**, 406–410.

Spielburg, P. I. (1940). Walking patterns of old people: Cyclographic analysis. In N. A. Bernstein (Ed.), *Investigations on the Biodynamics of Walking, Running and Jumping*, part II. Moscow: Central Scientific Institute of Physical Culture.

Statham, L. and Murray, M. P. (1971). Early walking patterns of normal children. *Clinical Orthopaedics and Related Research*, **79**, 8–24.

Stoffregen, T. A., Schmuckler, M. A. and Gibson, E. (1987). Use of central and peripheral optical flow in stance and locomotion in young walkers. *Perception*, **16**, 113–119.

Sutherland, D. (1984). *Gait Disorders in Childhood and Adolescence*. Baltimore, MD: Williams and Wilkins.

Sutherland, D., Olshen, R., Cooper, L. and Savio, L. (1980). The development of mature gait. *Journal of Bone and Joint Surgery*, **62A**, 336–353.

Taub, E. (1976). Movement in nonhuman primates deprived of somatosensory feedback. *Exercise and Sport Sciences Reviews*, **4**, 335–374.

Taub, E. and Berman, A. J. (1968). Movement and learning in the absence of sensory feedback. In: S. J. Freedman (Ed.), *The Neurophysiology of Spatially Oriented Behavior* (pp. 173–192). Homewood, NJ: Dorsey Press.

Thelen, E. (1984). Learning to walk: Ecological demands and phylogenetic constraints. In L. P. Lipsitt (Ed.), *Advances in Infancy Research*, vol. 3 (pp. 213 250). Norwood, NJ: Ablex.

Thelen, E. (1986a). Development of coordinated movement: Implications for early human development. In: M. G. Wade and H. T. A. Whiting (Eds), *Motor Skills Acquisition* (pp. 107–124). Dordrecht, Netherlands: Martinus Nijhoff.

Thelen, E. (1986b). Treadmill-elicited stepping in seven-month-old infants. *Child Development*, **57**, 1498–1506.

Thelen, E. (1988). Dynamical approaches to the development of behavior. In J. A. S. Kelso, A. J. Mandell and M. F. Schlesinger (Eds), *Dynamic Patterns in Complex Systems* (pp. 348–369). Singapore: World Scientific Publishers.

Thelen, E. (1989a). Evolving and dissolving synergies in the development of leg coordination. In S. A. Wallace (Ed.), *Perspectives on the Coordination of Movement* (pp. 259–281). New York: Elsevier.

Thelen, E. (1989b). Self-organization in developmental processes: Can systems approach work? In M. R. Gunnar and E. Thelen (Eds), *Systems and Development: The Minnesota Symposia on Child Psychology*, vol. 22 (pp. 77–117). Hillsdale, NJ: Erlbaum.

Thelen, E., Bradshaw, G. and Ward, J. A. (1981). Spontaneous kicking in month-old infants: Manifestations of a human central locomotor program. *Behavioral and Neural Biology*, **32**, 45–53.

Thelen, E. and Cooke, D. W. (1987). Relationship between newborn stepping and later walking: A new interpretation. *Developmental Medicine and Child Neurology*, **29**, 380–393.

Thelen, E. and Fisher, D. M. (1982). Newborn stepping: An explanation for a 'disappearing reflex'. *Developmental Psychology*, **18**, 760–775.

Thelen, E., Fisher, D. M. and Ridley-Johnson, R. (1984). The relationship between physical growth and a newborn reflex. *Infant Behavior and Development*, **7**, 479–493.

Thelen, E., Fisher, D. M., Ridley-Johnson, R. and Griffin, N. (1982). Effects of body build and arousal on newborn infant stepping. *Developmental Psychobiology*, **15**, 447–453.

Thelen, E., Kelso, J. A. S. and Fogel, A. (1987). Self-organizing systems and infant motor development. *Developmental Review*, **7**, 39–65.

Thelen, E., Skala, K. D. and Kelso, J. A. S. (1987). The dynamic nature of early coordination: Evidence from bilateral leg movements in young infants. *Developmental Psychology*, **23**, 179–186.

Thelen, E. and Ulrich, B. D. (1991). Hidden precursors to skill: A dynamical systems analysis of treadmill-elicited stepping during the first year. *Monographs of the Society for Research in Child Development*, Serial No. 223, vol. 56, No. 1.

Thelen, E., Ulrich, B. and Jensen, J. (1989a). An 'outside-in' approach to the development of leg movement patterns. In C. von Euler, H. Forssberg and H. Lagercrantz (Eds), *Neurobiology of Early Infant Behavior* (pp. 107–118). New York: Stockton Press.

Thelen, E., Ulrich, B. and Jensen, J. (1989b). The developmental origins of locomotion. In M. Woollacott and A. Shumway-Cook (Eds), *The Development of Posture and Gait Across the Lifespan* (pp. 25–47). Columbia: USC Press.

Thelen, E., Ulrich, B. D. and Niles, D. (1987). Bilateral coordination in human infants: Stepping on a split-belt treadmill. *Journal of Experimental Psychology: Human Perception and Performance*, **13**, 405–410.

Turvey, M. T., Shaw, R. E. and Mace, W. (1978). Issues in the theory of action: Degrees of freedom, coordinative structures and coalitions. In J. Requin (Ed.), *Attention and Performance*, vol. VII (pp. 557–595). Hillsdale, NJ: Erlbaum.

Ulrich, B. D., Jensen, J. L. and Thelen, E. (1991). Stability and variation in the development of infant stepping: Implications for control. In A. E. Patla (Ed.), *Adaptability of Human Gait: Implications for the Control of Locomotion*. Amsterdam: Elsevier.

Van der Straaten, J. H. M., Lohman, A. H. M. and Van Linge, B. (1975). A combined electromyographic and photographic study of the muscular control of the knee during walking. *Journal of Human Movement Studies*, **1**, 25–32.

Whitall, J. (1989). A developmental study of the interlimb coordination in running and galloping. *Journal of Motor Behavior*, **21**, 409–428.

Whiting, H. T. A. (1984). *Human Motor Actions: Bernstein Reassessed*. New York: North-Holland.

Winter, D. A. (1980). Overall principle of lower limb support during stance phase of gait. *Journal of Biomechanics*, **13**, 923–927.

Winter, D. A. (1983a). Biomechanical motor patterns in normal walking. *Journal of Motor Behavior*, **15**, 302–330.

Winter, D. A. (1983b). Moments of force and mechanical power in jogging. *Journal of Biomechanics*, **16**, 91–97.

Winter, D. A. (1984). Kinematic and kinetic patterns in human gait: Variability and compensating effects. *Human Movement Science*, **3**, 51–76.

Winter, D. A. (1989). Biomechanics of normal and pathological gait: Implications for understanding human locomotor control. *Journal of Motor Behavior*, **21**, 337–355.

Winter, D. A. and Robertson, D. G. E. (1978). Joint torque and energy patterns in normal gait. *Biological Cybernetics*, **29**, 137–142.

Wisleder, D., Zernicke, R. F. and Smith, J. L. (1990). Speed-related changes in hindlimb intersegmental dynamics during the swing phase of cat locomotion. *Experimental Brain Research* **79**, 651–660.

Woollacott, M., Debu, B. and Mowatt, M. (1987). Neuromuscular control of posture in the infant and child: Is vision dominant? *Journal of Motor Behavior*, **19**, 167–186.

Woollacott, M. H., von Hofsten, C. and Rosblad, B. (1988). Relation between muscle response onset and body segmental movements during postural perturbations in humans. *Experimental Brain Research*, **72**, 593–604.

Woollacott, M., Shumway-Cook, A. and Nashner, L. (1982). Postural reflexes and aging. In J. A. Mortimer (Ed.), *The Aging Motor System*, (pp. 98–119). New York: Praeger.

Woollacott M., Shumway-Cook, A. and Nashner, L. (1986). Aging and posture control: Changes in sensory organization and muscular coordination. *International Journal of Aging and Human Development*, **23**, 97–114.

Woollacott, M. H. and Sveistrup, H. (1992). Changes in the sequencing and timing of muscle response coordination associated with developmental transitions in balance abilities. *Human Movement Science*.

Yamashita, T. and Katoh, R. (1976). Moving pattern of point of application of vertical resultant force during level walking. *Journal of Biomechanics*, **9**, 93–99.

Yang, J. F., Winter, D. A. and Wells, R. P. (1990a). Postural dynamics in the standing human. *Biological Cybernetics*, **62**, 309–320.

Yang, J. F., Winter, D. A. and Wells, R. P. (1990b). Postural dynamics of walking in humans. *Biological Cybernetics*, **62**, 321–330.

Zarrugh, M. Y., Todd, F. N. and Ralston, H. J. (1974). Optimization of energy expenditure during level walking. *European Journal of Applied Physiology*, **33**, 293–306.

Zernicke, R. F., Schneider, K. and Buford, J. A. (1991). Intersegmental dynamics during gait: Implications for control. In A. E. Patla (Ed.), *Adaptability of Human Gait: Implications for the Control of Locomotion* (pp. 187–202). Amsterdam: Elsevier.

Chapter 7

Reaching and Grasping. Parallel Specification of Visuomotor Channels

M. Jeannerod
INSERM U94, Bron, France

1 INTRODUCTION

The present chapter deals with a fundamental aspect of visuomotor behavior: the generation and control of goal-directed arm movements during the action of reaching and grasping. This action combines two widely different types of motor behavior. Reaching is a primitively developed behavior for interacting with the external milieu; grasping is a highly achieved type of behavior, due to specialization of the hand in primates and humans. This difference in biological significance between the two behaviors is reflected at the level of their neural substrates and modes of control. Reaching is mostly affected by the proximal joints of the arm, and deals with spatial relationships of the objects and the body. Its function is to carry the hand at an appropriate location within extrapersonal action space. It must include mechanisms for computing the distance and direction of the target point in space. By contrast, grasping is a distal behavior effected by finger movements, which deals with intrinsic qualities of objects. The coordinate system in which grasping movements are generated therefore does not relate to the body, it relates to the object and the hand, irrespective (within limits) of the position of the hand in extrapersonal space.

Isolation of either component is artificial, however, although it may be convenient for the purpose of analysis. Reaching and grasping are functionally interrelated, such that reaching is a precondition for grasping and therefore for transporting, manipulating and transforming objects. Its purpose is to bring the specialized area of the hand into contact with objects, for acquiring and using object-related information. It therefore represents a discrete transitional stage within the continuous processing of the information provided by the hand during manipulation, for tactile recognition, tactile to visual cross-modal matching, etc. This process is essential for building up representations of objects.

Association of the two behaviors in most everyday actions makes their study fascinating, partly because it raises the point of how neural subsystems with such different biological functions can be coordinated and synchronized. The above

Handbook of Perception and Action, Volume 2
ISBN 0-12-516162-X

general considerations will therefore have implications for describing the kinematic properties of these components of the same action, and for studying their underlying mechanisms.

2 REACHING

Guiding the hand to the location of a target in extrapersonal space involves complementary mechanisms that combine to achieve accuracy – the ultimate goal of the movement. One of these mechanisms is directional coding, the function of which is to orient the arm toward a target located in body-centered space; another mechanism is amplitude coding, the function of which is to generate the proper dynamics along the spatial path selected for that movement. There are indications in the literature which suggest that direction and amplitude of a reaching movement are specified in parallel. Favilla, Henning and Ghez (1989), for example, measured reaction times of force impulses in response to targets of different amplitudes appearing in two possible directions. Their hypothesis was that, if specification of response amplitude required the prior specification of response direction, amplitude specification would be delayed until direction specification was complete. Alternatively, if amplitude specification could proceed without direction specification, its time course would be little affected by the concurrent need to specify direction. The results were definitely more in favor of the second expectation – that is, in favor of a concurrent specification of the two parameters for the same movement.

2.1 Neurophysiological Mechanisms Underlying Directional Coding of Reaching Movements

The mechanisms by which the central nervous system controls limb movements directed at objects within extrapersonal space must subserve simultaneously two functions: (1) the computation of the target position in body-centered visual space; and (2) the computation of the position of the moving limb with respect to that target. These mechanisms can only be studied in experiments where the study of neuronal responses to visual targets are combined with the study of the corresponding behavioral responses.

2.1.1 Parietal Cortex Mechanisms

Neurons coding for the direction of reaching arm movements were first found in the posterior part of monkey parietal cortex, where they belong to a broader category of neurons selectively activated during specific aspects of visuomotor behavior, such as reaching, manipulation, visual fixation or eye movement. Neurons related to reaching or manipulation were described by Hyvärinen and Poranen (1974) and by Mountcastle et al. (1975) in the parietal lobules, more specifically within areas 5 and 7. The cells described by Mountcastle et al. in both areas have no receptive field or other sensory properties in the visual or somatosensory modalities; instead, they discharge during active reach to objects of motivational interest (a piece of food, for example), or during active manipulation of these objects – hence the terminology of 'projection neurons' and of 'command functions' used by these authors to designate an unspecified reaching system. By contrast, Hyvärinen and Poranen (1974) considered that the cells responding to arm movement in area 7 had directional properties, in specifying reaching in a given direction of extrapersonal space. In their experiments, activation of such neurons required association of a visual stimulus and of a movement toward it. Neither presentation of the visual stimulus, nor execution of the movement alone were found sufficient conditions for firing these neurons. A population of neurons coding for movement direction was also found in parietal area 5 (Kalaska, Caminiti and Georgopoulos, 1983). Figure 7.1 shows maps of superior and inferior parietal lobules. The localization of reaching cells has been plotted on the cortical convexity, showing a dense concentration in subarea 7b.

Hyvärinen and Poranen (1974) and Mountcastle *et al.* (1975) both tended to assign the parietal cortex a role in generation of neural commands for movements directed at extrapersonal space. Other authors (e.g. Robinson, Goldberg and Stanton, 1978), however, considered that properties of the visuomotor neurons (especially a category of eye movement-related cells, the visual-fixation cells) could well be explained by 'passive' responses to visual stimuli. Accordingly, they proposed that area 7 is specialized in high-order sensory (visual) processing and has a predominant role in visual and visuopatial functions. In order to account for the fact that discharges of inferior parietal lobule neurons increase when movements are actively produced by the animal during presentation of the stimuli, they proposed the intervention of an additional 'attentional' mechanism. The cells fulfilling these criteria are concentrated in subarea 7a. It remains, as Lynch (1980) argued, that the fact that a given cell receives a sensory input does not preclude its participation in sensorimotor or even motor processes. Indeed, according to the conception of cooperating visual and proprioceptive mechanisms, it is critical that these parietal 'reaching neurons' receive the relevant inputs (visual, tactile, kinesthetic) for elaborating the representation of the movement and controlling its execution. Finally, new experiments by Andersen, Essik and Siegel (1985) have disclosed in area LIP (an area buried in the intraparietal sulcus, Figure 7.1), a population of cells that respond directionally to saccadic eye movements.

Other arguments as to the visuomotor function of the parietal cortex can be drawn from lesion experiments. One problem raised by posterior parietal lesions is to distinguish between impairments affecting spatial processes involved in goal-directed actions and impairments in visual processes, largely independent of goal-directed action and involved in the perception of spatial relationships between objects. It has been clearly established that large posterior parietal lesions do not affect complex visual discriminations (Blum, Chow and Pribram, 1950). According to Pohl (1973), lesions that produce impairments in spatial orientation (in the parietal cortex) are in a different location from those that produce impairment in nonspatial visual discrimination (in the inferotemporal cortex). More recently, Mishkin, Lewis and Ungerleider (1982) and Mishkin and Ungerleider (1982) showed that visual modality-specific spatial abilities are subserved by the pre-occipital zone, although the inferior parietal lobule would subserve a supramodal spatial ability to which the visual modality (as well as other modalities) would contribute. The effects of simultaneous ablation of the two areas cumulate in

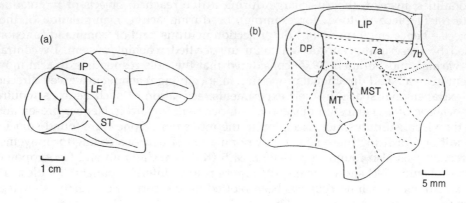

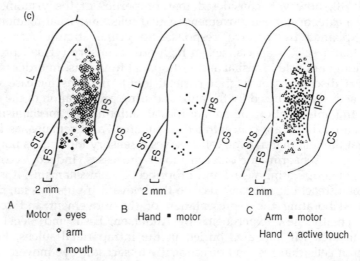

Figure 7.1. *The role of the posterior parietal cortex in controlling reaching. (a) The cortical zone located between the intraparietal sulcus (IP) and the lunate sulcus (L) has been outlined on the convexity of the right hemisphere in the monkey. LF: Lateral (sylvian) fissure. (b) Unfolding of this zone shows the parts of parietal cortex buried in the sulci. Areas DP, MT, MST, LIP, 7a and 7b participate in various aspects of reaching behavior [From Andersen and Gnadt, 1989.] (c) Lateral views of area 7, where neurons recorded during reaching movements have been projected. Note concentration of arm 'motor' neurons in the anterior half of area 7 (area 7a). CS: central sulcus; STS: superior temporal sulcus; IPS: intraparietal sulcus; FS: sylvian fissure. [From Hyvärinen, 1981.]*

producing spatial disorientation (Milner, Ockelford and Dewar, 1977; Mishkin *et al.*, 1982).

Studies focusing on the effects of inferior parietal lobule lesions on visuomotor behavior in the monkey have revealed highly specific impairments, including a reaching deficit first mentioned by Peele (1944). Reaching impairment following this lesion in the monkey is characterized by the fact that the animals misreach with

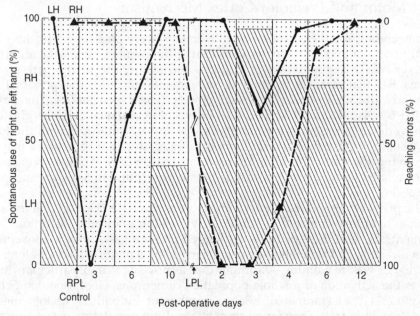

Figure 7.2. *Effects of posterior parietal lesion on reaching movements in the monkey. One monkey was tested during reaching for pieces of food. Before the lesion (control) both the left hand (LH) and the right hand (RH) performed with no errors. The monkey used preferentially his right hand (striped area). Following the right parietal lesion (RPL), only the left hand was affected. This hand was not spontaneously used, but when the monkey was forced to use it, a consistent misreaching was observed. Note reverse effect following left parietal lesion (LPL). [Results replotted from Faugier-Grimaud, Frenois and Stein, 1978.]*

their arm contralateral to the lesion in either part of the visual field (the 'hand effect') (Faugier-Grimaud, Frenois and Peronnet, 1985; Faugier-Grimaud, Frenois and Stein, 1978; Lamotte and Acuna, 1978; Hartje and Ettlinger, 1973). Their ipsilesional arm is usually not affected, although a 'visual field effect' (also involving misreaching with the ipsilesional arm within the contralesional field) has been obvserved by Stein (1978). Figure 7.2 displays the results of an experiment by Faugier-Grimaud *et al.* (1978), where a monkey was successively ablated in area 7 on both sides. Following the first lesion (on the right side), the animal misreached targets with the left, contralesional arm. After recovery from this deficit, which took less than 1 week, area 7 on the left side was lesioned. This lesion produced misreaching with the right arm and also, more transiently, with the left arm. Complete recovery was obtained 12 days following the second lesion. When spontaneous use of the hands was scored in this animal, it was found that before the lesion the monkey tended more often to use its left hand. After the right area 7 lesion, the monkey used first exclusively, then preferentially, its right hand. The reverse occurred after left-sided lesion. Finally, after complete recovery, the monkey recovered preferential use of the left hand.

Misreaching following parietal lesion consistently involves a systematic bias of reaches toward the side of the lesion, a fact which was reported by all the above-mentioned authors. Finally, the reaching deficit is more severe in the absence of visual feedback from the limb (e.g. in darkness) than under visual guidance.

2.1.2   Motor and Premotor Cortex Mechanisms

Neurons coding for the direction of movements were also found in the monkey cortical premotor and motor areas. Concerning the premotor areas, Gentilucci *et al.* (1988) described a population of neurons located in the lower part of area 6 (subarea F4) that fired in relation to movements affecting the proximal joints, particularly during reaching at visual objects. These neurons can be passively activated by visual stimuli located within reaching distance and also fire during arm movements directed to a particular space sector, congruent with the location of the visual receptive field. The authors have suggested that F4 neurons play a role in specifying the end-point area for reaching movements. Another population of neurons related to hand and finger movements was found in a distant subarea (see below).

In the primary motor area itself, Georgopoulos *et al.* (1982) found that the activity of single neurons changed in an orderly fashion with the direction of arm movements. Each of these neurons discharged preferentially prior to movements in a given direction and was therefore characterized by a preferred vector along which its discharge was maximum. Assuming that a movement in a particular direction involves the activation of a whole population of neurons, Georgopoulos, Schwartz and Kettner (1986) summated a large number of individual vectors measured during a reaching task. They found that the resulting population vector was a good predictor of the direction of movements.

Parietal (areas 5 and 7) and motor (areas 4 and 6) cortical mechanisms combine for selecting the proper movement direction as a function of the visual goal. The timing of movement-related neuronal discharges in the two cortical locations suggests that premotor and motor cortex neurons relate to movement initiation, whereas parietal neurons relate to its monitoring during execution.

2.2   Experiments Designed for Testing Directional Control Mechanisms of Reaching Movements

One way of studying directional control of goal-directed movements behaviorally is to introduce perturbations during their execution. Observation of the corrections generated in response to a perturbation (for example, an unexpected change in target location) can be a source of information for understanding the mechanisms underlying the central representations that steer the movement to its goal. The way the kinematics and the trajectory of the movement are reorganized in order to reach the new target, as well as the timing of this reorganization, should reflect the activity of neural structures involved in the various steps of this representation.

This approach, often referred to as the 'double-step' stimulation paradigm, has recently become quite popular for the study of sensorimotor coordination. It has been speculated that the perturbation probes the system at the level of preparation or execution of the movement which is currently activated at the time where it occurs. It this hypothesis is correct, then perturbing the movement at different times should produce different effects (see Jeannerod, 1990b). Indeed, the description of behavioral effects produced by double-step stimulation experiments will reveal strong differences between whether the second step (i.e. the change in target location) is presented prior to the movement, or during the movement itself.

2.2.1 Behavioral Effects of Perturbations Occurring During the Reaction Time of the Reaching Movement

In these experiments the change in target location is made to occur prior to the movement – that is, during the reaction time of the response to the first step. The second step is usually presented at fixed intervals with respect to the first (interstimulus interval, ISI). The conceptual framework for this approach was set more than 20 years ago by Megaw (1974) and by Gottsdanker (1973). According to the first author, the beginning of the movement should be influenced only by the first target step, and the response to the second step should appear later on, so that the corrected movement would be composed of two successive responses overlapping in time. Alternatively, the latter author postulated that the two responses combine and produce a corrected movement which would deflect from its onset the contribution of the second target step.

The more recent experiments have not completely solved this problem, although they have raised other critical issues on the nature of the corrective mechanism. Georgopoulos, Kalaska and Massey (1981), in the monkey, used ISI of 50–400 ms. They found that, when the movement started, it was first oriented in the direction of the first target and reoriented in the direction of the second target after a period of time which was a function of the duration of the ISI. In other words, the later the second step occurred, the longer the movement toward the first target lasted. According to the authors, the initial movement to the first target was a fragment of the control response that would have occurred if the target location had not changed. In addition, the time taken from the appearance of the second target to the change in direction of the movement was similar to the control reaction time for that target (i.e. between 200 and 300 ms).

These results were confirmed and expanded to humans by at least two groups of experimenters. Soechting and Lacquaniti (1983) found that the initial part of the movement was oriented in the direction of the first target, and that the change in direction occurred after a time that corresponded to one reaction time. These authors thus rightly adopted the Georgopoulos *et al.* conclusion that the aimed motor command is emitted in a continuous, ongoing fashion as a real-time process that can be interrupted at any time by the substitution of the initial target by a new one. The fact that the effects of this change on the ensuing movement appear without extra delays beyond the usual reaction time is an important result, because it implies that there is no refractory period in processing the input level: the movement trajectory can be corrected even if the second stimulus is given very soon after the first. Van Sonderen, Denier van der Gon and Gielen (1988) also confirmed that the reaction times to the change in target location were in the same range as those for single steps. Concerning the initial orientation of the movements, however, they reported that for a short ISI (e.g. 25–50 ms) the orientation of the first movement was a combination of the two target positions. For a longer ISI the arm was initially directed toward the first target, and then shifted abruptly in the direction of the second, as found by the previous authors.

The common finding in all three studies is that the perturbation generated by changing the location of the target during preparation of a movement directed toward that target cannot be corrected before a substantial delay has elapsed. This delay, which approximates the duration of one reaction time, is in any case longer than the minimum time required for vision to influence movements. It is likely that it relates to the time needed by the visual map to compute the position of the new target and to establish a new goal for the action. In other words, this type of perturbation would impinge upon the preparation of the movement at the time when the information contained in the visual map is being transferred into motor commands.

The amount of time needed to correct the trajectory of the movement should therefore relate to the timing of the transformations occurring at the level of this map. This point was illustrated by an experiment of Georgopoulos and Massey (1987). These authors requested subjects to perform reaching movements at various angles from the direction of a visual stimulus and found that reaction times of these movements increased linearly with the size of the angle. They proposed that this increase in reaction time was related to mentally rotating the movement vector until the angle of rotation corresponded to the angle of the required size. The rate of rotation was estimated by the authors to be around $400 \deg s^{-1}$.

Changes affecting the visual map where targets for visually directed movements are represented thus rely on a relatively slow mechanism, whereby the location of the target has to be recomputed and new motor commands have to be specified. These processes seem to be, at least partly, endowed with awareness of the subject. By contrast, as will be shown below, other mechanisms responsible for corrections of perturbations occurring at the time of the movement itself have a much shorter time constant, to the detriment of awareness of the corrections.

2.2.2   Behavioral Effects of Perturbations Time-Locked with the Reaching Movements

At variance with the experiments reported above, changes in target location can be made to occur time-locked with the onset of the reaching movements. In this situation, where the second step is conditional on the appearance of the movement triggered by the first step, the ISI is equal to the reaction time to the first step and therefore varies from trial to trial.

Such an experiment was performed by Pélisson *et al.* (1986; see also Goodale, Pélisson and Prablanc, 1986). The subjects' task was to point at visual targets with their unseen hand. The initial target steps were from midline to targets located between 20 and 50 cm. The second steps were of a smaller amplitude (e.g. from 30 to 32 cm, or 40 to 44 cm) but sufficiently large to make corrections of pointing clearly visible. The second steps, when present, were triggered by the onset of the ocular saccades which are normally present shortly before the hand begins to move (Biguer, Jeannerod and Prablanc, 1982; Prablanc *et al.*, 1979a). As demonstrated by Figure 7.3, the results showed that when second steps occurred subjects invariably corrected their hand trajectories in order to reach the final target positions. Yet, the duration of the corrected movements was not influenced by the perturbation, and was the same as that of control single-step movements directed at targets of the same locations (Figure 7.3a). In addition, the kinematic analysis of the movements showed that double-step trial movements did not differ from single-step trial movements (Figure 7.3b). Specifically, double-step trial movements showed no secondary accelerations, which suggests that corrections were generated without delay, as an online process. It would be interesting to know, by triggering the second step later and later in the movement, at which point secondary movements

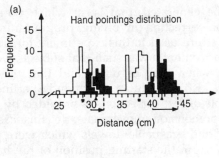

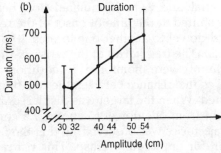

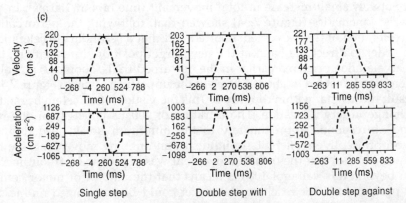

Single step   Double step with   Double step against

Figure 7.3. *Online corrections of arm direction during a double step pointing experiment. (a) Distribution of pointings directed at stationary and displaced targets. For a single step to 30 cm, the distribution of pointings represented by the white histogram (mean indicated by the star) undershoots the target. When the target is further displaced from 30 to 32 cm (double step), the distribution of pointings represented by the dark histogram (mean indicated by the filled triangle) undershoots the 32-cm target. Notice, however, that the distance between the star and the triangle is equal to the target shift, i.e. subjects fully correct their ongoing response. The same applies for a target shift from 40 to 44 cm, and for a target shift from 50 to 54 cm (not shown). (b) Duration of hand pointing movement (mean and standard deviations) versus amplitude of the final target position. When a target is displaced, for instance from 40 to 44 cm, the duration increases as compared with responses to the 40-cm single step, but the total duration corresponds (by extrapolating from the observed durations to 40 and 50 cm stationary targets) to the predicted duration of pointings to a stationary target appearing at 44 cm. Thus, no additional reaction time or extra processing time appears within the total duration to the double step stimulation, nor is it associated with a higher variability of movement duration. (c) Averaged velocity (upper row) and acceleration (lower row) profiles of pointing movements during single step or double step trials. Note lack of reacceleration in double step trials. [From Pélisson et al., 1986.]*

would begin to be generated, that is, at which point subjects would shift to a different mode of correction involving programming of a new movement. In addition, the procedure used in this experiment for triggering the second steps (at the onset of eye movements) was such that subjects were not aware of the changes in target location when they occurred and that the corrections were generated unconsciously (see also Bridgeman, Kirch and Sperling, 1981).

Another example of fast corrections is provided by the experiment of Paulignan *et al.* (1990) on prehension movements. In this case, the targets consisted of three-dimensional and graspable dowels which were placed on a concentric array at a fixed distance from the starting position of the hand. The dowels were made of transparent material, and were illuminated from below. In some trials the light could be suddenly shifted at the time of onset of the reaching movement, from the initially illuminated dowel to another one located 10 degrees to the right or to the left (perturbed trials). The trajectories of the wrist, of the tip of the index finger and of the tip of the thumb were monitored. In addition, the kinematics of the wrist movement, as well as the distance between the two fingertips (the size of the finger grip), were computed. When the target was displaced at the onset of the movement (by shifting the light from one dowel to another) a complex rearrangement of the wrist and finger trajectories was observed, so that the fingers were finally placed in the correct position for an accurate grasp. This rearrangement was effected with only a relatively small increase in total movement time (about 100 ms). Inspection of the wrist kinematics (Figure 7.4a) showed that, following the perturbation, the initial acceleration of the movement aborted and that a secondary acceleration took place in order to direct the hand at the new target position. Interestingly, the first peak in acceleration occurred earlier in the perturbed trials, about 105 ms following movement onset, instead of about 130 ms in the unperturbed ones (Figure 7.4b). The latter result means that within roughly 100 ms the visuomotor system began to react to the change in target location. The duration of 100 ms is less than one reaction time, and corresponds approximately to the minimum delay needed by visual and/or proprioceptive reafferents to influence an ongoing movement (see below). In addition, the fact that the overall movement was completed without increase in duration beyond this value of 100 ms means that the pattern of motor commands initially programmed for reaching the target could be rearranged online. Such a rearrangement implied not only redirecting the wrist toward the new target location, but also introducing new commands for keeping the orientation of the finger grip invariant with respect to the object. These results will be discussed again in Section 4.

Another result of this experiment, which reminds one of the findings by Goodale, Pélisson and Prablanc (1986) and Pélisson *et al.* (1986), was that, whereas the subjects were aware that the location of the target dowel had changed during the trial, they made an erroneous estimate of the time at which the change occurred: instead of seeing the change occurring immediately after movement onset, they saw it near the end of the movement trajectory, as their hand was coming close to the target. As in the Pélisson *et al.* experiment, the early motor reaction to the perturbation was dissociated from its perception by the subject. In both experiments, the motor system was able to detect the perturbation and to correct the movement trajectory, even though the information it used for this correction was not consciously available at the time the correction was made (Castiello, Paulignan and Jeannerod, 1991).

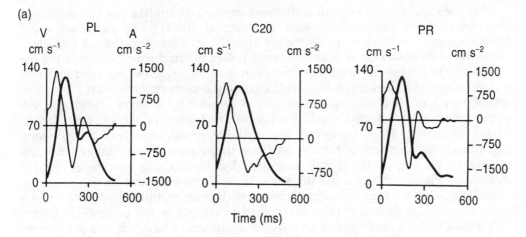

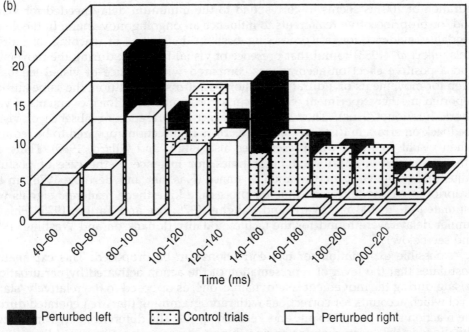

Figure 7.4. *Motor correction during perturbation of object position. (a) Kinematic pattern of prehension movements in perturbed trials. Three individual movements are shown. The movement shown in the middle of the figure corresponds to a movement directed at the 20-degree dowel in the control (unperturbed) condition (C20). The other two movements correspond to perturbed movements, when the dowel position is shifted to the left (PL) or to the right (PR). The thick line represents the arm velocity; the light line, the acceleration. Note fast deceleration and reacceleration following perturbations. (b) Time to peak acceleration in control and perturbed trials. Note shorter time to peak in perturbed trials. [Results from Paulignan et al., 1991a.]*

There are other examples, in a different context, of similar fast corrections in ongoing complex movements. Abbs and Gracco (1984) have described rapid compensation of perturbations applied to articulators during speech, in an experiment where the lower lip was unexpectedly pulled down during production of the phoneme /ba/. They showed that lip closure was nevertheless achieved and that the phoneme was correctly pronounced despite the perturbation. Such a compensation, which implied that lip closure was performed by a larger lowering of the upper lip, was thus effected within a delay compatible with the correct production of the phoneme. They suggested that this correction reflected an open-loop adjustment, independent of sensory feedback in the usual sense, but nevertheless relying on proprioceptive signals generated by the ongoing movement. Such a conception clearly fits into the definition of feedforward mechanisms given by Arbib (1981): 'A strategy whereby a controller directly monitors disturbances to a system and immediately applies compensatory signals to the controlled system, rather than waiting for feedback on how the disturbances have affected the system' (p. 1466).

The above experimental results, and particularly the fact that the first detectable difference between perturbed and nonperturbed movements occurred some 100 ms after the perturbation (at the time of the first acceleration peak), emphasize the rapidity of processing of movement-related information for online corrections. A duration of 100 ms seems to correspond to the minimum delay needed for visual and/or proprioceptive reafferents to influence an ongoing movement. In the visual modality, evidence for fast processing exists in the context of reaching for targets. Zelaznik et al. (1983) found that presence of visual feedback during the movement had a positive effect on accuracy, as compared with absence of visual feedback, even for movements of a duration as short as 120 ms. In addition, the same authors reported another experiment where accuracy was measured for movements of very short duration (70 ms). They found no effect of presence or absence of visual feedback on errors in distance, although errors in direction appeared to be reduced when visual feedback was present (see also Elliott and Allard, 1985). There are other examples of short visuomotor times, for instance in the case of postural adjustments following perturbation of stance (Nashner and Berthoz, 1978). In the proprioceptive modality, the time for processing kinesthetic reafferent signals was estimated at 70–100 ms (Evarts and Vaughn, 1978; Lee and Tatton, 1975). Finally, similar delays were found for the tactile modality (Johansson and Westling, 1987; and see below).

A possible explanation for fast corrections can be proposed. This explanation postulates that the level of representation of the action activated by perturbations arising during the movement is a 'dynamic' one, as opposed to the relatively 'static' level which accounts for corrections with reprogramming that are generated during the reaction time (see Prablanc and Pélisson, 1990). The difference between the two situations is that perturbations arising during the movement create a discrepancy between the visual signals related to the new target position and the incoming proprioceptive signals generated by the movement itself, which is not the case for perturbations occurring before the movement has started. In this context a dynamic representation can thus be considered as a network that would permanently monitor the movement-related reafferent input and compare it with the efferent motor signals. Any change in the target–limb spatial configuration would be encoded by the network as a deviation from the represented action, and would automatically (and therefore unconsciously) trigger reorganization of the commands sent to the execution level.

This mechanism, which represents a revised version of the classic corollary discharge model (e.g. Held, 1961), must operate at a level where the visual and the proprioceptive maps are interconnected, and where a comparison of position of the target relative to the body and position of the moving limb relative to the target can be made.

2.2.3 The Interaction of Vision and Proprioception during Visuomotor Coordination

Describing the mechanism by which visual and proprioceptive signals are matched is a key issue for understanding visuomotor coordination. The movement generator receives signals arising from static and dynamic proprioceptors, which provide positional sense for the relative joint angles. Proprioception, however, because it is limited to personal space and cannot signal limb position with respect to the target, must be calibrated by visual signals (Jeannerod, 1988, 1990b; Jeannerod and Prablanc, 1983). Figure 7.5 gives a simplified view of the mechanisms involved in the calibration of target position in visual space with respect to the body (visual map), and of the calibration of limb position with respect to the target (proprioceptive map).

Simple behavioral experiments demonstrate that vision of the limb prior to the movement plays an essential role in this mechanism. Prablanc and his colleagues compared the accuracy of hand pointing movements in two situations. In the first situation, where the hand remained permanently invisible to the subject, large

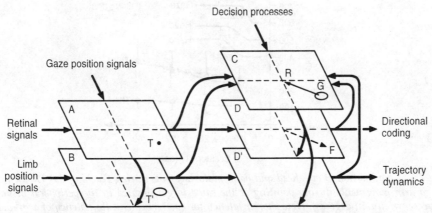

Figure 7.5. *A model for the central representation of goal-directed movements. The visuomotor map (A) encodes target position (T) in body-centered coordinates. Proprioceptive map (B) encodes limb position with respect to body and to target. Area T' represents the final position that the limb should reach in order to match target position. (C) Goal level: the goal (G) of the action appears as a local activation to the network. This activation is assumed to propagate to execution levels (D–D'). Signals arising from execution levels and from the periphery deactivate the goal level and restore its resting activity (R). Execution level (D–D') generates execution commands for movement direction and kinematics in order to drive the limb to its final position. [From Jeannerod, 1990a.]*

pointing errors were observed. By contrast, in the second situation where the hand was visible at rest before the movement and was masked as soon as the movement was started, the pointing performance was clearly improved, due to reduction of both the constant and the variable erors (Prablanc *et al.*, 1979b). This result demonstrates that visual information about the static position of the hand relative to the body and the target is sufficient for calibrating position sense, or in other words for matching the two maps with each other. There are no data available as to how often the proprioceptive map needs to be updated to keep in register with

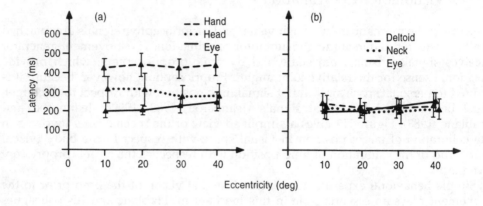

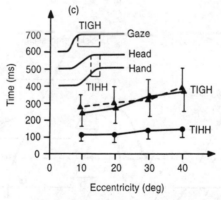

Figure 7.6. *Coordination of eye, head and hand motor systems during reaching. (a) Latency of eye, head and arm movements during pointing at the same target, located in the peripheral visual field (target eccentricity, in degrees). Note shorter latency for eye movement. (b) Latency of arm and neck EMG discharges compared with eye movement latency during the same reaching movements as in (a). Note clustering of latencies around the time of eye movement onset. (c) Time interval between end of gaze movements and end of hand movement (TIGH) with the head fixed (triangles, broken line) or free to move (solid line). Note consistent delay of 300 ms or more allowing foveation to occur before hand reaches the target. The black circles represent the delay between end of head movement and end of hand movement (TIHH). The delay of 100 ms allows time for head movement signals to influence hand movements. [(a) and (b) from Biguer, Jeannerod and Prablanc, 1985; (c) from Biguer, Prablanc and Jeannerod, 1984.]*

the visual map. The key experiment would be, by using the same paradigm, to expose the hand prior to the movement only on the first of a series of trials, and to measure on how many of the hand-unexposed subsequent trials the effect of visual exposure would last. According to Elliott and Madalena (1987), a 2 s delay between occlusion of premovement visual information and movement onset is sufficient for significantly increasing the pointing error. It can therefore be speculated that, without vision of the hand, the two maps will drift with respect to each other and positional sense will rapidly lose its calibration with respect to visual space.

An important mechanism for ensuring the superimposition of the two maps is that of foveation. During foveation, the gaze axis is aligned with the position of the target in space. Provided that the hand at its initial position is also visible at the same time, foveation will result in aligning the visual and prioprioceptive coordinate systems on the target position, before the hand movement starts. This is in fact achieved in normal reaching behavior by the coordination of eye, head and hand motor systems. Intrinsic delays are such that, during reaching movements directed at a target impinging on the peripheral retina, the eye movement always leads the sequence followed by the head movement, and finally by the hand movement (Figure 7.6a). The eye, head, hand sequence results from the pattern of muscular commands, whereby eye, neck and arm muscles begin to contract at the same time. Because of differences in inertial load, the interval between muscular commands and overt movements differs (Biguer, Jeannerod and Prablanc, 1982; Biguer, Prablanc and Jeannerod, 1984) (Figure 7.6b). Figure 7.6 also shows that the time interval between onset of gaze movement and completion of pointing movements directed at targets of different eccentricities ranges between 200 and 300 ms. Particularly, the time between end of head movement and completion of hand movement is about 100 ms. These delays are sufficient for signals generated by the gaze and/or the head movement to be used for improving hand movement accuracy (Biguer, Jeannerod and Prablanc, 1985). Further work by Biguer *et al.* (1988), studying the effects of vibrating neck muscles on localization of visual targets, is strongly suggestive of a role of neck proprioception in these directional mechanisms.

2.3 The Kinematic Coding of Reaching Movements

Another aspect of the control of reaching movements is specification of the correct kinematics along the path selected for getting to the target. Data concerning this aspect come almost exclusively from experiments in humans, which are part of a long and fruitful tradition in psychology (for reviews, see Georgopoulos, 1986; Jeannerod, 1988; Meyer *et al.*, 1990).

Specification of kinematics determines the timing of the movements and the respective durations of their acceleration and deceleration phases. Emphasis on the speed of the movements, as in pointing for example, will result in relatively symmetrical (bell-shaped) velocity profiles. By contrast, emphasis on accuracy, as in prehension, will produce slower movements with a longer deceleration phase and, therefore, an asymmetrical velocity profile. In addition, the kinematic pattern also depends on the task in which the subject is involved. This point is illustrated by the results of experiments where reaching movements are compared in different conditions of task constraint. A constraint is defined here as a variable that limits the manner in which movement control occurs. As an example, the target size can be considered as a movement constraint, such that movements aimed at small targets have velocity profiles distinctly different from those produced in attaining larger targets (Soechting, 1984).

The effects of such constraints on movement kinematics were tested by Marteniuk *et al.* (1987). In their experiment, the goal of reaching movements, as well as the required movement extent and accuracy, were systematically varied. Subjects were asked either to hit a target using the index finger, or to grasp a disk between the thumb and the index finger. Both targets and disks had the same sizes (2 or 4 cm) and were placed at distances of 20 or 40 cm from the resting position of the right hand. Movement time was longer during grasping than during hitting. Furthermore, according to 'Fitts' law', it increased in both cases as a function of difficulty of the task (as quantified by combining the target/disk width and the movement amplitude; see Fitts, 1954). Both types of movement had similar values of maximum velocity, and in both cases maximum velocity was higher with increasing target/disk width and with increasing movement amplitude. The most interesting difference between the two types of movement was the repartition of movement time into acceleration and deceleration. The peak velocity during hitting and during grasping was reached at about the same time, and the longer duration of grasping movements was due to a higher percentage of total movement time spent in the deceleration phase.

Marteniuk *et al.* (1987) also explored further the determinants of the movement kinematics by comparing grasping movements in two different situations. In both, the subjects had to grasp the disk as in the previous experiment; in one situation they had to throw it into a large container, and in the other they had to fit it tightly into a small container. Only the reaching parts of the movements were analyzed. This comparison was undertaken with the aim of exploring whether the context within which a movement is executed can affect its characteristics. Indeed, movement time was found to be longer for grasping movements executed prior to fitting than for movements executed prior to throwing. This lengthening in movement time was due to lengthening of the deceleration phase (Figure 7.7).

These data clearly indicate that planning and control of trajectories do not occur through the use of a general and abstract representation that would adjust movements for different task conditions, by simply scaling a basic velocity profile. Instead, higher-order factors such as representation of the goal, the context and also probably the knowledge of the result of the action seem to be able to influence not only duration and velocity, but also the intrinsic kinematic structure of the movements. These empirical findings represent limitations to the notion, implicit in several models of movement control (e.g. Meyer, Smith and Wright, 1982; Schmidt *et al.*, 1979), of a generalized motor program representing the elementary unit for the movements belonging to each given class of action.

An important problem arises as to how reaching movements are calibrated in amplitude to the target position. A long tradition, started by Woodworth (1899), has attributed an upmost importance to the role of visual feedback in adjusting movement amplitude and, more specifically, in triggering secondary 'correction' movements. The classic interpretation of Fitts' law (the fact that movement time increases linearly with the difficulty of the task) also implied that longer movement times were in fact due to the presence of secondary movements. Observations on

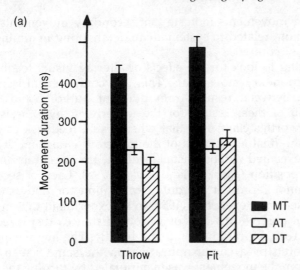

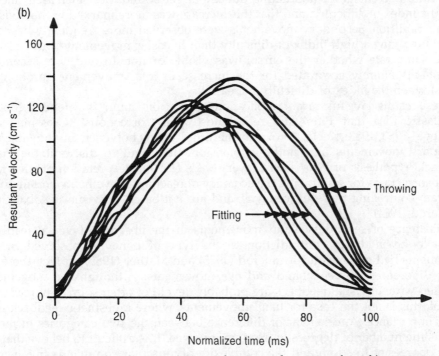

Figure 7.7. *Influence of task constraints on the temporal pattern of reaching movements. (a) Movements have been recorded during the action of grasping. On some trials subjects had to grasp the disk and throw it away. On other trials, they had to grasp the disk and fit it into a small box. These task constraints influenced both total movement duration (MT), which was longer in the fit condition, and the velocity profiles. In the throw condition, acceleration time (AT) was longer than deceleration time (DT), although the reverse was observed in the fit condition. (b) Representative velocity profiles in the two conditions. Note that time has been normalized to enable comparison. [Data from Marteniuk et al., 1987.]*

different types of reaching movements indicate that secondary movements might be a ubiquitous phenomenon, related to systematic undershooting in aiming tasks where terminal precision is required.

It may thus be interesting to look for the effects of altering visual feedback on the occurrence of these secondary movements. This is a controversial issue, first because of discrepancies between results from different authors, and second because of the implication of these results for the underlying hypothesis about movement control. Woodworth's claim was that when visual feedback cannot be used during movements the final adjustment of the trajectory is lacking. It is true that reaching movements executed without visual feedback are inaccurate and tend to undershoot the target position (e.g. Prablanc et al., 1979a). Lack of secondary movements, however, cannot represent the only explanation for undershooting. This problem was addressed by Meyer et al. (1988) in an experiment that involved reaching for targets of variable widths and of various distances displayed on a cathode-ray tube (CRT) screen, by rapidly rotating a handle. The angular position of the handle was monitored by a cursor appearing on the same screen as the targets. Visual feedback from the movement was manipulated by turning the cursor on or off (visible and invisible cursor conditions, respectively). It was found that error rate (percentage of hits falling outside target boundaries) increased linearly with the index of difficulty, and that this increase was more marked in the invisible cursor condition. Secondary movements were observed more frequently in movements involving a high index of difficulty than in easier movements, but occurred at the same rate whether the cursor was visible or not. In addition, secondary movements entirely accounted for the increase in total movement duration observed when the index of difficulty increased.

These results have important implications. On the one hand, they tend to confirm the classic idea that Fitts' law relies mostly on 'corrections' (Crossman and Goodeve, 1963/1983; Keele, 1968); on the other hand, however, in showing that secondary movements owe nothing to vision, they tend to discredit the visual feedback hypothesis of Fitts' law. Meyer et al.'s (1990) interpretation of such facts is that corrections for optimizing the accuracy of reaching movements pertain to the program controlling these movements, and are not based on visual feedback (see Jeannerod, 1984).

Persistence of secondary hand movements in the absence of visual feedback seems to be in direct contradiction to the type of behavior observed in eye movements by Prablanc and Jeannerod (1975) and Mather (1985). In fact, there are many differences between hand and eye movements. Although eye movements executed without visual feedback are probably devoid of other sources of reafferent control, this is not the case for hand movements, where kinesthetic feedback is of major importance. Another major difference between the two categories of movement is the number of degrees of freedom involved. It is difficult to believe that the many degrees of freedom and the complexity of muscular commands involved in a hand reaching movement could all be handled by visual feedback alone. Visual feedback relates to the end-point of the limb, but does not reflect the intrinsic aspects of the movement that have to be controlled for achieving accuracy. By contrast, a simple terminal feedback may be sufficient for controlling accuracy in ocular saccades. This difference might well explain why secondary movements are more dependent on visual feedback in eye movements than in arm movements (Jeannerod, 1986b).

It remains to be determined at which level of movement control vision acts to improve accuracy. Surprisingly, there are very few data concerning this point and very few investigators seem to have attempted a comparative kinematic analysis of movements executed in conditions where visual feedback is present or excluded. Carlton (1981) made high-speed cine-film analysis of movements executed under different degrees of visual feedback exclusion. The technique was such that a varying amount of the hand movement toward the target could be masked, but that terminal visual feedback was always available. Movement time was found to increase as a function of the amount of movement masked, due to a longer time spent by the hand near the target. This result shows that lack of visual feedback slows down the deceleration phase, by maintaining low velocity for a longer time before the stop. This effect, however, might be due not only to a lack of visual feedback *per se*, but could also reflect a systematic strategy of the subject to wait until error feedback becomes available at the end of the movement.

This section has focused on one aspect of motor control: the role of visual and proprioceptive signals in direction and amplitude coding. There are clearly many other possible mechanisms for controlling movements. For example, it has been proposed that limb positions would be defined by an equilibrium between forces (the load of the musculoskeletal apparatus, the viscoelastic properties of the muscles, etc). Assuming that these forces were encoded within the central nervous system, the arrest of a movement at the location of a target would be simply explained by a change in tonic activation of the agonist muscle. This would produce a change in the equilibrium point between forces and would displace the limb by the required amount, without a need for monitoring sensory feedback (for an

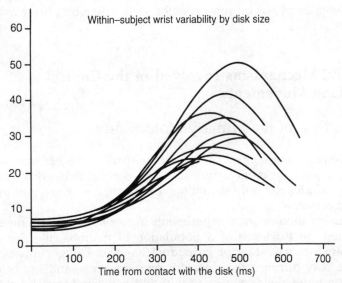

Figure 7.8. *Variability of arm path during reaching. Each line represents the variability, expressed as the standard deviation (in mm) with respect to the mean, of arm paths during reaching toward one of ten possible targets. Curves of variability are plotted as a function of time to contact, which implies that the zero value represents the end of the movement. Note low variability in the last 200 ms of the movements. [From Marteniuk et al., 1990.]*

example of this mode of control, see Bizzi *et al.*, 1984). An argument in favor of the equilibrium point hypothesis can be drawn from the study of variability of reaching movements. It has been shown by several authors that the spatial paths of movements directed at a given target vary from trial to trial (Marteniuk *et al.*, 1990; Paulignan *et al.*, 1991a). This variability, however, is not evenly distributed over the spatial path. It is maximum during the early part of the movement, and becomes very low as the hand approaches the target (Figure 7.8). This 'convergence' of trajectories at the object location is more suggestive of a mechanism guiding the end-point of the limb to the target, than of a detailed specification of the kinematics of each of the involved joints.

3 GRASPING

The function of grasping is to acquire objects with the purpose of manipulation, identification and use. Tool behavior is one of the possibilities offered by a fully developed hand, and must also be included in the function of grasping. The anatomy and physiology of the hand and its neural apparatus seem to have evolved across species along two main lines: the development of an opposable thumb and the development of independent finger movements, both properties sometimes collapsed under the term 'digital dexterity'. This section will include first a description of neurophysiological mechanisms related to hand and finger movements; these mechanisms are mostly concentrated within cerebral cortex. The second part of this section will include a description of grasping by the human hand, considered as the most achieved hand with regard to digital dexterity, with only a few references to more 'primitive' hands. Behavioral aspects of grasping will be studied with emphasis on sensorimotor, rather than on purely motor, aspects of the function.

3.1 Neural Mechanisms Involved in the Control of Hand Movements

3.1.1 The Role of the Primary Motor Cortex

Finger movements are controlled by highly specific mechanisms which seem to depend exclusively on cortical function. The cortical network involved in finger movements includes not only the motor cortex, but also areas within the premotor and parietal cortex.

In the primary motor cortex, experiments in monkeys performing a gripping task have revealed the existence of a population of neurons, the firing of which is directly related to activation of individual hand and finger muscles. First, these neurons fire only during execution of a precision grip, and not of a power grip, which demonstrates their connection with intrinsic hand muscles rather than with forearm muscles (Muir and Lemon, 1983) (Figure 7.9a, b). Second, the neurons burst with a short latency (about 11 ms) prior to muscle activation, which indicates a monosynaptic connection (Lemon, Mantel and Muir, 1986). Finally, each of these

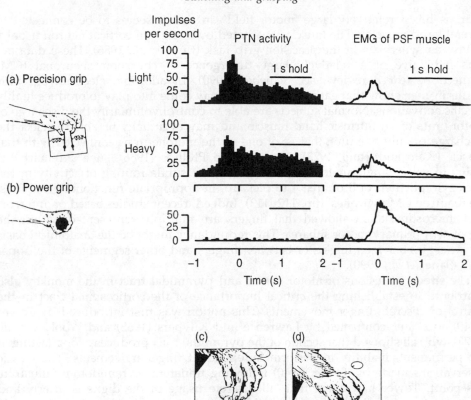

MONKEY #77-15

Figure 7.9. *Contribution of primary motor cortex to precision grip in the monkey. Upper part: (a) Left: Activity of a pyramidal tract neuron (PTN) during precision grip with two degrees of force (light and heavy). On the right: integrated EMG activity of an interosseus muscle partly controlled by the PTN. (b) During power grip, the neuron is not activated, which shows its selectivity for the precision grip. Zero value on time scale corresponds to onset of force exerted by the animal on the manipulandum. [From Muir and Lemon, 1983.] Lower part: effects of pyramidotomy on hand movements during extraction of food pellets from wells of different sizes. (c) After operation, only clumsy whole hand prehension is possible; the monkey cannot extract food from small wells. (d) After recovery, the affected hand shows the normal pattern of precision grip. [From Chapman and Wiesendanger, 1982.]*

neurons has a relatively large 'motor field', in that it seems to be connected to several hand muscles. The muscles facilitated by one given cortical neuron usually behave as synergists in the precision grip task (Buys et al., 1986). These data are thus indicative of a relatively large divergence of corticomotoneuronal (CM) connections (for a review, see Schieber, 1990). In addition, electromyographic results in man show that gating mechanisms may come into play to produce highly specific activations. Normal subjects are able to control voluntarily the discharge of motor units of an intrinsic hand muscle and may eventually be able to select the discharge of only one unit, that is, of one of the motoneurons connected with that muscle (Kato and Tanji, 1972). According to Phillips (1986), such a remarkable ability to select single motoneurons argues for a 'subtle routing of activity in the thick synaptic neuropil of area 4 to pick up, in appropriate functional groupings, the required CM neurones' (pp. 112–113). Indeed, recent studies based on intracortical microstimulation showed that fingers are multiply represented within the upper arm primary motor subarea. This redundancy might be the anatomical basis for synergies between fingers or between fingers and other segments of the upper limb (Sanes et al., 1990).

The effects of lesions of motor cortex and pyramidal tract in the monkey also contribute to establishing the critical importance of the corticospinal tract in the control of discrete finger movements. This notion was first introduced by Tower (1940) and later confirmed by Lawrence and Kuypers (1968) and Woolsey et al. (1972), who all showed that section of the pyramidal tract produces a long-lasting, if not permanent, inability to perform independent finger movements. The classic observations made by Tower (1940) following unilateral pyramidotomy illustrate this point. Tower had noted that 'all discrete usage of the digits is utterly and permanently abolished', specially in those actions where 'the digits are used separately as in the opposition of thumb and index to pick up small objects, or in fine manipulation of objects, or in separation of one digit from the others' (p. 55). This specific deficit was well illustrated by the impossibility for the animals to execute grooming or by their awkward attempts at grasping food:

> 'Instead of the normal movement which culminates in the opposition of thumb and index to pick up small objects,... the residual movement of the paretic arm is a highly stereotyped reaching-grasping act involving the entire body half, similar to the reaching-grasping act of the newborn monkey... The hand is brought down on the object in half pronation and scoops it into the ulnar side of the hand, unless, as frequently happens, the fist closes before reaching the objects.' (p. 56).

The degree of recovery from this deficit has been quantified in monkeys by Chapman and Wiesendanger (1982) following unilateral section of the pyramidal tract at the pontine level, and by Passingham, Perry and Wilkinson (1983) following unilateral lesion of the primary motor cortex. In the Chapman and Wiesendanger experiment, the animals' performance was scored in a Kluver board task, i.e. the number of pellets of food extracted from holes of different sizes and the time needed for clearing the board, were measured for each hand. The strategy utilized by the animals for grasping the pellets was found to be changed after pyramidotomy when the hand contralateral to the lesion was tested. Animals first used all four fingers for extracting the food – a strategy that was efficient only for the larger holes (Figure 7.9c, d). At a later stage (30 to 40 days after surgery), monkeys regained the ability to pry out the pellets from the smaller holes by using either the thumb or the index finger. Once extracted, the pellets could be grasped between the opposed thumb and index finger, but this precision grip remained weak and clumsy and the food was eventually dropped before reaching the mouth. Passingham *et al.* obtained very similar results, except that recovery was limited to reaching the board, and that the animals never recovered the normal use of wrist and fingers. Partial recovery of grip formation observed by Chapman and Wiesendanger might be explained by incompleteness of the pyramidal tract lesions.

Neonatal lesion of the corticospinal system corresponding to the hand area results in lack of development of the distal component of prehesion. Lawrence and Hopkins (1972, 1976) and Passingham *et al.* (1978, 1983) have shown that monkeys with complete unilateral ablation of area 4 performed during infancy never acquire a precision grip when tested later in adulthood. Precision grip in monkeys normally develops around the eighth postnatal month, i.e. by the time when maturation of the corticospinal tract is completed, as judged from the formation of cor- ticomotoneuronal synapses (Kuypers, 1962) and the level of excitability of mo- toneurons by motor cortex stimulation (Felix and Wiesendanger, 1971).

3.1.2 The Role of Cortical Areas Outside the Primary Motor Cortex

Other cortical areas, such as premotor areas and parietal areas, are also involved in controlling finger movements. In area 6 a specific population of neurons (in subarea F5) was found to be related to the execution of distal movements of either hand. The discharge of many of these neurons was influenced by the way in which the hand was shaped during the action: precision grip neurons, finger prehesion neurons, whole hand prehension neurons could be identified (Rizzolatti *et al.*, 1988). These neurons, however, are poorly sensitive to 'passive' visual stimuli, as opposed to the neighboring population of cells related to proximal joint movements (see above).

Posterior parietal areas also are involved in the control of finger movement. As shown by Sakata *et al.* (1985), neurons in monkey area 7 (in the posterior bank of the intraparietal sulcus) respond to complex visual stimuli, including moving stimuli of different sizes and orientations. More recently, the same authors found within the same part of area 7 (near subarea LIP) a population of neurons which are selectively activated during manipulation by the animal of objects of a given configuration (e.g. a push-button, a handle, etc). Neurons showed differential changes in activity with different objects. Some of them were 'motor dominant': they discharged during hand manipulation of one given object in the light and in the dark, and were not influenced by mere visual fixation of the object by the animal. Other neurons were more active during manipulation in the light ('visual and motor' neurons). Finally, another category of neurons were 'visual dominant': they were not activated during manipulation in the dark, and were as much influenced by visual fixation of the object as by its manipulation (Taira *et al.*, 1990). The authors' suggestion was that these neurons are able to integrate visual and motor signals related to object-oriented action, and might therefore represent the link between object properties and the corresponding motor commands.

It is thus not surprising that lesions of posterior parietal areas also affect the ability to shape the hand according to object size or configuration. Monkeys with such lesions are impaired in grasping and manipulating small objects. The hand remains open and the fingers remain stretched until palmar contact occurs with the object. Tactile cues then trigger an inadequate grasp, in which the object is seized between the palmar surface of the hand and the palmar surface of the finger (Brinkman and Kuypers, 1973; Faugier-Grimaud, Frenois and Stein, 1978; Haaxma and Kuypers, 1975). Similar observations in humans are reported in Section 6.

3.2 The Human Hand as a Grasping Apparatus

By using the criterion of stability of the grasp as a prerequisite for handling objects, Napier (1956) considered that human prehensile movements can be described along only two main motor patterns. 'If', Napier stated, 'prehensile activities are to be regarded as the application of a system of forces in a given direction then the nature of prehensile activity can be resolved into two concepts – that of *precision* and that of *power*' (p. 906). The precision and the power grip pattern can be used alternatively or in combination for almost every object. In other words, the pattern of the grip is not determined (solely) by the shape or the size of the object (e.g. a rod can be held with a precision grip as in writing, or a power grip as in hammering); it is the intended activity that is the main determinant of the type of grip for each given action. The two grips differ anatomically by both the posture of the thumb and the posture of the fingers. Precision grip is mostly characterized by opposition of the thumb to one or more of the other fingers. Opposition means that the thumb is abducted at the metacarpophalangeal and at the carpometacarpal joints, so that its pulpar surface is diametrically opposed to the pulpar surface of the other fingers. In power grip, the fingers are flexed to form a clamp against the palm, the thumb is adducted at the two joints, and there is no opposition between the thumb and the other fingers. The two types of grip have clearly different degrees of involvement in manipulative actions; only the precision handling allows movements of the object relative to the hand and movements of the object within the hand because of opposition of the thumb to the other fingers (Elliott and Connolly, 1984).

The patterns of neuromuscular innervation for the two types of grip seem to be very different. In power grip, fingers are flexed by powerful biarticular muscles, although during precision handling there is an interplay between flexion and extension. According to Landsmeer (1962), 'the interphalangeal joints can be flexed and extended only when the metacarpo-phalangeal joints remain extended, while the metacarpo-phalangeal joints can be flexed and extended only when the interphalangeal joints are flexed' (p. 169).

Precision grip with true opposition of the pulpar surfaces of the thumb and the index finger is considered as the top attribute of dextrous hands. The problem of whether this attribute is specific to the human hand or not is a matter for discussion. The Heffner and Masterton scale for ranking digital dexterity (Heffner and Masterton, 1975), based on anatomy of the hand, includes only humans in the topmost category, that with opposable thumb and precision grip (see also Napier, 1961). Recent work, based on fossil anatomical evidence, indicates that this category should be extended to remote predecessors of modern humans (e.g. *Paranthropus robustus*, 1.8 million years ago), which are credited with dextrous tool use behavior (Susman, 1988). The relative ratio of index finger length, as well as the position of the articulation of the thumb, have changed from a chimpanzee-like hand in *Australopithecus afarensis* (4 million years ago) to a modern human-like arrangement in *Homo erectus* (1.5 million years ago). It remains that the classification based on anatomy of the hand is probably underinclusive, and should be counterbalanced by a classification based on behavioral observation with emphasis on the capability for independent finger movements and for the use of tools. Tool use behavior is well known in apes like the chimpanzee and orang-utan (McGrew, 1989). Others, like the gibbon for instance, because of the small size of their thumb relative to their other fingers, perform handling of small objects by means of the pulp of the thumb and the side of the middle phalanx of the index finger. It should not be concluded from this difference that these animals are not capable of opposition: they can abduct their thumb and rotate it in front of their other fingers, but the shortness of the thumb prevents contact between the pulpar surfaces (Napier, 1960). More primitive monkeys like rhesus monkeys or baboons are also capable of accurate precision grips. Other still more primitive animals use whole hand prehension with a nonopposable thumb, a good example of which is given by behavioral observation of the squirrel monkey. In this animal, objects are reached with all the fingers in a slightly curved convergent position; in the later stage of the reach, the fingers diverge and straighten, closing in a scooping motion at contact with the object: the fingers frequently close to the palm with the distal and medial phalanges parallel to the palm, rather than curled around the objects as human fingers do (Fragaszy, 1983). Interestingly, this description of a primitive prehensile behavior can be applied almost without change to pathological prehension in humans following cortical lesions (see below).

3.2.1   Anticipatory Finger Posturing. The Pattern of Grip Formation

The type of grip that is formed by the hand in contact with the object represents the end-result of a motor sequence which starts well ahead of the action of grasping itself. The fingers begin to shape during transportation of the hand at the object location. This process of grip formation is therefore important to consider, because it shows dynamically how the static posture of the hand is finally achieved. No systematic investigation of this aspect of grasping (preshaping) seems to have been made until the film study by Jeannerod (1981). Examples of preshaping sequences are shown in Figure 7.10.

The pattern of grip formation is not an undifferentiated pattern: it is specified, at least in part, by the type of action in which the subject is engaged. Finger movements during preshaping contribute to the building of a specific spatial configuration, where the relative positions of the hand and the object to be grasped are constrained both by biomechanical factors and by higher-order visuomotor mechanisms for object recognition.

Preshaping first involves a progressive opening of the grip with straightening of the fingers, followed by a closure of the grip until it matches object size. The point in time where grip size is the largest (maximum grip size) is a clearly identifiable landmark which occurs within about 60–70% of the duration of the reach (see below) – that is, well before the fingers come into contact with the object (Jeannerod,

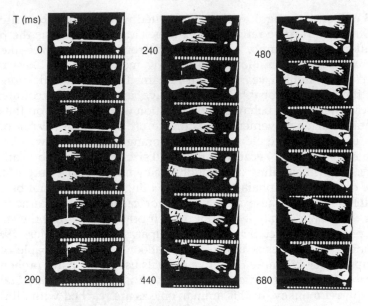

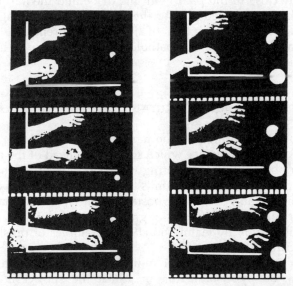

Figure 7.10. *Patterns of preshaping during human prehension. Upper part: decomposition of preshaping during a single prehension movement lasting 680 ms. Lower part: Comparison of preshaping during prehension of a small sphere (left) or a large sphere (right). Reconstructed from films taken at 50 frames per second. Note presence of a mirror in the rear allowing dorsal view of the hand.*

1981, 1984; see also Wallace and Weeks, 1988; Wing, Turton and Fraser, 1986). This biphasic opening–closure motor pattern might not be unique to humans: a few observations based on films during prehension in rhesus monkeys have revealed a closely similar opening of the grip followed by closure before contact with the object (unpublished results, courtesy of S. Faugier-Grimaud).

The amplitude of grip aperture during grip formation covaries with object size (Gentilucci *et al.*, 1991; Jeannerod, 1981, 1984; Marteniuk *et al.*, 1987, 1990; Wallace and Weeks, 1988; Wing and Fraser, 1983; Wing *et al.*, 1986). Marteniuk *et al.* (1990) found that for each increase of 1 cm in object size the maximum grip size increased by 0.77 cm (Figure 7.11a). Subjects use two different strategies for achieving this pattern. In the first strategy, the grip size increases at the same rate whatever the object size, with the consequence that maximum grip size is reached earlier in movement time for a small object than for a large object (Gentilucci *et al.*, 1991;

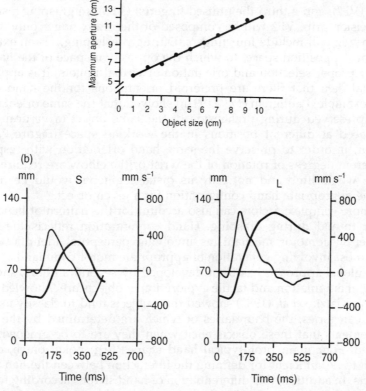

Figure 7.11. *Relationship of grip size to object size. (a) Maximum aperture of grip plotted against object size. [From Marteniuk* et al., *1990.] (b) Kinematic pattern of grip aperture in two prehension movements. On the left, movement directed to a small dowel (S); on the right, to a larger cylinder (L). Thick lines, change in grip size as a function of movement time; thin lines, rate of change (velocity) of grip size. Note maximum grip size reached earlier during prehension of small dowel. [From Paulignan* et al., *1991b.]*

Marteniuk *et al.*, 1990). For an example, see Figure 7.11b. By contrast, in other cases the rate of increase is faster for a large than for a small object, with the consequence that grip size peaks at the same time for both large and small objects. This second pattern corresponds to that described earlier by Jeannerod (1981). It seems that the only determinant for using either one of the two strategies is movement time, so that the subjects tend to equate the time to maximum grip aperture for large and small objects when movements become faster.

One possible explanation for the biphasic pattern of grip formation relates to the thumb–index finger geometry. Because the index finger is longer than the thumb, the finger grip has to open wider than required by object size, in order for the index finger to turn around the object and achieve the proper orientation of the grip. Indeed, the movement of the index finger contributes the most to grip formation, whereas the position of the thumb with respect to the hand tends to remain invariant (Wing and Fraser, 1983) (Figure 7.12a). The outcome of this motor pattern has been formalized by Arbib (1985), Iberall and Arbib (1990) and Iberall, Bingham and Arbib (1986). Their idea is that the basic elements of the hand are the 'virtual fingers', one of them being the thumb (VF1), another the finger(s) that oppose to the thumb (VF2), and a third the unused finger(s) (VF3). In grasping a small object with a precision grip, VF2 will be composed of the index finger only, whereas in power grip VF2 will include four fingers. During preshaping, vision extracts from the object an 'opposition space' to which the opposition space of the hand will be matched by proper selection and orientation of virtual fingers. It is apparent from experimental data that there are preferred orientations for the hand opposition space. For example, Paulignan *et al.* (1991a) showed that the same orientation of the hand was preserved during prehension of the same object (a vertical cylindrical dowell) placed at different positions in the working space (Figure 7.12b). This implies that, in order to preserve the same hand orientation with respect to the object, different degrees of rotation of the wrist or the elbow are required. In other words, the whole limb and not only its distal segments would be involved in building the appropriate hand configuration for a given object.

Other, more complex, factors can also account for the pattern of hand configuration prior to and during grasping. Hand configuration reflects the activity of higher-order visuomotor mechanisms involving perceptual identification of the object and those involving generation of appropriate motor commands. Accordingly, a more global approach has been developed by several authors, showing that preshaping, manipulation and tactile exploration of objects are 'knowledge-driven'. For instance, Klatzky *et al.* (1987) showed that subjects tend to classify usual objects into broad categories, the boundaries of which are determined by the pattern of hand movements that these objects elicit when they are to be grasped, used and manipulated. Four main prototypical hand shapes (e.g. poke, pinch, clench and palm) seem to be sufficient for defining the interaction between the hand and most usual objects. In addition, this differentiation of hand shapes according to the forms of objects is retained in preshaping during actual reaching (see also Lederman and Klatzky, 1990; Pellegrino, Klatzky and McCloskey, 1989). The same idea, that characteristics of reaching and grasping movements depend on prior knowledge gained from previous real world interactions with objects, has also been emphasized by Athenes and Wing (1990).

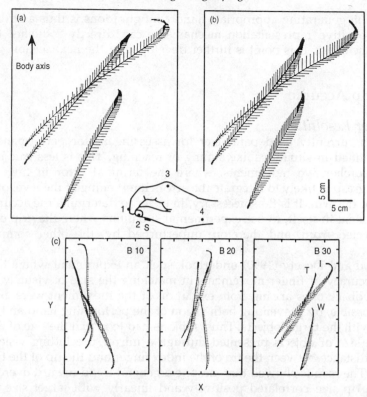

Figure 7.12. *Spatial path and variability of wrist, index finger and thumb during prehension movements in one normal subject. (a) Prehension of a small object. (b) Prehension of a larger object. (c) Prehension of the small object located at 10, 20 or 30 degrees (B10, B20 and B30, respectively) to the right of subject's midline. W, Trajectory of a marker located at the wrist level; T, at the tip of the thumb; I, at the tip of the index finger. Trajectories are sampled at 250 Hz and normalized over 10 trials. The horizontal and vertical bars represent the values of one standard deviation with respect to the mean trajectory, for each of the 100 normalized frames. The drawing of the hand in the middle of the figure shows the starting posture of the subject's hand. 1 and 2 indicate the index and thumb markers; 4, the wrist marker; S, start switch for triggering perturbations at onset of movement (see Figures 7.14 and 7.15). Note larger contribution of the index finger to the pattern of grip formation during preshaping. Also note relatively similar orientation of hand opposition despite differences in object size or location. [From Paulignan et al., 1991a.]*

These findings seem consistent with the fact that hand movements during grasping are largely predetermined by object-related visual input and by object affordance. Indeed, in normal subjects, both the biphasic pattern of grip formation (opening of the finger grip followed by anticipatory closure) and the coordination of the reaching and grasping components are correctly achieved in situations where the hand remains invisible to the subject. Similarly, the size of the maximum grip aperture correlates with the size of the object in the absence of visual feedback from the hand (Jeannerod, 1981, 1984). The fact that object-related visual input acts proactively in generating appropriate hand configurations is thus a strong indication that cognitive representation mechanisms can directly influence the motor control of the hand. This point is further developed in the next section.

3.2.2   Grip Accuracy

Visuomotor Resolution

Accuracy, a currently used parameter for assessing motor performance, can be easily quantified in situations like aiming or reaching. This is less true in the case of natural prehensive movements, where the terminal error in finger position during the grasp is likely to integrate the errors intervening at the level of the other segments of the arm. It is thus necessary, in order to determine the accuracy of the grip component in itself, to use experimental situations where the grip component is disconnected from, and therefore unperturbed by, the other components of prehension.

Jeannerod and Decety (1990) undertook such an experiment where they examined the accuracy of finger movements in matching the size of visually presented objects. Feedback cues arising from execution of the movement were excluded as much as possible, by preventing both vision of the performing hand and contact of that hand with the target objects. Thus, subjects had to match the size of their finger grip to the size of objects presented through a mirror precluding vision of their hand. The distance between the tip of the index finger and the tip of the thumb was measured. The results showed that, despite a general trend toward overestimation, the mean grip size correlated positively and linearly with target size with high correlation coefficients (Figure 7.13).

These results raise important issues concerning the accuracy of converting retinal signals related to object size into a finger posture, referred to here as 'visuomotor estimation'. First, it is interesting to compare the present results with those obtained in psychophysical experiments testing the subjective scaling of visual length or size. Hering (quoted by Marks, 1978) had proposed that the perceived length of a line should be proportional to its physical length, and should not follow a logarithmic function as is the case in the perception of other physical dimensions; this contention turned out to be true (Stevens and Guirao, 1963). The subjective scaling of area, however, has been found by several authors to be related to physical size by a power function with an exponent of 0.7–0.8 (Ekman and Junge, 1961; Stevens and Guirao, 1963). The discrepancy between subjective scaling of length and area might be related to the type of instructions given to the subjects. Teghtsoonian (1965) showed that if subjects were required to estimate the 'objective area' of circles (How large are the circles?) their judgements followed a linear relation to physical size, as was found for the lines. In contrast, if the task was to estimate the 'apparent size' of the same circles (How large do they look to you?), then their judgements followed a power function (exponent 0.76) with respect to physical size. The Jeannerod and Decety (1990) results, showing that visuomotor estimation of size is linearly related to target size, therefore suggest that motor programs actually 'read' objective size rather than apparent size.

The second point raised by the Jeannerod and Decety (1990) results is that the degree of precision attained in visuomotor estimation of size is lower than during the real movement of grasping objects. This difference may be explained by the fact

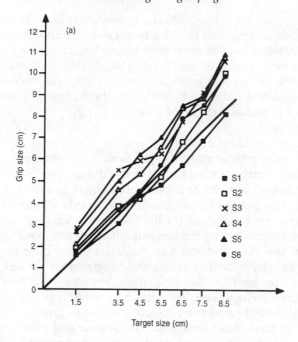

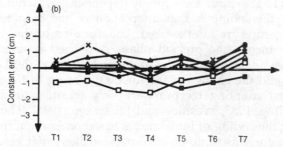

Figure 7.13. *Relationship of grip size to target size during matching the size of a visual object with the hand. (a) Values of grip size plotted against object size in six subjects (S1–S6). Note highly linear correlation. (b) Constant errors in matching the size of visual objects with the hand. Negative values indicate underestimation. Values of grip size corrected for finger size have been plotted in six subjects (S1–S6); T1–T7, target objects. [From Jeannerod and Decety, 1990.]*

that in the Jeannerod and Decety experiment visual feedback signals were lacking, although these signals are normally present during prehension. As already stressed in Section 2, it is a well-known general rule in motor control that accuracy of visually goal-directed movements deteriorates in conditions where visual feedback is either suppressed or degraded. Indeed, studies where accuracy of prehension was measured as the global outcome of natural coordinated reaching and grasping movements (i.e. where possible errors in grip formation cumulated with errors in execution of the other components of the movement) showed relatively large errors when visual feedback was prevented (Jeannerod, 1984) or in conditions of speeded performance (Wallace and Weeks, 1988). In order to explain the higher accuracy attained in pure visual scaling, one might also suggest that in this task subjects rely on the readout of analytic visual mechanisms (specialized for size, orientation, etc.), which are likely to be quite accurate. In contrast, during visuomotor estimation, subjects have to rely on mechanisms involved in the transformation of visual information into motor commands. It is likely that the complexity of this transformation involves many potential sources of inaccuracy.

Anticipatory Control of Grip Force

Finally, another aspect of grip accuracy is specification of grip force. This parameter also has to be, at least partly, specified in advance, during the preshaping phase, in order for the adequate force to be applied on the object at the onset of the grasp. Lifting an object implies a sequence of coordinated events where the grip force (to grasp the object) and the load force (to lift the object) vary in parallel. The grip force/load force ratio must exceed the slip ratio, itself determined by the coefficient of friction between the skin and the object surface. Changing the coefficient of friction (by using an object coated with sandpaper, suede or silk, for instance) changes the grip force, so that the load force remains invariant and the grip force/load force ratio increases when frictional forces decrease. By contrast, increasing the weight of the object results in an increase of both grip force and load force and an invariant grip force/load force ratio (Johansson and Westling, 1987).

The respective contributions of anticipatory mechanisms and of reflex adjustments to the accuracy of grip force have been extensively studied. It appears that the adaptive changes in grip force are strongly dependent on tactile afferent signals. A demonstration of this point is that adaptation of the grip force to friction disappears if the fingertips are anesthetized. The duration of the initial, isometric phase of lifting movements (the preload phase, $c.$ 100 ms) is sufficient for tactile afferents from the fast adapting receptors to come into play, the latency between the onset of the slip and the change in the force ratio being in the range of 75 ms. In addition, these fast adapting receptors are very sensitive to slip signals (see Johansson and Westling, 1987; Westling and Johansson, 1984). These signals may be used for updating the coding of initial forces based on internal representation of object properties, and for sensorimotor learning. It is likely that visual cues related to object size will also be used for building this representation.

4   THE COORDINATION OF REACHING AND GRASPING

The current model for explaining the coordination of actions involving simultaneously several motor components, like prehension, is that of parallel functional ensembles, characterized by specific input–output relationships, and specialized for generating each component of the action (see Jeannerod, 1981). During prehension, the reaching arm movement carrying the hand to the location of the target object is executed in parallel with finger movements that shape the hand in anticipation of the grasp. Thus, the input of the visuomotor channel specialized for grasping, for example, is tuned to visual object size, and its output is connected to distal muscles for generating a precision grip. The other channel specialized for the proximal aspect of the movement obviously must have a different structure and mode of activation. The experimental arguments suggesting that, in primates, the respective motor systems involved in reaching and grasping movements can be considered as separate modules have been reviewed in the neurophysiological sections of this chapter.

Theories involving parallel activation, however, are faced with the problem of how the different systems that are separately, and simultaneously, activated can be coordinated with each other in order to achieve the desired action. The fact that the two components of prehension are separate movements with different modes of organization, and belonging to different levels of visual processing, implies different timing. They must therefore be bound by a distinct coordination mechanism, so that transport of the hand and shaping of the fingers coincide in time, and the reach terminates exactly at the time when the fingers come in contact with the object. Indeed, most of the theories that account for multiple joint actions involve specific mechanisms for ensuring coordination of the components in the temporal and spatial domains (Arbib, 1981; Bernstein, 1967). Arbib's conception (see Iberall and Arbib, 1990) implies that the various motor schemas responsible for prehension (e.g. 'move the arm', 'orient', 'preshape', 'enclose object', etc.) are hierarchically organized within a broader coordinated control program which determines the order and the degree of activation of the schemas.

Such a coordination mechanism cannot be regulated by peripheral input. Activation of cutaneous afferents at the time of contact of fingers with the object would not be sufficient, despite the rapidity of tactile motor loops, to account for a proper timing of prehension. By extrapolating from the Johansson and Westling data (see above), a delay of 75 ms is needed for tactile signals to influence an ongoing movement. This means that, if the hand was still traveling at $1 \, \mathrm{m \, s^{-1}}$ at the time of contact, it would pass the object location by more than 7 cm before full stop. This would not be compatible either with the degree of accuracy required for grasping, nor with the observed spatiotemporal organization of the grasp. The alternative hypothesis, that coordination between the two components belongs to a preorganized functional temporal structure, will be examined in the following sections.

4.1 Spontaneous Temporal Covariation of the Two Components

A number of the experimental data reviewed in the previous sections point to a preorganized coordination of submovements during prehension. First, there is a possibility that cortical commands to the arm muscle might be arranged in synergies. Second, the fact that hand configuration remains invariant during the grasping of objects of the same shape at different spatial locations implies that not only distal segments but also proximal ones are involved in grip formation.

One way of studying the degree of coordination between the two components is to look for possible invariant relationships between kinematic landmarks of the respective trajectories of the involved limb segments during natural movements. It was shown by Jeannerod (1984) that the main kinematic landmark of the grip component–the time to maximum grip aperture–occurred at a fixed ratio of total movement time. In the Jeannerod paper, this ratio was between 75 and 80% of movement time in most subjects. Very similar values (72–82%) were found in a sample of adult subjects studied by von Hofsten and Rönnqvist (1988). This result was further replicated and expanded by Wallace and Weeks (1988) and Wallace, Weeks and Kelso (1990), who showed that the ratio of time to maximum grip/ movement time was remarkably stable despite large variations in movement time and speed, and despite different initial postures of the fingers. Such a temporal invariance, which is strongly indicative of functional coupling of the two components, will be shown to be preserved even in pathological conditions: when movement time is increased, the time to maximum grip increases by a corresponding amount; conversely, in conditions where grip formation is delayed or altered, a correlative lengthening of movement time is observed (see Section 6).

Another, more controversial, finding is also in favor of functional coupling. Jeannerod (1981, 1984) had observed that the time to maximum grip aperture was systematically correlated with the occurrence of secondary accelerations of the wrist movement. Later work by other authors, however, failed to replicate this result (e.g. Marteniuk et al., 1990). The explanation for this discrepancy may be that secondary accelerations are not always observed in prehension movements. Whereas they are clearly present during lowering of the hand toward the object in movements executed in the vertical plane (as in Jeannerod's experiments), they are absent in other types of prehension movements (e.g. performed in the horizontal plane). Finally, the search for other kinematic covariations between the two components has not been entirely successful until now. A correlation was occasionally found between the time of occurrence of the velocity peak of the transportation component and the time of occurrence of the maximum grip aperture (Marteniuk et al., 1990; Paulignan et al., 1990). This correlation was not observed in all subjects and, within subjects, was not present in all conditions. Another, more consistent correlation was found between the time of occurrence of maximum grip aperture and that of the peak deceleration of the wrist (Gentilucci et al., 1991).

4.2 Effects of Systematic Manipulation of One Component on the Kinematics of the Other

Another way of understanding the modalities of coordination between the two components of prehension is to examine the degree of stability of each given component when the other one is manipulated experimentally.

In an experiment where subjects had to grasp a dowel by performing reaching movements either at a normal speed or as fast as possible, Wing, Turton and Fraser (1986) found that maximum grip aperture was larger when the movement was faster. The authors interpreted this effect of movement speed on the grip component as an anticipatory error-correcting behavior. This result was partly confirmed by Wallace and Weeks (1988) in a series of experiments involving manipulation of error tolerance during grasping. Error tolerance boundaries were imposed on the grasp, with the corollary that the subjects had to regulate the duration of their movements in order to minimize their error. As predicted by Fitts' law, the duration of the movement was indeed a function of the accuracy demand. As an example, when the error tolerance was large (e.g. displacements of the objects by up to 7.5 cm were allowed during the grasp), the movement lasted 243 ms and the wrist velocity was 165 cm s^{-1}. By contrast, when the error tolerance was smaller (maximum object displacement allowed: 2.5 cm), movement duration increased up to 379 ms and the wrist velocity dropped to 117 cm s^{-1}. The interesting point was that, in the conditions where the movement duration decreased, the grip size tended to become larger by about 10%. Wallace and Weeks were able to demonstrate that the critical factor affecting grip size was movement duration, not movement speed: in manipulating simultaneously the two parameters (by instructing the subjects to perform movements of fixed durations directed at targets placed at different distances), they showed that increasing movement velocity without increasing movement duration was without effect on grip size. These results of Wallace and Weeks, along with those of Wing *et al.*, thus demonstrate that decrease in movement time (whether it is an indirect effect of larger error tolerance, or a consequence of instruction given to the subject) produces larger grip apertures.

Conversely, systematic changes of the grip component may affect the transportation component. Marteniuk *et al.* (1990) found prehension movements to last longer when the size of the object was smaller, due to lengthening of the deceleration phase of reaching. This finding is consistent both with the fact that movement time is generally a function of task difficulty, and with the fact that changes in total movement time are generally due to changes in duration of the deceleration phase (e.g. Marteniuk *et al.*, 1987; see also Section 2). Finally, in addition to affecting movement time, object size also affected the timing of the grip. Marteniuk *et al.* (1990) showed that the time to maximum grip aperture was a function of task difficulty, such that maximum grip size occurred earlier for smaller targets (but see Section 3.1 for another explanation of this result).

4.3 Effects of Perturbations Applied to One of the Components

Perturbing the input of a sensorimotor system is a commonly ued paradigm for probing the various functional levels of control of that system (Jeannerod, 1990b). In this section, the effects of unexpected changes in position or in size of the object prior to or during a prehension movement are examined. Change in position of the object will be considered as perturbing specifically the transportation component of the movement, whereas a change in size of the object will be considered as perturbing the grip component. The problem will be to determine to what extent a perturbation theoretically limited to one of the components will exert its effects on that component only, or whether it will also affect the other.

4.3.1 Perturbation of Object Location

As mentioned earlier (see Section 2), perturbations affecting the position of the object at the onset of the movement produce rapid corrections of the wrist trajectory, such that the object is correctly grasped with only a little increase in movement time (Paulignan *et al.*, 1990). A more complete analysis of these results, however, showed that the effects of object displacement were not limited to corrections affecting the transport component. The grip aperture was also affected. On most perturbed trials, the two components of prehension became kinematically coupled during corrective responses. The alteration of the wrist trajectory for reorienting the movement to the new target position was immediately followed

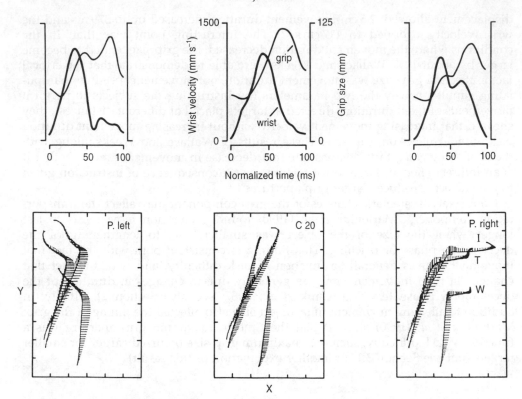

Figure 7.14. *Effects of sudden change in object position at the onset of prehension movements. This experiment was the same as that described in Figure 7.4. Upper row: kinematics of prehension during a movement directed at the central (20°) dowel (middle diagram) and during a perturbed-left and a perturbed-right movement (diagrams on the left and on the right, respectively). Thick line, velocity of the wrist; thin line, grip aperture. Data averaged on six subjects. Note corrections not only on wrist kinematics, as already shown in Figure 7.4, but also on grip kinematics. [From Paulignan* et al.,* 1990.] Lower row: spatial paths and variability of wrist, index finger and thumb in the same experiment. [From Paulignan* et al.,* 1991a.]*

(within about 50 ms) by a brief interruption of grip aperture, not required by the situation since object shape and size remained unchanged (Paulignan *et al.*, 1990, 1991a) (Figure 7.14). This finding was recently replicated by Haggard and Wing (1991). In their situation, the subject's arm was suddenly pulled back by a mechanical device during approach to the object. This perturbation triggered a rapid correction of the transport component, such that the arm was reaccelerated in order to reach for the object position. In about 70% of perturbed trials, the perturbation applied to the arm also provoked a reversal of grip aperture. As the change in grip formation occurred some 70 ms later than the change in transport, Haggard and Wing interpreted this coupling of the two components as an effect of a coordination mechanism. They proposed that (proprioceptive) information generated by the arm movement was used for stopping grip formation during the correction for the transport. In this way, the temporal coordination between the two components would be restored during the final phase of the movement.

Coordination of the two components would thus rely on comparison between information generated by each segmental movement, so that the corresponding motor commands could be modulated for minimizing the mismatch between components. One possible role in such a mechanism could be played by the C3–C4 propriospinal neurons, which are likely to receive proprioceptive signals generated by several segments of the same limb and to control the activity of the corresponding motoneuron pools. In addition, the propriospinal neurons receive visual input via a tectospinal route (Alstermark *et al.*, 1990). The prediction arising from this hypothetical mechanism is that peripherally deafferented subjects should lose the temporal coordination between transport and grasp and, in addition, would be unable to correct their prehension movements in response to perturbations of either object position or size. Although this prediction, to our present knowledge, has never been tested directly, there are a few indirect arguments against the 'spinal' hypothesis. Prehension movements were examined by Jeannerod, Michel and Prablanc (1984) in one patient (R.S.) with complete anesthesia (including loss of position sense) of one hand and forearm, due to a lesion of parietal cortex. While in this patient proprioceptive input was spared at the spinal level, her prehension movements were deeply disorganized and coordination between components was lost. This result indicates that mechanisms for temporal coordination between motor components during prehension should lie upstream with respect to the spinal cord, possibly at the cortical level (see below).

4.3.2   Perturbation of Object Size

Brisk changes in the size or shape of a graspable object are not easily produced. Paulignan *et al.* (1991b) used concentric objects made of a central dowel (diameter 1.5 cm) surrounded by a larger cylinder (6 cm). These objects were made of translucent material and were illuminated from below (see Paulignan *et al.*, 1991b). The light illuminating the dowel could be shifted below the cylinder, so that the cylinder now appeared to be illuminated. This created the impression of a sudden expansion of the dowel, without change in spatial location. The reverse effect (light shifted from cylinder to dowel), thus giving the impression of a shrinking of the cylinder, could also be produced. Perturbing object size at the onset of the movement clearly affected the grip component. If the perturbation consisted of increasing object size (from dowel to cylinder), the grip formation sized to the small object was interrupted and the grip aperture was reincreased in order to accommodate the large object. This correction in grip size began a relatively long time (330 ms) after the perturbation.

Response to the perturbation in object size, however, was not limited to the grip component. Total movement time was increased by over 170 ms in the small to large perturbation, and by about 85 ms in the large to small case. No change could be seen in the timing of kinematic landmarks of the transport component, at least during the first 300 ms, which means that the additional movement time was spent in the later part of the movement. Indeed, a long-lasting low-velocity phase was present in the transport component, so that the wrist virtually stopped at the vicinity of the object before the fingers came in contact with it (Figure 7.15).

Examination of the finger trajectories in the perturbed trials in the Paulignan *et al.* 1991b experiment revealed that the relative contribution of each finger to the grip

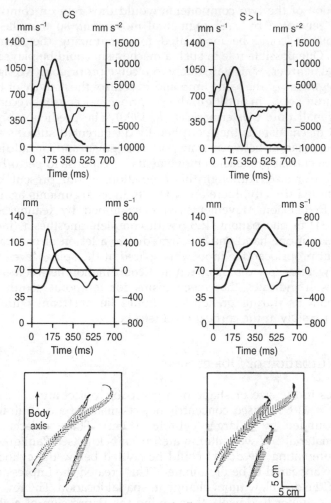

Figure 7.15. *Effects of sudden change in object size at the onset of prehension movements. Diagrams on the left: wrist kinematics (upper), grip kinematics (middle) and spatial path and variability (lower) of unperturbed movements directed at a small object. Diagrams on the right: the case of a sudden increase in object size at onset of movement. Note increase in duration of low velocity phase of wrist movement (upper), correction in grip size (middle) and reorganization of spatial path for increase in grip size (lower). Also note relatively late occurrence of the grip correction, as compared with early corrections in wrist trajectory during perturbation of object position (see Figures 7.5 and 7.14). [From Paulignan et al., 1991b.]*

pattern was changed with respect to unperturbed trials. In the normal condition, the contribution of the index finger to the grip was clearly larger than that of the thumb. In the perturbed trials, it appeared that the contribution of the thumb was increased (Figure 7.15). In addition, large rotations of the wrist were observed, which were not present in unperturbed conditions. These changes represent a remarkable example of 'motor equivalence', a concept which accounts for performing the same action by different means according to the conditions of execution.

Other examples of motor equivalence in hand movements have been described by Cole and Abbs (1987) during rapid pinch. These authors showed that over repetitions of this simple behavior the individual finger and thumb joints varied in their angular positions at the time of contact of the two fingers while the point of contact remained invariant. This was obtained by corresponding covariations of the finger paths. As already stated above, these quick changes in motor patterns responsible for motor equivalence seem to imply an encoding of the end positions of the limb segments with respect to the goal, rather than an encoding of detailed prescriptions for joint positions.

Taken together, the results of perturbation experiments, which show covariation of movements of the wrist and the fingers during corrections, create the impression of a synergy of the two components of prehension. Perturbation of object location, which should, in principle, affect the transport component only, also affects grip formation. Similarly, perturbation of object size affects not only grip formation, but also transport. A synergy, however, would have implied a strict temporal correlation of the components, which was not confirmed by statistical analysis of the data. Instead, the two submovements that compose prehension appear to be only loosely time-coupled. This pattern of coordination is reminiscent of the coordinative-structure concept, whereby independent musculoskeletal elements can become functionally linked for the execution of a common task, without implying structural relationships between them (Kelso *et al.*, 1980).

5 DEVELOPMENT OF REACHING AND GRASPING

Another justification for considering the proximal and distal components of prehension as separate (although coordinated) functional entities can be drawn from behavioral studies of the development of prehension in human infants and in young animals.

In babies, earlier studies have shown that finger posturing is lacking during reaching at visual objects until the age of approximately 20 weeks. According to Halverson (1931), inaccurate posturing is then observed but it is not until the age of 36–52 weeks that precision grip can be formed. More recent work, however, has shown that infants are able to make use of visual information for crude finger posturing earlier than previously suspected. According to Bruner and Koslowski (1972), infants 10–22 weeks of age may show coarsely adapted hand movements when they are presented with small graspable visual objects within reach. This is not the case for objects of a larger size, exceeding the grasping capability of the hand. Von Hofsten (1982) has shown that even younger infants (1 week old) may intercept the trajectory of moving objects and come into contact with them. These movements are first jerky and oscillatory, but they improve rapidly up to a point where two phases can be discerned, namely, an initial rapid arm extension lasting around 500 ms and then a series of stepwise smaller movements (von Hofsten, 1979). These reaching movements, however, are effected with a widely open hand without evidence of grip formation. It is only when the object has been touched that crude prehensile movements of the fingers can be observed. Von Hofsten and Rönnqvist (1988) reported a systematic study of the reaching and grasping pattern in infants of 5–6, 9 and 13 months of age. Displacements of the tip of the index

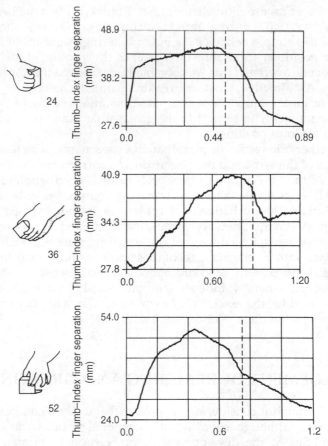

Figure 7.16. *Development of the motor pattern of grip formation in the human infant. The change in grip aperture as a function of time is shown in three representative movements in a 5-month-old (upper), a 9-month-old (middle) and a 13-month-old (lower). Dashed line represents contact with target-object. Note fully matured pattern with a clearly distinct maximum grip aperture at 13 months. [Fromvon Hofsten and Rönnqvist, 1988.]Drawings on the left represent typical hand postures during grasping in infants of corresponding ages (in weeks). [From Halverson, 1931.]*

finger and of the tip of the thumb were monitored during movements directed at spherical objects. It was observed that, in all three age groups, the hand opened during the reaching phase; but it was only in the 13-month-olds that the hand began to close in anticipation of the grasp. In the younger groups, the hand remained open until, or immediately before, contact with the object (Figure 7.16). This, according to von Hofsten and Rönnqvist, does not imply that closure of the fingers was triggered tactually, because the timing of the finger movements was compatible with a late, visually triggered, closure. Similarly, in the younger groups, the size of the maximum grip aperture was not systematically correlated with object size, whereas a significant correlation was found at 13 months. The general interpretation of these results was that visual anticipatory control of the hand by intrinsic object characteristic begins very early, but that the adult pattern is not met before at least 13 months. In addition, these results show that, in contradistinction to previous results (Bower, Broughton and Moore, 1970), the grip formation is systematically integrated with the reach from the earliest developmental stage.

It remains that the late occurrence of visually triggered hand shaping is controversial; some babies are reputed to show it within the first weeks of life (Bower, Broughton and Moore, 1970). Their movements, however, are of an immature style and they do not seem to be related to the presence of a visual object (Bower, Broughton and Moore, 1970; Trevarthen, 1982). In addition, although maximum finger opening seems to be related to the maximum extension of the wrist (hence suggesting a coordinated reaching and grasping pattern), they are much slower than adult movements. Trevarthen has suggested that finger movements observed in very young infants might represent the expression of a preformed proximodistal motor pattern (prereaching), which later will evolve into mature prehension (Trevarthen, 1984). Observations by Humphrey (1969) suggest that crude reaching and grasping movements might even be present in human fetuses, at an age when it may be assumed that only spinal motor centers are functional.

It is difficult to determine whether poor ability to adapt finger posture to the shape of a visual object in human infants is due to incomplete maturation at the input or the output levels of the visuomotor system that controls the movement. In favor of the input level, Di Franco, Muir and Dodwell (1978) observed that an infant at the prereaching stage will reach as actively for a two-dimensional picture of an object as for the real object. This observation, however, seems somewhat contradictory to that of Bruner and Koslowski (1972, see above), who showed that babies will attempt to reach only for objects of a graspable size. As for the output level, it is worth stressing the deleterious effects on hand shaping of early reflex reactions and synergies. In Twitchell's (1970) terms, the 'initial prehension appears more accidental than intentional' and 'the emergence of the instinctive avoiding response at the time of these early attempts at voluntary prehension causes ataxia of reach and overpronation of the hand'. Twitchell (1970) recognizes that dexterous prehension appears late and that small objects remain difficult for the infant to handle; 'the required thumb–fingers apposition does not appear until the grasp reflex can be fractionated during the second half-year of life'. Later, 'the instinctive avoiding response can contaminate activity and the fingers may abduct or dorsiflex too much as the hand is extended toward the object' (p. 33).

In order to discuss other possible justifications for the concept of a duality of motor mechanisms in prehension, it is tempting to relate the developmental time course of finger movements in children to the maturation of motor pathways. Accordingly, the late development of finger movements and the persistence of instinctive reactions might reflect immaturity of corticomotoneuronal synapses controlling independent hand and finger movements. It is known that pyramidal fibers continue to increase in diameter up to somatic maturity. In addition, it has been shown that the pyramidal tract myelinates relativity late in humans: myelination increases up to the eighth postnatal month, and seems to be complete at around the age of 1 year (Yakovlev and Lecours, 1967) or even 2 years (Langworthy, 1933). These results indicate that consistent formation of a precision grip during prehension of visual objects would be contemporary with the existence of a functional corticospinal tract. In humans, however, more data are needed to establish a precise anatomofunctional correlation.

As in children, very young monkeys develop goal-directed arm extension earlier than manipulative movements. Observations by J. Vauclair (personal communication, 1986) in the baboon showed that, during the first three postnatal weeks, the animal makes tentative unimanual reaches directed at visual objects. In these reaches, either hand is thrown in the direction of the food-target with the fingers fully extended (unspecified reaches, 75% of cases) and eventually achieves a palmar grasp (25% of cases). Palmar grasp develops at the expense of unspecified reaches, but precision grip does not appear until the seventh week after birth. Interestingly, it is only at the time when precision grip appears that the hand preference becomes detectable and that unimanual reaches become clearly lateralized.

In the monkey, dissociation between development of proximal and distal components of prehension does reflect immaturity of the corticomotoneuronal synapses that control independent hand and finger movements. According to Kuypers (1962), this pathway does not fully develop until the eighth month in macaques, and it is not until then that these animals can make a precision grip (see also Lawrence and Hopkins, 1976).

6 NEUROLOGY OF REACHING AND GRASPING

Lesions affecting the cortical network responsible for the action of prehension provide examples where the two components of this action can be dissociated. Effects of motor cortex and parietal cortex lesions will be reported and interpreted within the general framework of disconnection between critical zones devoted to visual and motor aspects of grip formation.

6.1 Effects of Pyramidal Lesion in Humans

Lesions involving motor cortical areas or their efferent pathways (as in hemiplegia following stroke, for instance) are of relatively frequent occurrence. In studying recovery from hemiplegia in patients with surgical resection of area 4, Hécaen and Ajuriaguerra (1948) had noticed that movements of the proximal joints recovered first, with a return to normal muscular force within 4–6 weeks. By contrast, fine and isolated finger movements appeared to be permanently lost in these patients. A recent reinvestigation of this dissociation by Lough *et al.* (1984) confirmed that patients with hemiplegia usually recover the shoulder–elbow synergy for transporting the hand near an object, provided the shoulder is passively supported against gravity, but that finger movements seem to remain indefinitely clumsy. During prehension, these patients do not shape their hand in anticipation of the grasp; the grasp is achieved with the palmar surface of the whole hand instead of the fingertips.

Besides adult hemiplegia, there are other pathological conditions where a specific alteration of finger movements can be studied more easily. One of these conditions is infant hemiplegia, a disease of unknown origin associated with malformation and/or lack of maturation at the cortical level within one hemisphere. It consists of spastic palsy of the limbs on one side, sometimes accompanied by mild mental disability. Interestingly, the hemiplegia is usually not noticed until the age of about 40 weeks, i.e. around the time that the hand normally becomes engaged in prehensile activities. At this early stage, the only noticeable deficit is disuse of the affected hand in manipulation normally requiring both hands. Spasticity may appear at a later stage (Twitchell, 1970).

Finger movements during prehension have been examined by Jeannerod (1986c) in two such patients aged 23 months and 5 years, respectively. In the younger patient, the affected (right) hand remained spontaneously unused. It was only when the normal hand was attached that the right hand could be teased, though with difficulty, to grasp objects. The normal hand appeared to shape incompletely with respect to the object, although the finger extension–flexion pattern was nonetheless clearly present. In addition, contact of the hand with the object triggered an immediate posturing of the fingers which ensured accurate grasping. By contrast, the affected hand remained exaggerately stretched throughout the duration of the movement, without any evidence of grip formation. Some posturing of the fingers occurred after contact with the object, resulting in a very incorrect and clumsy grasp. In the older child, the affected hand was used spontaneously – partly as a result of training and rehabilitation procedures continued for several years. Better cooperation of this patient allowed more complete analysis of her prehension movements. With her normal hand, she performed correct and accurate grips with a fully developed, adult-like pattern. Prehension with the affected hand differed from that of the normal hand only for what concerned the pattern of grip formation. The index finger was exaggerately extended and flexed incompletely, if at all, before contact with the object. In some examples, no finger grip formation could be detected, although the velocity profiles corresponding to the transportation components appeared relatively similar to those of the normal hand. The lack, or the abnormal character, of grip formation with the affected hand resulted in awkward and clumsy grasps of the objects which were occasionally dropped from the hand (Figure 7.17).

Effects of lesions involving larger aspects of motor cortex, or even one complete hemisphere (hemispherectomy), are also relevant to this point. One such case has been fully described in a paper by Müller *et al.* (1991). The patient, who had a left infantile hemiplegia, was operated on at age 18 years for right hemispherectomy. The right hemisphere presented a cystic cavitation involving part of the lower frontal gyrus, and the arm–face area of the primary somatosensory cortex, but no lesion was observed macroscopically in the primary motor cortex. When the patient was examined at age 50, she showed a clear distoproximal dissociation in motor functions with the left arm. Whereas actions performed with proximal segments – like fist clenching, wrist flexion–extension, elbow movements – were possible with only a mild hemiparesis, and shoulder movements were normal, she showed a consistent inability to move the fingers of the left hand individually. Motor tasks involving the fingers, like pencil shading, which were executed at the normal 5 Hz rate with the right hand, were slowed down to about 1 Hz with the left hand. In addition, these movements were irregular and inaccurate. The grasping component of prehension was found to be severely affected: the formation of hand aperture was disturbed and was limited to a crude flexion synergy of the hand and fingers. The patient could manage to hold only large objects.

These observations have important implications for the respective roles of motor pathways involved in reaching and grasping. In the patient described by Müller *et al.* (1991), where only ipsilateral corticomotoneuronal projections were likely to be

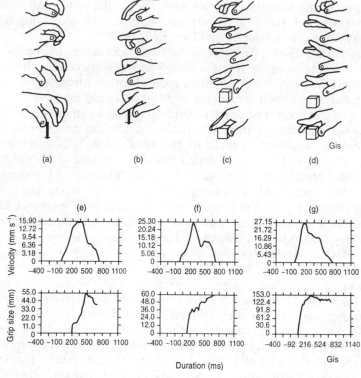

Figure 7.17. *Pattern of finger grip in one child with infant hemiplegia following neonatal damage of the left motor areas. Upper figure: (a) normal hand; (b), (c), (d) affected hand. Note hyperextension of index finger and poor independence of fingers during prehension. Redrawn from film. Lower figure: wrist velocity and grip size during: (e) one movement with the normal hand, and (f, g), two movements with the affected hand. Patient G.I.S., 5 years old. [From Jeannerod, 1986c.]*

preserved, a large restoration of proximal components was achieved, whereas finger movements were still very poor more than 30 years following the hemispherectomy.

6.2 Effects of Lesion of the Anterior Parietal Lobe

These lesions often involve somatosensory deficit, such as tactile anesthesia and loss of position sense. This deficit severely disturbs motor function, particularly that of the distal part of the limb. Typically, these patients show an inability to manipulate small objects and difficulties in making a pincer grip. Their exploratory finger movements during palpation of objects are slowed down with respect to normals: they cannot perform tasks involving fast repetitive movements like tapping, for example. Terminologies such as 'tactile paresis' or 'tactile apraxia' have been used to account for this motor impairment due to somatosensory deficit of central origin (Pause *et al.*, 1989).

Other aspects of grasping movements, like preshaping and grip formation, are also altered in such patients. This is illustrated by the case of a patient with an extensive lesion of primary parietal areas on the left side (case R.S., Jeannerod, Michel and Prablanc, 1984). Following the lesion, the patient suffered a complete anesthesia (including the loss of position sense) in the distal segments of the right arm. When R.S. was tested for simple motor tasks with that arm, she was found to be unable to perform normally. In the absence of visual control, only simple,

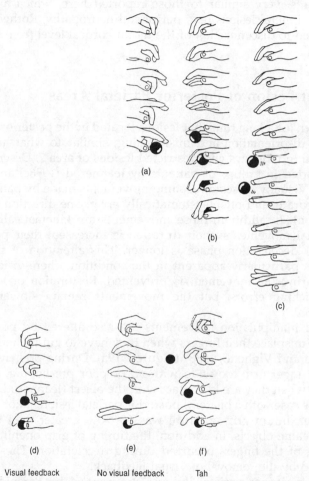

(a)

(b)

(c)

(d)   (e)   (f)

Visual feedback   No visual feedback   Tah

Figure 7.18. *Pattern of prehension movements in deafferented patients. Upper figure: patient R.S. with anterior parietal lobe lesion in the left hemisphere: (a) normal hand; (b), (c) affected hand. In (b), the hand is visible to the subject; note clumsy grasp without independent posturing of the fingers. In (c) the hand is not visible to the subject; note complete lack of grip formation. [From Jeannerod, Michel and Prablanc, 1984.] Lower figure: deafferentiation for kinesthetic sensations following a bulbar lesion in patient T.A.H. Prehension movements are normal under visual control (d) but they become impaired in the absence of visual feedback (e), (f). [From Jeannerod, 1986c.] Comparison of the two subjects suggests a role for the cortical level in the matching of visual and proprioceptive information controlling prehension.*

monoarticular movements could be executed, whereas more complex movements like prehension aborted after a few attempts. When visual control of the moving limb was made possible, complex movements remained abnormally slow and awkward (Figure 7.18). This observation is important because it emphasizes the role of cortical mechanisms in establishing the connection between visual and proprioceptive reafferences. Clearly, in this and other patients with somatosensory deficits of cortical origin, persistence of kinesthetic afferents at the cerebellar and spinal levels, and at the level of other subcortical structures, did not provide sufficient cues for maintaining correct motor control. This remark suggests that the distal impairments, very similar to those reported here, which are observed in patients with peripheral lesions (e.g. peripheral neuropathy; Rothwell *et al.*, 1982) must be attributed to disconnection of the motor cortical level from somatosensory information.

6.3 Effects of Lesion of Posterior Parietal Areas

It has been known for a long time that lesions located in the posterior parietal cortex produce spatial disorientation and misreaching, similar to what has been subsequently observed in monkeys with restricted lesions of area 7. Description of these effects was reported in groups of patients by Jeannerod (1986c) and Perenin and Vighetto (1988). Visually directed reaching movements made by patients with such lesions are inaccurate, and often systematically err in one direction (usually to the side of the lesion). In addition, these movements are kinematically altered with respect to normal movements: their duration is increased, their peak velocity is lower, and their deceleration phase is longer. This alteration of movement kinematics becomes particularly apparent in the condition where vision of the hand prior to and during the movement is prevented. Restoration of visual feedback reduces the reaching errors, but the movements remain slower than normal (Jeannerod, 1986b).

Grasping and manipulation movements are also altered by posterior parietal lesions. Patients misplace their fingers when they have to guide their hand visually to a slit (Perenin and Vighetto, 1988) (Figure 7.19a). During prehension of objects, they open their finger grip too wide with no or poor preshaping, and they close their finger grip when they are in contact with the object (Jeannerod, 1986c) (Figure 7.19b). In a single case with a bilateral posterior parietal lesion, Jakobson *et al.* (1991) observed that maximum grip aperture was 60–70% greater than that of normal controls for the same objects. In addition, the timing of grip opening was variable and reposturing of the fingers occurred during deceleration. These impairments were exacerbated by the removal of visual feedback.

Patients with posterior parietal lesions, as observed by Perenin and Vighetto (1988) and by Jeannerod (1986), had intact somatosensory control of their hand (no anesthesia, no loss of positional sense) and intact visuospatial functions (they could correctly localize objects visually). It may therefore be speculated, in accordance with the above remarks on the importance of the cortical level in regulating prehension movements (see Section 4), that lesions of these parietal areas produce disconnection of visual and proprioceptive inputs from each other at a level where they are supposed to cooperate for steering movements to their targets. This pathological disconnection will produce a condition where proprioceptive cues will

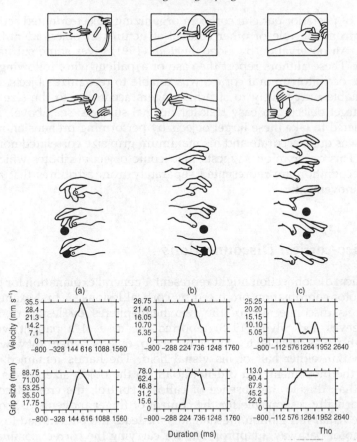

(a)

Velocity (mm s⁻¹)

35.5
28.4
21.3
14.2
7.1
0
-800 -328 144 616 1088 1560

(b)

26.75
21.40
16.05
10.70
5.35
0
-800 -288 224 736 1248 1760

(c)

25.25
20.20
15.15
10.10
5.05
0
-800 -112 576 1264 1952 2640

Grip size (mm)

88.75
71.00
53.25
35.50
17.75
0
-800 -328 144 616 1088 1560

78.0
62.4
46.8
31.2
15.6
0
-800 -288 224 736 1248 1760

113.0
90.4
67.8
45.2
22.6
0
-800 -112 576 1264 1952 2640

Duration (ms)

Tho

Figure 7.19. *Pattern of finger movements in patients with lesion of posterior parietal areas. Upper figure: errors in hand orientation toward a slit. [From Perenin and Vighetto, 1988.] Lower figure: prehension in a patient with a posterior parietal lesion on the right side. (a) Normal hand, (b) and (c) affected hand, with and without visual feedback, respectively. Note lack of finger posturing in (b) and reaching error in (c). Also note increase in duration of low-velocity phase of wrist movement in (c). [From Jeannerod, 1986c.]*

no longer be calibrated by visual cues, in other words where limb and object positions in space will no longer be matched with each other. In such a condition, the whole system has to shift from the optimal feedforward mode of motor control based on continuous updating of limb position by visual cues, to a substitutive and much less efficient mode based on peripheral feedback (see Jeannerod, 1988, 1990a). Visual feedback mechanisms can detect errors of the terminal segment of the limb relative to the object, but cannot carry information regarding joint angles or kinematics, which is likely to be necessary for establishing coordination between limb segments. In addition, corrections based on detection of terminal errors must be iterative in order to progressively reduce the error between the limb and the object. Experiments mentioned in Section 2, especially those involving fast corrections, clearly showed that such a slow mechanism would be inappropriate for controlling normal movements.

This role of posterior parietal cortex in organizing object-oriented action must be dissociated from the role of other cortical structures in object identification and recognition. An observation by Goodale *et al.* (1991) gives some substance to this dissociation. These authors report the case of a patient who, following a bilateral lesion of the occipitotemporal cortex, was unable to recognize objects. The patient was also unable purposively to size his fingers according to the size of visually inspected target objects (an easy task for normal subjects; see above). In contrast, when instructed to take these target objects by performing prehension movements, the patient was quite accurate and his maximum grip size correlated normally with object size. This observation suggests that iconic object attributes which are used for object recognition are represented separately from attributes that are used to control the movement.

6.4   Cortico-cortical Disconnections

Cortico-cortical disconnection might represent a general explanation for disruptions in sensorimotor coordination produced by cortical lesions. A first example of such a condition is disconnection of the two hemispheres by lesion of the corpus callosum. Jeeves and Silver (1988) reported the case of a patient with callosal agenesis, who was unable to correctly grasp objects when they were briefly presented within either half of his visual field. The hands remained wide open throughout the movement and did not adapt to the object size. Jeeves and Silver speculated that, due to the absence of callosal control, the crossed corticospinal pathway (normally responsible for the control of finger movements) could not be activated by visual recognition mechanisms. Instead, the patient had to rely on the ipsilateral motor pathway, inappropriate for carrying the correct commands.

A similar explanation, based on cortico-cortical disconnection, may apply to patients with lesions in the posterior part of parietal lobe, who present with limb apraxia. There are very few detailed studies of motor performance in such patients. Poizner *et al.* (1990) reported computer analysis of movements in a group of apraxic patients. The types of movement studied were movements of the subjects pretending to wind, erase, carve, etc. They found both spatial and temporal errors in relative placement of the limb segments. Spatial errors were characterized by improper orientation of the limb, predominating in the distal segments.

These results indicate that coordination between limb segments during goal-directed movements relies on a large cortical network involved in object identification, spatial localization and motor planning.

ACKNOWLEDGEMENTS

Thanks are due to Professor S. Keele (University of Oregon) for his comments on a previous version of this chapter. I also thank Dr G. P. van Galen and an anonymous referee for their critical remarks. This work was supported by INSERM (Paris), Université Claude Bernard (Lyon), and by a grant from the European Economic Communities (SC10177A).

REFERENCES

Abbs, J. H. and Gracco, V. L. (1984). Control of complex motor gestures: Orofacial muscle responses to load perturbations of lip during speech. *Journal of Neurophysiology*, **51**, 705–723.

Alstermark, B., Gorska, T., Lundberg, A. and Petterson, L. C. (1990). Integration in descending motor pathways controlling the forelimb in the cat. 16. Visually guided switching of target-reaching. *Experimental Brain Research*, **80**, 1–11.

Andersen, R. A., Essik, G. K. and Siegel, R. M. (1985). Encoding of spatial location by posterior parietal neurons. *Science*, **230**, 456–458.

Andersen, R. A. and Gnadt, J. W. (1989). Posterior parietal cortex. In R. Wurtz and M. E. Goldberg (Eds), *The Neurobiology of Saccadic Eye Movements* (pp. 315–335). Amsterdam: Elsevier.

Arbib, M. A. (1981). Perceptual structures and distributed motor control. In V. B. Brooks (Ed.), *Motor Control. Handbook of Physiology*, vol. II (pp. 1449–1480). Baltimore, MD: Williams and Wilkins.

Arbib, M. A. (1985). Schemas for the temporal organization of behavior. *Human Neurobiology*, **4**, 63–72.

Athenes, S. and Wing, A. M. (1990). Knowledge directed coordination in reaching for objects in the environment. In S. Wallace (Ed.), *Perspectives on the Coordination of Movement*. Amsterdam: North-Holland.

Bernstein, N. (1967). *The Coordination and Regulation of Movements*. Oxford: Pergamon Press.

Biguer, B., Donaldson, I. M. L., Hein, A. and Jeannerod, M. (1988). Neck muscle vibration modifies the representation of visual motion and detection in man. *Brain*, **111**, 1405–1424.

Biguer, B., Jeannerod, M. and Prablanc, C. (1982). The coordination of eye, head and arm movements during reaching at a single visual target. *Experimental Brain Research*, **46**, 301–304.

Biguer, B., Jeannerod, M. and Prablanc, C. (1985). The role of position of gaze in movement accuracy. In M. I. Posner and O. S. M. Marin (Eds), *Mechanisms of Attention. Attention and Performance*, vol. XI (pp. 407–424). Hillsdale, NJ: Erlbaum.

Biguer, B., Prablanc, C. and Jeannerod, M. (1984). The contribution of coordinated eye and head movements in hand pointing accuracy. *Experimental Brain Research*, **55**, 462–469.

Bizzi, E., Accorneo, N., Chapple, W. and Hogan, N. (1984). Posture control and trajectory formation during arm movement. *Journal of Neuroscience*, **4**, 2738–2744.

Blum, J. S., Chow, K. L. and Pribram, K. H. (1950). A behavioural analysis of the organization of the parieto-temporo-preoccipital cortex. *Journal of Comparative Neurology*, **93**, 53–100.

Bower, T. G. R., Broughton, J. M. and Moore, M. K. (1970). The coordination of visual and tactual inputs in infants. *Perception and Psychophysics*, **8**, 51–53.

Bridgeman, B., Kirch, M. and Sperling, A. (1981). Segregation of cognitive and motor aspects of visual function using induced motion. *Perception and Psychophysics*, **29**, 336–342.

Brinkman, J. and Kuypers, H. G. J. M. (1973). Cerebral control of contralateral and ipsilateral arm, hand and finger movements in the split-brain rhesus monkey. *Brain*, **96**, 653–674.

Bruner, J. S. and Koslowski, B. (1972). Visually pre-adapted constituents of manipulatory action. *Perception*, **1**, 3–14.

Buys, E. J., Lemon, R. N., Mantel, G. W. H. and Muir, R. B. (1986). Selective facilitation of different hand muscles by single corticospinal neurons in the conscious monkey. *Journal of Physiology*, **381**, 529–549.

Carlton, L. G., 1981. Processing visual feedback information for movement control. *Journal of Experimental Psychology: Human Perception and Performance*, **7**, 1019–1030.

Castiello, U., Paulignan, Y. and Jeannerod, M. (1991). Temporal dissociation of motor responses and perceptual awareness: a study in normal subjects. *Brain*, **114**, 2639–2655.

Chapman, E. and Wiesendanger, M. (1982). Recovery of function following unilateral lesions of the bulbar pyramid in the monkey. *Electroencephalography and Clinical Neurophysiology*, **53**, 374–387.

Cole, K. J. and Abbs, J. H. (1987). Kinematic and electromyographic responses to perturbation of a rapid grasp. *Journal of Neurophysiology,* **57,** 1498–1510.

Crossman, E. R. F. W. and Goodeve, P. J. (1963/1983). Feedback control of hand movements and Fitts law. Paper presented at the Meeting of the Experimental Society, Cambridge, 1963. Reprinted in *Quarterly Journal of Experimental Psychology* (1983), **35A,** 251–278.

Di Franco, D., Muir, D. W. and Dodwell, P. C. (1978). Reaching in very young infants. *Perception,* **7,** 385–392.

Ekman, G. and Junge, K. (1961). Psychophysical relations in visual perception of length, area and volume. *Scandinavian Journal of Psychology,* **2,** 1–10.

Elliott, D. and Allard, F. (1985). The utilisation of visual feedback information during rapid pointing movements. *Quarterly Journal of Experimental Psychology,* **37A,** 407–425.

Elliott, D. and Madalena, J. (1987). The influence of premovement visual information on manual aiming. *Quarterly Journal of Experimental Psychology,* **39A,** 541–559.

Elliott, J. M. and Connolly, K. J. (1984). A classification of manipulative hand movements. *Developmental Medicine and Child Neurology,* **26,** 283–296.

Evarts, E. V. and Vaughn, W. J. (1978). Intended arm movements in response to externally produced arm displacements in man. In J. E. Desmedt (Ed.), *Cerebral Motor Control in Man: Long-loop Mechanisms. Progress in Clinical Neurophysiology* (pp. 178–192). Basel: Karger.

Faugier-Grimaud, S., Frenois, C. and Peronnet, F. (1985). Effects of posterior parietal lesions on visually guided movements in monkeys. *Experimental Brain Research,* **59,** 125–138.

Faugier-Grimaud, S., Frenois, C. and Stein, D.G. (1978). Effects of posterior parietal lesions on visually guided behavior in monkeys. *Neuropsychologia,* **16,** 151–168.

Favilla, M., Henning, W. and Ghez, C. (1989). Trajectory control in targeted force impulses. VI. Independent specification of response amplitude and direction. *Experimental Brain Research,* **75,** 280–294.

Felix, D. and Wiesendanger, M. (1971). Pyramidal and nonpyramidal motor cortical effects on distal forelimb muscles of monkeys. *Experimental Brain Research,* **12,** 81–91.

Fitts, P. M. (1954). The information capacity of the human motor system in controlling the amplitude of movement. *Journal of Experimental Psychology,* **47,** 381–391.

Fragaszy, D. M. (1983). Preliminary quantitative studies of prehension in squirrel monkeys (*Saimiri sciureus*). *Brain Behavior and Evolution,* **23,** 81–92.

Gentilucci, D. M., Castiello, U., Scarpa, M., Umilta, C. and Rizzolatti, G. (1991). Influence of different types of grasping on the transport component of prehension movements. *Neuropsychologia,* **29,** 361–378.

Gentilucci, D. M., Fogassi, L., Luppino, G., Matelli, M., Camarda, R. and Rizzolatti, G. (1988). Functional organization of inferior area 6 in the macaque monkey. I. Somatotopy and the control of proximal movements. *Experimental Brain Research,* **71,** 475–490.

Georgopoulos, A. P. (1986). On reaching. *Annual Review of Neuroscience,* **9,** 147–170.

Georgopoulos, A. P., Kalaska, J. F., Caminiti, R. and Massey, J. T. (1982). On the relations between the direction of two-dimensional arm movements and cell discharge in primate motor cortex. *Journal of Neuroscience,* **2,** 1527–1537.

Georgopoulos, A. P., Kalaska, J. F. and Massey, J. T. (1981). Spatial trajectories and reaction times of aimed movements: Effects of practice, uncertainty and change in target location. *Journal of Neurophysiology,* **46,** 725–743.

Georgopoulos, A. P. and Massey, J. T. (1987). Cognitive spatial-motor processes. *Experimental Brain Research,* **65,** 361–370.

Georgopoulos, A. P., Schwartz, A. B. and Kettner, R. E. (1986). Neuronal population coding of movement direction. *Science,* **233,** 1416–1419.

Goodale, M. A., Milner, A. D., Jakobson, L. S. and Carey, D. P. (1991). Perceiving the world and grasping it. A neurological dissociation. *Nature,* **349,** 154–156.

Goodale, M. A., Pélisson, D. and Prablanc, C. (1986). Large adjustments in visually guided reaching do not depend on vision of the hand or perception of target displacement. *Nature,* **320,** 748–750.

Gottsdanker, R. (1973). Psychological refractoriness and the organization of step-tracking responses. *Perception and Psychophysics*, **14**, 60–70.

Haaxma, H. and Kuypers, H. G. J. M. (1975). Intrahemispheric cortical connections and visual guidance of hand and finger movements in the rhesus monkey. *Brain*, **98**, 239–260.

Haggard, P. and Wing, A. M. (1991). Remote responses to perturbation in human prehension. *Neuroscience Letters*, **122**, 103–108.

Halverson, H. M. (1931). An experimental study of prehension in infants by means of systematic cinema records. *Genetic Psychology Monographs*, **10**, 110–286.

Hartje, W. and Ettlinger, G. (1973). Reaching in light and dark after unilateral posterior parietal ablations in the monkey. *Cortex*, **9**, 346–354.

Hécaen, H. and Ajuriaguerra, J. de. (1948). Etude des troubles toniques, moteurs et végétatifs et de leur récupération après ablation limitée du cortex moteur et prémoteur. *Congrès des Médecins Aliénistes et Neurologistes*, 249–274.

Heffner, R. and Masterton, B. (1975). Variation in form of the pyramidal tract and its relationship to digital dexterity. *Brain Behavior and Evolution*, **12**, 161–200.

Held, R. (1961). Exposure-history as a factor in maintaining stability of perception and coordination. *Journal of Nervous and Mental Disease*, **132**, 26–32.

Humphrey, T. (1969). Postnatal repetitions of human prenatal activity sequences with some suggestions of their neuro-anatomical basis. In R. J. Robinson (Ed.), *Brain and Early Behavior* (pp. 43–84). London: Academic Press.

Hyvärinen, J. (1981). Regional distribution of functions in parietal association area 7 of the monkey. *Brain Research*, **206**, 287–303.

Hyvärinen, J. (1982). *The Parietal Cortex of Monkey and Man*. Berlin: Springer.

Hyvärinen, J. and Poranen, A. (1974). Function of the parietal associative area 7 as revealed from cellular discharges in alert monkeys. *Brain*, **97**, 673–692.

Iberall, T. and Arbib, M. A. (1990). Schemas for the control of hand movements: An essay on cortical localization. In M. A. Goodale (Ed.), *Vision and Action. The control of Grasping* (pp. 204–242). Norwood: Ablex.

Iberall, T., Bingham, G. and Arbib, M. A. (1986). Opposition space as a structuring concept for the analysis of skilled hand movements. In H. Heuer and C. Fromm (Eds), *Generation and Modulation of Action Patterns*, Exp. Brain Res. Series 15 (pp. 158–173).

Jakobson, L. S., Archibald, Y. M., Carey, D. P. and Goodale, M. A. (1991). A kinematic analysis of reaching and grasping movements in a patient recovering from optic ataxia. *Neuropsychologia*, **29**, 803–809.

Jeannerod, M. (1981). Intersegmental coordination during reaching at natural visual objects. In J. Long and A. Baddeley (Eds), *Attention and Performance*, vol. IX (pp. 153–168). Hillsdale, NJ: Erlbaum.

Jeannerod, M. (1984). The timing of natural prehension movements. *Journal of Motor Behavior*, **16**, 235–254.

Jeannerod, M. (1986a). Are corrections in accurate arm movements corrective? In H. J. Freund, U. Büttner, B. Cohen and J. North (Eds), *Progress in Brain Research*, vol. 64, (pp. 353–360). Amsterdam: Elsevier.

Jeannerod, M. (1986b). Mechanisms of visuomotor coordination. A study in normal and brain-damaged subjects. *Neuropsychologia*, **24**, 41–78.

Jeannerod, M. (1986c). The formation of finger grip during prehension. A cortically mediated visuomotor pattern. *Behavior and Brain Research*, **19**, 99–116.

Jeannerod, M. (1988). *The Neural and Behavioural Organization of Goal-Directed Movements*. Oxford: Oxford University Press.

Jeannerod, M. (1990a). The interaction of visual and proprioceptive cues in controlling reaching movements. In D. R. Humphrey and H. J. Freund (Eds), *Motor Control: Concepts and Issues* (pp. 277–291). New York: John Wiley.

Jeannerod, M. (1990b). The representation of the goal of an action and its role in the control of goal-directed movements. In E. L. Schwartz (Ed.), *Computational Neuroscience* (pp. 352–368). Cambridge, MA: MIT Press.

Jeannerod, M. (1990c). A hierarchical model for voluntary goal-directed actions. In J. C. Eccles and O. Creutzfeldt (Eds), *The Principles of Design and Operation of the Brain* (pp. 257–275). Rome: Pontificia Academiae Scientiarum.

Jeannerod, M. and Decety, J. (1990). The accuracy of visuomotor transformation. An investigation into the mechanisms of visual recognition of objects. In M. Goodale (Ed.), *Vision and Action. The Control of Grasping* (pp. 33–48). Norwood: Ablex.

Jeannerod, M., Michel, F. and Prablanc, C. (1984). The control of hand movements in a case of hemianaesthesia following a parietal lesion. *Brain, 107,* 899–920.

Jeannerod, M. and Prablanc, C. (1983). The visual control of reaching movements. In J. Desmedt (Ed.), *Motor Control Mechanisms in Man* (pp. 13–29). New York: Raven Press.

Jeeves, M. A. and Silver, P. H. (1988). The formation of finger grip during prehension in an acallosal patient. *Neuropsychologia, 26,* 153–159.

Johansson, R. S. and Westling, G. (1987). Signals in tactile afferents from the fingers eliciting adaptive motor responses during precision grip. *Experimental Brain Research, 66,* 141–154.

Kalaska, J. F., Caminiti, R. and Georgopoulos, A. P. (1983). Cortical mechanisms related to the direction of two dimensional arm movements. Relations in parietal area 5 and comparison with motor cortex. *Experimental Brain Research, 51,* 247–260.

Kato, M. and Tanji, J. (1972). Conscious control of motor units of human finger muscles. In G. G. Samjen (Ed.), *Neurophysiology Studied in Man.* Amsterdam: Excerpta Medica.

Keele, S. W. (1968). Movement control in skilled motor performance. *Psychological Bulletin, 70,* 387–404.

Kelso, J. A. S., Holt, K. G., Kugler, P. N. and Turvey, M. T. (1980). On the concept of coordinative structures as dissipative structures. I. Empirical lines of convergence. In G. E. Stelmach and J. Requin (Eds), *Tutorials in Motor Behavior,* (pp. 49–70). Amsterdam: North-Holland.

Klatzky, R. L., McCloskey, B., Doherty, S., Pellegrino, J. and Smith, T. (1987). Knowledge about hand shaping and knowledge about objects. *Journal of Motor Behavior, 19,* 187–213.

Kuypers, H. G. J. M. (1962). Corticospinal connections: Postnatal development in rhesus monkey. *Science, 138,* 678–680.

Lamotte, R. H. and Acuna, C. (1978). Defects in accuracy of reaching after removal of posterior parietal cortex in monkeys. *Brain Research, 139,* 309–326.

Landsmeer, J. M. F. (1962). Power grip and precision handling. *Annals of the Rheumatic Diseases, 21,* 164–170.

Langworthy, O. R. (1933). Development of behavior pattern and myelinization of the nervous system in the human fetus and infant. *Contributions to Embryology of the Carnegie Institution, 24,* 1–58.

Lawrence, D. G. and Hopkins, D. A. (1972). Development aspects of pyramidal control in the rhesus monkey. *Brain Research, 40,* 117–118.

Lawrence, D. G. and Hopkins, D. A. (1976). The development of motor control in the rhesus monkey. Evidence concerning the role of cortico-motoneuronal connections. *Brain, 99,* 235–254.

Lawrence, D. G. and Kuypers, H. G. J. M. (1968). The functional organization of the motor system in the monkey. I. The effects of bilateral pyramidal lesions. *Brain, 91,* 1–14.

Lederman, S. J. and Klatzky, R. L. (1990). Haptic object classification. Knowledge-driven exploration. *Cognitive Psychology, 22,* 421–459.

Lee, R. G. and Tatton, W. G. (1975). Motor responses to sudden limb displacements in primates with specific CNS lesions and in human patients with motor system disorders. *Canadian Journal of Neurological Science, 2,* 285–293.

Lemon, R. N., Mantel, G. W. H. and Muir, R. B. (1986). Corticospinal facilitation of hand muscles during voluntary movements in the conscious monkey. *Journal of Physiology, 381,* 497–527.

Lough, S., Wing, A. M., Fraser, C. and Jenner, J. R. (1984). Measurement of recovery of function in the hemiparetic upper limb following stroke: A preliminary report. *Human Movement Science, 3,* 247–256.

Lynch, J. C. (1980). The functional organization of posterior parietal association cortex. *Behavior and Brain Science, 3,* 485–498.

Marks, L. E. (1978). Multimodal perception. In C. Carterette and M. P. Friedman (Eds), *Handbook of Perception,* vol. VIII: *Perceptual Coding* (pp. 321–339). New York: Academic Press.

Marteniuk, R. G., Leavitt, J. L., Mackenzie, C. L. and Athenes, S. (1990). Functional relationships between grasp and transport components in a prehension task. *Human Movement Science, 9,* 149–176.

Marteniuk, R. G., MacKenzie, C. L., Jeannerod, M., Athenes, S. and Dugas, C. (1987). Constraints on human arm movement trajectories. *Canadian Journal of Psychology, 41,* 365–378.

Mather, J. A. (1985). Some aspects of the organization of the oculomotor system. *Journal of Motor Behavior, 17,* 373–383.

McGrew, W. C. (1989). Why is ape tool-use so confusing? In V. Standen and R. A. Foley (Eds), *The Behavioural Ecology of Humans and Other Mammals* (pp. 457–472). Oxford: Blackwell.

Megaw, E. D. (1974). Possible modification to a rapid on-going programmed manual response. *Brain Research, 71,* 425–441.

Meyer, D. E., Abrams, R. A., Kornblum, S., Wright, C. E. and Smith, J. E. K. (1988). Optimality in human motor performance: Ideal control of rapid aimed movements. *Psychological Review, 95,* 340–370.

Meyer, D. E., Smith, J. E. K., Kornblum, S., Abrams, R. A. and Wright, C. E. (1990). Speed–accuracy tradeoffs in aimed movements. Toward a theory of rapid voluntary action. In M. Jeannerod (Ed.), *Motor Representations and Control. Attention and Performance,* vol. XIII (pp. 173–226). Hillsdale, NJ: Erlbaum.

Meyer, D. E., Smith, J. E. K. and Wright, C. E. (1982). Models for the speed and accuracy of aimed movements. *Psychological Review, 89,* 449–482.

Milner, A. D., Ockelford, E. M. and Dewar, W. (1977). Visuospatial performance following posterior parietal and lateral frontal lesions in stumptail macaques. *Cortex, 13,* 350–360.

Mishkin, M., Lewis, M. E. and Ungerleider, L. G. (1982). Equivalence of parieto-precoccipital subareas for visuospatial ability in monkeys. *Behavior and Brain Research, 6,* 41–56.

Mishkin, M. and Ungerleider, L. G. (1982). Contribution of striate inputs to the visuospatial functions of parieto-preoccipital cortex in monkeys. *Behavior and Brain Research, 6,* 57–77.

Mountcastle, V. B., Lynch, J. C., Georgopoulos, A., Sakata, H. and Acuna, C. (1975). Posterior parietal association cortex of the monkey: Command functions for operations within extra-personal space. *Journal of Neurophysiology, 38,* 871–908.

Muir, R. B. and Lemon, R. N. (1983). Corticospinal neurons with a special role in precision grip. *Brain Research, 261,* 312–316.

Müller, F., Kunesch, E., Binkofski, F. and Freund, H. J. (1991). Residual motor functions in a patient after right-sided hemispherectomy. *Neuropsychologia, 29,* 125–145.

Napier, J. R. (1956). The prehensile movement of the human hand. *Journal of Bone and Joint Surgery, 38B,* 902–913.

Napier, J. R. (1960). Studies of the hands of living primates. *Proceedings of the Zoological Society of London, 134,* 647–657.

Napier, J. R. (1961). Prehensility and opposability in the hands of primates. *Symposia of the Zoological Society of London, 5,* 115–132.

Nashner, L. and Berthoz, A. (1978). Visual contributions to rapid motor responses during postural control. *Brain Research, 150,* 403–407.

Passingham, R. E., Perry, V. H. and Wilkinson, F. (1978). Failure to develop a precision grip in monkeys with unilateral neocortical lesions made in infancy. *Brain Research, 145,* 410–414.

Passingham, R. E., Perry, V. H. and Wilkinson, F. (1983). The long-term effects of removal of sensorimotor cortex in infant and adult rhesus monkeys. *Brain,* **106,** 675–705.

Paulignan, Y., McKenzie, C., Marteniuk, R. and Jeannerod, M. (1990). The coupling of arm and finger movements during prehension. *Experimental Brain Research,* **79,** 431–436.

Paulignan, Y., McKenzie, C., Marteniuk, R. and Jeannerod, M. (1991a). Selective perturbation of visual input during prehension movements. I. The effects of changing object position. *Experimental Brain Research,* **83,** 502–512.

Paulignan, Y., Jeannerod, M., McKenzie, C. and Marteniuk, R. (1991b). Selective perturbation of visual input during prehension movements. II. The effects of changing object size. *Experimental Brain Research,* **87,** 407–420.

Pause, M., Kunesch, E., Binkofski, F. and Freund, H. J. (1989). Sensorimotor disturbances in patients with lesions of the parietal cortex. *Brain,* **112,** 1599–1625.

Peele, T. L. (1944). Acute and chronic parietal lobe ablations in monkeys. *Journal of Neurophysiology,* **7,** 269–286.

Pélisson, D., Prablanc, C., Goodale, M. A. and Jeannerod, M. (1986). Visual control of reaching movements without vision of the limb. II. Evidence of fast unconscious processes correcting the trajectory of the hand to the final position of a double-step stimulus. *Experimental Brain Research,* **62,** 303–311.

Pellegrino, J. W., Klatzky, R. L. and McCloskey, B. P. (1989). Time course of preshaping for functional responses to objects. *Journal of Motor Behavior,* **21,** 307–316.

Perenin, M. T. and Vighetto, A. (1988). Optic ataxia: A specific disruption in visuomotor mechanisms. I. Different aspects of the deficit in reaching for objects. *Brain,* **111,** 643–674.

Phillips, C. G. (1986). *Movements of the Hand.* Liverpool: Liverpool University Press.

Pohl, W. (1973). Dissociation of spatial discrimination deficits following frontal and parietal lesions in monkeys. *Journal of Comparative and Physiological Psychology,* **82,** 227–239.

Poizner, H., Mack, L., Verfaellie, M., Rothi, L. J. G. and Heilman, K. M. (1990). Three-dimensional computer graphic analysis of apraxia. Neural representations of learned movements. *Brain,* **113,** 85–101.

Prablanc, C., Echallier, J. F., Komilis, E. and Jeannerod, M. (1979a). Optical response of eye and hand motor systems in pointing at a visual target. I. Spatio-temporal characteristics of eye and hand movements and their relationships when varying the amount of visual information. *Biological Cybernetics,* **35,** 113–124.

Prablanc, C., Echallier, J. F., Jeannerod, M. and Komilis, E. (1979b). Optimal response of eye and hand motor systems in pointing at a visual target. II. Static and dynamic visual cues in the control of hand movements. *Biological Cybernetics,* **35,** 183–187.

Prablanc, C. and Jeannerod, M. (1975). Corrective saccades. Dependence on retinal reafferent signals. *Vision Research,* **15,** 465–469.

Prablanc, C. and Pélisson, D. (1990). Gaze saccade orienting and hand pointing are locked to their goal by quick internal loops. In M. Jeannerod (Ed.), *Motor Representations and Control. Attention and Performance,* vol. XIII (pp. 653–675). Hillsdale, NJ: Erlbaum.

Rizzolatti, C., Camarda, R., Fogassi, L., Gentilucci, M., Luppino, G. and Matelli, M. (1988). Functional organization of area 6 in the macaque monkey. II. Area F5 and the control of distal movements. *Experimental Brain Research,* **71,** 491–507.

Robinson, D. L., Goldberg, M. E. and Stanton, G. B. (1978). Parietal association cortex in the primate. Sensory mechanisms and behavioral modulations. *Journal of Neurophysiology,* **41,** 910–932.

Rothwell, J. C., Traub, M. M., Day, B. L., Obeso, J. A., Thomas, P. K. and Marsden, C. O. (1982). Manual motor performance in a deafferented man. *Brain,* **105,** 515–542.

Sakata, H., Shibutani, H., Kawano, K. and Harrington, T. L. (1985). Neural mechanisms of space vision in the parietal association cortex of the monkey. *Vision Research,* **25,** 453–463.

Sanes, J. N., Soner, S. and Donoghue, J. P. (1990). Dynamic organization of primary motor cortex output to target muscles in adult rats. Long-term patterns of reorganization following motor or mixed peripheral nerve lesions. *Experimental Brain Research,* **79,** 479–491.

Schieber, M. H. (1990). How might the motor cortex individuate movements? *Trends in Neuroscience*, **13**, 440–445.

Schmidt, R. A., Zelaznik, H., Hawkins, B., Frank, J. S. and Quinn, J. T. (1979). Motor-output variability: A theory for the accuracy of rapid motor acts. *Psychological Review*, **86**, 415–451.

Soechting, J. F. (1984). Effect of target size on spatial and temporal characteristics of a pointing movement in man. *Experimental Brain Research*, **54**, 121–132.

Soechting, J. F. and Lacquaniti, F. (1983). Modification of trajectory of a pointing movement in response to a change in target location. *Journal of Neurophysiology*, **49**, 548–564.

Stein, J. (1978). Long-loop motor control in monkeys. The effects of transient cooling of parietal cortex and of cerebellar nuclei during tracking tasks. In J. Desmedt (Ed.), *Cerebral Motor Control in Man: Long-Loop Mechanisms* (pp. 107–122). Basel: Karger.

Stevens, S. S. and Guirao, M. (1963). Subjective scaling of length and area and the matching of length to loudness and brightness. *Journal of Experimental Psychology*, **66**, 177–186.

Susman, R. L. (1988). Hand of *Paranthropus robustus* from member 1, Swartkrans. *Science*, **240**, 781–784.

Taira, M., Mine, S., Georgopoulos, A. P., Murata, A. and Sakata, H. (1990). Parietal cortex neurons of the monkey related to the visual guidance of hand movements. *Experimental Brain Research*, **83**, 29–36.

Teghtsoonian, M. (1965). The judgement of size. *American Journal of Psychology*, **78**, 392–402.

Tower, S. S. (1940). Pyramidal lesion in the monkey. *Brain*, **63**, 36–90.

Trevarthen, C. B. (1982). Basic patterns of psychogenetic change in infancy. In T. G. Bever (Ed.), *Dips in Learning* (pp. 7–46). Hillsdale, NJ: Erlbaum.

Trevarthen, C. B. (1984). How control of movement develops. In H. T. A. Whiting (Ed.), *Human Motor Actions. Bernstein Reassessed* (pp. 223–261). Amsterdam: North-Holland.

Twitchell, T. E. (1954). Sensory factors in purposive movement. *Journal of Neurophysiology*, **17**, 239–252.

Twitchell, T. E. (1970). Reflex mechanisms and the development of prehension. In K. Connolly (Ed.), *Mechanisms of Motor Skill Development* (pp. 25–38). London: Academic Press.

van Sonderen, J. F., Denier van der Gon, J. J. and Gielen, C. C. A. M. (1988). Conditions determining early modification of motor programmes in response to changes in target location. *Experimental Brain Research*, **71**, 320–328.

von Hofsten, C. (1979). Development of visually directed reaching: The approach phase. *Journal of Human Movement Studies*, **5**, 160–178.

von Hofsten, C. (1982). Eye–hand coordination in the newborn. *Developmental Psychology*, **18**, 450–461.

von Hofsten, C. and Rönnqvist, L. (1988). Preparation for grasping objects: A developmental study. *Journal of Experimental Psychology: Human Perception and Performance*, **14**, 610–621.

Wallace, S. A. and Weeks, D. L. (1988). Temporal constraints in the control of prehensive movements. *Journal of Motor Behavior*, **20**, 81–105.

Wallace, S. A., Weeks, D. L. and Kelso, J. A. S. (1990). Temporal constraints in reaching and grasping behavior. *Human Movement Science*, **9**, 69–93.

Westling, G. and Johansson, R. S. (1984). Factors influencing the force control during precision grip. *Experimental Brain Research*, **53**, 277–284.

Wing, A. M. and Fraser, C. (1983). The contribution of the thumb to reaching movements. *Quarterly Journal of Experimental Psychology*, **35A**, 297–309.

Wing, A. M., Turton, A. and Fraser, C. (1986). Grasp size and accuracy of approach in reaching. *Journal of Motor Behavior*, **18**, 245–260.

Woodworth, R. S. (1899). The accuracy of voluntary movements. *Psychological Review Monograph Supplements*, **3**, 1–114.

Woolsey, C. N., Gorska, T., Wetzel, A., Erickson, T. C., Earls, F. J. and Allman, J. M. (1972). Complete unilateral section of the pyramidal tract at the medullary level in *Macaca Mulatta*. *Brain Research*, **40**, 119–123.

Yakovlev, P. I. and Lecours, A. R. (1967). The myelogenetic cycles of regional maturation of the brain. In A. Minkowski (Ed.), *Regional Development of the Brain in Early Life* (pp. 3–70). Oxford: Blackwell.

Zelaznik, H. N., Schmidt, R. A., Gielen, S. C. A. M. and Milich, M. (1983). Kinematic properties of rapid aimed hand movements. *Journal of Motor Behavior*, **15,** 217–236.

Chapter 8
Catching: A Motor Learning and Developmental Perspective

G. J. P. Savelsbergh*† and H. T. A. Whiting†

*Free University, Amsterdam, The Netherlands and
†University of York, UK

1 INTRODUCTION

Catching, as a spatially and temporally constrained action of a very precise nature (Alderson, Sully and Sully, 1974), has, not unnaturally, attracted considerable attention in the psychological literature from two perspectives: motor development and human performance/motor learning.

Historically, *motor development* research, going back at least as far as Gesell (1929), has been largely descriptive in nature and directed toward developmental changes in patterns of movement coordination with age, primarily as observed in phylogenetic skills such as walking, running, crawling, sucking, etc. In contrast, *motor learning* research has been largely addressed to theoretical questions using either narrowly constrained laboratory tasks or, on limited occasions, ontogenetic skills – such as driving a motor vehicle, typewriting or piloting an aircraft. Traditionally, these two areas of psychological endeavor have been kept distinct from one another. Such an artificial distinction has, however, been questioned: van Rossum (1987), for example, has advanced the thesis that 'practice' is a relevant aspect of motor development. He contends that the concept of skill acquisition should be centrally positioned in any theoretical model of motor development and has attempted to address the communality between motor learning and motor development by means of both a redefinition of terms and an elaboration of Schmidt's (1975) schema theory – particularly the concept of variability of practice.

More recently, Newell *et al.* (1989) pointed to the anomaly in distinguishing between the development of motor skills in the motor development literature – in which the acquisition of movement coordination has been a central concern – and the acquisition of skill in the motor learning literature where, at least in principle, the concern is similar. This artificial distinction, together with the kinds of skills studied in the two approaches – phylogenetic as against ontogenetic – rather than any inherent theoretical differences may account for the apparent anomaly. A further factor that may have given rise to the distinction is the tendency, in motor developmental studies, to focus attention on the concept of coordination (the

Handbook of Perception and Action, Volume 2
ISBN 0-12-516162-X

development of novel patterns of movement) and in motor learning on scaling changes within a particular movement pattern (Newell et al., 1989).

With these distinctions in mind, it might be expected that more common ground would be found between motor development and motor learning theorists when they choose to study similar skills. While this is less generally true, it is true for the skill of 'catching' although it has to be said that, in the context of motor development, the work on catching is sparse. For this reason, this chapter is divided into two main sections. In Section 2 a fairly coherent research line over the past 20 years – which can be categorized under the rubric *human performance/motor learning* – will be sketched out. This will be followed by Section 3 on the *development* of catching behavior in which there is much less coherency, but a number of interesting experimental lines which provide prospects for future work.

2 CATCHING: A HUMAN PERFORMANCE/MOTOR LEARNING PERSPECTIVE

It is a truism that experimental questions and paradigms reflect particular theoretical frameworks prevalent at the time. Examination of a particular research theme, such as 'catching behavior' is no exception and, when that theme persists over an extended period of time, it would not be surprising to discover a change both in the nature of the questions being asked as well as in the methodology being used in empirical work. The late 1960s saw a spate of experiments on interceptive actions such as 'catching' (Alderson, Sully and Sully, 1974; Sharp and Whiting, 1974, 1975; Whiting, Alderson and Sanderson, 1973; Whiting, Gill and Stephenson, 1970; Whiting and Sharp, 1973) conceived in the general framework of theories about information processing that were in vogue at that time. More specifically, the authors of these studies were concerned with the general question of the necessity of 'keeping the eye on the ball' in order to make successful one-handed catches. Such a question reflected concern about 'the amount' of information necessary on which to make decisions rather than on the 'nature' of that information *per se*. This orientation was in line with prevailing information processing notions, notably, that the human operator processes information in discrete samples, the basic concept being that input information is integrated over a period of time and processed as a single 'sample' or 'chunk'.

More generally, such approaches gave rise to the related concept of a 'perceptual moment' and the ensuing perceptual moment hypothesis[1] (Moray, 1970; Whiting, Gill and Stephenson, 1970) although there was little agreement among experimenters about the duration of such a moment. Those theorists who related the phenomenon to alpha rhythms (Murphree, 1954; Walter, 1950; White, 1963) considered it to be about 100 ms while, earlier, Ansbacher (1944) had deduced a value of 55 ms – a value similar to that obtained by Shallice (1964) using Michotte's (1963) data on the perception of causality. In discussing the psychological refractory period, Welford (1968) attempted to account for the grouping of signals that occur

---

[1]The implication here is that the brain processes information discontinuously in time, each operation lasting a 'moment' (Shallice, 1964). Such a concept has been termed by Stroud (1955) the 'perceptual moment' hypothesis.

in close temporal proximity by proposing a 'gate' which prevented subsequent signals entering the decision mechanism once it had started its computations. This 'gate', it was postulated, took an appreciable time to close: in the region of 80 ms. The possibility that such a moment is variable had been predicted by Stroud (1955), who suggested a range of 50–200 ms.

2.1 The Information Processing Approach to Catching

This was the conceptual framework that gave rise to the experiments mentioned above. An early pilot experiment involved a continuous ball-throwing and catching task (Whiting, 1967). Subjects were required to aim a ball attached by a string to the ceiling of the laboratory at a target (a small metal 'T'). After release, the ball continued on its elliptical flight path before being caught again by the subject and aimed, once again, at the target. Subjects performed a series of such repetitive actions for trial periods of one minute, the dependent variables being the accuracy of the aiming, the number of balls aimed and the total score (a product of number of balls and accuracy). Whiting (1967) was able to demonstrate that, once having had the opportunity to watch the ball *throughout* its trajectory while performing the skill, it was possible to maintain the standard of performance when, in later trials, opportunity for viewing the ball was spatially restricted (i.e. when sections of the trajectory were occluded according to a specific design).

A follow-up experiment (Whiting, 1968), using similar approaches, demonstrated the effect of training subjects under a series of restricted viewing conditions when, later, they were required to perform the skill without such restrictions. Training under some of the restricted viewing conditions was shown to be as effective as training without such restrictions. What was not clear from these experiments was whether what was learned in training was in fact carried over to the task in full light. This was the central question in a subsequent experiment (Whiting, 1970). Although the answer to this question is interesting, and will be returned to in later discussions about training, what was of more immediate interest was determining what subjects actually do when allowed reasonable freedom to develop their skill in a similar apparatus situation. To this end, subjects were given the choice, in an otherwise completely dark room, of viewing either the ball or the target to which it was aimed but not both at the same time. It was demonstrated that, as practice sessions progressed, subjects chose to watch the ball for less and less time before it reached the catching hand, i.e. they switched their direction of vision from ball to target earlier and earlier in the flight path of the ball. There were, however, marked individual differences in this respect.

From the point of view of coming to understand 'catching' *per se*, these earlier experiments had the limitation that they were confounded by the nature of the task, i.e. by the fact that the subjects themselves initiated the flight of the ball and thus had access to both *proprioceptive* and *efferent outflow* information about ball flight as well as the fact that an aiming (throwing) action, following on the catch, was also required. While these questions, in themselves, were potentially interesting, Whiting and his coworkers reverted to a paradigm in which only one-handed 'catching' of a ball – propelled towards them by a machine – was required.

Following on the findings of the previous experiments, and intrigued by the perceptual moment hypothesis, an attempt was made to determine whether there

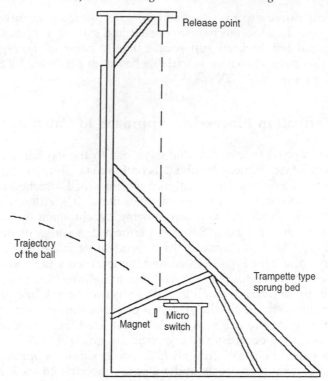

Figure 8.1. *Side elevation of apparatus.*

were critical time intervals for taking in flight information in ball-catching (Whiting, Gill and Stephenson, 1970). A solid perspex ball was caused to enter onto a parabolic flight path by means of a rather 'Heath-Robinson' type apparatus (Figure 8.1). An electronic device enabled the ball to be illuminated for predetermined temporal intervals of its flight path starting from the point in time at which it landed on the trampette (100, 150, 200, 250, 300 and 400 ms – the latter being the total flight time of the ball). Performance (Figure 8.2) – as indexed by number of successful catches – was shown to be better the longer the time that was available to view the ball. The possibility that sufficient information could be assimilated within one 'perceptual moment' seemed unlikely on the basis of these results. Once again, however, individual differences were apparent. Some subjects produced results under the 100 and 150 ms conditions that were remarkably good. Nine had catches of 9 or more (out of 20) under the 100 ms condition and 18 subjects achieved this level under the 150 ms condition. In retrospect, it has to be remarked here that subjects may well have been able to cope with more limited information if that information had been provided at a more appropriate time in the flight path of the ball. This issue will be picked up later.

Lamb and Burwitz (1988) attempted to replicate this experiment using a similar paradigm. While they were able to demonstrate improvement in catching perform-ance when viewing time was increased from 100 to 200 ms, no further improvement in performance was noted when the viewing time was increased to 300 or 400 ms. The results of this experiment, however, have to be considered in the light of

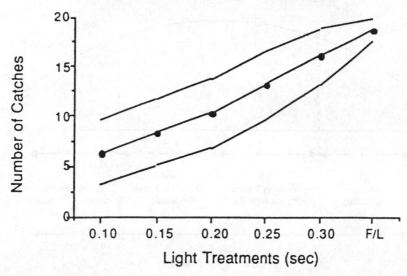

Figure 8.2. *Performance curve: combined means of all subjects (means + standard deviations). [After Whiting, Gill and Stephenson, 1970.]*

individual differences between 'good' and 'poor' catchers reported later in the chapter, as well as the methodological differences between their study and that of Whiting, Gill and Stephenson (1970) – in the former study, room lights were turned off for predetermined periods, whereas in the latter study only the ball was illuminated in an otherwise completely dark room.

It was at about this stage of the experimentation that Sharp joined Whiting as a research student. Having been nurtured in an information processing environment in Canada, it was perhaps not surprising that, having reviewed the previous set of experiments, he should come to the conclusion that a potentially important confounding was possible in the experimental paradigm being used. In increasing the amount of time for which subjects are able to see the ball, one also restricts the amount of time for which they are *not* able to see the ball. It might well be that the period of time for which they do not see the ball is necessary for the processing of information obtained during the viewing periods. To investigate this possibility the experimental paradigm illustrated in Figure 8.3 was designed, a tennis ball projection machine being used in place of the apparatus previously developed in the laboratory.

In Figure 8.3, DP represents the variable period for which the room was in darkness from the moment of ball projection to the moment at which the room was first illuminated. VP represents the time interval for which the room, and hence the ball, was illuminated; OP and LP represent the remainder of time for which the ball was occluded in flight. The distinction between OP (an independent variable) and LP (a constant time interval) is conceptual (since both are, in effect, occluded periods), necessitated by the fact that the period of occlusion following on VP cannot have an effect right up to the moment of ball–hand contact. There is, in fact, an interval preceding this moment (designated LP) – equivalent to a central nervous system latency plus movement time – during which, in classic information processing terms, any change in the stimulus conditions can have no effect on the response

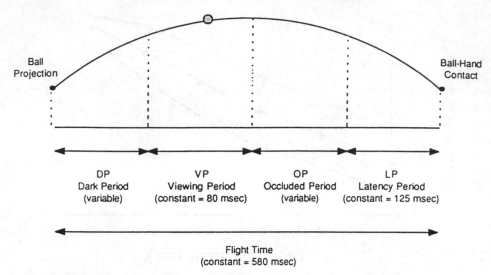

Figure 8.3. *Schematic representation of the experimental paradigm.*

of subjects. This interval was taken to be constant and shown to be in the region of 125 ms. Hence the effective occluded period – the variable of interest – is the interval between light offset and the beginning of LP.

In 1973, Whiting and Sharp demonstrated, in an experiment in which VP was kept constant at 80 ms but in which the occluded period OP was varied between 0 and 360 ms, that success in ball-catching is significantly affected by the temporal extent of the occluded period following a constant viewing time (80 ms) of the ball flight (Figure 8.4). Thus, this confirms Sharp's contention of the importance of the occluded period in catching behavior and reinstates the possibility that a 'percep-

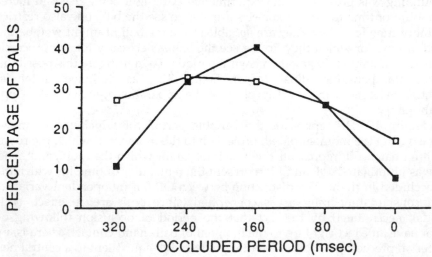

Figure 8.4. Percentage of all deliveries caught (—□—) and located (—■—) *as a function of occluded period. [After Whiting and Sharp, 1973.]*

tual moment' (if one wished to think in those terms) of 80 ms – at an appropriate point of time in the trajectory of the ball – could provide sufficient information on which to make a catching action.

The decline in performance between OP = 160 ms and OP = 320 ms suggests that subjects experience increasing difficulty when they have to predict ball flight over successively longer intervals of time. Such an interpretation found support in the then topical idea of the decay of information in immediate memory. If, however, the OP effect was due solely to prediction limitations, performance would have been expected to increase as OP changed from 160 to 0 ms. As the trend was, in fact, the reverse, an alternative answer was sought. When sight of the ball is available only late in its trajectory, subjects do not have sufficient time to process the necessary flight information and to translate their perception of the ball's flight into an appropriate response pattern.

In a subsequent experiment, the results of which are illustrated in Figure 8.5, Sharp and Whiting (1974) manipulated both OP and VP, demonstrating that both variables and their interaction were significant sources of variation. Generally, the effect of VP diminished as OP was extended. When OP was zero, increases in VP were followed by significant improvement in catching success until VP was 120 ms. Presumably, increasing VP within this range provided subjects with more time in which both to extract visual information and to select an appropriate response. Unfortunately, it was not possible to differentiate between these processes but it was notable that an increase in VP of as little as 20 ms could facilitate the entire process.

That this experiment left much unexplained was apparent from the fact that even under the most favorable conditions (VP = 160 ms; OP = 80 ms) subjects still only caught about 45% of the balls whereas in full light (the criterion for acceptance as a subject) the catches were nearer 100%.

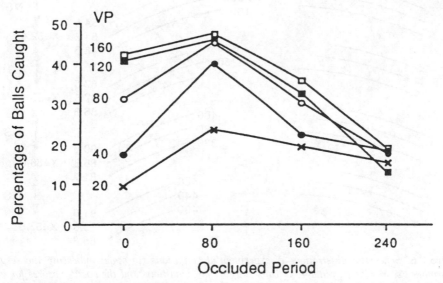

Figure 8.5. *Percentage number of balls caught as a function of viewing and occluded period. VP, viewing period. [After Sharp and Whiting, 1974].*

In a subsequent experiment, Sharp and Whiting (1975) extended the range of VP, OP and DP (Figures 8.6 and 8.7). They demonstrated that catching success was a discontinuous function of total time (VP + OP) up to about 120 ms, where a plateau is apparent, and from 240 up to 320 ms where a second plateau is reached.

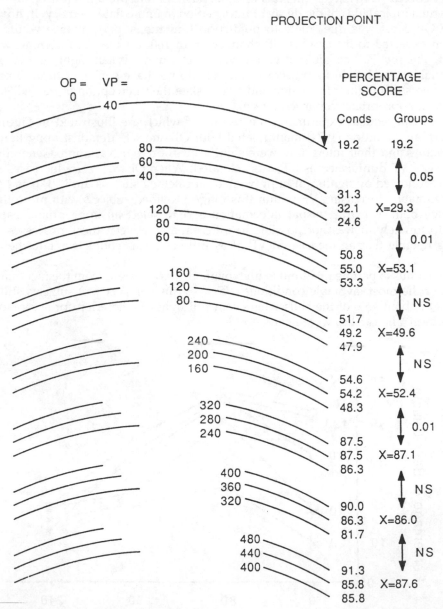

Figure 8.6. *Schematic illustrations of experimental conditions (to scale) indicating the respective performance scores (as percentages of balls caught) for conditions and the average scores for groups of conditions with the same total time (OP + VP). NS, not significant; OP, occluded period (ms); VP, viewing period (ms).*

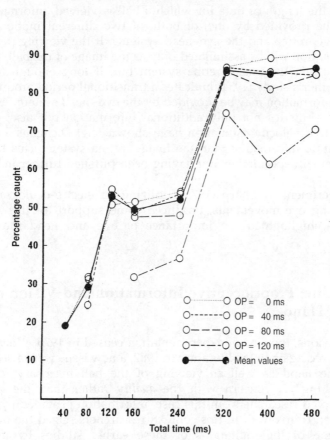

Figure 8.7. *Catching performance as a function of total time at each level of occluded period (OP).*

The former reflects the findings of the previous experiment and the latter demonstrates how, by extending the total time available for handling information, performance can be raised from around 50% to around 90% of balls caught.

This performance discontinuity was discussed as being linked to the notion of 'quality' of the visual image in information processing terms (Aaronson, 1967). In this respect, increasing the viewing period beyond a certain value (120 ms in the present case) may not provide any more information or a 'better' representation of the ball's flight until a further stage is reached. This was a notion discussed by Sharp and Whiting (1974) and in the earlier study of Whiting, Gill and Stephenson (1970), in which the concept of a critical viewing period was linked to the perceptual moment hypothesis. Such an explanation was, however, dismissed as being too speculative. Instead, a second hypothesis – related to eye movements (measured in this study) – was invoked. Thus, the discontinuity was discussed in terms of motion perception and a transition in processing from the image–retina system to the eye–head motion detecting system. The normal eye movement response to a moving object involves an initial reaction time and then a saccade to meet the object. At this point, if the object's velocity is not too high, the eyes begin tracking with smooth pursuit thereby maintaining a stable retinal image. Thus, dependent upon the length of time for which a ball is viewed, information about its motion may be provided by one, or both, of two different motion detection systems: the image–retina and the eye–head systems. If the viewing period is too short, then information will be assimilated only as the image of the ball 'paints' the retina and, hence, via the image–retina system but, if long enough for pursuit tracking (Westheimer's study (1954) indicates a transitional period around 200 ms), then additional information may be provided by the eye–head system. Apparently, the latter system provides not only additional information but also, as several studies of subjective velocity estimation have shown (e.g. Dichgans and Brandt, 1972), more accurate information than the image–retina system. This hypothesis, however, must remain speculative, not having been pursued further in a catching context.

A further experiment by Sharp (1975), utilizing an electro-oculographic technique for recording eye movements, produced some support for this hypothesis and, in addition, highlighted the importance of eye and head movement in ball-catching skills.

2.2　A New Line: Proprioceptive Information and Vision of the Catching Hand

For pragmatic reasons, this line of experimentation ceased in 1975. When the topic of catching appeared again in the literature in 1982, a new issue was raised, namely: is viewing of the hand as well as viewing of the ball necessary for efficient one-handed catching? A concern with the *quality* rather than the *quantity* of information occupied researchers – in this case, information provided by the active body member (hand) involved. In this context, researchers seized the opportunity to overcome some of the limitations of these earlier studies by utilizing as dependent variables, in addition to the number of balls caught, the number of spatial and temporal errors. The potential usefulness of such a refinement of analysis was appreciated in the literature as early as 1970 and received limited experimental attention from Whiting, Gill and Stephenson (1970):

> 'It must also be pointed out that in this experiment the task was to catch the ball. The quality of the catch was immaterial. In other situations in which, for example, the task involves doing something with the ball after it has been caught, the quality of the catch might well affect the efficiency with which the subsequent part of the task is carried out. Watching the ball for longer periods of time prior to its entering the hand might well influence the quality of the catch.' (Whiting, Gill and Stephenson, 1970, p. 271)

It was this kind of consideration that gave rise to the high-speed film analysis of catching by Alderson, Sully and Sully (1974). They demonstrated how the coordination of the interceptive action of catching demands conformity to rather severe spatiotemporal constraints. Their analysis emphasized two kinds of catching error: position and grasp (spatial and temporal), the former being defined as a failure of the hand to make contact with the ball in the region of the head of the metacarpals and the latter as a failure to close the hand at the correct time, even though the ball does in fact make contact with the hand in the metacarpal region. Overall, their analysis suggested (when subjects begin with their catching hand by their side) a

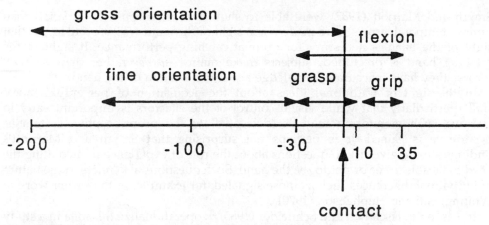

Figure 8.8. *The events in catching. [After Alderson, Sully and Sully, 1974.]*

gross spatial orientation of the catching hand some 200 ms prior to the catch, followed by a fine orientation some 50 ms later and, finally, a grasp and hold action which begins some 32–50 ms before the completion of the catching action (Figure 8.8).

Given that the study of Alderson, Sully and Sully (1974) has often been cited in the literature, it is worth drawing attention to the fact that only one ball velocity was used, $10 \, \mathrm{m \, s^{-1}}$, so that the generality of the analysis must await further evidence from studies in which a range of ball velocities is used.

It was Smyth and Marriott who, in 1982, initiated the new line of inquiry in posing the question as to whether sight of the hand was necessary for optimal catching performance. Such a question had, however, been raised some years earlier, albeit in the context of *reaching* and *grasping* rather than *catching*, by other experimenters. The assumption, then, was that corrections made during the course of reaching movements are based upon information arising from a comparison between the position of a 'seen' hand and a 'seen' target (Beggs and Howarth, 1972; Carlton, 1981; Keele and Posner, 1968). Thus, an initial ballistic movement of the reaching limb is, in its later trajectory, guided by dynamic visual feedback (Beaubaton and Hay, 1986). These findings, in developmental terms, have to be considered in the light of the demonstration by Whiting and Cockerill (1974) that, in a ballistic aiming task (propelling a small trolley up an inclined plane), children between the ages of 6 and 19 years were more accurate with vision of the target only than with vision of the hand only.

A similar rationale is seen to underlie the work of Smyth and Marriott (1982). Their thesis was that as articular proprioception is normally considered to provide accurate information about limb position, particularly in ball skills in which the eyes are thought to be occupied with tracking the ball, prevention of sight of the catching hand should, in principle, have no detrimental effect on catching performance. In their study, Smyth and Marriott (1982) excluded vision of the hand in a catching task–similar to that utilized by Sharp and Whiting–by means of a matt black perspex screen attached to the side of the subject's head, which, effectively, also prevented sight of the ball for the last approximately 150 ms. They also included a control condition in which a 'see-through' perspex screen was used.

Smyth and Marriott (1982) were able to show that more position (spatial) than timing (temporal) errors were made when sight of the hand was prevented, i.e. that sight of the hand is necessary for optimal catching performance. If sight of the catching hand is precluded, subjects make mainly *spatial* rather than *temporal* errors – they have inaccurate knowledge about the location of the hand.

In the light of traditional ideas about the acquisition of perceptual motor skill – particularly that while visual control of the effectors is important early in learning such monitoring may be 'delegated' to the proprioceptive system as experience is gained – it is perhaps not surprising that Smyth and Marriott's findings should give rise to questions about the role of experience in mediating the need to be able to see or not to see the hand. Such questions also relate to the nature of individual differences such as those signaled, for example, in the earlier work of Whiting, Gill and Stephenson (1970).

It was left to Fischman and Schneider (1985) to operationalize this idea in a study utilizing a similar paradigm to that of Smyth and Marriott (1982), but it is worth reporting that in their study the distance between ball projection machine and subject was 9.4 m (compared with 7 m in Smyth and Marriott, 1982) and horizontal ball projection velocity was $10.8 \, \text{ms}^{-1}$ (compared with an estimated $8.2 \, \text{ms}^{-1}$ in Smyth and Marriott, 1982). Unlike, the studies of Sharp and Whiting (1974, 1975), in both the Smyth and Marriott (1982) and Fischman and Schneider (1985) studies subjects started with their catching hand at their side rather than in the catching position itself. Thus, in the terms of Alderson, Sully and Sully (1974), both a gross and a fine orientation of the hand was necessary. Fischman and Schneider (1985) used as subjects so-called experts: baseball and softball players (experiment 1) and novices (experiment 2). Their study, it was claimed, provided some support for Smyth and Marriott's (1982) contention that sight of the hand is necessary for succcessful one-handed catching. This claim was based on their demonstration – in experiment 1 – that catching performance without an opaque screen being present was better than with a screen. There are, however, a number of reasons why their findings do not necessarily support the contention of Smyth and Marriott (1982) with respect to the necessity of viewing the hand (Whiting, 1986). In the first place, Fischman and Schneider (1985) failed to include a control condition involving a transparent screen despite the fact that Smyth and Marriott (1982) had shown this to have a detrimental effect on performance. That this may not be too serious an omission is apparent from subsequent studies in which no differences between screen conditions have been shown (e.g. Whiting, Savelsbergh and Faber, 1988). It may be that the differences signaled by Smyth and Marriott (1982) have more to do with the type of screen being used, i.e. attached or not attached to the head (head movements, as such, might have more serious consequences in their study). In addition, it has to be noted that the experimental populations in the two studies were very different. Any comparisons made in this respect, therefore, should be based only on the results of the second experiment of Fischman and Schneider (1985).

A particularly interesting difference found in the Fischman and Schneider study (1985), in contrast to that of Smyth and Marriott (1982), was more temporal than spatial errors when vision of the hand (and to some extent the ball) was obscured by an opaque screen. The fact that in both studies subjects were unable to see their catching hand at all in some of the conditions leaves open the question: if it is necessary to see the hand, at what stage in the trajectory of the ball is that necessary?

In both studies, subjects were able to see the ball but not the hand until a period between 150 and 200 ms (the 'latency period') prior to ball–hand contact. During the latter period, they could see neither ball nor hand. Fischman and Schneider's (1985) proposition that losing sight of the ball during the latency period affects the positioning phase of novice catchers but not of experienced ones, even if true, needs to be qualified since in the study by Alderson, Sully and Sully (1974) the gross positioning (at least) of the hand takes place some 200 ms prior to ball–hand contact. If anything, therefore, it is the fine orientation that takes place 150–200 ms before contact which is affected. No distinction is made by either Smyth and Marriott (1982) or Fischman and Schneider (1985) between these two spatial parameters. Further qualifications would be necessitated by the findings of Sharp and Whiting (1975) – previously addressed. Subjects in that experiment (unselected university students), of similar status to those used in the Smyth and Marriott (1982) study and in the second experiment of Fischman and Schneider (1985), were not able to see their catching hand under any of the conditions (since the room was in darkness) for, at least, the last 200 ms of ball flight. Nevertheless, under the block of conditions in which subjects could view the ball for periods of 480, 440 or 400 ms (see Figure 8.6) their catching successes were 91.3, 85.8 and 85.8%, respectively – equivalent to those obtained by Smyth and Marriott (1982) under normal catching conditions and, under the 480 ms condition, close to the performance of Fischman and Schneider's (1985) experts.

A further critique to be leveled at the Fischman and Schneider (1985) study is that they confound their (so-called) cultural differences with in-task differences in catching ability. The point is made in a study by Whiting, Alderson and Sanderson (1973) in which no significant differences could be demonstrated in one-handed catching under restricted viewing conditions between cricketers (expert catchers?) and noncricketers (inexpert catchers?). When, however, the two groups of subjects were reclassified on the basis of a task-specific measure (one-handed catching within the laboratory task-setting) into three ability groups, significant differences in catching performance between the ability groups under *restricted* viewing conditions were apparent.

Pursuing similar lines of inquiry to those of Smyth and Marriott (1982) and Fischman and Schneider (1985), Diggles, Grabiner and Garhammer (1987) – using a similar paradigm, except that their subjects were seated – claim to have shown, in accordance with Smyth and Marriott (1982), that occluding vision of the catching arm results in more errors, specifically more position errors. This finding was shown to be true for both skilled and unskilled subjects: a finding which, they suggest, indicates that both groups process information, visual and proprioceptive, in a qualitatively similar fashion. It should, however, be noted (Whiting and Savelsbergh, 1987) that in no way could the findings of this research enable statements to be made about information processing qualities. An interpretation of their individual differences finding (based on skill level) was marred in the same way as that of Fischman and Schneider (1985), i.e. subjects were classified on the basis of some external criterion (sport achievement) rather than on the basis of a within-task criterion without demonstrating that there was, necessarily, a significant relationship between the two.

The above picture is further confounded by a recent report of von Hofsten (1987) which maintains – contrary to Smyth and Marriott (1982), Fischman and Schneider (1985) and Diggles, Grabiner and Garhammer (1987) – that viewing the catching hand during the catching act does not seem to improve performance. This standpoint would seem to be based on the recently published work of Rosengren, Pick and von Hofsten (1988). In a similar ball projection paradigm to that used in the studies reported above, sight of the ball–in an otherwise dark room–was provided by means of luminous paint. Similarly, sight of the hand could be manipulated by the wearing (or not) of a white cotton work glove painted with dots of luminous paint at the wrist and finger joints. A number of other visual conditions (similar to those of Savelsbergh and Whiting, 1988) were also used in this experiment. An added advantage, from a generalization point of view, was the use of a combination of ball velocities (8.6 and 6.7 m s^{-1}) and projection angles (50 cm to the left, 50 cm to the right and directly on the center line of the subject's body, at both shoulder and waist height). The results obtained led Rosengren, Pick and von Hofsten (1988) to conclude that vision of one's hand does not aid in performance of the catching task.

It should be commented that catching luminous balls, in an otherwise dark room, introduces other confounding factors such as figure–ground relationships and environmental structure. In fact, Rosengren, Pick and von Hofsten (1988) demonstrated the facilitatory effect of the presence of a 'minimal visual frame' in the field of view on catching performance. The way in which such an enhancement of the visual environment would improve catching performance is open to a number of possible interpretations. From a cognitive viewpoint, for example, it could have to do with a facilitation of velocity perception. Thompson (1982) demonstrated that perceived velocity is dependent upon stimulus contrast, suggesting that this has important implications for velocity judgements in the real world as well as in laboratory experiments.

Taken together, the experiments discussed in this section, while interesting, are by no means conclusive–there remain a number of incomplete answers (Whiting, Savelsbergh and Faber, 1988). The question as to whether or not sight of the hand is necessary for optimal catching remains unclear since in the experiments reported a number of confounding factors make unequivocal answers impossible. Not the least of these is the determination of the composition of subject groups when attention is to be focused on individual differences, and the methods by which prevention of the sight of the hand is maintained. Figure–ground relationships in the different experimental set-ups might also account for some of the putative differences shown–particularly with respect to the study by Rosengren, Pick and von Hofsten (1988). However, in as far as the latter experiments would wish to invoke the detection of a 'time to contact' (tau[2]) information variable rather than the perception of velocity *per se*, the question here might be rephrased in terms of the effect of figure–ground contrast on the detection of 'tau'.

In an attempt to address some of these issues, Whiting, Savelsbergh and Faber (1988) carried out a pilot study in which a task-specific criterion was used to classify subjects into groups of 'good' and 'poor' catchers. The basic paradigm was similar to that of the studies discussed in the previous section. The methodologies of both Smyth and Marriott (an occluding screen; 1982) and Rosengren, Pick and von Hofsten (luminescent balls; 1988) (based on the limited methodology reported in von Hofsten, 1987) were used for different groups of subjects and two video cameras (at right angles to one another) were used in order to provide information about spatial and temporal errors. Whiting *et al.* were able to provide tenuous

---

[2]See page 478 for an explanation of tau.

support for the need of 'poor' catchers *only* to view the hand – they were shown to make more spatial errors when not allowed to view their catching hand than did 'good' catchers. In this way, they demonstrated that classifying subjects on the basis of a task-specific criterion of performance leads to a more refined qualification of Smyth and Marriott's findings. The most interesting finding of this study, however, was the apparent trend toward poorer performance on all three dependent variables (number of catches, spatial and temporal errors) as the environment became successively degraded, i.e. in going from a full light condition where sight of the hand was prevented by an opaque screen, to the condition where only hand or hand and ball, illuminated by ultraviolet light, was/were visible (Table 8.1).

Rosengren, Pick and von Hofsten (1988) report a similar effect of varying the amount of visual information on performance although their 'composite points' dependent variable did not allow separate analyses of spatial and temporal errors. The latter finding – of an effect on catching performance of degrading the environment in the studies of Whiting, Savelsbergh and Faber (1988) and of Rosengren, Pick and von Hofsten (1988) – raises the interesting question whether it is preventing sight of the hand *per se* that is responsible for the detrimental effects found or whether it is the successive degradation of the environment, of which preventing sight of the hand may be an aspect.

Table 8.1. *Means and standard deviations (SD) of catches (out of 30); position and grasp errors, under the five conditions for good and poor catchers. [After Whiting, Savelsbergh and Faber, 1988]*

	Good (n=15)		Poor (n=14)	
	Mean	**SD**	**Mean**	**SD**
Catches				
Test	29.29	0.961	19.22	4.146
TS	28.26	1.870	17.35	7.890
BS	26.86	3.159	18.35	5.943
UVHB	24.80	5.185	9.71	7.269
UVB	22.60	5.475	7.21	6.104
Position errors				
Test	0.06	0.25	4.42	3.10
TS	0.80	0.94	6.21	4.62
BS	1.20	1.56	8.28	4.14
UVHB	3.00	3.50	12.57	5.47
UVB	4.13	3.99	15.50	4.76
Grasp errors				
Test	0.53	0.64	4.64	3.20
TS	0.93	1.28	6.14	4.57
BS	0.86	1.35	3.35	2.59
UVHB	2.20	2.07	8.21	4.75
UVB	3.26	1.98	6.28	3.73

Test, in full light; TS, transparent screen in full light; BS, black screen in full light; UVHB, in dark with hand and ball visible; UVB, in dark with ball visible.

Comparing the results of conditions in which – in addition to the luminous ball – a visual frame, a visual frame and luminous hand, and luminous hand with no luminous frame were present, Rosengren *et al.* were able to show that performances under the two conditions that included the visual frame were significantly better than when only the hand was visible. In this way, they effectively answered this question in favor of the effects of degrading the environment. They had not, however, been able to show whether the effect was indexed by *spatial* or by *temporal* errors. To pursue this issue, Savelsbergh and Whiting (1988) replicated the Whiting *et al.* (1988) experiment utilizing a more efficient UV lighting system and a more objective assessment of the kind of errors made by subjects under the restricted light conditions. The latter was achieved by having subjects verbally report errors made under the environment light conditions. These could be compared with the more objective video records. On average, the specification accuracy was shown to be 83.62% – giving a reasonable degree of confidence in the verbal report of subjects under the environment 'dark' conditions. The following eight experimental conditions were utilized

Environment illuminated:
(1) N: Normal (full light) catching conditions.
(2) TS: Transparent screen – a flexible plastic screen (1.20 × 0.25 × 0.002 m) adjusted to the height of the subject, extending forward 25 cm to the side of the face. The screen made loose contact in the glenohumeral region of the subject. It was attached to two vertical strings (separated by a distance of 25 cm) which were fixed to the ceiling and to a heavy wooden bar on the ground which assured that they remained taut.
(3) OS: Opaque screen – as for the TS condition, an opaque (black) screen being substituted for the transparent screen.
(4) ST: Only the strings remained hanging, the foremost of these being in the subject's field of view. (Since conditions including strings alone as an external frame of reference were not shown to have any significant effect on performance, the rationale for their usage will not be discussed here.)

Environment dark:
(5) UVHB: Both hand and ball illuminated by a UV light in an otherwise completely dark room.
(6) UVHB + ST: Ball, hand and foremost string illuminated by UV light.
(7) UVB: Ball only illuminated by UV light.
(8) UVB + ST: Ball and foremost string illuminated by UV light.

The classification of subjects and the results are illustrated in Table 8.2. This shows the way in which subjects were assigned to groups on the basis of a within-task criterion (catching a ball in full light, 20 trials) applied on three successive occasions. The results confirm the large difference between the groups as well as the stability (over days) of the rating 'good' and 'poor' catchers.

The results presented in Table 8.3 both confirmed and qualified the previous findings of Smyth and Marriott (1982) with respect to an increase in the number of spatial errors – for 'poor' catchers only – when sight of the hand is precluded. They also confirm the previous speculations of Whiting, Savelsbergh and Faber (1988) that degrading the environment leads to a decrement in performance for both

Table 8.2. *Means and standard deviations (SD) of successful catches (out of 20) for both groups of catchers. [After Savelsbergh and Whiting, 1988]*

	Good (*n*=12)		Poor (*n*=10)		
Test	Mean	SD	Mean	SD	Statistics
1	19.58	0.49	10.70	3.95	7.35*
2	19.41	0.86	11.90	3.70	6.50*
3	19.75	0.43	13.80	2.27	8.46*

*Significant at 5% level.

Table 8.3. *Means of successful catches (out of 20) and number of spatial and temporal (grasp) errors under the eight conditions for 'good' and 'poor' catchers. [After Savelsbergh and Whiting, 1988]*

	Good (*n*=12)			Poor (*n*=10)		
Condition	Catches	Spatial errors	Temporal errors	Catches	Spatial errors	Temporal errors
ST	19.58	1	1	13.30	25	41
N	19.75	0	3	13.80	29	33
TS	19.83	1	2	13.10	29	41
OS	18.75	7	9	11.00	48	40
UVHB	18.75	6	9	10.40	38	58
UVB	17.58	12	17	8.30	57	59
UVHB+ST	17.91	8	17	10.90	41	43
UVB+ST	17.66	13	15	8.80	52	52
Total		48	73		319	367

ST, string illuminated; N, normal (full light) conditions; TS, transparent screen; OS, opaque screen; UVBH, in dark with hand and ball visible; UVB, in dark with ball visible; UVHB+ST, ball, hand and foremost string illuminated; UVB+ST, ball only illuminated.

'good' and 'poor' catchers (a distinction that was not possible in the Rosengren *et al.*, 1988, study). Since this was demonstrated for both the dependent variables 'number of catches' and 'frequency of temporal errors', it is likely that the former is merely reflecting the latter since spatial errors were not shown to be significantly affected by degrading the environment.[3] If this interpretation is accepted, there remains the problem of explaining the significant effect of not being able to see the hand on the number of catches made. For the 'poor' catchers, this would clearly seem to reflect the consequence of their making more spatial errors when the sight of the hand was occluded. For the 'good' catchers, the evidence is less clear-cut, since they did not make significantly more errors under this condition. It has to be

[3]However, the *P*-value of 0.084 showed a clear tendency that catching in the dark caused more spatial errors than catching in the light.

noted, however, that the actual number of spatial errors for 'good' in comparison to 'poor' catchers is very small.

It would seem justified on the basis of these findings, therefore, to conclude that occluding sight of the catching hand and degrading the environment produce separate, additive effects on performance. There is little support for speculation by Whiting, Savelsbergh and Faber (1988) that these two conditions may be reducible to the one effect of degrading the environment *per se*.

The finding of an effect of degrading the environment on the making of temporal errors is a vexed one in its own right and has to be seen in the light of Lee's (Lee and Young, 1986) concept of 'tau' – a specification of the time to contact of a moving object derived (directly) from the inverse of the relative rate of dilation of the closed optical contour generated in the optical array by the approaching object, rather than from the processing of positional, velocity and acceleration information derived from the flight of the ball. The argument is, in this respect, a default argument since it would not seem possible to demonstrate convincingly that subjects (catchers) use tau rather than computing time to contact from perceived distance and velocity. It does seem more 'plausible' an interpretation of skilled timing, however, as Lee *et al.* (1983) suggest. McLeod, McLaughlin and Nimmo-Smith (1986) make the additional point that a computation influenced by a range of cognitive inputs (e.g. position, velocity, acceleration) will inevitably lead to trial-to-trial variability in the time taken to perform it because the process will concatenate the variability of inputs.

If the tau explanation is invoked in the context of these results, a problem arises since no direct evidence would appear to be available for an effect of manipulating figure–ground relationships on the ability to make use of tau. Related evidence is, however, available from a study by Koslow (1985), who showed that the greater the contrast between stimulus and background, the farther away from the background the stimulus appeared to be. Translated to the 'environment dark' conditions in the above experiment, the ball should appear to be closer to the subject than it actually is. Why such a subjective phenomenon should have precedence over the more objective 'time to contact' variable tau is, at the moment, unclear.

The answer may be found by applying the methodologies utilized in published studies on the effect of contextual variation on velocity perception in the context of questions about the pick-up of tau. This might prove to be a profitable line of enquiry. Schiff (1965), for example, in his studies of optical 'looming' effects, points out that the difference between approach to and of an object becomes optically ambiguous in only a few special cases – as when a form is magnified against a uniform untextured background, e.g. clear sky. Thompson (1982), albeit using the movement of sine wave gratings, showed, at temporal frequencies below 8 Hz, that a decrease in contrast reduces apparent velocity. Gogel and McNulty (1983) showed perceived velocity to be a function of reference mark density. This is explained in terms of the increasing contribution of relative motion cues to the perception of visual speed as a function of the average separation (or average adjacency) of the moving point from surrounding reference marks.

While this kind of experiment from a tau perspective had not been reported in the literature up to 1988, the experiments of Savelsbergh and Whiting (1988) and of Rosengren, Pick and von Hofsten (1988) give rise to two more recent lines of development in the literature on catching about which there is much to say. In the first place, the earlier experiment of Whiting (1968), which showed the potentially positive effect of training in the dark (with only the ball visible) on performance when transferred to normal light, focuses attention on the question of changeover following experience, from visual to kinesthetic monitoring. This was supported by Rosengren *et al.*'s (1988) finding of a positive increment in performance following training in the dark. Second, the effect of degrading the environment on temporal errors, while calling for additional studies, suggested other experiments that merited priority before returning to this important question. These two further lines of development will be discussed in the context of concepts derived from ecological psychology.

2.3 Ecological Perspective on Catching

2.3.1 Spatial and Temporal Information Sources

An ecological perspective on the control of catching assigns primary importance to the fact that, for successful catching of a ball traveling on a relatively unpredictable trajectory, all the necessary information on which the spatial positioning and timing of the grasp of the hand is made must, by definition, be available in the optic array. The narrow time window within which the grasp has to be initiated for successful catching to occur dictates that the performer must, somehow, have access to predictive temporal information.

2.3.2 Predictive Temporal Source

The approach of a ball can be considered to give rise to an expanding optical array. Experimental work by Schiff had, earlier, shown that expanding shadow projections evoked avoidance behavior in rhesus monkeys (Schiff, Caviness and Gibson, 1962), adult fiddler crabs and 2-week-old chickens (Schiff, 1965). Bower, Broughton and Moore (1970b) reported defensive behavior of 10-day-old infants elicited by approaching objects giving rise to optical expansion (see also Ball and Tronick, 1971; Bower, 1972, 1974; Yonas *et al.*, 1977). It was Lee (1976, 1980), however, who demonstrated that the pattern of optical expansion, brought about by the relative approach between the actor and the environmental structure of interest, contained predictive temporal information. This information – the inverse of the relative rate of dilation of the closed optical contour of a surface generated in the optic array – specifies a first-order temporal relationship between actor and environment, namely, the remaining time to contact if the speed of relative approach were to remain constant. The expanding optical projections in the aforementioned studies thus specified imminent collision and, therefore, evoked avoidance behavior. However, the inverse of the relative rate of dilation, denoted 'tau' (Lee, 1976, 1980) is useful not only in avoidance behavior but also in circumstances such as the regulation of gait during the run-up phase of the long jump (Lee, Lishman and Thomson, 1982), the folding of the wings by gannets diving into the sea (Lee and Reddish, 1981), the jumping up to punch a falling ball (Lee *et al.*, 1983) and the directed striking of a table-tennis ball (Bootsma, 1988).

Of special interest is the study by Lee *et al.* (1983) because it demonstrated that the behavior of subjects was consistent with gearing of their actions to tau and not

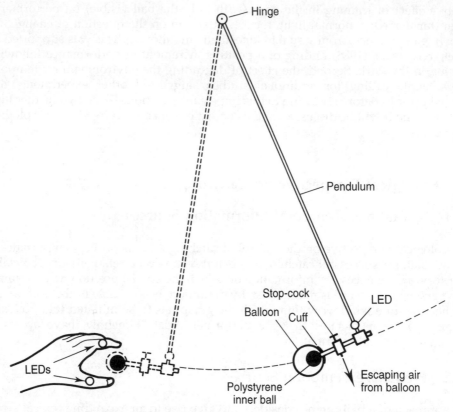

Figure 8.9. *The position of the light-emitting diodes (LEDs) on the hand and on the pendulum, and how the balls and 'deflating ball' were attached to the pendulum. [From Savelsbergh, Whiting and Bootsma, 1991.]*

to the real time to contact in the case of a discrepancy between the two – brought about by a nonconstant relative approach. Thus, tau appears to be a likely candidate for the timing of the initiation (and guidance) of the grasp in ball-catching. As the ball approaches, its image on the retina expands and the inverse of the relative rate of dilation directly specifies time to contact and, therefore, when to initiate the grasp. Evidence for the use of tau in catching was provided by Savelsbergh, Whiting and Bootsma (1991) in an experiment which required one-handed catching of a ball on a spatially predictable path. Subjects were required to catch a luminous ball attached to a pendulum (no spatial uncertainty) in a totally dark room (Figure 8.9).

Three ball sizes were used and randomized over trials. Two of these were 5.5 and 7.5 cm in diameter. A third ball could be made to change its diameter during flight from 7.5 to 5.5 cm. By using this third deflating ball, the provision of nonveridical information – in the sense that the time to contact of the approaching ball is not consistent with the rate of optical dilation – was achieved. The results showed that the time of appearance of the maximal closing speed was significantly later for the deflating ball than for the balls of constant size as a result of an overestimation of (absolute) time to contact. Even more important was the finding

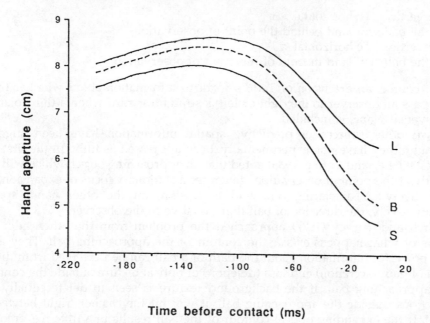

Time before contact (ms)

Figure 8.10. *The adjustments of the mean aperture of the hand for large (L), small (S) and 'deflating ball' (B) in the last 200 ms (sample 200 Hz). [After Savelsbergh, Whiting and Bootsma, 1991.]*

that fine adjustments to the aperture of the hand occurred not only for the ball of constant size but also for the deflating ball, even though subjects were (apparently) unaware (verbal report) of its 'behaviour' (Figure 8.10).

The subtlety of the tuning demonstrated in this experiment points to a closely coupled perception–action system, rather than some prestructured action pattern.

Interesting as these results proved to be, from a catching point of view it has to be appreciated that it is not only temporal precision that is necessary; spatial precision – in the sense of getting the hand into the right place and, of course, at the right time – is also a prerequisite. Has an ecological approach anything further to contribute in this respect?

2.3.3 Predictive Spatial Information

A series of experiments by Todd (1981) demonstrated that subjects can accurately predict whether an approaching object, simulated on a computer screen, following a parabolic flight path, will land in front of or behind them, even when only part of the ascending flight path can be followed. Todd demonstrated that such information is specified by the ratio (the 'Todd number') of two time to contact components, i.e. time to contact with the vertical (longitudinal) plane through the point of observation and time to contact with the horizontal (sagittal) plane through the point of observation. When the Todd number (Turvey and Carello, 1988) is varied, the following predictions can be made:

Tc vertical/Tc horizontal = 1
    the ball will land at the point of observation;

Tc vertical/Tc horizontal > 1
   the ball will land behind the point of observation;
Tc vertical/Tc horizontal < 1
   the ball will land in front of the point of observation.

Of course, an extension of Todd's work to information about whether the ball will pass an observer to the right or left is straightforward when a third plane, the transversal plane, is included.

Two other sources of predictive spatial information have been suggested, although they have not, experimentally, been addressed as fully. In the first place, Lee (1980; Lee and Young, 1986) noted that an approaching object, which will arrive exactly at the point of observation, generates a stationary focus of expansion in the optic array. A displacing center of expansion, on the other hand, specifies, quantitatively, the direction of ball flight relative to the observer.

Fitch and Turvey (1977) approached the problem from the other side, i.e. in terms of what happens *outside* the contour of the approaching ball. They argued that powerful information about the path of a ball can be perceived from different rates of gain (accretion) and loss (deletion) of optical texture outside the contour of the approaching ball. If the background texture is seen to delete equally in all directions outside the approaching ball, it will hit the catcher 'right between the eyes'. If the expanding optical contour of the ball results in a differing amount of deletion of background texture, the direction of ball flight, relative to the observer, is therein, quantitatively, also specified. Thus, while Todd's and Lee's analyses indicate that predictive spatial information is available from within the expanding optical contour of an approaching ball, Fitch and Turvey (1977) argue that the provision of a textured background enriches the information content of the optic array. Note that, in situations where no textured background is available, it should still be possible, according to Todd's and Lee's analyses, to make correct predictions about the direction of ball flight. This was confirmed in the training experiments of Savelsbergh (1990).

2.4   Training of Catching Behavior in a Degraded Environment

In one of their series of studies, Rosengren, Pick and von Hofsten (1988) demonstrated a significant increment in performance for a selected group of subjects (the better performers) when they were required to catch an extended sequence of balls ($n = 72$) in the dark (with only the luminous ball being visible). By means of a control condition in which subjects were required to stand in the dark for a similar period of time as the other subjects spent on catching (20 min), before carrying out a test (24 trials) in the dark room with only a luminous ball available, they were able to demonstrate that time spent in the dark *per se* does not result in any significant decrement in performance—at least within the period of time investigated. While these positive training effects are suggestive, it should be noted that Rosengren, Pick and von Hofsten (1988) used only relatively short periods of training within a single training session. Davids and Stratford (1989) also showed catching performance increments following longer periods of catching experience in which vision of the hand was prevented by an opaque screen in an otherwise light room. Experience (training) comprised 240 catching trials spread over a period of 3 days.

Neither of these training studies, however, looked at the effect of training under degraded environmental conditions (opaque screen or luminous ball/hand) on performance when subjects were *transferred into a full light condition*, thus leaving open questions about the practical relevance of such training effects and whether they are temporary or more long term. A transfer study of this kind (Whiting, 1968) was introduced earlier, albeit using a continuous ball throwing and catching task. Unfortunately, potentially confounding factors in that study prevented categorical statements about training effects being made.

With the limitations of these experiments in mind, Savelsbergh (1990) attempted to extend the findings by addressing the question of whether training under environmentally degraded conditions leads to improved performance when transferred into normal lighting conditions. In the first experiment of the series 17 subjects, matched on the basis of catching performance in full light, were divided into an 'environment light' ($n = 9$) and an 'environment dark' ($n = 8$) group. Following a further pre-test in full light (used both to confirm the selection as well as to provide baseline information) subjects were required, over a 3-day period, to continue training either in full light (environment light) or with only a luminous ball visible in an otherwise dark room (environment dark). The paradigm used required, on each day, a pre-test in full light (for both groups of subjects) followed by three training sessions (3×30 trials – either in the dark with only a luminous ball available or in full light) followed by a post- (transfer) test in full light (for both groups of subjects). The results are presented in Table 8.4.

An analysis of the results gave rise to two important findings. First, the subjects who trained in the dark showed increments in performance (in the dark) for each of the training days. Moreover, these increases were cumulative over days. Second, significant positive transfer effects for the environment dark group when changing at the end of each day's training sessions to performing (the test session) in full light (Figure 8.11) were found as well as significant negative transfer effects when changing at the beginning of each day's training sessions from the full light condition (pre-test) to the dark training conditions (Figure 8.12).

Unfortunately, in this study only the dependent variable number of successful catches was used so that it was difficult to pinpoint to what, precisely, the training effects could be attributed.

With respect to the performance increments following on training in the dark with only a luminous ball visible, however, circumstantial evidence points to an improvement in spatial accuracy. Davids and Stratford (1989) – previously discussed – using an extended series of trials ($n = 240$), demonstrated that it is the ability to spatially position the arm correctly in the line of flight of the ball which improved with task experience (training). Grasp (temporal) errors remained constantly high over trial blocks within conditions, i.e. they were not amenable to training which involved occlusion of vision of the catching hand.

Provisionally, the positive and negative transfer effects were attributed to a facilitation/inhibition of temporal accuracy provided by the presence or absence of a structured environment. It will be recalled that the Savelsbergh and Whiting (1988) study demonstrated that degrading the environment produced decrements in performance as indexed by an increase in temporal errors.

In a second of this series of experiments, Savelsbergh (1990) partially replicated the design of the first experiment, albeit using squash rather than tennis balls during the training sessions. Following a pre-test to establish that subjects were, indeed, relatively poor catchers, training took place over a period of 2 days. A

Table 8.4. *Means and standard deviations (in parentheses) of successful catches (out of 30) for each training session and post-test for each day for the 'environment light' and 'environment dark' groups*

	Environment light (n=9)		Environment dark (n=8)	
Day 1				
Pre-test	6.66	(4.47)	5.25	(5.00)
Training 1	8.00		3.37	
Training 2	9.22		4.25	
Training 3	8.33		4.62	
Post-test	8.44	(6.24)	8.62	(7.17)
Day 2				
Pre-test	7.55	(6.49)	9.00	(7.29)
Training 1	8.44		7.12	
Training 2	10.22		6.62	
Training 3	8.55		6.87	
Post-test	8.88	(7.79)	14.00	(8.44)
Day 3				
Pre-test	10.33	(7.90)	11.37	(4.44)
Training 1	9.55		10.50	
Training 2	11.33		11.00	
Training 3	9.55		10.25	
Post-test	10.55	(5.18)	14.37	(6.09)

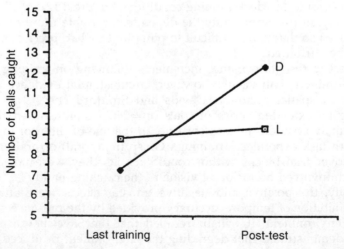

Figure 8.11. *The transfer effect from last training session to post-test. The significant second-order interaction training group × transfer. D, 'environment dark' training group; L, 'environment light' training group.*

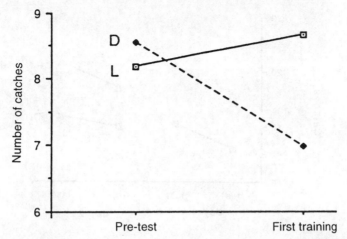

Figure 8.12. *The transfer effect from pre-test to the first session to post-test. The second-order interaction training group × transfer. D, 'environment dark' training group; L, 'environment light' training group.*

training day comprised 5 blocks, each of 30 trials, with a rest period of 2 minutes between blocks. The dependent variables (following Rosengren, Pick and von Hofsten, 1988) were:

(1) The number of balls caught (per block of 30 trials).
(2) The number of complete misses (per block of 30 trials).
(3) The total number of points scored (2 points for a successful catch, 1 for a touch but not caught, and 0 points for a complete miss) per block of 30 trials.

The results are given in Figure 8.13.

The results confirm the effect of training in the dark – with significantly more balls being caught at the end of the training days than at the beginning. Given the demonstration that, over training days, there was a significant reduction in the number of balls missed, Savelsbergh (1990) confirms the previous tentative conclusion that training in the dark leads to increased spatial accuracy. This does not, however, deny that such training effects may manifest themselves also in other ways. This could not be demonstrated with the design used.

What about the positive and negative transfer effects shown in the previous experiment? In an attempt to clarify the speculative conclusion that these effects could be attributed to a facilitation/inhibition of temporal accuracy, a third experiment was carried out. In the design used, it was important to bear in mind that transferring from dark to light and vice versa had an effect on whether or not the hand could be seen. Subjects from experiment 2 ($n = 29$) were divided, on the basis of their catching scores at the end of day 2, into four (transfer) groups of similar mean catching ability, the so-called:

H(and) group ($n = 7$); V(isual)F(rame) group ($n = 7$);
D(ark) group ($n = 7$); and L(ight) group ($n = 8$).

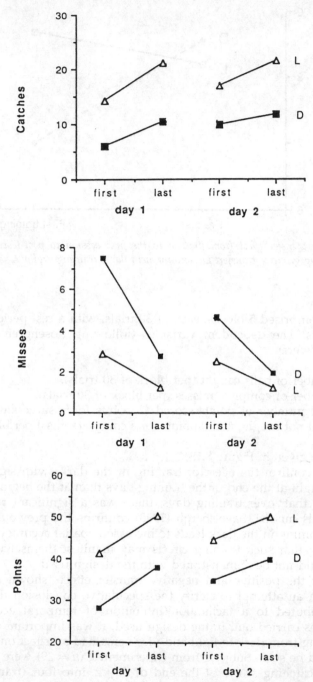

Figure 8.13. *Mean performances for the dependent variables: number of catches, misses and points over the 2 days of training. D, 'environment dark' training group; L, 'environment light' training group.*

The basic apparatus set-up was that of experiment 2. The visual frame (VF group) was constructed from a plastic-coated metal network (1.20 m wide × 1.85 m high) painted with luminescent paint (mesh 5 × 5 cm^2).

Subjects were required to perform 2 blocks of 30 trials in the dark (with only the ball visible)–training trials. This was followed by a rest interval of 2 minutes and, then, 3 blocks of 30 trials under one of the four transfer conditions (H, VF, D, L). Results are presented in Figure 8.14.

Analyses were carried out, separately, for the dependent variables (caught, misses, total number of points). The findings show a positive transfer effect–on all three dependent variables–when changing from performing in the dark to performing in the 'light' under two of the four conditions (H and L). There was no significant difference in this respect between the H and the D groups. A positive transfer effect from training in the dark to performing with vision of the hand and ball (H) or under the full light condition (L) for the dependent variable misses implies an improvement in the accurate positioning of the hand following on practice in the dark. An apparent anomaly was the decrement in performance when moving from the dark to the visual frame (VF) condition for all three dependent variables.

The purpose of this experiment was to provide more information about the effect on catching behavior, after a period of training in the dark, of two potential sources of information: the *hand* and/or a *structured environment*. The significant positive transfer effect for the dependent variable *number* of *misses* when transferring from training in the dark to performing with only the hand and ball visible (H) or to a full light condition (L) supports the idea that being able to see the hand, for subjects at this (relatively low) level of performance, does have a positive effect on performance. However, the fact that the transfer effect was so much more pronounced for the group who transferred into full light (L) for the dependent variables *number of points* and *number of catches* suggests that this is not the only advantage that being in the light contributes. This effect would appear not to be attributable to the modest, but significant, decrease in the number of misses alone, but suggests also (following on the findings of Savelsbergh and Whiting, 1988) an increment in temporal accuracy. If this explanation is accepted, there remains the anomaly of the negative effects reported when subjects transferred from training in the dark to performing with a visual frame of reference (VF). How is this anomaly to be explained? The significant negative effect on the number of *misses* when transferring from training in the dark to performing under the visual frame condition suggests that this condition affects the spatial positioning of the hand in a detrimental way. Why this should be so is not entirely clear.

In the first place, it is worth noting that Rosengren, Pick and von Hofsten (1988) also used a visual frame in their experiments. They found that the facilitation of the frame was rather minimal–but not negative, as in the present experiment. They also raise the question as to why the frame does not help more, offering the possible answer that it has to do with the fact that the frame is all in one plane, i.e. does not extend very far into the peripheral visual field. A fourth experiment run in order to examine the effect of different frames showed that a frame had no or only minor enhancing effects on catching (for elaborated discussion, see Savelsbergh, 1990; Savelsbergh, Whiting and Pijpers, 1992).

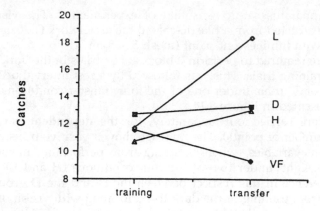

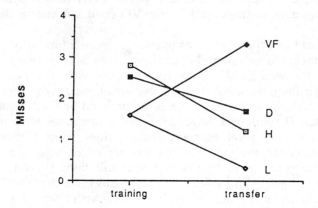

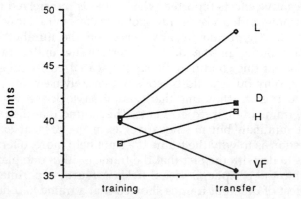

Figure 8.14. *Mean performances for the dependent variables: number of catches, misses and points for the training and transfer trials. D, 'environment dark' training group; L, 'environment light' training group; VF, visual frame group; H, hand group (hand and ball visible).*

While the results of these experiments lend credence to the idea – stemming from ecological psychology – that all the necessary information is, indeed, available in the ball, the corollary that it is, then, simply a matter of becoming sensitive to the relevant information' does not necessarily follow. While one of the interpretations of the findings is that training in the dark leads to subjects becoming more sensitive to the relevant information, Regan (1986; Beverley and Regan, 1973) has put forward an alternative explanation. This explanation is in terms of specific sensitivities of the human visual system – position in depth and orientation being two of these. In these terms, the major effect of training is on improving the subject's ability to use the visual machinery rather than on improving that machinery *per se*. More specifically, Beverley and Regan (1973) pointed out that:

'the relative velocity of the two retinal images provides a precise cue to the direction of motion in depth, and suggested that the brain might be organised to take advantage of this geometrical fact'.

A ball moving sideways produces retinal images that move at the same speeds in the same direction whereas a ball that will hit the head produces retinal images moving in opposite directions. The ratio of the retinal image velocities uniquely specifies the direction of motion in depth. This ratio is very sensitive when the trajectory passes near to the head (Regan, 1986). Thus, subjects, even when training in the dark, have access to information about stereoscopic motion in depth and position in depth.

This line of experimentation clearly gives rise to important theoretical questions which await empirical support. Such work is ongoing in a number of laboratories.

We return now to the second line of development signaled earlier. In so doing, it has to be recognized that in the more recent experimental work reported above on catching, particularly that over the past 3 years, recourse has been made to explanatory concepts like *direct perception* and *perception–action coupling* – concepts that are central to ecological psychology (Gibson, 1966, 1979; Turvey, 1977, 1990). Such concepts have given rise to new strategies for approaching problems of this kind and to the posing of a variety of new questions.

3 CATCHING: A DEVELOPMENTAL PERSPECTIVE

In the late 1920s and early 1930s, a number of descriptive studies (Gesell, 1929; Halverson, 1931) were addressed to the development of infant manual control. Halverson (1931) provided a detailed statistical record of infant prehension. He observed different styles of reaching or approaches to a cube by infants aged between 16 and 52 weeks. There was a clear shift in style of reaching at approximately 7 months of age. Immature, ballistic style reaching gave way to visually guided, indirect reaching which indicated ongoing corrections to the trajectory path. At a later age, direct reaching subsequently predominated.

At the time infants start developing reaching behavior for stationary objects (16–20 weeks) they will also successfully reach for moving ones: from about 18 weeks of age onward, infants are able to catch an object that moves at $30 \, \mathrm{cm \, s^{-1}}$ (von Hofsten and Lindhagen, 1979). In the case of reaching for moving objects, perception of space and motion, the coordination of hand motion and object motion, and the ability to predict an object's future location are all necessary abilities for success. Empirical evidence comes from a series of experiments conducted by von Hofsten and his coworkers (von Hofsten, 1980, 1982, 1983, 1984; von Hofsten and Lindhagen, 1979), in which children were placed in a semireclining infant seat and an attractive, colorful object traveled in front of them in a horizontal arc at about chest level. The object appeared either from the left-hand side or from the right-hand side of the child. Speed and distance of the object to the child were varied. Age of the infants, across all these studies, varied from 4 days to 9 months.

The von Hofsten studies demonstrated that infants were able to anticipate the future location of a moving object. Eight-month-old babies when presented with objects traveling in a horizontal arc at $60 \, \text{cm s}^{-1}$ demonstrated considerable catching competence. Some of them even caught objects moving at 90 and $120 \, \text{cm s}^{-1}$ at a variety of positions in front of them. It was suggested by von Hofsten that the infants used a strategy that consisted of an approach component and a tracking component – both play a role in the control of the movement of the hand in relation to an object. In the von Hofsten and Lindhagen (1979) study, the infants seemed to display their catching sophistication by not automatically reaching toward the object – independent of its approaching speed. The infants 'knew' whether a catch was possible or not. When the object was approaching with a high velocity no catching attempt was made.

These findings are in line with the results of a more recent pilot study carried out by Savelsbergh, Jongmans and Hopkins (1989). The question in this study was whether the position of the approaching object would affect with which hand infants would catch the object. For example, when the object approached from the left, would the infant use the left hand? The procedure was as follows (see Figure 8.15). The three infants, aged 2.5, 5 and 10 months, sat in a semireclining seat and an attractive yellow foam-plastic ball, with a tuft of red, blue, green and black cotton strings on top of it, was placed in the infant's hand (left and right separately) to familiarize him/her with the object. Two conditions were presented. In the static condition, the ball was placed on a table in front of the child within reaching distance at three different positions: at the midline of the infant's body, 10 cm to the left or 10 cm to the right. This condition required *reaching* behavior of the infant. The second (dynamic) condition required *catching* behavior of the infant. Here the ball, attached to a pendulum, was made to approach the infant at chest level, from three similar positions as in the static condition. In contrast to the von Hofsten studies, the ball approached the infant directly in the frontal plane. The time-window (the time available to make contact with the object) was therefore much more limited. The findings are reported in Table 8.5.

A clear difference as to whether or not an attempt was made is to be noticed between the two youngest infants in the *static* condition and between the two youngest and the oldest infant in the *dynamic* condition. The infant of 2.5 months showed only reaching behavior – when the ball was situated in front or to the right – and no catching behavior. The infant of 5 months showed reaching *and* catching behavior, but the frequency of the catching was less than that of the 10-month-old and was more dependent on the position from which the ball was made to approach. The 10-month-old infant did not appear to have any problems.

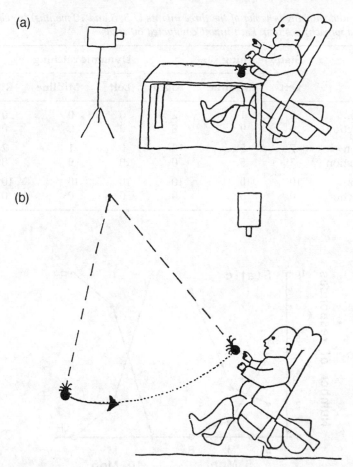

Figure 8.15. *The infants sat in a semireclining chair. (a) In the static condition the ball was placed on a table in front of the child within reaching distance at three different positions: at the midline of the infant's body, 10 cm to the left or 10 cm to the right. (b) In the dynamic condition the ball was attached to a pendulum.*

By means of a questionnaire, the hand preference of parents and grandparents was determined: all appeared to be right-handed. Figure 8.16 shows which hand the infants (5 and 10 months old) used in order to reach or catch for the different ball positions. Based on the questionnaire results, it seems safe to assume that the infants, if not already, will become right-hand preferent. This is probably why the 5-month-old infant used his right hand more and reached and caught more balls at the midline and right side position. The 10-month-old infant, in contrast, showed a right-hand preference only when the ball was situated at the midline and right side; for the left side the left hand was used. Despite the fact that only three infants were involved in this pilot study, the findings support the contention of von Hofsten and Lindhagen (1979) that infants seem able to make accurate 'judgements' about their own possibilities, e.g. when an object approaches from the left side use the left arm: when the ball moves too fast, no catching behavior is possible.

Table 8.5. *Reaching and catching behavior of the three infants (2.5, 5 and 10 months) in relation to the ball (approach) position. Each infant conducted 60 trials*

Age (months)		Static reaching			Dynamic catching		
		Left	Midline	Right	Left	Midline	Right
2.5	Reaction	0	1	2	0	0	0
	No reaction	10	9	8	0	0	0
5	Reaction	7	5	10	0	1	2
	No reaction	3	5	0	10	9	8
10	Reaction	10	10	10	10	10	10
	No reaction	0	0	0	0	0	0

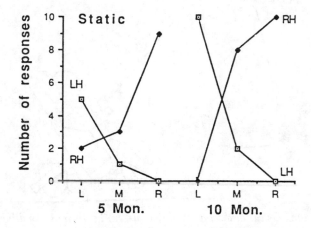

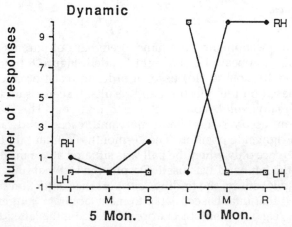

Figure 8.16. *The number of reaches (static) and catches (dynamic) for the infants aged 5 and 10 months, for the left (LH) and right hand (RH).*

Table 8.6. *(A) Percentages of successful catches and locations for the age groups 7, 10 and 13 years. [From Alderson, 1974.] (B) Percentages of successful catches and locations for the ages 8–13 years. [From Starkes, 1986.] (C) Percentages of successful catches for boys (M) and girls (F) of the age groups 9/10, 11/12 and 13/14.*

A			B		C		
(Alderson, 1974)			(Starkes, 1986)		(Savelsbergh and Whiting, unpublished data)		
Age (years)	Catches (%)	Locations	Age (years)	Catches (%)	Age (years)		
7	7	61					
			8	54			
			9	79	9/10	F	33.3
10	45	79	10	90		M	72.5
			11	92	11/12	F	47.0
			12	98		M	42.0
13	83	73	13	100	13/14	F	83.0
						M	76.0

Laszlo and Bairstow (1985) found that by the age of 1 year infants have acquired the ability to:

(1) Visually fixate stationary objects and visually accommodate objects at different distances.
(2) Reach for, and grasp, stationary and moving objects with a direct and economical reach.
(3) Reach out to stationary objects with only intermittent visual monitoring of the object.
(4) Anticipate impending contact, as the hand moves toward the object.
(5) Control reaching movements to stationary or moving objects that are planned and adapted to the particular circumstance.

For the age period 1–12 years there is a dearth in the literature with respect to catching behavior. Both Starkes (1986) and Alderson (1974) reported an increase in catching ability between, respectively, 8 and 13 years ($n = 56$) and 7 and 13 years ($n = 15$). Alderson's results showed that, with increasing age, children's ability to position the hand – as indexed by the percentage of correct locations – becomes more accurate (Table 8.6, column A).

Based on predictions made from earlier laboratory experimentation on motion perception, Alderson hypothesized that the prediction ability of 10- and 13-year-old boys would be sufficiently well developed for them to perform a simple one-handed catch in accordance with the adult temporal model, but that 7-year-olds would initiate flexion later than their elders, the degree of lateness being great enough to reduce their catching efficiency. High-speed film analyses of the catching behavior of children within these three age categories (13-year-olds: $n = 15$; 10-year-olds: $n = 13$; 7-year-olds: $n = 15$) showed a trend toward increasing accuracy with advancing age in both the spatial (confirmed in Starkes' experiment, 1986) and temporal components of a one-handed catch. It is interesting to note that some of the 7-year-olds found the task too difficult and would have preferred to have caught with two hands. For those 7-year-olds who did accomplish the requirements, it seemed that their major difficulty was in terms of temporal prediction of the grasping action. They initiated the flexion movement significantly later than the 10- and 13-year-old children. It should be noted, however, that the 7-year-olds still showed a surprisingly high degree of anticipatory behavior, their average positive error being only 20 ms. No differences in spatial accuracy were found between the 10- and the 13-year-old children.

Table 8.6, column C, provides unpublished data from the present authors concerning the one-handed catching behavior of a group of 64 children. Here, a ball projection machine delivered tennis balls with a mean velocity of $6.8\,\mathrm{m\,s^{-1}}$, at an angle of 30 degrees, from a height of 1.25 m. This ball velocity lies toward the upper end of estimates for indoor games, which Laszlo and Bairstow (1985) suggest is between 1.5 and $7.5\,\mathrm{m\,s^{-1}}$. Performance clearly increases with age.

Laszlo and Bairstow (1985) investigated the two-handed catching behavior of children between 6 and 12 years of age. Children were required to stand 3 m away from the end of a chute. The task was to catch a ball rolled down the chute. Setting the chute at different angles enabled different ball velocities to be created. By the age of 10–11 years (0.8 misses out of 40 balls) the children had reached an adult level of performance (0.4 misses out of 40 balls).

It should be noted that the developmental studies described so far have focused on the *goal per se* – catching or reaching for a ball. To this extent they are more akin to the studies from the motor learning literature discussed in Section 2. They make the point that the motor learning/motor development distinction is perhaps artificial and largely reflects the preference of the researcher for a particular kind of question.

A kinematic analysis of the arm movement in one-handed catching by children aged 9–13 years was carried out by Savelsbergh and van Santvoord (1989). This pilot study was in line with the coordination studies prevalent in the motor development literature. The central question was the way in which the elbow angle changes in relation to the shoulder angle. By digitizing – frame by frame (0.04 s) – three points on the arm (wrist, elbow and shoulder) and one reference point on the hip, displacement measures of the elbow and shoulder angle were obtained. In Figure 8.17, by way of example, the catching behavior of 4 of the 12 subjects involved is illustrated.

The mean approach velocity of the ball was $6.8\,\mathrm{m\,s^{-1}}$ and ball flight time was about 1.5 s (the ball left the machine at frame 1). The figure indicates that the shortening of the elbow angle starts between 900 and 1300 ms before hand–ball contact. The shoulder angle starts to extend *before* the elbow angle has 'stabilized' (indicated by arrows in Figure 8.17). This was the case in all 12 subjects and was independent of their catching ability. It is also clear from the figure that the angles continue to change right up to hand–ball contact rather than the hand 'stabilizing' and 'waiting' for the ball. What is to be seen is a relatively smooth continuous action adjusted to the approach of the oncoming ball. However, these findings are preliminary and it would be interesting to have more data on the kinematics of the catching arm in relation to different age groups and different ball velocities. This kind of data collection is ongoing by the present authors.

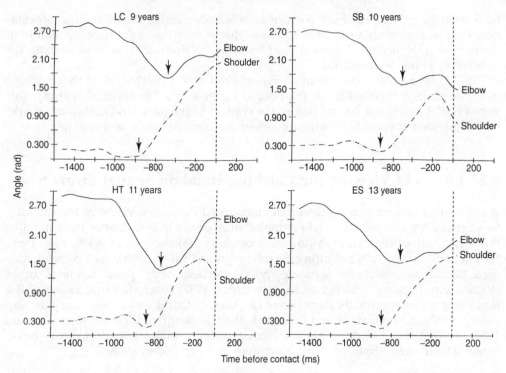

Figure 8.17. *The kinematic analyses for the elbow and shoulder angles (the dashed line indicates hand–ball contact).*

4 CONCLUSIONS

The bulk of the research discussed in this chapter takes as its departure point the fact that catching requires relatively precise temporal and spatial predictions. A failure to meet these requirements gives rise to two kinds of error: temporal and spatial.

4.1 Effect of the Length of the Viewing Time

While information about the trajectory of the ball is essential to successful catching, it is not necessary to view the entire ball trajectory. Prediction on the basis of prior information obviously plays a role and, in any case, information appearing late in the trajectory would have no steering function (Whiting, 1967). With a viewing period of 100–150 ms subjects (in the experiments of Whiting and his coworkers) reached a remarkably good performance level. This level was improved when viewing time was extended beyond 200 ms. Further extensions of the viewing time – to 300 and 400 ms – had little effect on catching performance. However, when vision of the ball was provided too early or too late in the flight path of the ball, and therefore the occluded period became too long (longer than 364 ms) or too short (shorter than 205 ms), catching performance was decreased. Based on this information later experiments were able to show that it was the 'total time' available (a combination of occluded period and viewing period) that was important for optimal catching performance.

The 'deflating ball' experiment of Savelsbergh et al., (1991) showed that catchers do, indeed, gear their action to the optical variable tau. However, this study also showed that in the last 200 ms before the contact of the hand and ball (particularly in the monocular condition) adjustments of the hand aperture still took place.

4.2 Effects of Viewing the Catching Hand on Spatial Errors

A number of experiments reviewed demonstrated that when vision of the catching hand is prevented unskilled catchers make more errors in positioning their hand in the flight path of the ball than do skilled catchers (Savelsbergh and Whiting, 1988; Smyth and Marriott, 1982; Whiting, Savelsbergh and Faber, 1988). As a consequence of a failure adequately to separate 'good' catchers from 'poor' catchers, other studies (e.g. Diggles, Grabiner and Garhammer, 1987) concluded that vision of the hand was necessary for all categories of catchers, or that it was unnecessary for any category of catcher (Davids and Stratford, 1989; Rosengren, Pick and von Hofsten, 1988), or that the absence of such information led to more temporal errors being made (Davids and Stratford, 1989; Fischman and Schneider, 1985).

4.3 Environmental Effects on Spatial and Temporal Predictions

Studies carried out by Rosengren, Pick and Hofsten (1988) and by Savelsbergh and Whiting (1988; Whiting, Savelsbergh and Faber, 1988) demonstrated that degrading of the environment by reducing the information available leads to an increase in catching errors. Under conditions in which only the ball (luminous) was visible in an otherwise dark room, Savelsbergh and Whiting (1988) showed that more spatial and temporal errors were made by both 'poor' and 'good' catchers. After extensive training (Savelsbergh and Whiting, 1992) in a totally dark room (the hand was not visible), however, where only a luminescent ball was visible, 'poor' catchers improved their positioning of the catching hand. From an ecological perspective, the ball must have provided spatial information to the subjects. The effect on the temporal errors in the dark is new (Savelsbergh and Whiting, 1988; Whiting, Pick and von Hofsten, 1988) and very interesting with respect to time to contact judgements. It is unclear why subjects should make more timing errors in the dark when the ball is visible and, consequently, the optical expansion pattern can be perceived. A possible explanation is that the subjects use a multisource strategy which is matched to the available information. A corollary to such an explanation might be that learning to make use of a particular source of information simply needs a long period of practice!

An enhancing effect on temporal and spatial precision was found when subjects moved from a dark environment (only ball visible) to a light environment. With respect to the temporal improvement: several studies of time to contact judgements – where the absence and presence of background grids were investigated

(McLeod and Ross, 1983; Schiff and Detweiler, 1979) – showed no enhancing effects of less, or more, structured environments. However, it should be noted that these studies were not *catching* experiments and, furthermore, the last 2 s of the path of the approaching object were not shown. The study of Savelsbergh *et al.* (1993) showed, however, that the last 200 ms play a role in catching behavior although the precise way in which the presence of an enriched background provides useful information during that time is not known. Some information in this respect is provided in the study by Rosengren, Pick and von Hofsten (1988) – already referred to – in which the presence or absence of a luminescent visual frame in a totally dark room was shown to affect catching performance. This frame appeared to enhance body stability and, hence, catching performance. (The effect of the environment on body stabilization has already been shown in the experiments of Lee and Lishman, 1977.)

4.4 Developmental Effects

The maturation of the nervous system imposes the most severe constraints on the development of reaching and grasping in the first year (von Hofsten, 1989). Already at an age of 18 weeks, infants reach for moving objects. The studies of von Hofsten and his coworkers (von Hofsten, 1980, 1982, 1983, 1984; von Hofsten and Lindhagen, 1979) showed that infants demonstrated considerable catching competence and at the age of 1 year reaching and grasping of moving objects become direct and economic.

There is a dearth of studies in the literature with respect to catching in the age period 1–12 years. Laszlo and Bairstow (1985), in one of the few studies available, focused on two-handed catching by children in the age range 6–12 years and found that catching ability reached adult level at the age of approximately 11 years. Corroboratory evidence is provided by the high-speed film analyses of Alderson (1974) which showed that, at the age of 10 years, positioning of the catching hand in the path of the ball (spatial accuracy) reached adult level.

ACKNOWLEDGEMENT

This paper was written while G. J. P. S. held a fellowship from the Commission of the European Communities for Science, Research and Development.

REFERENCES

Aaronson, D. (1967). Temporal factors in perception and short-term memory. *Psychological Bulletin*, **73**, 130–144.

Alderson, G. J. K. (1974). The development of motion prediction ability in the context of sports skills. Unpublished PhD Thesis, Department of Physical Education, University of Leeds, UK.

Alderson, G. J. K., Sully, D. L. and Sully, H. G. (1974). An operational analysis of a one-handed catching task using high speed photography. *Journal of Motor Behavior*, **6**, 217–226.

Ansbacher, H. L. (1944). Distortion in the perception of real movement. *Journal of Experimental Psychology*, **34**, 1–23.

Ball, W. and Tronick, E. (1971). Infants' responses to impending collision: Optical and real. *Science*, **171**, 812–820.

Beaubaton, D. and Hay, L. (1986). Contribution of visual information to feedforward and feedback processes in rapid pointing movement. *Human Movement Sciences*, **5**, 19–34.

Beggs, W. D. A. and Howarth, C. I. (1972). The accuracy of aiming at a target. Some further evidence for a theory of intermittent control. *Acta Psychologica*, **36**, 171–177.

Bernstein, N. A. (1967). *The Coordination and Regulation of Movements*. London: Pergamon Press.

Beverley, K. I. and Regan, D. (1973). Evidence for the existence of neural mechanisms selectively sensitive to the direction of movement in space. *Journal of Physiology*, **235**, 17–29.

Bootsma, R. J. (1988). The timing of rapid interceptive actions. PhD Thesis. Amsterdam: Free University Press.

Bower, T. G. R. (1972). Object perception in infants. *Perception*, **1**, 15–30.

Bower, T. G. R. (1974). *Development in Infancy*. San Francisco, CA: W. H. Freeman.

Bower, T. G. R., Broughton, J. M and Moore, M. K. (1970a). Demonstration of intention in the reaching behaviour of neonate humans. *Nature*, **228**, 679–681.

Bower, T. G. R., Broughton, J. M. and Moore, M. K. (1970b). The coordination of visual and tactual input in infants. *Perception and Psychophysics*, **8**, 51–53.

Bruce, V. and Green, P. (1985). *Visual Perception. Physiology, Psychology and Ecology*. Hillsdale, NJ: Erlbaum.

Carlton, L. G. (1981). Processing visual feedback information for movement control. *Journal of Experimental Psychology*, **7**, 1019–1030.

Davids, K. and Stratford, R. (1989). Peripheral vision and simple catching: The screen paradigm revisited. *Journal of Sports Sciences*, **7**, 139–152.

Dichgans, J. and Brandt, T. (1972). Visual–vestibular interaction and motion perception. *Bibliographia Ophthalmologica*, **82**, 327–338.

Diggles, V. A., Grabiner, M. D. and Garhammer, J. (1987). Skill level and efficacy of effector visual feedback in ball catching. *Perceptual and Motor Skills*, **64**, 987–993.

Fischman, M. G., and Schneider, T. (1985). Skill level, vision and proprioception in simple one-handed catching. *Journal of Motor Behavior*, **17**, 219–229.

Fitch, H. L. and Turvey, M. T. (1977). On the control of activity: Some remarks from an ecological point of view. In D. Landers and R. Christina (Eds), *Psychology of Motor Behavior and Sport*. Champaign, IL: Human Kinetics.

Gesell, A. (1929). Maturation and infants behavior pattern. *Psychological Review*, **36**, 307–319.

Gibson, J. J. (1966). *The Senses Considered as Perceptual Systems*. Boston, MA: Houghton-Mifflin.

Gibson, J. J. (1979). *The Ecological Approach to Visual Perception*. Boston, MA: Houghton-Mifflin.

Gogel, W. C. and McNulty, P. (1983). Perceived velocity as a function of reference mark density. *Scandinavian Journal of Psychology*, **24**, 257–265.

Halverson, H. M. (1931). An experimental study of prehension in infants by means of systematic cinema records. *Genetic Psychology Monographs*, **10**, 107–285.

Keele, S. W. and Posner, M. I. (1968). Processing of visual feedback in rapid movements. *Journal of Experimental Psychology*, **77**, 155–158.

Koslow, R. E. (1985). Peripheral reaction time amd depth perception as related to ball color. *Journal of Human Movement Studies*, **11**, 125–143.

Lamb, K. L. and Burwitz, L. (1988). Visual restriction in ball-catching: A re-examination of earlier findings. *Journal of Human Movement Studies*, **14**, 93–99.

Laszlo, J. I. and Bairstow, P. J. (1985). *Perceptual Motor Behaviour: Development and Assessment and Therapy*. New York: Holt, Rinehart and Winston.

Lee, D. N. (1976). A theory of visual control of braking based on information about time-to-collision. *Perception*, **5**, 437–459.

Lee, D. N. (1980). Visuo-motor coordination in space–time. In G. E. Stelmach and J. Requin (Eds), *Tutorials in Motor Behavior*. Amsterdam: North-Holland.

Lee, D. N. and Lishman, J. R. (1977). Visual proprioceptive control of stance. *Journal of Human Movement Studies*, **1**, 87–95.

Lee, D. N., Lishman, J. R. and Thomson, J. A. (1982). Regulation of gait in long jumping. *Journal of Experimental Psychology: Human Perception and Performance*, **8**, 448–459.

Lee, D. N. and Reddish, D. E. (1981). Plummeting gannets: A paradigm for ecological optics. *Nature*, **293**, 293–294.

Lee, D. N. and Young, D. S. (1986). *Experimental Brain Research*, vol. 15: *Gearing Action to the Environment*. Berlin: Springer.

Lee, D. N., Young, D. S., Reddish, D. E., Lough, S. and Clayton, T. M. H. (1983). Visual timing in hitting an accelerating ball. *Quarterly Journal of Experimental Psychology*, **35a**, 333–346.

McLeod, P., McLaughlin, C. and Nimmo-Smith, I. (1986). Information encapsulation and automaticity: Evidence from the visual control of finely-timed actions. In M. Posner and O. Malin (Eds), *Attention and Performance*, vol. 11. Hillsdale, NJ: Erlbaum.

McLeod, R. W. and Ross, H. E. (1983). Optic-flow and cognitive factors in time-to-collision estimates. *Perception*, **12**, 417–423.

Michotte, A. (1963). *The Perception of Causality*. London: Methuen.

Moray, N. (1970). *Attention: Selective Processes in Vision and Hearing*. London: Hutchinson.

Murphree, O. D. (1954). Maximum rates of form perception and the alpha rhythm: An investigation and test of current nerve net theory. *Journal of Experimental Psychology*, **48**, 57–61.

Newell, K. M., Kugler, P. N., van Emmerik, R. E. A. and MacDonald, P. V. (1989). Search strategies and the acquisition of coordination. In S. A. Wallace (Ed.), *Perspectives on the Coordination of Movement*. Amsterdam: Elsevier.

Prablanc, C., Echallier, J. F., Komilis, E. and Jeannerod, M. (1979). Optimal response of eye and head motor system in pointing at a visual target: I. Spatio-temporal characteristics of eye and hand movements and their relationships when varying the amount of visual information. *Biological Cybernetics*, **35**, 113–124.

Prablanc, C., Pelisson, D. and Goodale, M. A. (1986). Visual control of reaching movements without vision of the limb. I. Role of retinal feedback of target position in guiding the limb. *Experimental Brain Research*, **62**, 293–302.

Regan, D. M. (1986). The eye in ball games: Hitting and catching. *Proceedings of Conference on Vision and Sport*. Haarlem: De Vriesenborch.

Rosengren, K. S., Pick, H.L. and von Hofsten, C. (1988). Role of visual information in ball catching. *Journal of Motor Behavior*, **20**, 150–164.

Savelsbergh, G. J. P. (1990). *Catching Behaviour*. Meppel, Netherlands: Krips Repro.

Savelsbergh, G. J. P., Jongmans, M. and Hopkins, B. (1989). Reik- en vanggedrag bij babies. [Reaching and catching in infants.] Internal report, Faculty of Human Movement Sciences, Free University, Amsterdam.

Savelsbergh, G. J. P. and van Santvoord, A. A. M. (1989). Bewegingsanalyse van de arm bij eenhandig balvangen van kinderen in de leeftijd van 9–13 jaar. [Movement analysis of the limb in one-handed catching in 9- to 13-year-old children.] Internal report, Faculty of Human Movement Sciences, Free University, Amsterdam.

Savelsbergh, G. J. P. and Whiting, H. T. A. (1988). The effect of skill level, external frame of reference and environmental changes on one handed catching. *Ergonomics*, **31**, 1655–1663.

Savelsbergh, G. J. P. and Whiting, H. T. A. (1992). The acquisition of catching under monocular and binocular conditions. *Journal of Motor Behavior*, **24**, 320–328.

Savelsbergh, G. J. P., Whiting, H. T. A. and Bootsma, R. J. (1991). 'Grasping' tau! *Journal of Experimental Psychology: Human Perception and Performance*, **17**, 315–322.

Savelsbergh, G. J. P., Whiting, H. T. A. and Pijpers, R. J. (1992). The control of catching. In J. J. Summers (Ed.), *Approaches to the Study of Motor Control and Learning*. Dordrecht: North-Holland.

Savelsbergh, G. J. P., Whiting, H. T. A., Pijpers, R. J. and Santvoord, van A. A. M. (1993). The visual guidance of catching. *Experimental Brain Research, 93,* 146–156.

Schiff, W. (1965). Perception of impending collision: A study of visually directed avoidance behaviour. *Psychological Monographs, 79,* no. 604.

Schiff, W., Caviness, J. A. and Gibson, J. J. (1962). Persistent fear responses in rhesus monkeys to the optical stimulus of 'looming'. *Science, 136,* 982–983.

Schiff, W. and Detweiler, M. L. (1979). Information used in judging impending collision. *Perception, 8,* 647–658.

Schmidt, R. A. (1975). A schema theory of discrete motor skill learning. *Psychological Review, 82,* 225–260.

Shallice, T. (1964). The detection of change and the perceptual moment hypothesis. *British Journal of Statistical Psychology, 17,* 113–135.

Sharp, R. H. (1975). Skill in fast ball games: Some input considerations. Unpublished PhD Thesis, Department of Physical Education, University of Leeds, UK.

Sharp, R. H. and Whiting, H. T. A. (1974). Exposed and occluded duration effects in a ball-catching skill. *Journal of Motor Behavior, 3,* 139–147.

Sharp, R. H. and Whiting, H. T. A. (1975). Information-processing and eye-movement behaviour in ball catching skill. *Journal of Human Movement Studies, 1,* 124–131.

Smyth, M. M. and Marriott, A. M. (1982). Vision and proprioception in simple catching. *Journal of Motor Behavior, 14,* 143–152.

Starkes, J. L. (1986). Catching and spatially locating a ball in flight: Variables underlying their development. *Perceptual and Motor Skills, 63,* 1275–1286.

Stroud, J. M. (1955). The fine structure of psychological time. In H. Quastler (Ed.), *Information Theory in Psychology*. Illinois: Free Press.

Thompson, P. (1982). Perceived rate of movement depends on contrast. *Vision Research, 22,* 377–380.

Todd, J. T. (1981). Visual information about moving objects. *Journal of Experimental Psychology: Human Perception and Performance, 7,* 795–810.

Turvey, M. T. (1977). Preliminaries to a theory of action with reference to vision. In R. Shaw and G. Bransford (Eds.), *Perceiving, Acting and Knowing: Towards an Ecological Psychology*. Hillsdale, NJ: Erlbaum.

Turvey, M. T. (1990). The challenge of a physical account of actions: A personal view. In H. T. A. Whiting, O. G. Meijer and P. C. W. van Wieringen (Eds), *The Natural-physical Approach to Human Movement*. Amsterdam: Free University Press.

Turvey, M. T. and Carello, C. (1988). Exploring a law-based ecological approach to skilled action. In A. M. Colley and J. R. Beech (Eds), *Cognition and Action in Skilled Behaviour*. Amsterdam: North-Holland.

van Rossum, J. H. A. (1987). Motor development and practise. PhD Thesis. Amsterdam: Free University Press.

von Hofsten, C. (1980). Predictive reaching for moving objects by human infants. *Journal of Experimental Child Psychology, 30,* 369–382.

von Hofsten, C. (1982). Eye–hand coordination in the newborn. *Developmental Psychology, 18,* 450–461.

von Hofsten, C. (1983). Catching skills in infancy. *Journal of Experimental Psychology: Human Perception and Performance, 9,* 75–85.

von Hofsten, C. (1984). Developmental changes in the organization of prereaching movements. *Developmental Psychology, 20,* 378–388.

von Hofsten, C. (1987). Catching. In H. Heuer and A. P. Sanders (Eds), *Perspectives on Perception and Action*. Hillsdale, NJ: Erlbaum.

von Hofsten, C. (1989). Mastering reaching and grasping: The development of manual skills in infancy. In S. A. Wallace (Ed.), *Perspectives on the Coordination of Movement*. Amsterdam: North-Holland.

von Hofsten, C. and Lindhagen, K. (1979). Observations on the development of reaching for moving objects. *Journal of Experimental Child Psychology*, **28**, 158–173.

Walter, W. G. (1950). The functions of electrical rhythms in the brain. *Journal of Mental Science*, **96**, 1–31.

Welford (1968). *Fundamentals of Skill*. London: Methuen.

Westheimer, G. (1954). Eye movement responses to a horizontally moving visual stimulus. *Archives of Ophthalmology*, **53**, 932–941.

White, C. T. (1963). Eye movement, evoked responses and visual perceptions: Some speculations. In A. F. Sanders (Ed.), *Attention and Performance*. Amsterdam: North-Holland.

Whiting, H. T. A. (1967). Visual Motor Co-ordination. Unpublished PhD Thesis, University of Leeds, UK.

Whiting, H. T. A. (1968). Training in a continuous ball throwing and catching task. *Ergonomics*, **11**, 375–382.

Whiting, H. T. A. (1970). An operational analysis of a continuous ball throwing and catching task. *Ergonomics*, **13**, 445–454.

Whiting, H. T. A. (1986). Isn't there a catch in it somewhere? *Journal of Motor Behavior*, **18**, 486–491.

Whiting, H. T. A., Alderson, G. J. K. and Sanderson, F. H. (1973). Critical time intervals for viewing and individual differences in performance on a ball-catching task. *International Journal of Sport Psychology*, **4**, 155–166.

Whiting, H. T. A. and Cockerill, I. M. (1974). Eyes on hand–eyes on target?. *Journal of Motor Behavior*, **6**, 27–32.

Whiting, H. T. A., Gill, B. and Stephenson, J. (1970). Critical time intervals for taking in flight information in a ball-catching task. *Ergonomics*, **13**, 265–272.

Whiting, H. T. A. and Savelsbergh, G. J. P. (1987). Catch as catch can. *Perceptual and Motor Skills*, **65**, 353–354.

Whiting, H. T. A., Savelsbergh, G. J. P. and Faber, C. M. (1988). Catch questions and incomplete answers. In A. M. Colley and J. R. Beech (Eds.), *Cognition and Action in Skilled Behaviour*. Amsterdam: North-Holland.

Whiting, H. T. A. and Sharp, R. H. (1973). Visual occlusion factors in a discrete ball catching task. *Journal of Motor Behavior*, **6**, 11–16.

Yonas, A., Bechtold, A. G., Frankel, D., Gordon R. F., McRobert G., Norcia A. and Sternfels, S. (1977). Development of sensitivity to information for impending collision. *Perception and Psychophysics*, **21**, 97–104.

Chapter 9

Speaking

Carol A. Fowler

Dartmouth College and Haskins Laboratories, New Haven, USA

1 INTRODUCTION

Language users can speak understandably about almost anything, and they can do so almost anywhere. Moreover, the sequences of words composing their utterances can be novel in the experience both of the speaker and of the hearer. All that is required for novel utterances to be understood, roughly, is a competent speaker and a competent listener. A theory of the speaker's competence helps to define the problem of speech motor control. Consider, for example, the problem of sequencing that arises from the linguistic requirement, if understandable utterances are allowed sometimes to be novel, that sentences and words have an internal structure. Comprehension of novel utterances by hearers is possible because utterances universally are composed of familiar parts; that is, all utterances are composed of words that, ideally, are in the lexicon of the hearer as well as of the speaker. More than that, the familiar words of a novel utterance are ordered or otherwise marked according to syntactic conventions of the language, and the syntactic conventions allow the hearer to identify the roles of words in the utterance. Thereby they allow the listener to know the roles of the words' referents in the event being talked about – even if the listener has not witnessed the event or anything much like it.

To enable understandable communication about almost anything, languages need to have large, expandable lexicons of familiar words. And for lexicons to be large and expandable, with all of their component words pronounceable, words of the lexicon must have an internal structure. Words of spoken languages universally are composed of a relatively small number (11 to 141 across the languages in a recent survey; Maddieson, 1984) of meaningless parts that I will call variously phonemes, phonological or phonetic segments, or consonants and vowels. These meaningless components of words have attributes called 'features' that relate in some way to vocal tract behaviors or postures of the articulators of the vocal tract.

Hockett (1960) referred to this dual, ruleful layering of language units – that is, the ruleful ordering of meaningful words in sentences, and of meaningless consonants and vowels in words – as 'duality of patterning'. It is universal to human languages and, Hockett speculated, unique to them. Unique or not, it establishes as a major problem for talkers one of realizing units of the language in their proper sequence.

Handbook of Perception and Action, Volume 2
ISBN 0-12-516162-X

Notice that this is not a problem characteristic of every activity we perform. In basic activities, such as walking, breathing and chewing, there is sequencing but the sequencing is not arbitrary with respect to the physical implementing system. Accordingly, there are no misordering errors in these activities (that is, for example, we never inadvertently inhale twice in succession without exhaling in between). We do make action errors other than spoken ones (Norman, 1981; Reason, 1979), but error-prone actions like speech, and unlike breathing, walking and chewing, are those whose sequencing is arbitrary from the perspective of the implementing physical system.

Not only is there an ordering problem in speech but, in addition, the problem is not alleviated very much for the talker by environmental constraints on sequencing. To enable discussion of almost anything almost anywhere, the behaviors of the talker that implement a spoken communication must, to a considerable degree, be unconstrained by the environmental setting. Or, to put it more positively, to a very great degree, constraints on the serial vocal tract activities that realize a syntactically coherent linguistic message must come from a continuously changing speech plan.

The foregoing discussion of the structure of language is quite familiar perhaps, but in this instance familiarity does not imply any considerable depth of understanding. Despite a near consensus that words and phonemes are real constituents of the language, there is no consensus yet as to their essential properties or as to the media (neural, articulatory, acoustic) in which they can be manifest. Likewise, although theorists are well aware of the serial ordering problem for speakers, they have not reached consensus on how the problem is solved by talkers.

In the review that follows, I will focus on both general issues: the nature of units of spoken language and the means by which they are ordered in speech production. I will restrict the review largely to Hockett's lower of the dual tiers of language. That is, I will not consider how talkers choose what to say, or to any great degree how they select words to say or achieve syntactically acceptable utterances. Rather, given an intent by a talker to produce a particular sequence of words, I will consider what the essential properties of a planned string of words may be and how the plan is implemented as a sequentially ordered activity of the vocal tract.

In the next two major sections of the chapter, I will contrast two theoretical proposals concerning the nature of consonants and vowels. The proposals lead to quite different perspectives on speech activity and on the relationship it bears to those units of the language. A fourth section of the review will examine certain prosodic properties of utterances that emerge when sequences of phonological segments are realized as sequentially ordered, dynamical activities of the vocal tract.

I will introduce each section by describing relevant theories of language structure proposed in the field of linguistics. While foci of linguistic investigation are in some ways far removed from those of investigations of speech-motor control, there are important intersections. One occurs because speech-motor theorists have largely guessed that the units of the language identified in linguistic theory – with the essential attributes that linguists have ascribed to them – will turn out to be the units of the language that talkers aspire to utter. (However, see Kelso, Tuller and Saltzman, 1986, and also Moll, Zimmermann and Smith, 1977, who criticize this approach.) Accordingly, linguistic theories – particularly of phonology – are influential in shaping the form that theories of language and speech production have taken and in shaping the relationship that theorists see between planned units of the language and vocal tract activity. By introducing each section on the nature of linguistic units in this way, I am attempting to place two contrasting approaches to a theory of speech production in the context of theories of phonology that have informed them.

More than that, while Kelso *et al.* and Moll *et al.* may be correct that the units of the language as described by some *particular* linguistic theory do not aptly characterize the structure of activity in the vocal tract, in my view it is highly implausible that the elements of the language that language users know – that is, the ones that linguistic analyses attempt to uncover – are independent of the activities that implement them. For that reason, I consider it a mistake to study speech production and to develop hypotheses as to the larger organizations characteristic of vocal tract activity for speech in ignorance of the findings of linguistic phonological theories.

Linguistic investigations of systematic properties of spoken utterances uncover structure at a scale that direct observation of the detail of vocal tract activity may mask. That is, the systematicities may be characteristic of vocal tract activity, but if investigators do not know what to look for they may be difficult to see in the wealth of detail that direct observation of the vocal tract uncovers. In short, I include a description of linguistic phonological theories both because these perspectives have been influential in shaping speech production theories and because they should be influential.

2 'LINEAR' PHONOLOGIES AND RELATED APPROACHES TO THEORIES OF LANGUAGE AND SPEECH PRODUCTION

2.1 Linear Phonologies

Linguistic analysis reveals that words have an internal structure. They are composed at least of consonants and vowels. In different amounts and arrangements, consonants and vowels can be shown exhaustively to compose the tens of thousands of words of a language. In addition, they participate as individuals in phonological rules of the language, including rules of insertion, deletion and reordering. None of this evidence is obtained by studying words realized by activities of the vocal tract, and so none of it implies necessarily that these units of the language are units of speech activity or even of speech planning by the talker. If they are nonetheless units of the language, what is their status *vis à vis* speakers and hearers? Since the language itself exists only in so far as speakers and hearers know and use it, if consonants and vowels are units of the language, they must at least be units in the language user's *knowledge* of the language. This generally is the status accorded them in virtue of their roles in the lexicons of languages. They are said to be components of a language user's 'competence' – an idealized speaker–hearer's knowledge of the language that 'provides the basis for actual use of the language by a speaker–hearer' (Chomsky, 1965, p. 9).

To the extent that behavioral evidence converges with linguistic evidence to suggest that words composed of consonants and vowels are components of real language users' plans for an utterance, then there is evidence that components of competence do provide the 'basis for actual use of the language'. However, from this perspective, separate questions concern the units of vocal tract activity – if any – their nature, and their relationship to units of planning and competence. Units of the language users' competence may or may not be analogous in form to units of vocal tract activity; they may or may not stand in 1 : 1 correspondence to them.

Linear phonologies have been labeled 'linear', after the fact, to reflect the perspective they take on consonants and vowels as elements of language users' competence. In general, until the middle 1970s different theories of phonology that influenced theories of speaking agreed that consonants and vowels are constellations of simultaneous attributes called 'features'. Because the attributes are simultaneous, vertical slices drawn metaphorically through a word serve to isolate the individual feature constellations of individual consonants and vowels of the word. Theories that ascribe to this 'absolute slicing hypothesis' (Goldsmith, 1976) are 'linear' phonologies.

In *The Sound Pattern of English* (Chomsky and Halle, 1968), the consonants and vowels of a word are represented as columns of features. For Chomsky and Halle, features refer largely to articulatory correlates of the consonants and vowels. A partial representation of the features in 'but' follows:

[b]	**[ʌ]**	**[t]**
− vocalic	+ vocalic	− vocalic
+ consonantal	− consonantal	+ consonantal
− high	− high	− high
− back	+ back	− back
− low	− low	− low
+ anterior	− anterior	+ anterior
− coronal	− coronal	+ coronal
+ voice	+ voice	− voice
− continuant	+ continuant	− continuant

Chomsky and Halle (1968) identify two functions that features serve in the language. One is 'classificatory': features give distinct lexical entries distinct representations, and they do so in a way that reflects natural groupings of phonological segments as determined by the segments' participation in phonological processes of the language. To serve this function, consonants and vowels of words in the lexicon are represented, as above, by a list of binary-valued features. A second function is to reflect the phonetic capabilities of language users – that is, to reflect any distinction between pairs of speech sounds that a careful listener can hear and transcribe in a speech utterance. To serve that function, features are represented as continuous scales rather than as binary-valued.

In linear phonologies, words of the lexicon may have an internal structure superordinate to the phonological segment that will receive occasional mention below. Some words are composed of a stem and one or more affixes (in English, either a prefix or a suffix); other words, called 'compounds', may be composed of a pair of stems (e.g. 'greenhouse'); still others may be composed of just one stem. Another sublexical unit, the syllable, is not identified as a significant unit in the phonology of Chomsky and Halle (1968).

2.2 Approaches to a Theory of Speech Planning and Production from this Perspective

2.2.1 Introduction

Syntactic constructions span several words. Accordingly, building one requires planning, and one major set of questions that needs to be addressed in a theory of speaking concerns the nature of planning processes and the nature of the planned units. *A priori*, one might guess that finding answers to this set of questions will be more difficult than finding answers to questions concerning the units of vocal tract activity itself, because the latter are public while the former are largely covert. However, considerably more progress has been made in sorting out *planning* processes and units than in sorting out *executed* units of speech.

There are several reasons for this unexpected reversal. First, linguistic theory as just outlined ascribes properties to units of speech, phonological segments in particular, that preclude segments' realization as such in vocal tract activity. Also, speech activity itself does not invite segmentation into any obvious units other than, perhaps, the individual motions of individual articulators. When units of the linguistic message failed to show up in vocal tract activity, researchers were at a loss as to what *else* they ought to look for. It took changes in linguistic theory on the one hand and, on the other hand, new perspectives on vocal tract actions before progress could be made. But both developments are new, and progress is limited. These developments are described in Section 3.

On the other side, significant advances have been made in understanding planning for speech. It turns out that planning is not wholly covert and that the units of planning that reveal themselves in behavior do, in large part, conform to expectations derived from linear phonological theories.

The most important single source of evidence concerning planning is provided by spontaneous errors that talkers make when they speak. This evidence, augmented recently by experimental elicitation of errors (Baars, Motley and MacKay, 1975; Dell, 1980; Shattuck-Hufnagel, 1986, 1987) or by word games (Treiman, 1983) that require manipulation of parts of words, allows a fairly coherent story to be written about units of planning and about planning operations themselves. In the following sections, I will review the recent literature on speech errors and summarize the conclusions it permits concerning processes of planning.

Although the focus of this chapter is on speaking considered as production of words, themselves composed of phonological segments, the following review includes consideration of planning events upstream of that. Full appreciation of the order that phonological errors exhibit requires putting them in the context of other errors produced, apparently, at other phases of planning that are equally ordered, but respect different ordering constraints.

2.2.2 Definition of Errors

Talkers make a variety of mistakes when they speak. They may lose their train of thought, revise a sentence in midstream, or produce a disfluency that a phonetician would have difficulty transcribing. Alternatively, they may chronically pronounce a word in a way that listeners identify as erroneous, or produce a sentence that listeners consider ungrammatical but that the talker does not. These are not the kinds of error that researchers have used to investigate planning in speaking. Critical errors for that purpose are fluent departures from an utterance as the talker intended to produce it. Sometimes the talker's intentions are obvious; sometimes talkers correct themselves.

The following general kinds of error are most common (for more complete taxonomies, see Dell, 1986, and Shattuck-Hufnagel, 1979; the following examples of errors are from Crompton, 1982; Dell, 1986; Fromkin, 1971; Garrett, 1980a, b; and Shattuck-Hufnagel, 1979, 1983). One segment of an utterance may be replaced by another. Sometimes the replacing elements may come from the intended string (a *contextual substitution*) or else they may come from elsewhere (a *noncontextual substitution*). Three kinds of contextual substitution are common. In anticipations, an element later in the intended string substitutes for an earlier element ('sky in the sky' for 'sun in the sky'; 'leading list' for 'reading list'). Perseverations are complementary. A segment is substituted for a later one ('class will be about discussing the class' for 'class will be about discussing the test'; 'beef needle soup' for 'beef noodle soup'). In some quite remarkable errors, called *exchanges*, segments swap places ('I left the briefcase in my cigar', 'emeny'). Examples of noncontextual substitutions, in which the substituting segment is not the intended string, are 'Pass the salt' for 'Pass the pepper' and 'Bob McGord' for 'Bob McCord'.

In addition to substitution errors, segments can be added to a string, deleted from it or shifted. In a *shift* error, a segment moves from one location in the string to another ('something all to tell you' for 'something to tell you all'; 'point outed' for 'pointed out'). Finally, two words apparently competing for the same slot in a sentence can blend ('clarinola' for 'clarinet' and 'viola').

Although there are complications, generally it appears that the units that participate in speech errors are discrete units of linguistic theory. Most commonly, units are phonemes, words and morphemes. According to Shattuck-Hufnagel (1987), 40% of all errors in the corpus collected by her and by Garrett (1980a, b) are errors involving single whole consonants and vowels. Very rarely among the error types outlined above are there clear instances of feature errors ('glear plue sky') or errors involving linguistically incoherent sequences. Syllables, which are not assigned a role in the phonological theory of Chomsky and Halle, appear as units in speech errors no more commonly in Shattuck-Hufnagel's (1983) corpus than do CV or VC sequences (where C is an oral consonant and V is a vowel) that do not constitute whole syllables. Even so, syllables play a role in speech errors as outlined below.

2.2.3 What can be Learned from the Errors?

The units of language performance that errors reveal are not, necessarily, units of vocal tract activity. Although errors may be called 'slips of the tongue', they cannot arise in vocal tract activity. When a talker says: 'I left the briefcase in my cigar', he or she has anticipated a whole word three slots earlier in the sentence than its intended location. Moreover, the word – a noun – has been moved into the next closest slot in which a noun belongs. Such an error cannot be an error at the level of motor activity. Presumably, it arises in processes that plan – that is, construct – the intended communication prior to utterance.

Some conclusions that errors do warrant are that utterances are planned, there are planned units, and planned units correspond quite closely to units of linguistic competence as outlined by linear phonologies. Components of a speech utterance that can be arranged differently in different sentences, or words that can substitute one for the other in the language, are just the ones that emerge as discrete and autonomous in spontaneous errors of speech production.

Speech errors are more informative still, because they appear to provide information about the nature and ordering of planning processes in speaking. In particular, evidence suggests both a progressive narrowing of the planning domain and a shift from a focus on content and grammatical roles of words to a focus on surface grammatical form and then to a focus on phonological word shape.

Exchanges of whole words and of phonemes are informative in this regard. Whole-word exchanges can occur over fairly long surface distances in a sentence. In particular, they are very likely to cross syntactic phrase boundaries (81% of the time according to Garrett, 1980a). In contrast, words involved in phoneme exchanges span a syntactic phrase boundary just 13% of the time in Garrett's count.

An interpretation of these differences is that planning in which words are selected to serve some grammatical or propositional role spans several syntactic phrases while planning that focuses on words' labels has a considerably narrower domain. Further, word exchanges tend to be between words of the same syntactic class (85% of the time according to Garrett's count, 1980a), while phoneme exchanges occur between words of the same (39%) or different (61%) syntactic classes apparently indifferently. As described more fully below, constraints on phoneme exchanges are largely phonological. This suggests another shift that accompanies the narrowing of the planning domain. The focus of planning shifts from one on words as conveyers of content to one on words as phonological labels.

Evidence that there may be an in-between planning phase is provided by some 'stranding errors' in which two stems exchange, stranding their suffixes (e.g. 'I thought the park was trucked' from Garrett, 1980b). These look like whole-word exchanges in the sense that sequences of consonants and vowels that can stand alone exchange. However, the stranding exchanges in question occur over short distances and frequently involve exchanges of words from different grammatical categories: 70% of stranding exchanges occur within a syntactic phrase and 57% involve stems from different grammatical classes.

In respect to those properties, these stranding exchanges look almost like phoneme errors; however, the conditions under which the two kinds of error occur are quite different. When single phonemes misorder, the substituting and replaced segments are featurally similar. (They are identical with respect to the features 'consonantal' and 'vocalic'.) Consonantal substitutions move to the same location relative to the vowel of its new syllable (before it or after it) that it occupies relative to the vowel in the intended syllable. Moreover, the contexts of the consonants' and vowels' new and intended slots are featurally similar. In short, constraints on phoneme errors are phonological, while those on stranding errors are not to any obvious degree.

That word substitutions appear to occur in two varieties also points at least to two distinct phases of utterance planning. In one kind ('salt' for 'pepper'), substitutions are semantically similar to their targets, but not noticeably similar phonologically. In another kind ('apartment' for 'appointment'), the relationship is just the reverse. (Substitutions in the latter category are called 'malapropisms' by Fay and

Cutler, 1977.) It is as if the talker accesses the lexicon twice: once to search using semantic criteria for words to fill appropriate sentential roles and then later using phonological criteria to find utterable word labels.

A final source of information on the phasing of planning processes is provided by 'accommodations'. Consider the following errors (from Garrett, 1980b):

(1) 'I don't know that I'd hear one if I knew it' (for 'I don't know that I'd know one if I heard it').
(2) 'Even the best team losts' (for 'Even the best teams lost').

In the first error, 'know' and 'hear' exchange, and 'hear' strands its past-tense marker. Interestingly, when 'hear', pronounced /hʒ/ in the intended string, moves, it is pronounced /hiyr/ appropriately for its new location. (Letters enclosed in slashes represent phonological segments. A list of symbols likely to be unfamiliar appears in the Appendix.) Also, 'know' plus the stranded affix together are pronounced, not 'knowed' but 'knew'. The accommodations of 'hear' and 'know' to their new settings are lexically dependent. 'Heard' and 'knew' are irregular pasts; they cannot be undone and done respectively without consulting the lexicon. But now consider the second error. Here, the plural morpheme shifts from 'team' to 'lost.' It, too, shows an accommodation but the accommodation is not lexically dependent. The accommodation that the error does show is in the pronunciation of the plural morpheme. Whereas it is pronounced /z/ in 'teams' it is pronounced /s/ after 'lost'. This follows a rule for pronunciation of plural morphemes following /m/ (and most other voiced sounds) versus /t/ (and most other voiceless sounds), but it is insensitive to the fact that 'losts' is not a word.

One possibility, of course, is that some talkers (or some talkers sometimes) consult the lexicon to monitor for errors while others (or the same talkers other times) do not. A different generalization appears to fit the collection of errors of these two types, however. Stranding exchanges that occur over long distances, and shifts (or stranding exchanges: 'the park was trucked') that occur over short distances, may take place during different phases of sentence planning during which talkers are sensitive to different properties of a planned sentence. As the planning domain progressively narrows, focus shifts from grammatical and semantic properties to phonological ones, and from sensitivity to lexical properties to sensitivity only to fully systematic phonological properties of the language.

2.2.4 Slot and Filler Theories: Garrett and Shattuck-Hufnagel

Garrett (1980a, b) has proposed a model that takes an early representation of an utterance in which words and their sentential roles are specified into another, surface structure, representation in which words are ordered as they will be spoken and are appropriately inflected. Shattuck-Hufnagel (1979, 1983) suggests how words of a sentence are encoded phonologically for utterance. I will briefly review both proposals and then describe an important revision by Dell (1980, 1986, 1988).

Garrett calls the two representations that he proposes talkers construct *functional* and *positional*. A functional representation assigns sentential roles to words (or to their underlying semantic contents). Essentially, it represents the meaning of the utterance that that talker intends to convey in a fully transparent fashion. A positional representation orders words and assigns affixes to them in accordance with the syntactic constraints of the language.

Two major kinds of error may occur as the functional representation is assembled. As the lexicon is searched, a wrong word may be selected and, because the search is sensitive to content and grammatical form, substitutions will be semantically similar to targets and will be from the same syntactic category (e.g. 'salt' for 'pepper'). A second error may occur as words are assigned to sentential roles in the functional representation. For example, two nouns selected for different roles may be exchanged ('I left the briefcase in my cigar').

As the functional representation is formed, a positional 'frame' is also under construction. For insertion into the surface structure frame, the lexicon is searched once more, this time for word labels – that is, sequences of phonological segments that label the word contents inserted into the functional representation. Word substitutions can occur in this search as well, but these now are promoted by phonological similarity.

The frame itself is composed of affixes ('past tense', 'plural') and function words (closed-class words such as 'of', 'the'). Function words and affixes are considered part of the relatively fixed frame on empirical grounds. Each behaves differently from content words in its participation in speech errors. Function words do not generally participate in speech errors at all, and exchanging words and even phonemes jump over them. As for affixes, they are sometimes 'stranded' ('the park was trucked'). If they move, they shift, and they shift only a short distance ('the best team losts'). Garrett suggests that stranding errors occur as word labels are inserted into the positional frame. Apparently, the insertion process generally proceeds syntactic phrase by syntactic phrase; accordingly, errors occur largely within syntactic phrases. Yet the insertion process is rather insensitive to the form classes of inserted words; word exchanges over these short distances frequently violate form class.

As for shift errors, they are not really shifts of the bound morphemes, according to Garrett; rather, bound morphemes are part of the fixed positional frame. Instead, shifts involve misinsertions into the frame such that, for example, in 'even the best team losts' a pair of content words is inserted into the single slot before the plural morpheme.

Explaining phonological segment errors appears to require a model closely analogous to the content frame account of the 'positional level' representation proposed by Garrett. Recall some characteristics of phonological segment errors. They occur in the same varieties as word errors. That is, they appear as anticipations, perseverations, exchanges, as substitutions with no source in the planned utterance, as additions and as deletions. Conditions that promote phonological segment errors are phonological. Substituting and replaced segments are featurally similar and the slots into which substituting segments move have contexts similar to those of their source slots if any; these two contexts are featurally similar, and may even include some of the same consonants or vowels. In addition, consonants move to the same position in a syllable – before the vowel or after it – as they occupy in their source locations.

Exchange errors (e.g. 'it's *past fassing*') provide one major source of evidence favoring a content frame (slot filler) account of planning at the level of phonological segments. Like anticipations, they establish that words are planned for production in advance of their articulation. But they have an additional, quite remarkable, characteristic. In an exchange, if segment B substitutes for A in A's slot, then A substitutes for B in B's slot. How can that be explained except by supposing that words to be produced are specified as a frame of consonant and vowel slots and separately as a pool of phonological fillers for the slots? If B moves to A's slot and so has been used ahead of its time, instead of a deletion occurring at B's location – this never happens according to Shattuck-Hufnagel – the leftover A appears there.

Shattuck-Hufnagel (1979, 1983) proposes that phonological planning involves building a frame for a string of words to be produced. The frame specifies a sequence of slots for consonants and vowels. Lexical entries for words to be produced supply a pool of consonants and vowels to serve as slot fillers. The frame specifies featural attributes of the segments to fill the slots and a 'scan-copier' searches the pool of consonants and vowels for appropriate fillers. Fillers are appropriate if they have the right features and they occur in a context of segments with features like those surrounding the slot to be filled.

As it fills a slot with a segment, the scan-copier deletes the used segment from the pool. An exchange error occurs, then, when the scan-copier picks a wrong segment for one slot and eliminates it from the pool. Because it makes its selections based on the featural attributes of the segment to fill the slot, an erroneously picked segment is likely to be featurally similar to the target segment. Having selected a wrong segment for insertion into the frame and having eliminated it from the pool, the scan-copier has little choice but to use the left-over segment to fill the slot left empty by the earlier error. If the scan-copier makes two errors – if it selects a wrong segment for a slot and then neglects to eliminate it from the pool – then an anticipation occurs. Perseverations occur when a segment is used correctly, but is not deleted from the pool; the scan-copier then chooses that segment over the correct one to fill a later slot. Substitutions that have no source in the pool of fillers may reflect copying errors from filler pool to frame.

Shattuck-Hufnagel's account of phonological-segment level planning is attractive in at least two ways. First, it explains errors at this level analogously to Garrett's explanation of similar errors on words. Second, the account does a good job of explaining errors that occur and in explaining why nonoccurring errors fail to occur.

A major puzzle that the model raises, however, concerns the need for serial ordering of phonological segments of words in speech planning. There is an excellent reason why planning for the serial ordering of words must occur in speech production. It is precisely the reason offered at the very beginning of the chapter for why novel utterances are produceable and understandable. People routinely produce sequences of familiar words, ordered and affixed according to the syntactic conventions of the language, that they have never produced before. Presumably language users have very few stored sentences. Essentially all sentences are constructed for production.

Clearly, this is not true of words. Words are the familiar parts of which novel utterances are composed. They are produced over and over again with, of course, the same ordering of their component consonants and vowels. So the question remains: Why should speech production planning include a phase during which the phonological segments of words are ordered for output?

The only answer in the theory to the question why phonological segments must be redundantly ordered in speech planning seems to be that they must be or else speech errors would not appear as they do. Obviously this is unsatisfactory. If the only function of the scan-copy process were to create phoneme errors of speech, talkers would avoid the process. An alternative perspective on the errors and so on the answer to the question is provided by Dell's important revisions to the model, considered next.

2.2.5 Dell's Model

Appealing aspects of the models of Garrett and Shattuck-Hufnagel are that the units of planning they propose are, with the exceptions noted, those of accepted linguistic theory. Also, to a considerable degree, the models generate errors as a natural product of processes of speech planning. That is, the models are not, for the most part, designed to produce errors: they are designed to produce speech.

Unappealing aspects of the model are just those aspects that appear to be there only to explain error patterns. They include, most notably, the two retrievals of words from the lexicon in Garrett's model, needed to explain why some word substitutions are semantically motivated and others are phonologically motivated, and the reordering of already ordered phonemes in Shattuck-Hufnagel's model.

Slightly subtler empirical problems with the model led Dell (1980, 1986, 1988; Dell and Reich, 1980, 1981; see also, MacKay, 1982, 1987; Stemberger, 1985) to an important change in perspective on speech planning and to a new model. The change in perspective retains many central aspects of the models of Garrett and Shattuck-Hufnagel, but it eliminates (or motivates) unappealing attributes just described, and handles the data somewhat better.

The subtle failures of the slot filler models derive from their strict modularity. At the functional level of representation, the system is blind to phonological properties of words, but is sensitive to content and sentential role. When errors occur, they are exchanges between words of a common syntactic class or semantically similar word substitutions. At the positional level and beyond, the system is blind to content, increasingly blind to syntactic category and increasingly sensitive to phonological form. Accordingly, for example, phoneme errors frequently create nonwords, and misorderings occur between words that may differ in parts of speech. This characterization approximately fits the data, but it fails in detail.

Word targets and their substitution errors that are classified as meaning-based are more similar phonologically than are the same words randomly repaired (Dell, 1980; Dell and Reich, 1981). Although focus on semantic attributes of words may predominate when those word errors occur, the planning system is not wholly blind to the phonological properties of words. On the other side, although phoneme errors do often lead the talker to produce nonwords, there is a significant bias for them to create real words both in spontaneous errors (Dell, 1980; Dell and Reich, 1981) and in laboratory induced errors (Baars, Motley and MacKay, 1975). It seems that during a phase of planning for the serial ordering of phonemes, even though phonological properties predominate in promoting errors, the planning system is not wholly blind to lexicality and content.

How can a system be mostly modular, or modular with leaks? Dell suggests one way. Modularity is realized in part by frames of the sort that Garrett and Shattuck-Hufnagel propose. In Dell's model, there are three frames: surface syntax, words and syllables. Words are inserted into syntactic slots, morphemes into word slots and syllable constituents (currently isomorphic with single phonological segments in the model as simulated) into syllable frames. Selection of contents for the frames takes place in the lexicon, which has a special structure.

Dell (see also McClelland and Rumelhart, 1981) proposes a connectionist system in which the lexicon is a hierarchical network of units. Levels of the hierarchy include words, morphemes, syllable constituents, phonemes and features. The lexicon is a network in the sense that there are bidirectional excitatory linkages between each superordinate unit and its subordinate constituents on the next level down.

When 'activation' spreads through the lexicon, it spreads along the linkages. Accordingly, if a word, say 'swimmer', is activated because a talker intends it to be part of a sentence, activation spreads from the word 'swimmer' to its component morphemes, 'swim' and '-er'. From there, activation spreads upward from the component morphemes to each word of the lexicon having the morphemes as components. (In turn, those activated words activate their component morphemes, and so on.) Activation also spreads from activated morphemes downward in turn to their component syllable constituents, phonemes and features. The same principles of spreading operate everywhere, so that each activated phoneme sends activation downward to its features and upward to each word that contains the phoneme. Each feature activates any phoneme that contains it. Chaos, it seems.

The chaos is constrained or even regulated, however, by the process of inserting contents into frames. Figure 9.1 shows how speech production planning works in the model. The talker intends to say 'some swimmers sink'. Activation from the 'idea' for the message is not modeled except that it activates relevant words. Activation spreads from the words as described.

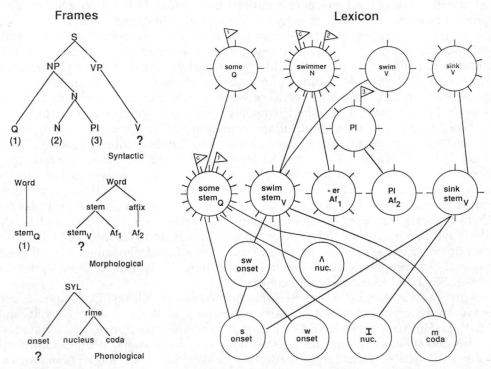

Figure 9.1. *Dell's model of language production including a connectionist lexicon and, to the left, a set of frames for constructing a sentence. See text for further explanation. [Adapted from Dell, 1986.]*

In the course of planning, talkers build a surface structure frame for the utterance. For each slot in the frame to be filled by a word, they build a word frame with slots for each morpheme. Finally, a syllable frame is constructed for each syllable of each morpheme.

The frame for 'some swimmers sink' specifies a quantifier for the first word slot. In the lexicon, the quantifier with the highest level of activation is selected to fill the slot. Most of the time that is the intended quantifier because it received initial activation from the intended message idea. (In the figure, a word in the lexicon is tagged with an order tag when it has been 'inserted' into the frame; accordingly, 'some' has been tagged with the number 1.) When the quantifier is picked, its activation level is set to zero, but it soon rebounds because its similar neighbors are active and will reactivate it.

The frame next calls for a noun and the selection process continues with the noun having the highest activation being selected for insertion. To construct the word frame, the tagged quantifier in the lexicon is designated the 'current node'. By virtue of that, it is given additional activation and its word frame is built. After some period of time to allow spreading to occur (and the amount of time varies with rate of talking), a morpheme of the appropriate sort (stem or affix) for the first available slot is selected; the selected morpheme is the one of the appropriate sort that has the highest activation. Now the next word in the syntactic frame is designated the current node at that level, while the just-selected morpheme is current at its level. This allows its syllable frame(s) to be built.

Insertions take place at three levels in the lexicon: words, morphemes and phonemes (not distinguished from syllable constituents). Errors take place during the insertion process; accordingly, only words, morphemes and phonemes will serves as units in errors.

Errors can occur in just one way. They occur if a unit, appropriate for the frame slot being filled, but not the intended filler, is more highly activated at the time of insertion than is the intended unit. This will happen sometimes because of the spreading process in the lexicon.

At the word level, a substitution error will occur if an unintended word of the appropriate syntactic class for the to-be-filled slot in the syntactic frame has higher activation than the intended word. Words that will be activated include other intended words for the utterance. Accordingly, sometimes exchanges, anticipations and perseverations will occur. On other occasions, a word not in the intended string may be highly activated to the extent that it is semantically and/or phonologically similar to the intended word.

An exchange occurs in the following way. At the time A's slot is to be filled in the frame, a word of the intended utterance, B, is more highly activated than A, and so B is selected to fill A's slot. Having been selected, B's activation level is set to zero, but it soon begins to rebound because its similar neighbors are active and activate it anew. When B's slot is to be filled, A may be more active than B, because B's activation level has been set to zero. Therefore A is selected and the error is an exchange. If B has rebounded and surpassed A, then B is selected and the error is an anticipation. (Notice that this predicts a change in the relative frequencies of exchanges and anticipations as speech rate increases; at fast rates, exchanges will be relatively more likely than at slow rates, because at fast rates B will not have time to rebound after being set to zero. Dell (1986) has found the appropriate interaction between speech rate and error type in an experiment in which phoneme errors are induced.)

Stranding errors ('the park was trucked', 'some sinkers swim') occur during insertion of morphemes into word frames, while phoneme errors occur during insertion of phonemes into syllable frames. These latter errors show a lexical bias because of the spread of activation from words through morphemes to phonemes. Substitutions are featurally similar because of the bidirectional spread of activation for phonemes to features. The contexts of misordering phonemes are similar because words that provide similar contexts for different phonemes will activate each other via their shared phonemes and features.

Dell has simulated a small lexicon and insertion process on the computer at the level of phonological selection. In general, it produces phoneme errors of the right sort in the right proportions. In addition, it shows a lexical bias in phoneme errors. More interestingly, perhaps, the model makes some unexpected predictions that are borne out by the simulation.

One, already mentioned, is the change in the ratio of exchange to anticipation errors as speech rate changes. A second is that the lexical bias will be reduced as speech rate increases, because there is less time for spreading of activation through the lexical network. A striking prediction is that low frequency words that are homophones of function words will inherit the resistance of function words to participation in speech errors.

Garrett (1980a) had included function words in the positional frame largely because function words very rarely participate in speech errors. Dell ascribes the resistance of function words to error to their high frequency. In his lexicon, words have resting activation levels that increase with their frequency of production. In effect, a talker is chronically prepared to produce words that are produced frequently. Words with already high activation levels most readily become the most highly activated words when insertion rules select words for insertion into the syntactic frame. Therefore, slips are rare on function words. Low frequency homophones of function words will inherit function words' error resistance to a considerable degree because they share the same syllables, phonemes and features.

Research shows that low frequency words are more likely to participate in speech errors both in spontaneous errors (Stemberger and MacWhinney, 1986) and in experimentally elicited errors (Dell, 1990). However, the frequency difference vanishes for function words as compared to their low frequency homophones (Dell, 1990).

In short, Dell's model preserves the appealing features of Garrett's and Shattuck-Hufnagel's models, and it eliminates (or perhaps motivates) the less appealing aspects of those models. Dell's model does not yet offer a reason why word onsets are so vulnerable to error. (However, Dell (1990) suggests that an adjustment to the model, such that the process of phoneme insertion into the syllable frame is made more serial and less parallel than it is currently, might give rise to an initialness effect.)

2.3   Performance of the Speech Plan

A conclusion from the collection of data and theory on speech errors is that units of competence as suggested by linguistic theories, and of planning as suggested by data from speech errors, are closely convergent. This means that elements that behave autonomously in language systems serve as autonomous units of speech planning as well. This is certainly good news. Language systems evolve and change during communicative interactions among speakers. They are, at least in part, fossilizations of consistent aspects of those interactions. Accordingly, it seems that the units of those systems should converge with units that talkers use in planning to speak.

The whole picture changes, however, when we turn from speech planning to speech production. Barring evidence to the contrary, one might expect to find a fairly direct relationship between planned phonological segments (the final planning stage in the models above) and activities of the vocal tract. Also, because planning units seem to correspond so closely to linguistic units, one might expect to see the feature columns of Chomsky and Halle's linear phonology realized in some fashion in the vocal tract.

Neither expectation is met, however. There is no neat correspondence between planned units and vocal tract activity and, indeed, correspondence is progressively more difficult to find the lower in the planning hierarchy the unit. That is, it is harder to find phonological segments in vocal tract activity than to find words, even though one might expect it to be the final planning stage that drives motor activity.

Before looking at vocal tract activity and its relationship to units of planning and of language competence, I provide an overview of the physical systems used to produce speech.

2.3.1 The Respiratory System, the Larynx and the Vocal Tract

Four anatomical systems are centrally involved in speech (Figure 9.2); they are: the respiratory system, the larynx, the nasal cavity and the oral cavity. The latter two constitute the *vocal tract*. Articulators in the oral cavity include the velum (the soft palate), the jaw, the upper and lower lips, and the tongue. To a degree, the tongue tip and the dorsum or tongue body are independently controlled.

Generally, speech is produced on an expiratory airflow and the respiratory cycle is modified during speech so that it occupies a considerably greater part of a breathing cycle than it does in vegetative breathing. The larynx, seated on the trachea, houses the vocal folds, which provide the primary sound source in speech. During voiced sounds, the vocal folds are approximated (adducted); while for unvoiced sounds, they are abducted. The adducted folds periodically stop the flow of air from the lungs from passing into the vocal tract. When the vocal folds stop the airstream, pressure builds up beneath them ('subglottal pressure'), and eventually the pressure blows the folds apart. The folds quickly close again, leading to another cycle of subglottal pressure build-up and release. During voiced phonemes, the vocal folds open and close periodically, cyclically releasing puffs of air into the vocal tract. The puffs of air contain energy at the frequency at which the vocal folds open and close (the 'fundamental frequency' or f_0 of voice) and, at successively lower intensities, at harmonics of the fundamental.

Vowels are produced with no obstruction to the airstream. They are distinguished one from the other largely by the positioning of the tongue body in the oral cavity. In high (or 'close') vowels, the tongue body is close to the palate, either toward the front of the mouth (as in /iy/) or toward the back (/uw/). In low ('open') vowels, the jaw is lowered so that the tongue body does not approach a

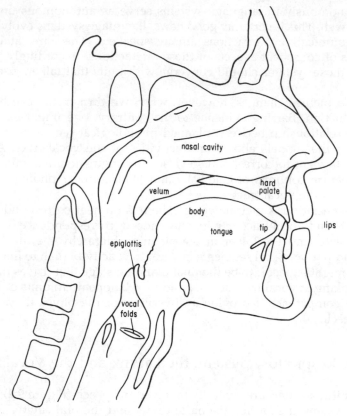

Figure 9.2. *A model of the vocal tract.*

point of constriction with the palate. Some vowels are produced with rounding of the lips (e.g. /uw/ or /ow/ in English); others are produced with lips retracted (/iy/). The movements of the tongue and the rounding or protrusion of the lips create cavities of different sizes and shapes in the vocal tract. In /uw/, a high back vowel, the cavity in front of the tongue body is long, while the back cavity is short; in the production of /iy/, the front cavity is short and the back cavity is long.

For vowels, the vocal tract serves as a filter for the acoustic energy produced at the laryngeal source. The cavities of the vocal tract have characteristic resonances ('formants') that depend on their lengths, and acoustic energy outside of the resonances is attenuated, yielding bands of energy in the vicinity of each formant.

Consonants are produced by obstructions to the airstream, for example at the lips (/b/, /p/, /m/) or at the hard palate using the tongue tip (/t/, /n/, /s/). During stop consonants (in English, /b, p, d, t, g, k/) the airflow is stopped temporarily and noise is produced at the point of constriction as the constriction is released. During fricatives (/s/, /z/, /f/, /v/, for example) an articulator closely approaches a fixed structure of the vocal tract, but leaves a narrow channel through which the airstream passes and becomes turbulent. During nasal segments, the velum lowers to allow air to pass through the nasal cavity, which serves as a resonator of fixed length.

2.3.2 Articulatory Dynamics

How do activities of the vocal tract realize a speech plan? In the last stage of planning, according to models reviewed earlier, phonemes are ordered for production. In linear phonologies, phonemes are bundles of simultaneous featural attributes. Were the relationship between linguistic competence and plan, and between plan and behavior, simple then one might expect to see speakers adopt successive postures of the vocal tract, each posture manifesting the set of featural attributes of a feature column. Short rests between postures might signal a morpheme boundary while longer rests signal a word boundary. Of course, because the vocal tract is a physical system, it cannot shift instantaneously from posture to posture. Accordingly, between postures one should see transitional phases.

However, vocal tract activity for speech looks nothing like that. During fluent speech, there are essentially no intervals in time when postures of the vocal tract are held. Relatedly, vocal tract activity cannot be partitioned into intervals that count as achievement of the features of a phoneme and others that count as transitions between phonemes. During speech, a great many different things go on at once; activities relating to the realization of a single phoneme are not synchronized, and activities for different phonemes overlap. Consider an instance in which it is possible to identify a feature (nasality) with a vocal tract movement (lowering the velum). One might expect the point of maximum lowering – or perhaps the point in lowering when air begins to pass through the nasal cavity (nasal coupling) – to count as achievement of the feature, [+nasal]. Accordingly, that point in time should coincide with achievement of the oral constriction for the nasal consonant if the 'absolute slicing' hypothesis is to hold for speech production. But it need not. Krakow (1988) has found that the point of maximum lowering of the velum for syllable final /m/ considerably precedes achievement of lip closure for /m/. The feature [+nasal] appears to be phase shifted relative to those that lip closure realizes, and it overlaps with gestures for a preceding vowel.

This overlap is known as 'coarticulation', and it is pervasive in speech. Coarticulation ensures that absolute slicing (temporal slicing in speech production) will never serve to isolate all and only movements associated with individual phonemic segments. Nor, for that matter, will 'spatial slicing'. In general, it is not possible to identify a movement of an articulator with one and only one phoneme. For example, closing movements of the jaw for a consonant such as /b/ are less extensive in the neighborhood of an open vowel than in the neighborhood of a close vowel (Sussman, MacNeilage and Hanson, 1973), and jaw height during closure is lower for /b/ before /a/ than for /b/ before /iy/ (cf. Keating, 1990). The consonant and vowel make overlapping demands on the jaw and the movement of the jaw reflects a compromise.

As MacNeilage and Ladefoged (1976) point out, initial reaction in the 1960 s to the discovery of the pervasiveness of context-conditioned variability of vocal tract movements owing to coarticulation was that coarticulation reflects mechanical constraints on vocal tract actions. The speech plan reflects an ideal that the vocal tract cannot realize, because it is a physical system. In fact, however, mechanical constraints cannot explain most of coarticulation, in part because much of it, like velum lowering for a nasal consonant, is *anticipatory* in direction.

Whatever the source of coarticulatory variability, it appears to create a considerable mismatch between, on the one hand, the characterization of phonological segments in linear phonologies and even in speech plans and, on the other hand, the behavior of the vocal tract. How is the apparent mismatch to be handled?

According to MacNeilage and Ladefoged (1976): 'This has led ... to an increasing realization of the inappropriateness of conceptualizing the dynamic processes of articulation itself into discrete, static, context-free linguistic categories such as "phoneme" and "distinctive feature"' (p. 90).

This does not mean that these linguistic categories should be abandoned entirely, however: 'Instead it seems to require that they be recognized even more than before as too abstract to characterize the actual behavior of the articulators themselves. They are, therefore, at present better confined to primarily characterizing earlier premotor stages of the production process, as revealed by speech errors, and to reflecting regularities at the message level (Fant, 1962) of the structure of language, such as those noted by phonologists' (p. 90).

Other investigators have expressed a similar view. For example, Kelso, Saltzman and Tuller (1986) write that: 'a final implication of the view presented here is that "segments" or phonological units as typically defined by linguists may not be relevant to the speech production system' (p. 46).

If the units apparently *are* relevant to speech planning, but apparently are not relevant to the speech production system, then where are we? One interpretation of this state of affairs is that there is, simply, a distinction between segments in the minds of language users and public behaviors of speakers. Hammarberg (1976) seems to hold this view: 'Segments cannot be objectively observed to exist in the speech signal nor in the flow of articulatory movements ... [T]he concept of segment is brought to bear *a priori* on the study of physical–physiological aspects of language' (p. 355).

This is unfortunate if true, because it considerably complicates the path of a communicative exchange. Speakers plan to produce a message consisting of words, themselves composed of sequences of consonants and vowels. But if consonants and vowels like that are not able to make public appearances in the vocal tract then they cannot structure the acoustic speech signal. Listeners must be like paleontologists (as Neisser, 1967, suggests) – who, finding small bone fragments, reconstruct an entire dinosaur; that is, listeners must use the acoustic signal as a collection of fragmentary hints as to the phonological word labels of a talker's intended linguistic message. Perhaps that is the way it is; perhaps not, however.

A different reason for the mismatch between the phonological segments of linguistic theory and vocal tract actions, as described by production researchers, may be that phonological segments of linear phonologies do not accurately represent real phonological segments of languages. It may be relevant that, while some of their properties are validated by speech errors, not all of them are.

Speech errors seem to reveal the following attributes of phonemes. They are somewhat autonomous, and their featural attributes are cohesive. Phonological segments are featurally distinctive. They are serially ordered in words.

Apparently, there is nothing in this characterization that requires the featural realization of phonemes not only to be cohesive, but also to be simultaneous in the way they are represented in the feature columns of linear phonologies. If cohesion can be achieved in some way other than by simultaneity, then the absence of synchrony in realization of the features of produced consonants and vowels does not separate planned from produced segments. Nor is there anything about planned segments that precludes temporal overlap in their realization as long as any overlap preserves the autonomy of each phonological segment and its ordering relative to neighbors. If phonemes need not be seen as discrete sequences of simultaneous features in a speech plan, is it possible that they need not be seen that way in the languages user's 'competence' either? That is, is the absolute slicing hypothesis any more required for the work that phonemes do in phonologies than for the work they do in speech plans? Recent developments of 'nonlinear' phonologies (Browman and Goldstein, 1986; Clements, 1985; Goldsmith, 1976) suggest that it is not; indeed, absolute slicing is not even tenable. These new phonologies help to reduce the chasm between phonological segments of linguistic competence and vocal tract behaviors by eliminating the absolute slicing constraint. They are reviewed briefly in Section 3.

Another reason for the mismatch between phonological segments as components of linguistic competence or of speech plans and as vocal tract activity is likely to be that we are not looking at vocal tract activity in a way that best reveals talkers' coordinations and controls. Coarticulation occurs, and so there is considerable overlap of movements associated with different phonological segments and context-conditioned variability of movement. Is there any way of looking at activity like this and recovering a phonological segmental structure?

In 1970, MacNeilage proposed a shift in perspective that looked promising. He proposed that a context-free articulatory correlate of a phonological segment be found in 'spatial targets' achieved in the vocal tract. Even though a target may be approached in different ways depending on its predecessor target, the target itself might be an invariant attribute of a segment. Similar proposals have been offered to explain equifinality in performance of pointing tasks (Bizzi and Polit, 1979; see also Fel'dman and Latash, 1982) and eye–head movements (Bizzi and Polit, 1979). MacNeilage proposed specifically that target muscle lengths are set by the gamma motoneurons of the nervous system that innervate muscle spindles. This should lead to movements toward the target muscle lengths and so toward invariant postures of the vocal tract articulators, independent of their starting positions.

In its specific proposals that invariant spatial targets represent articulated phonemes and that targets are achieved by setting target muscle lengths via the gamma system and muscle spindles, the theory is wrong. When a talker achieves bilabial closure for /b/, for example, the point in space where closure is achieved (relative, say, to the teeth) changes depending on the jaw's contribution to closure. In turn, those different spatial locations imply different lengths of muscles associated with jaw and lip locations.

Although the theory is wrong in its particular form, it is right in one important respect. For at least some attributes of some phonemes, an abstract invariant is achieved in the vocal tract whenever those attributes are planned and executed. When bilabial stops are produced, the lips close; when alveolar stops are produced, the tongue tip achieves contact with the hard palate; when velar stops are produced, the tongue body achieves contact with the soft palate. Possibly, there is a measure of invariance in speech production despite the context-conditioned variability introduced by coarticulation. The invariance is even more abstract and less particular than MacNeilage envisaged in 1970. New theoretical approaches in the domain of speech production attempt to make use of invariants like this. The approaches are described in Section 3.

If we discount, at least for the present, the possibility that there simply are irreconcilable incompatibilities between structure in speech activity and in the phonological competences and speech plans of language users, we can look for ways to eliminate apparent incompatibilities and so to bring the domains closer together. As MacNeilage and Ladefoged (1976) point out, making revisions to theory should be a two-way street. The phonologies of languages perhaps need developing with attention to the nature of vocal tracts that will realize speech. Theories of speech production need developing with attention to the essential properties of phonological segments (possibly: autonomous, cohesive distinctive attributes, serially ordered) that must be realized somehow in vocal tract activity if phonological segments are to make public appearances. On both sides, theorists must be open to recognizing old conceptualizations as conceptualizations, not as truths about phonological segments, about coarticulation and vocal tract activity and about the possible relationships between the realms of knowing (competence), planning and doing. Section 3 attempts to chart such rapprochement as linguistic theories and theories of speech production have been able to attain to date.

3 NONLINEAR PHONOLOGIES AND ANOTHER LOOK AT SPEECH PRODUCTION

Chomsky and Halle (1968) acknowledge as a major shortcoming of their work its inattention to the 'intrinsic content' of phonetic features (that is, inattention to their physical implementations). In large part, Chomsky and Halle's theory represented phonology as an imposition of a formal system on the vocal tract, the capabilities of which did not shape the formal system. The fact that simultaneous realization of the features of a phoneme is not possible for a vocal tract was not a reason to exclude that manner of representing phonological segments.

As Chomsky and Halle acknowledged, that is not a wholly realistic approach. There are clear indications, both in the segmental inventories of languages and in systematic processes in which the segments participate, that language structure develops with considerable regard for vocal tract capabilities and dispositions.

For example, Locke (1983) reports that the most common consonants in languages of the world are also most commonly transcribed in the babbles of prelinguistic infants – even of deaf infants. Lindblom (1986) has shown that two principles, maximization of perceptual distinctiveness and minimization of articulatory complexity, jointly do a good job of predicting the composition of phonemic–segmental inventories of languages of the world.

As for phonological processes, as MacNeilage and Ladefoged (1976) point out, they sometimes resemble physiological constraints or dispositions. Their example is the tendency in most languages that have been studied (Chen, 1970; Flege, 1988; Mack, 1982; Raphael, 1975) for vowels to be durationally longer before voiced than voiceless consonants. The reason for this is not entirely understood. However, it appears to reflect, in part, the faster closing gestures for voiceless than for voiced consonants (Chen, 1970; Summers, 1987). In turn, this difference may reflect the need to achieve a tighter seal during voiceless closures, which are associated with higher intraoral pressures than voiced closures (Lubker and Parris, 1970). In some languages including English, however, the vowel duration difference is considerably greater than can be explained by the difference in closing velocities (Chen,

1970; Flege, 1988; Flege and Port, 1981; Mack, 1982). In these languages the vowel duration difference, that may be a byproduct of different closing gestures for voiced and voiceless consonants, has been elevated into the phonology of the language as a regular process ('rule'). The rule has apparently in some way been 'triggered' (MacNeilage and Ladefoged, 1976) by the corresponding physiological disposition.

If segment inventories and phonological processes reflect articulatory capabilities, then an approach to phonology that largely ignores the vocal tract is likely to be unrealistic. Next, I briefly describe recent approaches to a theory of phonology that may be more realistic in this regard.

3.1 Nonlinear Phonologies and the Articulatory Phonology of Browman and Goldstein

A problem for representation of phonemes as feature columns arises in instances in which features have a scope smaller or larger than a single column. Consider the feature [+nasal], present in English in /m/, /n/ and /ŋ/. Some languages have so-called 'prenasalized' or 'postnasalized' consonants. Whereas most features of these segments span the whole segment's extent, nasality does not. In prenasalized stops, the first part of the consonant is nasalized, while the remainder is not. Postnasalized stops have the opposite pattern. Because prenasalized and postnasalized consonants have the duration of a single segment, are featurally identical across the segment except in respect to nasality, and have the distribution of single consonants (that is, they occur in contexts where clusters of consonants are otherwise not permitted; see Anderson, 1976), they are identified as single consonants, not as a sequence of two. However, there is no satisfactory way to represent the change in the nasal feature part-way through the segment in a linear phonology.

In other languages, nasality poses a different kind of problem for linear phonologies. These languages exhibit 'nasal harmony' in which a single nasal feature extends over more than one feature column. In the language Gokona (Hyman, 1982), if the first consonant of a word is nasal, all of the segments of the word are nasalized, or if not, but a word-internal vowel is a nasal vowel, every segment after the vowel must be nasalized. In another language, Terena (van der Hulst and Smith, 1982), the first person possessive is signaled by a spreading of nasality that begins at the left edge of a word and spreads until stopped by an obstruent consonant. The obstruent becomes a prenasalized obstruent. That is, the nasality extends half-way into its 'feature column' (so that [owoku] ('his house') becomes [õwõŋgu] ('my house')).

These instances in which a feature's span is either less or more than a whole column are not restricted to cases involving the feature [nasal]. In tone languages, tones may likewise have a span that is less or more than a whole segment (Goldsmith, 1976), as can various vocalic features in languages with diphthongs or vowel harmony.

One implication of these observations is that columns of simultaneous features cannot represent all of the relationships among the featural attributes of the segments of a word. A second is that, when two features have different domains, they are manifesting a measure of independence or autonomy that a phonology will need to capture.

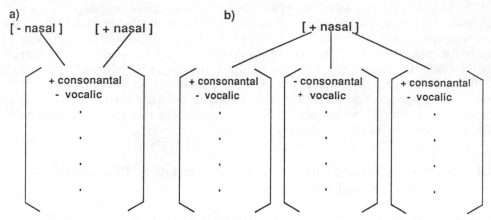

Figure 9.3. *An autosegmental tier for the nasal feature to capture: (a) postnasalized consonants, and (b) nasal harmony.*

A way to express the independence of the feature [+nasal] in languages with postnasalized stops might be as in Figure 9.3a; and in languages with nasal harmony as in Figure 9.3b.

Phonologies that adopt notations like this, in which some features occupy different ('autosegmental') tiers from others, and so may have different domains of influence, are nonlinear or autosegmental phonologies.

It is of interest, however, to go beyond the language-specific representations of Figure 9.3 to develop a 'universal' phonology – that is, a phonological system that expresses the *possibilities* for autonomy among features rather than expressing just the ones that are highlighted in the phonologies of just a particular language being studied.

The development of an 'articulatory phonology' by Browman and Goldstein (1986; 1990; see also, Clements, 1985; Sagey, 1986) reflects an understanding that possibilities for autonomy are set by the character of the vocal tract. By the same token, possible 'features' are determined in part by possible vocal tract actions, and the theory of articulatory phonology also makes an effort to identify its primitives with possible (and actual) vocal tract behaviors in speech.

In Browman and Goldstein's theory, fundamental units are not phonemes or features, but 'gestures'. They are linguistically significant goal-directed actions in the vocal tract defined by: (1) the *end-effector* of the action (for oral constrictions for consonants and vowels, the end-effector is the articulator that makes the constriction); and (2) by values of parameters of a dynamical equation that describes the appropriate action. For oral constriction gestures, the parameter values define a constriction in the appropriate location, and of the appropriate degree (closed for stops, a narrow opening for fricatives, etc.), and a final value ('stiffness' or *k*) regulates rate of approach to the constriction. In addition to gestures for oral constrictions, there are gestures of the velum to open the velar port for nasal consonants or vowels and to raise it for oral ones, and there are gestures of the glottis (that is, vocal fold gestures) to voice or devoice a segment of speech.

Although gestures are identified in part by their end-effectors, the movements that realize oral constrictions are achieved not only by the end-effector itself, but by supporting articulators as well. Accordingly, gestures to realize values of vocal tract variables, such as the appropriate tongue tip (=end-effector) constriction degree, often imply coordinated involvement of more than one articulator (in the example, the tongue and the jaw).

Consonants and vowels are realized by one or more gestures. For example, /m/ involves an oral constriction gesture and a gesture of the velum; /p/ shares its constriction gesture with /m/, but it lacks the gesture of the velum and includes a devoicing gesture.

The set of gestures possible for the vocal tract during speech has an implicit hierarchical structure that derives from the structure of the vocal tract itself. That structure displayed in Figure 9.4 also implies different degrees of autonomy among gestures and different likelihoods of gestures being grouped in phonological processes or in other classifications of segments.

In place of successive feature columns to represent words, Browman and Goldstein substitute a 'gestural score' such as that in Figure 9.5 for the word 'Tom.'

The association lines between 'root nodes' in the figure and gestural parameters reflect a clustering among the gestures associated with the initial consonant, vowel and final consonant of a word, but also reflect the temporal relationships among the gestures. (Notice, for example, that the glottal devoicing gesture for /t/ does not coincide wholly with the oral constriction gesture. Rather, it is offset to ensure aspiration of the consonant on release.) The wide bracketing of the vowel's gesture reflects its coarticulatory span, while the association lines from the root node to the gesture give its serial order.

Now let us return to the incompatibilities between phonological knowledge as characterized by a linear phonology and vocal tract activity for speech and consider how they have been reduced by this new phonological theory. In fact, they have been considerably reduced. In the new theory, gestures are inherently dynamic not

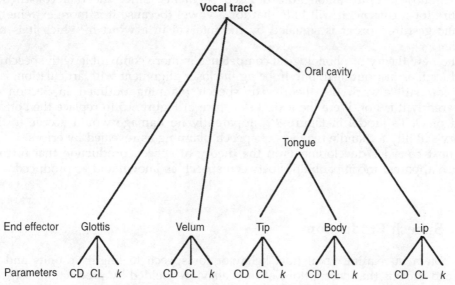

Figure 9.4. *The hierarchical structure of gestures. CD, constriction degree; CL, constriction location; k, stiffness value. [Adapted from Browman and Goldstein, 1990.]*

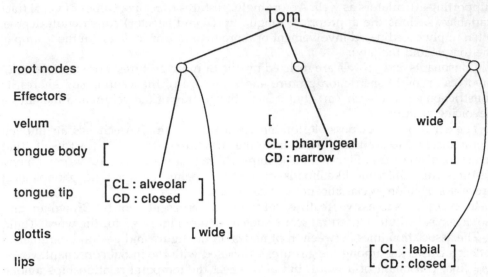

Figure 9.5. *A gestural score for 'Tom'. CD, constriction degree; CL, constriction location.*

static, and they are movements that actually occur in the vocal tract. In addition, the gestures of a consonant or vowel are not necessarily simultaneous and they can overlap with gestures of other segments. In the theory, cohesion among gestures of a consonant or vowel is specified, but not by simultaneity as it is in Chomsky and Halle's theory. The association lines indicate that there is cohesion, but the means by which the vocal tract can achieve it are not specified; that is left to the vocal tract. Likewise, lines to root nodes specify the serial order of segments, but they do not disallow overlap among the ordered segments. Since the oral constriction gesture for a consonant will hide that for a vowel (because it is more extreme), a vocalic gesture's order is signaled by the interval in a word in which it is not hidden.

The new theory of phonological competence is more compatible with speech as produced, as just outlined, but, in being in closer alignment with articulation, is it less compatible with the theories of speech planning outlined in Section 2? Apparently it is not. Were the lexical structure in Figure 9.5 to replace the bottom third of Dell's model in Figure 9.1, apparently no damage would accrue to the theory's ability to handle the facts of speech planning as revealed by errors.

I next consider developments in the theory of speech production that further reduce apparent incompatibilities between speech as known and as produced.

3.2 Speech Production

A problem in relating vocal tract behavior for speech to linguistic units and to planned units is that descriptions of the behaviors yielded by production research tend to be too fine-grained. That is, they are not behaviors at the scale of individual phonemes or even their features. Instead, observations of the vocal tract generally are of muscle activity or of movements of the individual articulators. However, neither individual muscles nor even individual articulators produce individual phonetic segments, or, for the most part, their features. Moreover, both muscle activity (MacNeilage and DeClerk, 1969) and movements of individual articulators (Sussman, MacNeilage and Hanson, 1973) are context-sensitive, reflecting converging influences of multiple phonetic segments. Thus, not only is the scale wrong, but the specificity of relationship between behavior and message unit is also absent.

Despite that, however, at a different level of description, there is specificity at least between some attributes of consonants and vowels and activity of the vocal tract. For example, as noted earlier, talkers always achieve lip closure for /b/, /p/ and /m/. Even though movements of the three articulators that achieve bilabial closure – the upper lip, the lower lip and the jaw – are context-sensitive, their joint action is invariant.

That there is a lack of invariance at a fine-grained level of analysis, but invariance (for at least some features of some phonetic segments) at a more coarse-grained level implies that somehow goals at the coarser-grained level are constraining finer-grained events (Fowler *et al.*, 1980; cf. Pattee, 1973; Weiss, 1941). It is as if, in bilabial closure, the jaw and lips are being regulated so that they can do whatever else they are disposed to as long as one thing they do is jointly to achieve lip closure.

Constraints like this imply coordination among articulators that respect the constraint. In turn, coordination implies a lack of independence among articulators and so a loss of freedom of movement. Except in producing bilabial obstruents, the jaw and lips are not required to achieve lip closure and they are free to move in ways that will not achieve it. Crucially, when freedom is lost, it is not lost in a hit or miss way. Rather, it is given up precisely to achieve some coarse-grained goal. Loss of independence at a finer level of description of a system brings about coherent functioning at a more macroscopic scale.

Examples like that of bilabial closure imply that there is a real coarse-grained level of organization of the speech system that may allow a closer mapping between vocal tract activity and the units it supposedly realizes. That level is macroscopic enough at least to encompass constraints on groups of articulators to achieve such ends as bilabial closure. Evidence supports the idea that there is such a level of organization.

3.2.1 Vowel Production with Bite Blocks and the Theory of Predictive Simulation

Speakers sometimes talk with a pipe or pencil between their teeth. Although the speech they produce is audibly distinct from speech produced without an obstruction that immobilizes the jaw, it is highly intelligible. Considerations of intelligibility aside, would a speaker choose to speak with a pipe or pencil between the teeth were that to require an entire reorganization of normal means of controlling the articulators? But how can immobilization of the jaw not require a reorganization, given that the jaw is normally quite active in speech? Possibly reorganization is not required because the speaker's means of controlling the articulators for speech include implementing 'constraints' of the sort considered briefly above, and these constraints build in the means by which a pipe may be compensated for. They build in compensations for jaw immobility not because pipe speech is anticipated, but because coarticulatory influences on the jaw must be handled.

In 1971, Lindblom and Sundberg published findings which suggested that speakers can produce acoustically normal or near-normal vowels with a bite block clenched between the teeth that not only immobilized the jaw but immobilized it in a position uncharacteristic for the vowels being produced. A great many replications and extensions of this experiment have been reported (e.g. Folkins and Zimmermann, 1981; Fowler and Turvey, 1980; Lindblom, Lubker and Gay, 1979; Lindblom *et al.*, 1987). The results are clear: vowels produced with a bite block are near-normal articulatorily (Gay, Lindblom and Lubker, 1981), acoustically (Lindblom, Lubker and Gay, 1979) and perceptually (Lubker, 1979).

Lindblom, Lubker and Gay (1979) offer an explanation for speakers' remarkable abilities to compensate. They suggest that phonetic segments are specified in memory as a set of sensory goals (see also Perkell, 1980). Associated with the goals are motor commands for achieving them in the absence of perturbation, coarticulatory or otherwise. Were the motor system for speech wholly 'open-loop' – that is, uninfluenced by feedback from the periphery – these motor commands would not realize the sensory goals for the vowel most of the time, because coarticulating segments would change the effects of the motor commands at the articulatory periphery. Were the motor system wholly 'closed loop' – that is, sensitive to, and regulated by, feedback – these effects of coarticulation could be undone, but only after they had already had their deleterious effects on vowel production. Predictive simulation was proposed as an improvement on open- and closed-loop modes of motor control.

In the predictive simulation system, effects of stored motor commands on the ongoing movements of articulators are simulated using sensory feedback as information about the current state of the vocal tract. Discrepancies between stored sensory goals and simulated sensory consequences of the motor commands are used to adjust the motor commands so that they will achieve the stored sensory goals for the vowel. A system like this will compensate for coarticulatory influences in the vocal tract and also for a bite block that immobilizes the jaw.

The model makes one prediction that has not yet been tested on bite block vowels, but that has been tested on perturbed consonants: it is that compensation should not be possible for perturbations introduced after movement toward the segment's target has begun. That is, once the revised motor commands have been allowed to affect the vocal tract, the system should behave either in an open-loop or in a closed-loop fashion. Perturbations after that will either go uncorrected or else they will be corrected after errors occur. This prediction is unconfirmed for consonant production.

3.2.2 Consonant Production and Synergies

A perturbation applied to the jaw or lower lip during achievement of bilabial closure that pulls the articulator away from its direction of travel does not prevent lip closure for a bilabial consonant (Abbs and Gracco, 1984; Folkins and Abbs, 1975, 1976; Gracco and Abbs, 1985; Kelso *et al.*, 1984). Rather, short-latency compensatory responses occur in the perturbed articulator as well as in the other articulators that contribute to closure so that their joint goal (bilabial closure in the example) is achieved. As in the research using a bite block, compensation is not complete; lip closure may be achieved with less compression of the lips than on unperturbed trials (Abbs and Gracco, 1984) and slightly later than on unperturbed trials (by about 25 ms in the research of Folkins and Abbs, 1975). However, the lips do close, and a successful bilabial consonant is produced.

In this research, in contrast to research on bite block vowels, perturbations are transient and they are applied during an ongoing closure movement for a consonant. In terms of the predictive simulation model, the perturbations are applied after motor commands for realizing a sensory goal have been revised and allowed to affect vocal tract movements. Yet compensation occurs and it may begin to occur within 20–30 ms of the perturbation (Kelso *et al.*, 1984). That compensation occurs at all under these conditions appears incompatible with the predictive simulation model. However, even if the model were modified to allow changes at the periphery to bring about further modification to motor commands, 20–30 ms of latency is an implausibly short time to allow for a new simulation and revision to the commands.

Evidence suggests that, even though the origin of compensation must be low level (that is, not too many synapses away from the periphery), the compensations are functional. Shaiman and Abbs (1987) show that when an articulator not involved in a closing movement is perturbed (when the upper lip is perturbed during closing for /f/), the closing response is no different from that on unperturbed trials. Compatibly (Kelso *et al.*, 1984), when an articulator that is involved in closing is perturbed (the jaw in alveolar closure), compensatory movements are not observed in articulators uninvolved with closure (the lips in the example).[1]

What kind of system could implement a constraint spanning more than one articulator that achieves coarse-grained closure goals? A system with these capabilities is a *synergy* (Gelfand *et al.*, 1971) or *coordinative structure* (Easton, 1972). As Lee (1984) points out, these terms have been used either specifically to refer to a system implemented in the peripheral nervous system and musculature that produces a goal-directed action or else more generally and loosely to refer to a system implemented anywhere that explains systematic macroscopic patterning in behavior. Obviously, the first definition is the stronger one and it is the one intended here. It includes classically defined reflexes, but also, more interestingly, neuromuscular systems that are established transiently for a purpose.

Properties of synergies, according to Lee (1984), include activation of the same set of muscles (not always supraliminally) for execution of the same goal-directed action, constrained temporal sequencing or phasing of muscle actions in repeated performances of the goal-directed action and scaling of the properties of the synergy over changes, say, in rate or magnitude of the movements composing the action. I would add one more, and that is short-latency adaptive responses to perturbation, evident in muscle activity and movement.

All of these characteristics are evident in locomotion (for a review, see Grillner, 1981). However, at least some properties may be evident as well in less fundamental, less evolutionarily primitive, actions such as intentional arm movements (scaling: Kelso, Southard and Goodman, 1979; stereotyped muscle action: Cordo

---

[1]Kelso *et al.* (1984) did observe some extra activity of the orbicularis oris muscle following perturbation of closing during /z/ of /baez/. However, it was not accompanied by kinematic changes in lip activity.

and Nashner, 1982; perturbation: Bizzi and Polit, 1979) or finger movements in typing (Terzuolo and Viviani, 1979).

All have been observed or at least hinted at in speech as well. Muscle actions of the jaw during speech are stereotyped at least in the sense that they are evident in speech produced with a bite block – that is, with the jaw immobilized – as in unconstrained speech (Folkins and Zimmermann, 1981). Actions of the jaw, upper lip and lower lip also exhibit a strict relative temporal ordering in opening gestures (Gracco and Abbs, 1986). Finally, muscle activity (Tuller, Kelso and Harris, 1982) and articulatory movements (Ostry, Keller and Parush, 1983) scale systematically with changes in rate of speech or in stress, as if an invariant system were undergoing simple changes in biomechanical parameters such as equilibrium length or stiffness (Ostry, Keller and Parush, 1983).

The speech system under perturbation also has properties characteristic of synergies. They use lower-level parts flexibly to achieve invariant larger-scale ends in a changing environment and despite perturbation. If the findings from the perturbation research in the speech literature are properly interpreted as revealing use of synergies in speech production, then it is a good guess that synergies are widely used there. The perturbation research shows that constriction gestures for bilabial, labiodental and alveolar obstruents exhibit short-latency compensation for perturbation. It would be surprising if constrictions for other consonants were achieved in some other way. In addition, synergies can account for findings that fostered the predictive simulation account. Possibly, vocalic constrictions, no less than consonantal ones, are achieved by synergies of the vocal tract.

This conclusion is rather momentous in two respects. First, it highlights the fact that there is order in vocal tract behavior at the scale at least of gestural attributes of phonemes. Second, the order in vocal tract behavior corresponds very closely to gestural primitives of Browman and Goldstein's articulatory phonology. Conclusions that there is a fundamental mismatch between elements of linguistic competence and articulatory behavior have been premature. They are considerably weakened by nonlinear phonological theories that attend to the physical characteristics of phonetic segments, and by a more appropriate perspective on vocal tract activity that reveals its macroscopic order.

3.2.3   Saltzman's Task Dynamics Model: Intragestural Coordination

Saltzman and his colleagues (Saltzman, 1986; Kelso, Saltzman and Tuller, 1986; Saltzman and Kelso, 1987; Saltzman and Munhall, 1989) identify synergies in action with nonlinear dissipative dynamical systems more generally (see also Kugler, Kelso and Turvey, 1980; Kugler and Turvey, 1987). Saltzman and Munhall define synergies as 'task-specific and autonomous (time-invariant) dynamical systems that underlie a motion pattern's emergent form as well as its adaptive stability'. In the theory, and in the model of speech production that simulates speaking, the macroscopic invariants (e.g. tract variables such as constriction locations and degrees) of a phonetic gesture serve as 'point attractors' in the vocal tract that cause movement toward the attractor regardless of the current state of the vocal tract and despite perturbation. Dynamic systems are like mass-spring systems, in which a spring, when displaced, approaches its rest position regardless of the direction or extent of displacement.

In speech, movement takes place variably in articulators that compose a synergy for realizing values of those tract variables. Each relevant articulator's contribution to achievement of tract variable values depends on other demands on the articulator imposed by its participation in other synergies that are simultaneously at work in the vocal tract. Saltzman (1986; Saltzman and Kelso, 1987) has successfully modeled achievement of bilabial closure using point attractor dynamics. More importantly, he has modeled effects of an online perturbation that freezes the jaw during closure. Despite the perturbation, the model's 'lips' close without requiring any changes in planned dynamical parameter values. Possibly a weakness in the implementation of the task dynamics model to date is that its 'synergies' are not organizations in the vocal tract neuromusculature *per se* but in a model vocal tract whose actions are seen as driving the vocal tract. From my, perhaps naive, perspective, this may add an intermediary that might be unnecessary were the organization inherent in the peripheral nervous system and musculature – as it apparently is, in the bilabial closure synergy, uncovered by the perturbation experiments described earlier.

3.2.4   Coordination of Gestures for a Consonant or Vowel

Despite the promise of an account of speech production in terms of vocal tract synergies, there remain larger-scale problems of coordination that are not handled by the constriction-producing synergies so far considered. Not all consonants and vowels are exhaustively characterized by their constrictions. Some consonants are unvoiced, and have an associated devoicing gesture of the vocal folds; some phonetic segments are nasalized and have an associated lowering gesture of the velum; some vowels are 'rounded' and have an associated rounding gesture of the lips. There are subtler vocal tract actions as well that I will not consider.

The relationships among the gestures for a consonant or vowel are not well understood. In articulatory phonology, they are represented by association lines to a common 'root node' (see Figure 9.5), and it seems likely that the association is reflected in some way in the vocal tract. Otherwise there would be no way of guaranteeing that, for example, the devoicing gesture of the larynx is timed appropriately with respect to the constriction gesture for an unvoiced consonant. Possibly, synergies for a constriction gesture, and for any other gestures for the same phonetic segment, themselves are subsumed under a larger synergistic organization responsible for maintaining their coordinative relationship. The literature does not yet show this convincingly, however. I briefly review what is known about the relationships among gestures of a segment.

Unvoiced Consonants
Devoicing gestures of the larynx are achieved by abduction then adduction of the vocal folds. In many contexts (for example, generally syllable-initially in English), unvoiced consonants are breathy or aspirated. Producing aspiration requires that the vocal folds be open upon release of the consonantal constriction. Indeed, Löfqvist (1980) reports that the peak opening of the vocal folds occurs very close to release of a voiceless consonant. Furthermore, a linear relationship between onset of closure and peak glottal opening is maintained over variations in rate of speaking and stress that ensures the appropriate time relationship between release

and the devoicing gesture. That a systematic relationship is maintained over variation in stress and rate implies a coordinative relationship between the gestures. This is further suggested by a finding reported by Munhall, Löfqvist and Kelso (1986). Munhall *et al.* applied a perturbation to the lower lip just before oral closure for /p/. The perturbation delayed achievement of oral closure and also delayed the devoicing gesture correspondingly.

Nasalized Consonants

It has been reported (Moll and Daniloff, 1971) that lowering of the velum for a nasal consonant anticipates other gestures for the consonant to a variable extent that depends on the number of vowels preceding the consonant. This observation is taken as evidence for a particular theory of coarticulation known as *feature spreading* (Daniloff and Hammarberg, 1973; see also, Henke, 1966). In a feature-spreading theory, coarticulation is a phonetic or even phonological (Hammarberg, 1976, 1982) process whereby certain features of a segment spread to any neighboring segments that are unspecified for the feature. (While oral consonants are specified [−nasal], English vowels are unspecified for nasality because changing the value of the nasality feature of a vowel in a word never changes the word from one into another.)

A different theory of coarticulation (coarticulation as 'coproduction': Fowler, 1980; or, more specifically, *frame theory*: Bell-Berti and Harris, 1981) holds that coarticulation is not a phonological process at all;[2] instead, it reflects the way that segments are serially ordered in the vocal tract. There is, then, no coarticulatory process by which features of one segment spread to other segments (although, as noted earlier, individual languages may have phonological processes, such as vowel and nasal harmony, in which features spread). Instead, coarticulation is a process of temporally overlapping the articulation of neighboring segments in an utterance. In these theories, if the velum lowers during a vowel before a nasal consonant, it is not because the vowel has acquired a new featural attribute, but because production of the vowel and consonant overlap. According to frame theory (Bell-Berti and Harris, 1981), anticipatory lowering of the nasal consonant retains its affiliation to a nasal consonant and anticipates oral constriction for the consonant by an invariant time interval regardless of the number of vowels preceding the nasal consonant.

How can such a theory be entertained in the light of evidence such as that reported by Moll and Daniloff (1971)? In fact, the data from this and other research are not very clear. Bladon and Al-Bamerni (1982) cite five published reports favoring feature spreading, four favoring frame theory, one with an ambiguous outcome and their own findings which suggest to them that there are two coarticulatory styles that speakers choose between. More importantly, however, Bell-Berti (1980) shows that none of the research up to the time of her review is interpretable. It is well known that vowels are associated with different characteristic postures of the velum depending on vowel height (Moll, 1962) and with lower positions of the velum than occur during oral consonants. When researchers report

---

[2]This is not to say that the sound inventories of languages have no influence on coarticulatory extent and patterning (Boyce, 1988; Manuel, 1987; Manuel and Krakow, 1984). Languages may constrain the extent to which coarticulation can cause the acoustic consequences of producing a segment to resemble the acoustic product of some other segment of the inventory.

lowering of the velum just after the C in a CVN and a CVVN sequence (where C is an oral consonant, V a vowel and N a nasal consonant), and so an earlier onset of lowering in CVVN, they are almost certainly confusing the lowering gesture from C to the first V with onset of lowering for N. According to frame theory, when those confounding influences are eliminated, lowering of the velum for the nasal consonant begins an invariant interval before oral constriction.

Although I think that frame theory provides a more realistic perspective on the relationshipship between the two gestures for a nasal consonant than does feature spreading theory, its claim of temporal invariance between onsets of the two gestures is almost certainly too strong. It would be surprising if manipulation of rate of speaking and of stress were not to change the temporal interval between the gestures. However, if the interval varies systematically with other temporal intervals associated with nasal consonant production (as the timing of the devoicing gesture does in research by Löfqvist and Yoshioka, 1984), then frame theory's claim of an affiliation between the gestures of a nasal consonant would be supported. There is at least one other source of variability in the relationship between the gestures, however. Krakow (1988, 1989) shows that lowering of the velum begins earlier and reaches maximum lowering earlier for syllable-final than for syllable-initial nasal consonants. Within each syllable position, the timing of maximum velum lowering and the oral constriction gesture is quite stable, however.

Rounded vowels

The same controversy, between feature spreading and frame theory, occurs in the literature on lip rounding. There are reports that lip rounding anticipates rounded vowel onset to an extent that varies with the number of preceding consonants (Benguerel and Cowan, 1974; Sussman and Westbury, 1981), and that it anticipates vowel onset by a fixed interval (Bell-Berti and Harris, 1979). As for nasality, estimates of the anticipation of lip rounding have been contaminated, here by the occurrence of lip muscle activity (Gelfer, Bell-Berti and Harris, 1982) and movement (Boyce, 1988) for consonants preceding the rounded vowel. Gelfer *et al.* find that onset of lip muscle activity (orbicularis oris) anticipates a vowel increasingly the longer the string of consonants before the vowel, whether the vowel in question is or is not rounded! When consonant-related activity is eliminated from sequences in which rounded vowels are produced, the onset of rounding for the vowel is invariant over consonant strings of lengths greater than one.

Here, as in the research on anticipation of nasality for a nasalized consonant, frame theory appears to handle the data better than feature spreading theory. This conclusion is supported as well by findings of a 'trough' in lip rounding movements and in muscle activity during a consonant string between two rounded vowels (Bell-Berti and Harris, 1974; Boyce, 1988; Perkell, 1986). If the feature [+rounding] were to spread to any consonants before a rounded vowel, then there should be no trough.

If there is an invariant timing relationship between rounding and the constriction gesture for a rounded vowel, then there must be some coordinative relationship between the two gestures. Most likely, however, the interval between the gestures will prove not to be invariant over variation in rate of speaking and stress, and an important question will be whether it bears some systematic relationship to other intervals involving the two gestures over these manipulations.

Intergestural Sequencing in Task Dynamics

In Saltzman's model, gestures have associated 'activation coordinates'. These provide values for the influence over time that a gesture exerts on the vocal tract. The time at which a gesture's activation level becomes positive is determined by the gestural score of Browman and Goldstein's model. Saltzman and Munhall do not consider this solution to the sequencing problem satisfactory, and they suggest an alternative that I will consider shortly.

3.2.5   Coarticulation of Constriction Gestures

The foregoing review examined coordination of gestures for a given consonant or vowel. I turn now to sequencing of gestures for neighboring consonants and vowels in an utterance.

Although there is some disagreement as to when movements toward vowels begin in a V_1CV_2 sequence (compare Gay, 1977, and the investigators cited just below), in at least some circumstances, they begin early enough to affect the acoustic speech signal during the closing transition from V_1 to C (Öhman, 1966). In a V_1CdCV_2 sequence, the malleable /d/ vowel may be strongly influenced by both flanking Vs (e.g. Fowler, 1981a,b). Examination of tongue movements during V_1CV_2 sequences suggest that, when the C does not involve the tongue body anyway, the tongue may move smoothly from V_1 to V_2. (These movements may be reduced or blocked when the tongue body is used to produce the consonant; Recasens, 1984.) This has led some investigators to conclude that vowel production is, where possible, continuous during speech (Fowler, 1980; Öhman, 1966; Perkell, 1969).[3] If so, and if movements toward V_2's constriction gesture can occur very early, it may imply that consonants in a sequence bear the major responsibility for preserving the serial order of consonants and vowels in a planned sequence.

Spatial Overlap in Speech

Sometimes overlapping gestures make competing demands on the same articulators. One possible outcome is that multiple influences on a common articulator are wholly independent and they simply sum at the periphery. Some kinds of overlap do look like that. For example, the position for the jaw during /b/ closure is lower if a coarticulating vowel is open than if it is closed (cited in Keating, 1990). Similarly, raising of the velum continues throughout a string of oral obstruents so that the position of the velum is higher during the second /t/ in a /ts#st/ sequence than in a /t#t/ sequence (Bell-Berti, 1980). Finally, Boyce (1988) found additive effects of rounding for vowels and lip movements associated with conson-

---

[3]Here is another example, possibly, of the phenomenon of 'triggering' discussed by MacNeilage and Ladefoged (1976), in relation to the findings of near-universal differences in vowel duration before voiced and voiceless consonants and of phonologization of the difference in a few languages. Many languages, perhaps all, show vowel-to-vowel coarticulation (see references in the text). However, a few languages (including, for example, Turkish, Hungarian and Yawelmani – an American Indian language of California) have phonological processes known as 'vowel harmony' in which, roughly, the vowels of a word are required to share a phonetic feature(s). For example, in Yawelmani a vowel is rounded ([+back]) if preceded by a vowel in the same word that is rounded and matched in height (Kenstowicz and Kisseberth, 1979).

ants. In fact, however, independence of influences is probably not generally realistic, as Saltzman and Munhall (1989) note. For example, while the jaw is susceptible to vocalic influences during /b/, it is not, or is less so, during /s/ (Keating, 1990). Accordingly, there must be a way to suppress vocalic influences in that context – in the task dynamics model, this is accomplished by 'blending rules' that have gesture-specific and phoneme-specific parameter values. There is, as yet, no systematic investigation of varieties of 'blending' in natural speech.

Serial Ordering of Consonants and Vowels

How does a talker know when to start producing the gestures of a segment? Are initiations timed as if by a clock (cf. 'comb' models of sequencing; Bernstein, 1967; Kozhevnikov and Chistovich, 1965) or are they triggered by information from the periphery signaling that it is time (cf. 'chain' models), or is there some third way? Each extreme model has deficiencies. In the speech literature, one recent proposal is a variant of a chain model.

Kelso and Tuller (1987) suggested that sequencing might depend on a phasing rule. For example, if a vowel's gesture is defined as spanning a 360-degree cycle, then a following consonant might be initiated at some fixed phase angle of the cycle (say after 200 degrees). Initial findings were supportive of the view; however, more recent findings (Nittrouer *et al.*, 1988) are not. Accordingly, the details of sequencing in speech are still not understood.

In Dell's (1986) model, recall that sequencing is achieved by giving a 'current node' extra activation as compared to activation assigned to later elements in a planned sequence. The lowest level of the language at which his model applies this sequencing is that of individual phonemes of a word. Therefore, the model will not give rise to temporally staggered gestures of a phoneme or to coarticulation more generally. With Figure 9.4 above substituted for Dell's lowest level, syllabic frame, gestural sequencing might be achieved by means of the gestural score. Indeed, as briefly noted earlier, that is how gestural sequencing is achieved currently in the task dynamics model.

However, Saltzman and Munhall (1989) do not find that solution satisfying, apparently because, whereas intragestural coordination is a product of the dynamics of the speech system, intergestural sequencing by this account is not. They intend to incorporate a version of Jordan's (1986) model for serial dynamics into the task dynamics model to replace the gestural score.

Briefly, in Jordan's model, learned sequences are trajectories through a 'state space' that, over learning, become 'attractors'. In contrast to the point attractors that cause realization of constrictions for consonants and vowels, however, these are trajectories that attract other less well-learned trajectories to it. A trajectory through a state space, in turn, determines successive values for output units in the model, and these values determine actions of the system. In task dynamics, the succession of positive activation values for gestures will be determined by the succession of positive values for different output units.

This kind of system allows learning of arbitrary orderings of a small inventory of elements and, to a large extent, that is exactly the task for a child acquiring a lexicon of words. In the model, learning a planned sequence occurs as an output sequence is compared to a 'teacher' sequence. Errors in the form of discrepancies between the output and teacher sequences are propagated back through the system and are used to change the weights on linkages between units in the network.

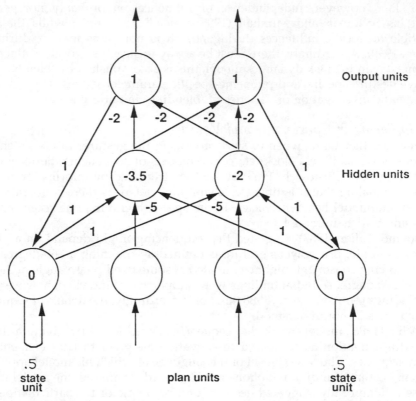

Figure 9.6. *A network consisting of two plan units, two state units, two hidden units and two output units. With the biases (value printed in the circles) and weights (values on the linkages) shown, and with plan units [1,0], the network will produce a sequence AAAB, where A is output [1,1] and B is [0,0]. Outputs are binary, taking on a value 1 if the net input to the unit is positive and 0 if it is negative. If the plan is [0,1], the network produces AB. [From Jordan, 1986.]*

Eventually, in the presence of a plan to perform a sequence, the output sequence matches that of the teacher. (See Figure 9.6 for a sample network that has learned to produce two different sequences in the presence of different plans.)

A remarkable property of Jordan's model is that ordered consonants and vowels of a learned sequence coarticulate without being explicitly instructed to. Coarticulation develops during the learning process as the model learns to match certain specified output values of the teacher. Output values for the segments of a word are determined by a plan for the word (a different one for each word, in which serial ordering of elements is not specified explicitly) and by changing values of state units in the system. Plan units and state units determine values of 'hidden units', which in turn determine values of output units (Figure 9.6). State values change over time, and their next value in a trajectory is determined by their previous value and by the just-computed output values. Therefore, successive values of state units are similar and they produce similar outputs. Accordingly, as learning proceeds, coarticulatory effects of an output tend to spread bidirectionally.

3.3 Concluding Remarks

A major aim of this section was to show that the phonologies of languages may be conceptualized in such a way that the fundamental units of language do not have characteristics that vocal tracts are physically incapable of realizing, and that vocal tract activity can be shown to exhibit macroscopic patterning at a scale commensurate with that of the fundamental units of language. Neither adjustment in point of view threatens the close correspondence uncovered in Section 2 between units of the language and units of a speech plan.

Some researchers have begun to believe that organizations for intentional activity are achieved in ways not unlike self-organizing processes in other dynamic systems. Possibly, then, synergies are examples of dynamic systems as Saltzman and his colleagues suppose. A major unresolved problem is still (cf. Lashley, 1951) to understand how speakers achieve largely accurate ordering of linguistic elements in speech. Jordan's approach to the problem appears quite successful and, according to Saltzman and Munhall, largely compatible with their own dynamic approach to modeling speech production more generally. It remains to be determined to what extent both of these models realistically reflect speaker's manners of implementing synergies and of ordering them sequentially.

There remains a different kind of mismatch between 'competence' and 'performance' that may, in the minds of many investigators, render an effort to equate linguistic units and produced units irrelevant. It is a view that phonological segments are inherently mental categories, where 'mental' means products of and residing in the mind of an intelligent organism.

This point of view is represented in the literature (Hammarberg, 1976, 1982; Repp, 1981). If it has merit, then any attempt to equate units of the language with physical activity of the vocal tract is a sort of category error. In my opinion, however, the view is fundamentally in error.

The claim is that phonological segments as known are mental things and those as uttered are physical things, and so they are things of fundamentally different kinds. This is not quite right, however. If there are phonological categories in the mind, they must have some physical (e.g. neurological) instantiation in the brain, and so they are physical things as well as mental ones. More importantly, however, public activities that communicate linguistic messages to listeners may also be seen as mental (psychological, intelligent) things as well as physical ones. As Ryle points out (1949), intelligent actions have two aspects: they are physical actions, but they are also intelligent. Accordingly:

> 'When a person talks sense aloud, ties knots, feints or sculpts, the actions which we witness are themselves the things which he is intelligently doing, though the concepts in terms of which the physicist or physiologist would describe his actions do not exhaust those which would be used by his pupils or his teachers in appraising their logic, style or technique. He is bodily active and he is mentally active, but he is not being synchronously active in two different "places" or with two different "engines". There is one activity, but it is one susceptible of and requiring of more than one explanatory description.' (p. 51).

A different argument also suggests that linguistic utterances as known and performed are not different kinds of things. When theorists conclude that speech activity fails to achieve linguistic units, they are taking the view that units of competence are primary and units of performance are derived. That is, what we do when we speak is a pale, not-entirely-true, reflection of what we know about the language and of what we plan to say. But an alternative view is that the relationship is reversed, both in the ontogeny of the individual and in its mature form. We know what units are autonomous in the language because they are used autonomously by native speakers when they talk. That is, competence (what we know) is derived from what we do and what we experience other members of our language community doing. (By analogy, there are such things in the world as chairs that we may come to know by experience. If it is true that we come to have a category corresponding to 'chairs' in memory, it is because there is such a category in the world that we have come to recognize. Chairs in the world are primary; what we know of them is derived.) Because what we know of language is derived from what we do and what we experience other members of a language community doing – indeed, because competence is knowledge of the essentials of language performance – the elements in each domain can, it seems, be the same kinds of things (but see, for example, Chomsky, 1986, for a wholly different point of view).

4 Prosodic Structure in Speech

The acoustic speech signal exhibits considerably more systematicity than the vocal tract activities considered so far will generate. In the domain of fundamental frequency (f_0), talkers produce utterances with an intonational melody. In addition, in at least some styles of speech, f_0 falls gradually throughout a sentence or phrase. Further, each content word of the language has at least one stressed syllable – that is, a syllable apparently produced with greater respiratory and articulatory effort (Lehiste, 1970) than other syllables so that it is longer, more intense, its vowel spectrally less centralized and its f_0 increased over an unstressed syllable consisting of the same phonological segments. In addition, syllables or groups of stressed and unstressed syllables (stress feet) are supposed to be produced rhythmically so that the one constituent or the other (that is, the syllable or the stress foot) is approximately isochronous in syllable- and stress-timed languages, respectively. Whether or not there is such a tendency is controversial (see, for example, Allen, 1975; Classe, 1939; Dauer, 1983; Ohala, 1970). However, it is the case, at least, that in many languages a syllable's vowel is shortened increasingly as consonants are added to the syllable (Fowler, 1983; Lindblom and Rapp, 1973) and a stressed vowel is shortened as unstressed syllables are added to the foot (Fowler, 1981a). Finally, apart from these shortenings (Rakerd, Sennett and Fowler, 1987), languages show lengthenings ('final lengthening'; Klatt, 1976) and pauses at the ends of phrasal constituents that correlate at least approximately with the syntactic depth of the boundary (Cooper and Paccia-Cooper, 1980). Oddly, however, the units that lengthenings and pauses delimit are only approximately syntactic (Gee and Grosjean, 1983).

As Fudge (1969) suggests, there are two kinds of hierarchical constituency in speech. There is the morphosyntactic grouping of phonemes into morphemes, morphemes into words and words into syntactic phrases. In addition, there is a phonological or prosodic hierarchy of phonemes into syllables, syllables into stress feet and stress feet into larger phrasal groupings.[4] Interestingly, the units of the first hierarchy misorder in speech errors while the units of the latter do not.[5] Nor, for the most part, are the prosodic groupings indicated in writing systems, while morphosyntactic ones often are. Gee and Grosjean's characterization of the prosodic organization as 'performance structures' is probably apt.

Even though prosodic structures may emerge uniquely in spoken utterances, they are not necessarily automatic consequences of vocal tracts producing speech. For example, intonation contours vary across utterances, and certain 'tunes' are associated with certain speaker attitudes or intended meanings.

In linguistics, metrical phonologies characterize the prosodic patterning best. I will briefly review this kind of phonological theory first as it characterizes stress and then as it has been applied to intonation.

4.1 Metrical Phonology[6]

4.1.1 Stress

The two syllables of any disyllabic word differ phenomenally in prominence or degree of stress. In the word 'return' the second syllable is more prominent than the first; in 'reason' the first is the more prominent. In metrical phonology, that relationship of prominence is expressed as follows (Liberman and Prince, 1977):

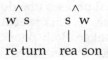

where s marks the stronger of the two 'tree branches' and the w the weaker. In longer words, too, one syllable stands out as most prominent or strongest; of the remaining syllables, some may appear very weak ('reduced') while others may be intermediate in prominence between the strongest and the weakest. For example, the third syllable in 'anecdotal' is strongest, the first is next strongest while the

---

[4]In MacKay's (1987) recent theory of speech production, the phonological hierarchy is the bottom part of a single hierarchical strucure that includes the morphological hierarchy as the top part. However, for two reasons, this is an error. First, consider the interface between the hierarchies. In MacKay's model, morphemes are superordinate to syllables. However, while there are some morphemes that can be said to be composed of one or more syllables (e.g. 'dog', 'carpet'), there are also syllables that are composed of morphemes ('grew', 'walks'). Second, and analogously, there are phonological groupings (stress feet, phonological and intonational phrases) larger than the syllable that are not necessarily coextensive with larger morphosyntactic units.

[5]This is not to say that talkers make no suprasegmental errors. They may impose phrasal stress on the wrong word or produce an inappropriate intonation contour (Cutler, 1980). It is only to say that the metrical units themselves do not misorder.

[6]The following is a composite of perspectives offered by Hayes (1982), Liberman and Prince (1977), Selkirk (1980a,b) and van der Hulst and Smith (1982).

other syllables are weak. Its metrical structure is as follows:

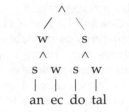

Such a tree structure suggests that there are at least three groupings of syllables: one in which pairs of syllables contrast in relative prominence, one in which syllables are grouped into larger constituents (stress feet) which themselves differ in prominence, and one in which feet are grouped into words.

Above the word, analogous rules can assign relative prominence to words of a sentence (see, for example, Selkirk, 1980a,b). In Selkirk's account (but see Selkirk, 1984), there are two hierarchical levels above the word: the 'phonological phrase' and the 'intonational phrase'. In the sentence: 'The absent-minded professor has been avidly reading about the latest biography of Marcel Proust,' there are four phonological phrases (with right edges after 'professor', 'reading', 'biography' and 'Proust'). These are not all syntactic groupings ('has been avidly reading' is not), but they do tend to group words into a structure of which the final word is the 'head' of a syntactic phrase. (The head of a noun phrase is a noun, that of a verb phrase is a verb, etc.) Intonational phrases (the domain of an intonational tune) are groupings of phonological phrases. Selkirk speculates that these groupings may be selected fairly freely by the speaker. Both phonological phrases and intonational phrases assign s to right branches of their trees. This is compatible with a general tendency for speakers to place newer and more foreground information later in a sentence (Gee and Grosjean, 1983); by making right branches prominent, newer or otherwise foreground information will be highlighted by being assigned pitch accents, for example.

Whereas at lower levels of the tree structure, prominence is realized as stress accent, at the higher levels it is realized by accents of an intonation contour (Beckman, 1985).

4.1.2 Intonation

Intonation contours are continuous, during voiced parts of an utterance. However, in the phonological accounts under consideration (Liberman, 1975, Pierrehumbert, 1980), intonational tunes are composed of sequences of discrete tones (low, middle and high in Liberman, 1975; low and high in Pierrehumbert, 1980, and in most subsequent accounts). Pitch accents composed of tones are aligned to prominent syllables; the intonation contour is interpolated and smoothed from prominent syllable to prominent syllable.

Languages may have characteristic tunes – that is, particular sequences of pitch accents and boundary tones that express a speaker's attitude or intended meaning. Possible tunes are generated by rule.

4.2 Why is there a Prosodic Organization Distinct from a Syntactic One?

Stress accents on words ensure that content words receive some measure of prominence for the listener. (Function words tend to be de-stressed.) Larger groupings that elevate the prominence of selected words allow particular words, and so particular parts of the communicative message, to be highlighted. Which words of an utterance are to be highlighted will have to do not only with the syntactic structure of the sentence, but also with the speaker's particular intent in uttering the sentence. The prosodic structure allows a measure of freedom in the talker's performance to augment what can be conveyed by the words in their syntactic groupings.

4.3 Speech Production Once Again: Prosodic Structures

In the final several sections, I will review evidence for four prosodic constituencies in speech production: syllables, stress feet, phonological phrases and intonational phrases. Questions are whether they manifest themselves at all in speech performance and if so how, what kinds of constituents they are and, in cases where proposals have been offered, how they make their way into speech performance.

4.3.1 Syllables

Syllables may have their foundations in the jaw cycle. The jaw is a major articulator for speech that cycles open and closed. Canonically, syllables are closing–opening cycles of the jaw. However, even if that is the ultimate source of syllables in speech, in languages they are more than closing and opening gestures of the jaw. Languages differ in the syllable structures they permit; all languages allow CV syllables, but many disallow complex structures such as the CCCVCC structure of the word 'strength' in English. Even so, the jaw cycle does manifest itself cross-linguistically in a universal tendency for syllables to respect a 'sonority hierarchy' such that consonants in a syllable order themselves so that they increase in vowel-likeness the closer they are to the vowel. (For example, the order of /t/ and /r/ is /tr/ before the vowel and /rt/ after it.) A consequence is that the jaw opens smoothly toward the vowel, rarely reversing direction, and smoothly closes after the vowel (Keating, 1983).

Syllables require mention in theories of phonology for several reasons. In some languages with phonological length distinctions (so that V:, a long vowel otherwise identical to V, counts as a distinct vowel from V, and C: is distinct from C), syllable structure constraints require that a syllable containing V: must be followed by C, not by C: while a syllable containing V is followed by C: (see, for example, Lehiste, 1970). In many instances, syllable structure constrains the application of a phonological process in the language. For example, according to Kahn (1976), in so-called r-less dialects of English, /r/s are dropped unless they are syllable-initial. Therefore, /r/s in 'car' and 'carpet' are dropped, while those in 'carry' and 'rack' are not.

Likewise, phonological theories require that syllables be assigned an internal structure. In 'quantity-sensitive' languages, syllable weight determines whether a syllable can be metrically strong; weight is determined in most quantity-sensitive languages by the number of consonants in the syllable 'rhyme' (the vowel and final consonants) or by the syllable nucleus (the vowel alone). Rarely is the syllable onset (the prevocalic consonants) relevant to a determination of metrical strength (but see Davis, 1988). For these languages, anyway, this suggests a hierarchical structure of the syllable into onset and rhyme, and of the rhyme into nucleus and final consonants ('coda'). This structure is supported on other grounds as well, such as the relative strength of sequencing restrictions on phonemes within and between these syllable constituents (Fudge, 1969).

I am unaware of any convincing evidence that syllables or syllable constituents are autonomous performance units, however. Although they may constrain the movement of phonemes in errors as described earlier (that is, consonants that misorder in speech errors tend to maintain their position relative to the vowel), they do not misorder in speech errors as phonemes and words do, for example.

Another place in which syllables appear in descriptions of systematic speech behavior is in descriptions of systematic influences on vowel duration. Lindblom, Lyberg and Holmgren (1981) conclude that, in Swedish, syllable structure affects vowel duration in that a vowel shortens progressively as consonants are added to the vowel either before or after it (see also Fowler, 1983, for English). As Lindblom *et al.* point out, this may be seen as a compensatory shortening effect as if the talker were attempting to maintain a constant syllable duration regardless of the number of segments in the syllable. However, as they also point out, as an attempt to maintain syllable isochrony, it is feeble. Shortening of the vowel in the presence of neighboring consonants is far smaller than the duration of the consonants themselves. Syllable isochrony is not maintained. In any case, there is reason to doubt that this is an effect of syllable structure. In the data presented by Lindblom *et al.*, vowels shorten even if the added consonants are in a syllable adjacent to it. Hence the shortening may not index syllable structure at all.

I have suggested that it is an acoustic-durational manifestation of coarticulatory overlap of the vowel by the neighboring consonants (Fowler, 1983). Consistent with that interpretation, Fowler *et al.* (1986) found no evidence of *articulatory* shortening of opening for a vowel as consonants are added to its syllable rhyme; jaw lowering for the vowel has about the same duration and extent regardless of the size of the coda. Instead, Fowler *et al.* found an earlier onset of jaw raising for the consonants in the coda.

Treiman (1983, 1984, 1986) has found considerable evidence that speakers are sensitive to syllable structure. In her research, subjects learn word games that require them to split off parts of syllables and recombine them. If the game requires them to split off the onsets of syllable pairs from their rhymes and to create new syllables consisting of the onset of one syllable attached to the rhyme of the other, they learn the game faster and with fewer errors than if a different parsing is required that violates syllable constituents. For syllable-final, but not syllable-initial, consonants, the difficulty of games that violate their constituency varies with the sonority of the consonants. That is, syllable-final games requiring either V/CC or VC/C partitionings were about equally difficult if the postvocalic consonant was a nasal, intermediate in sonority. Games requiring a V/CC partitioning were considerably easier than those requiring VC/C splits if the postvocalic consonant was an obstruent (a stop or a fricative). Finally, VC/C games were actually easier than V/CC games if the postvocalic consonants were the highly sonorous liquids, /l/ or

/r/. It is not yet evident, however, what makes consonants in the coda more cohesive with the vowel than consonants in the onset, or what makes more sonorous consonants – but possibly only those in the coda – more cohesive with the vowel than less sonorous ones.

In short, although there are hints that the syllable has some reality in speech planning and performance – as a structure that constrains the movement of consonants in speech errors and as a structure otherwise affecting the cohesiveness of consonants with the vowel – its role in speech production is far from clear.

4.3.2 Stress Feet

Syllables may be built on one kind of cycle, the closing and opening of the jaw, while stress feet realize another kind of rhythmicity – an approximate alternation of stressed and unstressed syllables. However, the stress rhythm, if there is one, has a less obvious foundation in dispositions of the vocal tract than the syllabic rhythm.

The stress foot manifests itself in speech in two ways: as an inclination on the part of speakers to alternate stressed and unstressed syllables and as a tendency to shorten stressed syllables when a foot is more than monosyllabic (or else perhaps a tendency to lengthen stressed syllables when a foot is monosyllabic; e.g. Bolinger, 1963, 1981). In fact, these may be joint reflections of a common stress-alternation tendency.

As for the tendency to alternate stressed and unstressed syllables, Kelly and Bock (1988) find that nonsense words with two stressable syllables are likely to be pronounced with trochaic stress (strong–weak) rather than iambic stress (weak–strong) when they are preceded by an unstressed syllable and followed by a stressed one; the tendency to use a trochaic rhythm is significantly reduced (but not reversed) when the preceding stress context is weak and the following one is strong.

Compatibly, disyllabic verbs have been found to be more likely (in spontaneous speech) to be followed by syllabic inflections (that is, inflections such as -ing for verbs or -es, pronounced /Iz/, for nouns) than disyllabic nouns (Kelly, 1988). Moreover, in an experiment in which disyllabic nonwords occurred in contexts where they served as verbs, they were more often produced with iambic stress if they ended in /d/ and took an -ed suffix (pronounced /Id/) than if they were identical except that they ended in a consonant after which -ed is pronounced /d/ or /t/.

A different manifestation of the stress foot in speech behavior is the occurrence of stressed syllable shortening when feet are more than monosyllabic. This occurs for words spoken in isolation (Lehiste, 1972) as well as words in context, among at least speakers of Swedish (Lindblom and Rapp, 1973), English (Fowler, 1981a) and Dutch (Nooteboom, 1973). The same pattern is considerably weaker in Italian (Vayra, Avesani and Fowler, 1984) – ostensibly a 'syllable-timed' language, rather than a stress-timed language (even though at least some investigators consider Italian to have a left-dominant stress foot structure; Nespor and Vogel, 1979). In Swedish and English, which have left-dominant feet, comparable shortening of a stressed syllable is not observed when an unstressed neighbor is in a different stress foot – that is, when they precede the stressed syllable (Fowler, 1981a; Lindblom and Rapp, 1973). In English, in at least some contexts, the shortening is correlated with coarticulatory overlap (Fowler, 1981a); to the extent that an unstressed syllable coarticulates with a stressed syllable, the stressed syllable is shortened by the unstressed syllable. Coarticulation and shortening may be independent indices of the greater cohesion between a stressed syllable and the immediately following unstressed syllable than between a stressed syllable and a preceding unstressed syllable or a final unstressed syllable in a trisyllabic foot. Alternatively, as I suggested above for shortening of vowels by consonants, the acoustic shortening may be a manifestation of coarticulatory overlap.

The shortening of stressed by unstressed syllables has been seen as an indication that talkers may be attempting to maintain isochrony of stress feet ('stress-timing'; for reviews, see Dauer, 1983; Fowler, 1977). However, as many researchers have pointed out, the small amount of shortening of the vowel does not come close to compensating for duration of an unstressed syllable added to a foot (e.g. the duration of 'speedy' is longer than that of the word 'speed' even though the first syllable in 'speedy' is shorter than that in 'speed').

Edwards and Beckman (1988) looked at these findings differently: they considered that the monosyllabic foot lengthened, rather than that the disyllabic foot shortened. They found that the jaw opening phase of a stressed syllable in a monosyllabic (as compared to a disyllabic) foot is lengthened relatively less than the closing phase so that the point of maximum opening of the jaw (and so the prominence peak for the vowel of a prominent syllable) occurs relatively earlier in the monosyllabic foot. They ascribed the lengthening to the presence of a stress clash. That the lengthening accomplishes a relative backward shift of the prominence peak of the vowel suggests that lengthening is a way of shifting the prominence peak of a stressed syllable back away from that of a following stressed syllable and alleviating the stress clash that way rather than by shifting stress off the first syllable altogether.

The foregoing review reveals at least a tendency to alternate strong and weak syllables and in addition, perhaps, a stronger degree of cohesion, in two languages with left-dominant feet, between stressed syllables and following unstressed ones than between stressed syllables and preceding unstressed ones. It does not reveal a reason for the alternations to occur, nor a function for the stress foot.

An entirely different perspective on the stress foot is provided by the work of Sternberg, Monsell and their colleagues (Monsell, 1986; Sternberg et al., 1978, 1980). These investigators designed an experimental procedure to study 'motor programming' in speech and typing. In the procedure as applied to speech, subjects were given a list of words to say as rapidly as they could. However, there was a considerable (several seconds) delay between list presentation and a signal to begin producing the list. The subjects' latencies to begin the utterance and their utterance durations provided the main measures in the experiments.

Because talkers know in advance what they will be saying, their latencies do not reflect a choice between utterance alternatives; the task measures 'simple reaction time'. Moreover, to the extent that it is possible to construct a speech plan in advance of its execution, subjects have the information and the time needed to construct one before the response signal is presented. Even so, the subjects' latencies to begin the utterance vary systematically with the number of things to say: a list of five-digit names is initiated later than a list of three-digit names, for example. Remarkably, the function relating latency to utterance length defined by the number of things to say is linear with a slope that is stable over different utterance compositions (e.g. digit names, days of the week). However, the function is linear with a stable slope only if the number of things to say is counted in stress feet, not in syllables, words or phrases (Monsell, 1986; Sternberg *et al.*, 1978, 1980). The linearity of the relationship means that each addition of a stress foot to a list of things to say adds a constituent amount of time (around 12 ms) to response latency.

Another remarkable finding of this research that has shaped its interpretation by Sternberg and his colleagues concerns the function relating total utterance duration to number of stress feet in the utterance. The duration function is not a straight line; rather, it is a quadratic function (that is, of the form $y = ax^2 + bx + c$, where y is utterance duration and x is the number of stress feet in the utterance). That the function is a quadratic means that the slope of the function increases by a constant amount as more stress feet are added to the utterance. That is, the more there is to say, the more slowly the components of the utterance are produced. Interestingly, the increase in slope (the coefficient of the x^2 term) is the same as the slope of the latency function (about 12 ms).

How can the collection of findings be explained? An intuitive idea is that the heavier the load on the system, the slower it works. One elaboration of this idea has been tested and ruled out. The elaboration is that the load in question is a 'processing' load in a system with a limited 'processing capacity'. That interpretation was ruled out in an experiment by Sternberg *et al.* (1978), in which talkers were given a list of digits to remember while producing another utterance as rapidly as possible after a response signal. The digit load was meant to require processing capacity and hence to increase latency and utterance duration if limited processing capacity were behind the latency and duration functions. However, the digit load had essentially no effect on the latency and duration functions even though subjects did well recalling the digits.

Sternberg *et al.* offer the following interpretation of their findings. The stress foot is the unit into which consonants and vowels of the words in the utterance list are packaged for execution. Subjects construct a motor program or plan in advance of the response signal consisting of the words of the utterance packaged into stress feet. When the response signal is presented to initiate the utterance, they must *retrieve* the first stress foot, *unpack* it into its parts and execute a *command* process to initiate vocal tract activity. To produce the whole utterance, they successively retrieve, unpack and command production of successive stress feet in the utterance. The retrieval process is sensitive to the number, but not the size, of stress feet, while the other two processes are sensitive to the size of each stress foot, but not the number of stress feet in the utterance. This can explain why, for example, the slope of the latency function is sensitive only to the number of stress feet, but not to their compositions.

The retrieval phase of plan execution is identified as a serial search through a buffer consisting of the stress feet to be produced. Because latency to speak increases with the number of things to be said, it must be supposed that the search does not proceed, say, left to right in a buffer in which stress feet are arrayed in the order, left to right, in which they will be said. Either the search order or the order of items in the buffer, or both, must be different from the to-be-uttered order. Morever, that the slope of the latency function has the same value as the coefficient of the squared term of the duration function implies that the buffer does not shrink as the utterance proceeds. If the talker has produced three of five stress feet in a sequence, to find the fourth the retrieval mechanism must still search through a buffer containing five stress feet. Otherwise, the latency to produce successive items in the utterance would shrink and overall the coefficient of the squared term of the duration function would be smaller than that of the latency function.

The latency to begin talking will also be affected by the time to unpack the first item in the sequence. The duration of the first stress foot will be determined by the duration of its command process (the more vocal tract gestures to be initiated, the longer the stress foot). The interword interval will be affected by the retrieval time for the next item and its unpacking time. In fact, those variables affect the entire interval consisting of the duration of the second syllable of a disyllabic stress foot and the interword interval. Accordingly, Sternberg et al. propose that the final part of a stress foot is allowed to continue during retrieval and unpacking of the next stress foot.

The model involves stages that, intuitively, are parts of motor planning and execution, and it accounts extraordinarily well for the data. However, at least one aspect of the model – its retrieval mechanism – is implausible. Why should the retrieval mechanism search elements in an order different from their to-be-produced order? Why would a talker not order items to be produced in their planned serial order? Dell's (1986) model offers a possible answer to these questions. In that model, the 'order' of to-be-produced items is their location in the lexicon. To signal their planned order in an utterance, they are assigned order tags. It is not difficult to imagine a retrieval mechanism more or less as described by Sternberg et al. searching among the order tags to find the appropriate unit to output. However, there are several difficulties with this attempted merger of Dell's lexicon and the motor plan of Sternberg et al. One is that sequences such as 'Monday Monday Monday Monday' and its subsets yield the same latency and duration functions as sequences such as 'Monday Friday Wednesday Tuesday' and its subsets. Yet in Dell's model, all the order tags for the 'Monday' sequences would be on the same word node. A second difficulty is that there is an incompatibility of units. Dell's units must be morphosyntactic while those of Sternberg et al. have been shown not to be. A third difficulty is that stress feet do not misorder in speech, but a retrieval mechanism of the sort proposed by Sternberg et al. seems unlikely to be infallible.

Rosenbaum, Kenny and Derr (1983; see also Rosenbaum, 1985) point out that the qualitative outcome reported by Sternberg et al. can be captured in an entirely different way than Sternberg et al. propose if elements in the to-be-uttered sequence are ordered and are hierarchically organized into a binary branching tree. In the model proposed by Rosenbaum et al., executing the first element in the sequence to be uttered requires that a pointer traverses a binary branching hierarchy from the top node to the leftmost terminal element. The more nodes in the tree that must be traversed, the longer the traversal time and so the longer the latency to output the first item in the string. In turn, the longer the string, the more nodes in the tree; accordingly, latency will correlate with string length. Outputting the next element after the first requires that the pointer move upward from the leftmost terminal element to the node from which that element and the next one branch and then move down from there to the terminal for the second element. In general, outputting any next element involves moving the pointer from one terminal element to the next by traveling along the tree branches that connect them. The more elements in the string, the more branches and nodes in the tree and so the longer, on average, it will take to get from terminal element to terminal element.

Accordingly, execution of the string will slow with string length. In addition, the model predicts differences within the string in interresponse time, with short times between elements 1 and 2 and between 3 and 4, for example, and the longest times between elements that bisect the string. To my knowledge, these predictions are untested.

This model has an advantage over that of Sternberg *et al.* in not having to suppose that elements to be produced in a given order are unordered from the perspective of the retrieval mechanism. It has the same disadvantages, however, of failing to rationalize the units that make up terminal elements of the tree and of lacking face plausibility. Why are string elements stress feet rather than morpho-syntactic units? Why shift from the syntactic tree (which need not be symmetrical and binary branching) to a binary branching one? What does the tree accomplish other than to slow down the output process (over a process that simply reads out elements of the string left to right)?

Having expressed some skepticism with the way that Sternberg *et al.* explain their data, and over the alternative account of Rosenbaum *et al.*, I have to confess that I do not know a better way. A place to look for an account, however, may be in the direction of the capacity account that Sternberg *et al.* tested and rejected. They rejected an idea that the latency and duration functions might be caused by limitations on central processing capacity by showing that extra demands on processing capacity (a memory load) did not affect response functions. Alternative-ly, however, perhaps the limitations are downstream of any pool of central processing capacity. Perhaps the limits are on a general pool of energy resources available to produce an utterance. As a first approximation, imagine that an inspiration makes available a pool of resources for producing an utterance on a single breath group. The more there is to say, the more limited the resources available for each unit to be uttered. Effects of unstressed syllables are not noticed because they require negligible expenditures from the resource pool. Reductions in resources affect time to initiate production of stressed syllables. If demands on the respiratory system were an important factor, then manipulating the sizes of inspirations or composing utterances of phonetic segments that deplete the air supply rapidly or slowly (e.g. /f/ versus /m/; see Gelfer, Harris and Baer, 1987) should affect the latency and duration functions where manipulations of memory load would not.

4.3.3   Phonological and Intonational Phrases

Phrasings above the foot are signaled in several ways. Three related ones are a tendency to lengthen syllables at a phrase boundary, a tendency to mark the boundary with a pause, and a tendency for cross-word phonological processes (such as palatalization as in 'did you' becoming 'didja') to be blocked. In addition, intonational phrases are the domains of a coherent intonational melody or tune and of a gradual decrease in fundamental frequency known as 'declination'.

Lengthenings, Pausing and Blocking of Cross-Word Effects
Even when speakers are reading, and so need not decide what to say next, they distribute pauses or other indices of slowing and braking unevenly in their speech utterances. The pauses are not randomly distributed, however.

Cooper and Paccia-Cooper (1980), in an extensive series of experiments, examined the distribution of pauses, lengthening and blocking of cross-word phonological effects in a variety of sentences that were read aloud. They manipulated the syntactic structure of otherwise similar sentences and found a close relationship between surface syntactic structure and the distribution of pausing, lengthening and blocking. In general, the more important the syntactic boundary, the longer the pause, the greater the lengthening of syllables on the 'left' side of the boundary and the greater the likelihood of blocking a cross-word phonological effect. They found no evidence that these three variables patterned differently. Presumably, all are indices of a slowing that serves to break an utterance into phrases.

To predict relative pause duration, amount of lengthening or probability of blocking at each word boundary in a sentence, Cooper and Paccia-Cooper proposed a complicated 14-step algorithm applied to each word boundary in the sentence. They recognized that the algorithm was not a realistic candidate for talkers to use to generate pausing and lengthening, however, and so it remained an unanswered question how and why the durational measures vary as they do in speech.

Gee and Grosjean (1983) tested the descriptive adequacy of the algorithm of Cooper and Paccia-Cooper as well as another proposed by Grosjean, Grosjean and Lane (1979) on a variety of spoken sentences. Although both algorithms explained a considerable proportion of the variation in pause durations, neither came close to explaining all of it, and neither constituted a realistic performance model for talkers.

Gee and Grosjean determined that more of the variance in pausing can be explained if domains between pauses are metrical, not syntactic, phrases. They proposed a new procedure that operates largely left to right in a sentence, producing pauses after each phonological phrase and longer pauses after phonological phrases that end an intonationl phrase. The new algorithm, besides explaining more of the variance than earlier ones, does constitute a more realistic performance model than the others, because it does not require that the talker have a whole sentence planned in order to determine how long to pause at each word boundary.

It is worth asking whether talkers *intend* to mark phonological and intonational phrases with pauses and lengthenings or whether these (and the blocking of cross-word phonological processes) are natural manifestations of occasional slowing of vocal tract activity as talkers pause to plan ahead. My guess is that the answer is 'a little of both'. On the one hand, it is probably not serendipitous that talkers mark phrase edges with *lengthenings*, with lengthenings especially on the left sides of the boundaries and with pauses that block cross-word processes. Many languages have been reported to exhibit final lengthening, while I am aware of no languages reported to show systematic final shortening. On the other hand, the patterns of lengthenings reported by Cooper and Paccia-Cooper and by Gee and Grosjean may be too systematic to reflect brakings to plan ahead, particularly since the talkers in these experiments are reading, not speaking spontaneously. My guess is that patterns of slowing have their origins in talkers' need to pause to plan ahead. Because talkers may plan coherent stretches of speech all at once, they are inclined to pause at phrase boundaries. Accordingly, the pauses and lengthenings provide information to listeners concerning the phrase structure of a sentence. More than that, the pausings tend to occur after phonological and intonational phrases and hence after 'heads' of syntactic phrases. This may help to set off or point to the heads of phrases for the listener. Because the pauses and lengthenings are informative in these ways, talkers may tend to supply them even when they do not need to pause to plan. This may constitute another example of the 'triggering' phenomenon discussed for the example of vowel length variation and following consonant voicing by MacNeilage and Ladefoged (1976; and see the introduction to Section 3). Systematic variation having a dispositional origin in the vocal tract that is, therefore, common to most languages, may be exaggerated, stylized and incorporated in the phonologies of some languages to serve a communicative function.

Intonation and Declination

Intonational melodies are patternings of the fundamental frequency (f_0) of the talker's voice; f_0 is sensitive to several variables in speech: two important ones are transglottal pressure and the tension of the vocal folds. Transglottal pressure is the difference in air pressure above and below the vocal folds. The larger the pressure difference, the higher f_0, other things being equal. In turn, a major way for talkers to influence transglottal pressure is by increasing or decreasing the pressure below the vocal folds (subglottal pressure or P_s) by pushing more or less air out of the lungs. As for tension of the vocal folds, increasing the tension will increase f_0, other things being equal. A major way to increase vocal fold tension is to contract the cricothyroid muscle of the larynx; a major way to decrease it is to relax that muscle. (In lower frequency ranges, the 'strap' muscles of the larynx may be used to lower f_0 actively.)

In 1967, Lieberman proposed a theory of intonation according to which there are two basic melodies: the 'unmarked breath group' and the 'marked breath group'. In the former, f_0 simply tracks P_s during an expiration. According to Lieberman (see also Ladefoged, 1967), P_s is flat throughout an utterance until a final fall at the end. Therefore, f_0 is flat with a final fall utterance (or phrase) at the end. The marked breath group is similar except that the final fall in f_0 caused by the final fall in P_s is counteracted by an increase in laryngeal tension. Generally, this will cause a final rise in f_0 characteristic of yes/no questions. Lieberman recognized that contours may be more complex than the marked and unmarked breath groups. Accordingly, he proposed a feature, prominence, that could be used to accent a particular word in a sentence that the talker wanted to emphasize. In the theory, prominence is implemented by an increase in subglottal pressure.

Lieberman's theory proved quite controversial, fueling the 'lungs versus larynx' controversy (Ohala, 1978). Most controversial was Lieberman's view that pitch accents in an intonational melody are implemented by an increase in P_s. Currently, the prevailing view is that pitch accents are implemented by tensing and relaxing laryngeal muscles that stretch or shorten the vocal folds.

There is at present no psychological theory of intonational performance, and so no theory explaining how intonational melodies are produced. However, Liberman and Pierrehumbert (1984) suggest that they do not require extensive preplanning; rather, as for pausing and lengthening, they can be implemented left to right as phrases are uttered. In their view, as noted, the intonational melody, between which speakers interpolate, constitute a sequence of discrete pitch accents (approximately, Lieberman's prominence feature).

Despite general disconfirmation of Lieberman's view that intonational accents are imposed by the respiratory system, there is probably a role for systematic variation in respiratory activity in implementing an f_0 contour. Many researchers, beginning with Pike (1945; see also Breckenridge, 1977; Cohen, Collier and t'Hart, 1982; Cohen and t'Hart, 1965; Maeda, 1976), have noticed a tendency in some styles of speech (but not all; see Lieberman *et al.*, 1985; Umeda, 1982) for f_0 to decline over the course of an interval of speech, probably an intonational phrase. Cohen and t'Hart (1965) coined the word 'declination' to refer to the fall in f_0.

The reason for declination in speech has been controversial. An intuitive reason for the fall is the reduction in lung volume between inspirations. One factor that affects P_s is the elastic recoil force of the expanded lungs. That force diminishes over the course of an expiration as the lungs deflate; other things being equal, so should P_s and f_0. Other things are not equal, of course. Expiratory muscles are increasingly recruited during an expiration to offset the fall in P_s because of lung deflation (Weismer, 1985). As I already noted, Ladefoged (1967) and Lieberman (1967) both report that P_s is flat until the final fall at the end of a breath group. Convinced that a decline in P_s could not account for declination, some researchers (Breckenridge, 1977; Ohala, 1978) concluded that declination is implemented by tensing and then relaxing muscles of the larynx that first stretch the vocal folds and then allow them gradually to shorten.

If declination is implemented by laryngeal action of this sort, then it must not be a dispositional feature of speech, but rather an intentionally implemented one. Cooper and Sorenson (1981) proposed an elaborate model for implementing declination under the assumption that talkers do intentionally impose it on their utterances. In the model, speakers estimate how long a sentence will be in seconds and they estimate when, in seconds from utterance onset, each intonational peak of the sentence will occur. Using these estimates, talkers apply a 'topline rule' to select f_0 values for the accent peaks.

The model has been criticized on a variety of grounds. It does not rationalize declination. That is, it offers no reason why talkers would implement the fall; they appear to engage in considerable computation for no apparent purpose. Moreover, the theory does not offer any insight into why declination occurs so commonly across languages (for a review, see Cooper and Sorenson, 1981). Declination occurs in most languages where it has been sought; I am aware of no languages found to exhibit some other systematic global contour shape. Simon (1980) recommends that dispositional accounts of declination be pursued in favor of this model of declination as an intentional imposition. In any case, the model does not fit the data well (Pierrehumbert and Liberman, 1982) – a fact that was somewhat masked for Cooper and Sorenson, who applied a defective means of estimating the model's fit. In addition, a simpler model, still supposing that declination is intentionally imposed, can fit the data at least as well without having to claim that f_0 contours are preplanned on a second-by-second basis (Liberman and Pierrehumbert, 1984). According to this model, speakers step f_0 down a fixed proportion of its current value at each accent.

Has an account of declination as a dispositional consequence of respiratory changes during an expiration in fact been disconfirmed? In my view, it has not been entirely. Some such account has an advantage over others as well in explaining why declination occurs so commonly across languages.

Early suggestions that P_s is flat over an utterance are not supported by later studies. Collier and Gelfer (1984) and Gelfer (1987; Gelfer, Harris and Baer, 1987) report an exponential fall in P_s over the course of a sentence that the decline in f_0

tracks quite closely. Moreover, in their data, the magnitude of the fall in P_s can explain all of the fall in f_0 except, occasionally, at the very beginning of the contour, where the starting f_0 may be increased sometimes by activity of the cricothyroid muscle (Collier, 1987).

This does not mean that declination is wholly unregulated by talkers. The fall in P_s is not a simple reflection of lung deflation because, as noted, expiratory muscles are recruited increasingly during an utterance to offset the effects of the decline in the recoil force of the lungs. Apparently they often do not offset the reduction of the recoil force entirely. Why not? Possibly, they do not because talkers intend f_0 to decline and that is how they implement declination. Alternatively, they may only offset effects of reduction in the recoil force on P_s enough to ensure sufficient transglottal pressure for phonation out to the end of an utterance (cf. Collier, 1987). Within that constraint, they allow P_s to fall as the lungs deflate, and they allow f_0 to fall with it. The latter account has the advantage of explaining why declination occurs so commonly across languages. The former account may have some validity as well, however.

As noted, talkers may tense the cricothyroid contour initially, possibly to exaggerate the contour for listeners. Second, some languages, including English, may have downstepping intonational melodies in which declination appears in an exaggerated and stylized form. Declination may represent yet another example of 'triggering' whereby a universal, dispositional, behavioral systematicity is elevated in stylized form into the phonologies of some languages, perhaps because it provides useful information to listeners here, in delimiting phrases.

5 CONCLUDING REMARKS

I have proposed that, at the levels on which I have focused, speaking occurs in two major phases: planning and performance. In planning, morphosyntactic units of an utterance – words, morphemes and phonemes – are ordered into syntactic phrases. They make themselves evident as planning units, because they occasionally misorder and they do so in characteristic ways that rule out a hypothesis that the misorderings reflect mistakes in the motor realization of speech.

Recent progress by linguists and speech production researchers has gone a considerable way toward disconfirming a generally held view that linguistic units as components of linguistic competence are not realized or even realizable in the vocal tract, because units of competence have properties, such as discreteness and context independence, that are incompatible with physical systems such as the vocal tract. The work of disconfirming the hypothesis has proceeded in two directions. Linguists have begun to focus on the previously neglected 'intrinsic content' of phonetic segments. Gestural rather than abstract featural primitives have helped to yield linguistic units ostensibly designed to be uttered. As for speech production theorists, they have stepped back from the details of vocal tract activity and found a level of more coarse-grained order. The order is achieved by coordinative structures or synergies that Saltzman and his colleagues identify with dynamic systems more generally. It appears that the smallest synergies at work in the vocal tract during speech implement the smallest, that is gestural, components of a planned utterance.

Despite the fundamental correspondence I claim for units of competence, planning and performance, something new does arise in speech performance. The something new is the grouping of words into metrical phrases – a grouping that is not apparent in speech planning as revealed by speech errors. Ostensibly the new grouping arises in each performance as a talker chooses to highlight certain content words in a sentence. The words are highlighted by pitch accents on them, and the phrases in which they participate are set off by lengthenings and pausing. These highlightings may themselves require some planning but they can, according to current viewpoints, be output largely left to right as the morphosyntactic speech plan is uttered.

APPENDIX

Unfamiliar Symbols for Phonemic and Phonological Segments

Symbol	Example
/a/	box
/ɝ/	bird
/I/	bit
/iy/	beed
/ow/	boat
/uw/	boot
/ŋ/	king

Symbol	Interpretation
~	nasality
V:, C:	length

ACKNOWLEDGEMENTS

The preparation of this manuscript was supported by NICHD Grant HD 01994 and NINCDS Grant NS-13617 to Haskins Laboratories.

REFERENCES

Abbs, J. and Gracco, V. (1984). Control of complex gestures: Orofacial muscle responses to load perturbations of the lip during speech. *Journal of Neurophysiology*, **51**, 705–723.

Allen, G. (1975). Speech rhythm: Its relation to performance universals and articulatory timing. *Journal of Phonetics*, **3**, 75–86.

Anderson, S. (1976). Nasal consonants and the internal structure of segments. *Language*, **52**, 326–345.

Baars, B., Motley, M. and MacKay, D. (1975). Output editing for lexical status from artificially-elicited slips of the tongue. *Journal of Verbal Learning and Verbal Behavior*, **14**, 382–391.

Beckman, M. (1985). *Stress and Nonstress Accent*. Dordrecht, The Netherlands: Foris Publications.

Bell-Berti, F. (1980). Velopharyngeal function: A spatio-temporal model. In N. Lass (Ed.), *Speech and Language*, vol. 4 (pp. 291–316). New York: Academic Press.

Bell-Berti, F. and Harris, K. (1974). More on motor organization of speech gestures. Haskins Laboratories Status Reports on Speech Research, No. SR37/38, pp. 9–20.

Bell-Berti, F. and Harris, K. (1979). Anticipatory coarticulation: Some implications from a study of lip rounding. *Journal of the Acoustical Society of America*, **65**, 1268–1270.

Bell-Berti, F. and Harris, K. (1981). A temporal model of speech production. *Phonetica*, **38**, 9–20.

Benguerel, A.-P. and Cowan, H. (1974). Coarticulation of upper lip protrusion in French. *Phonetica*, **30**, 41–55.

Bernstein, N. (1967). *Coordination and Regulation of Movement*. London: Pergamon Press.

Bizzi, E. and Polit, A. (1979). Characteristics of the motor programs underlying visually evoked movements. In R. Talbott and D. Humphrey (Eds), *Posture and Movement* (pp. 169–176). Amsterdam: Mouton.

Bladon, A. and Al-Bamerni, A. (1982). One stage and two stage temporal patterns of coarticulation. *Journal of the Acoustical Society of America*, **72**, S104 (Abstract).

Bolinger, D. (1963). Length, vowel, juncture. *Lingustics*, **1**, 1–29.

Bolinger, D. (1981). *Two Kinds of Vowels, Two Kinds of Rhythm*. Bloomington, IN: Indiana University Linguistics Club.

Boyce, S. (1988). The influence of phonological structure on articulatory organization in Turkish and English: Vowel harmony and coarticulation. PhD Thesis, Yale University.

Breckenridge, J. (1977). Declination as a phonological process. Bell Laboratories Technological Memorandum, Murray Hill, NJ.

Browman, C. (1978). Tip of the tongue and slip of the ear: Implications for language processing. *UCLA Working Papers in Phonetics*, No. 42.

Browman, C. and Goldstein, L. (1986). Towards an articulatory phonology. *Phonology Yearbook*, **2**, 219–252.

Browman, C. and Goldstein, L. (1990). Articulatory gestures as phonological units. *Phonology*, **6**, 201–251.

Chen, M. (1970). Vowel length variation as a function of the voicing of the consonant environment. *Phonetica*, **27**, 129–158.

Chomsky, N. (1965). *Aspects of the Theory of Syntax*. Cambridge, MA: MIT Press.

Chomsky, N. (1986). *Knowledge of Language: Its Nature, Origin and Use*. New York: Praeger.

Chomsky, N. and Halle, M. (1968). *The Sound Pattern of English*. New York: Harper.

Classe, A. (1939). *The Rhythms of English Prose*. Oxford: Blackwell.

Clements, G. N. (1985). The geometry of phonological features. *Phonology Yearbook*, **2**, 225–252.

Cohen, A., Collier, R. and t'Hart, J. (1982). Declination: Construct or intrinsic feature of speech pitch. *Phonetica*, **39**, 254–273.

Cohen, A. and t'Hart, J. (1965). Perceptual analysis of intonation patterns. *Proceedings of the Fifth International Congress of Acoustics* (A. 16). Liege, Belgium.

Collier, R. (1987). F_0 declination: The control of its setting, resetting and slope. In T. Baer, C. Sasaki and K. Harris (Eds), *Laryngeal Function in Phonation and Respiration* (pp. 403–421). Boston, MA: College-Hill Press.

Collier, R. and Gelfer, C. (1984). Physiological explanation of f_0 declination. In M. P. R. van den Broecke and A. Cohen (Eds), *Proceedings of the Tenth International Congress of Phonetic Sciences* (pp. 354–360). Dordrecht, The Netherlands: Foris Publications.

Cooper, W. and Paccia-Cooper, J. (1980). *Syntax and Speech*. Cambridge, MA: Harvard University Press.

Cooper, W. and Sorenson, J. (1981). *Fundamental Frequency in Sentence Production*. New York: Springer.

Cordo, P. and Nashner, L. (1982). Properties of postural adjustments associated with rapid arm movement. *Journal of Neurophysiology*, **47**, 287–302.

Crompton, A. (1982). Syllables and segments in speech production. In A. Cutler (Ed.), *Slips of the Tongue and Language Production* (pp. 73–108). Amsterdam: Mouton.

Cutler, A. (1980). Errors of stress and intonation. In V. Fromkin (Ed.), *Errors in Linguistic Performance: Slips of the Tongue, Ear, Pen and Hand* (pp. 67–80). New York: Academic Press.

Daniloff, R. and Hammarberg, R. (1973). On defining coarticulation. *Journal of Phonetics*, **1**, 239–248.

Dauer, R. (1983). Stress timing and syllable timing reanalyzed. *Journal of Phonetics*, **11**, 51–62.

Davis, S. (1988). Syllable onsets as a factor in stress rules. *Phonology*, **5**, 1–20.

Dell, G. (1980). Phonological and lexical encoding in speech production: An analysis of naturally occurring and experimentally elicited slips of the tongue. PhD Thesis, University of Toronto.

Dell, G. (1986). A spreading-activation theory of retrieval in sentence production. *Psychological Review*, **93**, 283–321.

Dell, G. (1988). The retrieval of phonological forms in production: Tests of predictions from a connectionist model. *Journal of Memory and Language*, **27**, 124–142.

Dell, G. (1990). Effects of frequency and vocabulary type on phonological speech errors. *Language and Cognitive Processes*, **5**, 313–349.

Dell, G. and Reich, P. (1980). Toward a unified theory of slips of the tongue. In V. Fromkin (Ed.), *Errors in Linguistic Performance: Slips of the Tongue, Ear, Pen and Hand* (pp. 273–286). New York: Academic Press.

Dell, G. and Reich, P. (1981). Stages in sentence production. *Journal of Verbal Learning and Verbal Behavior*, **20**, 611–629.

Easton, T. (1972). On the normal use of reflexes. *American Scientist*, **60**, 591–599.

Edwards, J. and Beckman, M. (1988). Articulatory timing and the prosodic interpretation of syllable duration. *Phonetica*, **45**, 156–174.

Fant, G. (1962). Descriptive analysis of the acoustic aspects of speech. *Logos*, **5**, 3–17.

Fay, D. and Cutler, A. (1977). Malapropisms and the structure of the mental lexicon. *Linguistic Inquiry*, **8**, 505–520.

Fel'dman, A. and Latash, M. (1982). Interaction of afferent and efferent signals underlying joint position sense: Empirical and theoretical approaches. *Journal of Motor Behavior*, **14**, 174–193.

Flege, J. (1988). The development of skill in producing word-final English stops: Kinematic parameters. *Journal of the Acoustical Society of America*, **84**, 1639–1652.

Flege, J. and Port, R. (1981). Cross-language phonetic interference: Arabic and English. *Language and Speech*, **24**, 125–146.

Folkins, J. and Abbs, J. (1975). Lip and jaw motor control during speech: Responses to resistive loading of the jaw. *Journal of Speech and Hearing Research*, **18**, 207–220.

Folkins, J. and Abbs, J. (1976). Additional observations on responses to resistive loading of the jaw. *Journal of Speech and Hearing Research*, **19**, 820–821.

Folkins, J. and Zimmermann, G. (1981). Jaw-muscle activity during speech with the mandible fixed. *Journal of the Acoustical Society of America*, **69**, 1441–1445.

Fowler, C. (1977). *Timing Control in Speech Production*. Bloomington, IN: Indiana University Linguistics Club.

Fowler, C. (1980). Coarticulation and theories of extrinsic timing. *Journal of Phonetics*, **8**, 113–137.

Fowler, C. (1981a). A relationship between coarticulation and compensatory shortening. *Phonetica*, **38**, 35–50.

Fowler, C. (1981b). Production and perception of coarticulation among stressed and unstressed vowels. *Journal of Speech and Hearing Research*, **46**, 127–139.

Fowler, C. (1983). Converging sources of spoken and perceived rhythms of speech: Cyclic production of vowels in monosyllabic stress feet. *Journal of Experimental Psychology: General*, **112**, 386–412.

Fowler, C., Munhall, K., Saltzman, E. and Hawkins, S. (1986). Acoustic and articulatory evidence for consonant–vowel interactions. *Journal of the Acoustical Society of America*, **80**, S96 (Abstract).

Fowler, C., Rubin, P., Remez, R. and Turvey, M. (1980). Implications for speech production of a general theory of action. In B. Butterworth (Ed.), *Language Production, I: Speech and Talk* (pp. 373–420). London: Academic Press.

Fowler, C. and Turvey, M. (1980). Immediate compensation for bite-block vowels. *Phonetica*, **37**, 306–326.

Fromkin, V. (1971).The nonanomalous nature of anomalous utterances. *Language*, **47**, 27–52.

Fromkin, V. (Ed.) (1973). *Speech Errors as Linguistic Evidence*. The Hague: Mouton.

Fudge, E. (1969). Syllables. *Journal of Linguistics*, **5**, 253–286.

Garrett, M. (1980a). Levels of processing in sentence production. In B. Butterworth (Ed.), *Language Production I: Speech and Talk* (pp. 177–220). London: Academic Press.

Garrett, M. (1980b). The limits of accommodation. In V. Fromkin (Ed.), *Errors in Linguistic Performance: Slips of the Tongue, Ear, Pen and Hand* (pp. 263–271). New York: Academic Press.

Gay, T. (1977). Cinefluorographic and electromyographic studies of articulatory organization. In M. Sawashima and F. Cooper (Eds), *Dynamic Aspects of Speech Production* (pp. 85–102). Tokyo: University of Tokyo Press.

Gay, T., Lindblom, B. and Lubker, J. (1981). Production of bite-block vowels: Acoustic equivalence by selective compensation. *Journal of the Acoustical Society of America*, **69**, 802–810.

Gee, P. and Grosjean, F. (1983). Performance structures: A psycholinguistic and linguistic appraisal. *Cognitive Psychology*, **15**, 411–458.

Gelfand, I. M., Gurfinkel, V., Tsetlin, M. and Shik, M. (1971). Some problems in the analysis of movements. In I. Gelfand, V. Gurfinkel, S. Fomin and M. Tsetlin (Eds), *Models of the Structural–Functional Organization of Certain Biological Systems* (pp. 329–345). Cambridge, MA: MIT Press.

Gelfer, C. (1987). A simultaneous physiological and acoustic study of fundamental frequency declination. PhD Thesis, CUNY.

Gelfer, C., Bell-Berti, F. and Harris, K. (1982). Determining the extent of coarticulation: Effects of experimental design. Paper presented at the 103rd meeting of the Acoustical Society of America, Chicago.

Gelfer, C., Harris, K. and Baer, T. (1987). Controlled variables in sentence intonation. In T. Baer, C. Sasaki and K. Harris (Eds), *Laryngeal Function in Phonation and Respiration* (pp. 422–435). Boston, MA: College-Hill Press.

Goldsmith, J. (1976). *Autosegmental Phonology*. Bloomington, IN: Indiana University Linguistics Club.

Gracco, V. and Abbs, J. (1985). Dynamic control of the perioral system during speech: Kinematic analyses of autogenic and nonautogenic sensorimotor processes. *Journal of Neurophysiology*, **54**, 418–432.

Gracco, V. and Abbs, J. (1986). Variant and invariant characteristics of speech movements. *Experimental Brain Research*, **65**, 156–166.

Grillner, S. (1981). Control of locomotion in bipeds, tetrapods and fish. In V. B. Brooks (Ed.), *Handbook of Physiology: Motor Control* (pp. 1179–1236). Baltimore, MD: Williams and Wilkins.

Grosjean, F., Grosjean, L. and Lane, H. (1979).The patterns of silence: Performance structures in sentence production. *Cognitive Psychology*, **11**, 58–81.

Hammarberg, R. (1976). The metaphysics of coarticulation. *Journal of Phonetics*, **4**, 353–363.

Hammarberg, R. (1982). On redefining coarticulation. *Journal of Phonetics*, **10**, 123–137.

Hayes, B. (1981). A metrical theory of stress rules. PhD Thesis, MIT.

Hayes, B. (1982). Extrametricality of English stress. *Linguistic Inquiry*, **13**, 227–276.

Henke, W. (1966). Dynamic articulatory modeling of speech production using computer simulation. PhD Thesis, MIT.

Hockett, C. (1960). The origin of speech. *Scientific American*, **203**, 89–96.

Hyman, L. (1982). The representation of nasality in Gokona. In H. van der Hulst and N. Smith (Eds), *The Structure of Phonological Representations*, Part I (pp. 111–130). Dordrecht, The Netherlands: Foris Publications.

Jordan, M. (1986). *Serial Order: A Parallel Distributed Processing Approach*. Institute for Cognitive Science, University of California, San Diego.

Kahn, D. (1976). *Syllable-based Generalizations in English Phonology*. Bloomington, IN: Indiana University Linguistics Club.

Keating, P. (1983). Comments on the jaw and syllable structure. *Journal of Phonetics*, **11**, 401–406.

Keating, P. (1990). Mechanisms of coarticulation: The window model of coarticulation: Articulatory evidence. In J. Kingston and M. Beckman (Eds), *Papers in Laboratory Phonology I: Between the Grammar and the Physics of Speech* (pp. 451–470). Cambridge: Cambridge University Press.

Kelly, M. (1988). Rhythmic alternation and lexical stress differences in English. *Cognition*, **29**, 107–138.

Kelly, M. and Bock, K. (1988). Stress in time. *Journal of Experimental Psychology: Human Perception and Performance*, **14**, 389–413.

Kelso, J. A. S., Saltzman, E. and Tuller, B. (1986). The dynamical perspective on speech production: Data and theory. *Journal of Phonetics*, **14**, 29–56.

Kelso, J. A. S., Southard, D. and Goodman, D. (1979). On the coordinating of two-handed movements. *Journal of Experimental Psychology: Human Perception and Performance*, **5**, 229–238.

Kelso, J. A. S. and Tuller, B. (1987). Intrinsic time in speech production: Theory, methodology and preliminary observations. In E. Keller and M. Gopnik (Eds), *Motor and Sensory Processes in Language* (pp. 203–222). Hillsdale, NJ: Erlbaum.

Kelso, J. A. S., Tuller, B. and Saltzman, E. (1986). The dynamical perspective on speech production: Data and theory. *Journal of Phonetics*, **14**, 29–60.

Kelso, J. A. S., Tuller, B., Vatikiotis-Bateson, E. and Fowler, C. (1984). Functionally-specific articulatory cooperation following jaw perturbations during speech: Evidence for coordinative structures. *Journal of Experimental Psychology: Human Perception and Performance*, **10**, 812–832.

Kenstowicz, M. and Kisseberth, C. (1979). *Generative Phonology*. San Diego, CA: Academic Press.

Klatt, D. (1976). The linguistic uses of segment duration in English: Acoustic and perceptual evidence. *Journal of the Acoustical Society of America*, **59**, 1208–1221.

Kozhevnikov, V. and Chistovich, L. (1965). *Speech: Articulation and Perception*. Washington, DC: Joint Publications Research Service, No. 30, p. 543.

Krakow, R. (1988). *Articulatory Organization and the Structure of Words and Syllables*. Meeting of the American Speech and Hearing Association.

Krakow, R. (1989). The articulatory organization of syllables: A kinematic analysis of labial and velar gestures. PhD Thesis, Yale University.

Kugler, P., Kelso, J. A. S. and Turvey, M. (1980). On the concept of coordinative structures as dissipative structures, I. Theoretical lines of convergence. In G. Stelmach and J. Requin (Eds), *Tutorials in Motor Behavior* (pp. 3–47). Amsterdam: North-Holland.

Kugler, P. and Turvey, M. (1987). *Information, Natural Law and the Self-Assembly of Rhythmic Movements*. Hillsdale, NJ: Erlbaum.

Ladefoged, P. (1967). *Three Areas in Experimental Phonetics*. London: Oxford University Press.

Lashley, K. (1951). The problem of serial order in behavior. In L. Jeffress (Ed.), *Cerebral Mechanisms in Behavior* (pp. 112–136). New York: John Wiley.

Lee, W. (1984). Neuromotor synergies as a basis for coordinated intentional action. *Journal of Motor Behavior*, **16**, 135–170.

Lehiste, I. (1970). *Suprasegmentals*. Cambridge, MA: MIT Press.

Lehiste, I. (1972). The timing of utterances and linguistic boundaries. *Journal of the Acoustical Society of America*, **51**, 2018–2024.

Liberman, M. (1975). The intonational system of English. PhD Thesis, MIT.

Liberman, M. and Pierrehumbert, J. (1984). Intonational invariances under changes in pitch range and length. In M. Aronoff and R. Oehrle (Eds), *Language Sound Structure* (pp. 157–233). Cambridge, MA: MIT Press.

Liberman, M. and Prince, A. (1977). On stress and linguistic rhythm. *Linguistic Inquiry*, **8**, 249–336.

Lieberman, P. (1967). *Intonation, Perception and Language*. Cambridge, MA: MIT Press.

Lieberman, P., Katz, W., Jongman, A., Zimmerman, R. and Miller, M. (1985). Measures of the sentence intonation of spontaneous speech in American English. *Journal of the Acoustical Society of America*, **77**, 649–657.

Lindblom, B. (1986). On the origin and purpose of discreteness and invariance in sound patterns. In J. Perkell and D. Klatt (Eds), *Invariance and Variability of Speech Processes* (pp. 493–510). Hillsdale, NJ: Erlbaum.

Lindblom, B., Lubker, J. and Gay, T. (1979). Formant frequencies of some fixed-mandible vowels and a model of speech-motor programming by predictive simulation. *Journal of Phonetics*, **7**, 147–161.

Lindblom, B., Lubker, J., Gay, T., Lyberg, B., Branderud, P. and Holmgren, K. (1987). The concept of target and speech timing. In R. Channon and L. Shockey (Eds), *In Honor of Ilse Lehiste* (pp. 161–181). Providence, RI: Foris Publications.

Lindblom, B., Lyberg, B. and Holmgren, K. (1981). *Durational Patterns of Swedish Phonology: Do They Reflect Short-term Memory Processes?* Bloomington, IN: Indiana University Linguistics Club.

Lindblom, B. and Rapp, K. (1973). *Some Temporal Regularities of Spoken Swedish*. Papers in Linguistics from the University of Stockholm, No. 21, pp. 1–59.

Lindblom, B. and Sundberg, J. (1971). Acoustical consequences of lip, tongue, jaw and larynx movement. *Journal of the Acoustical Society of America*, **50**, 1166–1179.

Locke, J. (1983). *Phonological Acquisition and Change*. New York: Academic Press.

Löfqvist, A. (1980). Interarticulator programming in stop production. *Journal of Phonetics*, **68**, 792–801.

Löfqvist, A. and Yoshioka, H. (1984). Intrasegmental timing: Laryngeal–oral coordination in vowel–consonant production. *Speech Communication*, **3**, 279–289.

Lubker, J. (1979). The reorganization times of bite block vowels. *Phonetica*, **36**, 273–293.

Lubker, J. and Parris, P. (1970). Simultaneous measurements of intraoral pressure, force of labial contact, and labial electromyographic activity during production of the stop-consonant cognates. *Journal of the Acoustical Society of America*, **47**, 625–633.

Mack, M. (1982). Voicing-dependent vowel duration in English and French: Monolingual and bilingual production. *Journal of the Acoustical Society of America*, **71**, 173–178.

MacKay, D. M. (1982). The problem of flexibility, fluency, and speed–accuracy trade-off in skilled behavior. *Psychological Review*, **84**, 483–506.

MacKay, D. M. (1987). *The Origin of Perception and Action*. New York: Springer.

MacNeilage, P. (1970). Motor control of serial ordering of speech. *Psychological Review*, **77**, 182–196.

MacNeilage, P. and DeClerk, J. (1969). On the motor control of coarticulation in CVC monosyllables. *Journal of the Acoustical Society of America*, **45**, 1217–1233.

MacNeilage, P. and Ladefoged, P. (1976). The production of speech and language. In E. Carterette and M. Friedman (Eds), *Handbook of Perception: Language and Speech* (pp. 75–120). New York: Academic Press.

Maddieson, I. (1984). *Patterns of Sounds*. Cambridge: Cambridge University Press.

Maeda, S. (1976). A characterization of American English intonation. PhD Thesis, MIT.

Manuel, S. (1987). Acoustic and perceptual consequences of vowel-to-vowel coarticulation in three Bantu languages. PhD Thesis, Yale University.

Manuel, S. and Krakow, R. (1984). Universal and language-specific aspects of vowel-to-vowel coarticulation. Haskins Laboratories Status Reports on Speech Research, No. SR 77/78, pp. 69–87.

McClelland, J. and Rumelhart, D. (1981). An interactive activation model of context effects in letter perception. Part I: An account of basic findings. *Psychological Review*, **88**, 375–407.

Moll, K. (1962). Velopharyngeal closure on vowels. *Journal of Speech and Hearing Research*, **5**, 30–77.

Moll, K. and Daniloff, R. (1971). Investigation of the timing of velar movements during speech. *Journal of the Acoustical Society of America*, **50**, 678–684.

Moll, K., Zimmermann, G. and Smith, A. (1977). The study of speech production as a human neuromotor system. In M. Sawashima and F. S. Cooper (Eds), *Dynamic Aspects of Speech Production* (pp 107–127). Tokyo: University of Tokyo Press.

Monsell, S. (1986). Programming of complex sequences: Evidence from the timing of rapid speech and other productions. In H. Heuer and C. Fromm (Eds), *Experimental Brain Research Series*, vol. 15: *Generation and Modulation of Action Patterns* (pp. 72–86). Berlin: Springer.

Munhall, K., Löfqvist, A. and Kelso, J. A. S. (1986). Phase-dependent sensitivity to perturbation reveals the nature of speech coordinative structures. *Journal of the Acoustical Society of America*, **80**, S38.

Neisser, U. (1967). *Cognitive Psychology*. New York: Appleton-Century-Crofts.

Nespor, M. and Vogel, I. (1979). Clash avoidance in Italian. *Linguistic Inquiry*, **10**, 467–482.

Nittrouer, S., Munhall, K., Kelso, J. A. S., Tuller, B. and Harris, K. (1988). Patterns of interarticulatory phasing and their relation to linguistic structure. *Journal of the Acoustical Society of America*, **84**, 1653–1661.

Nooteboom, S. (1973). The perceptual reality of some prosodic durations. *Journal of Phonetics*, **1**, 25–45.

Norman, D. (1981). Categorization of action slips. *Psychological Review*, **88**, 1–15.

Ohala, J. (1970). Aspects of the control and production of speech. UCLA Working Papers in Phonetics, No. 15.

Ohala, J. (1978). Production of tone. In V. Fromkin (Ed.), *Tone: A Linguistic Survey* (pp. 5–39). New York: Academic Press.

Öhman, S. (1966). Coarticulation in VCV utterances. *Journal of the Acoustical Society of America*, **39**, 151–168.

Ostry, D., Keller, E. and Parush, A. (1983). Similarities in the control of the speech articulators and the limbs: Kinematics of tongue dorsum movements in speech. *Journal of Experimental Psychology: Human Perception and Performance*, **9**, 622–636.

Pattee, H. (1973). The physical basis and origin of hierarchical control. In H. Pattee (Ed.), *Hierarchy Theory: The Challenge of Complex Systems* (pp. 71–108). New York: Braziller.

Perkell, J. (1969). *Physiology of Speech Production: Results and Implications of a Quantitiative Cineradiographic Study*. Cambridge, MA: MIT Press.

Perkell, J. (1980). Phonetic features and the physiology of speech production. In B. Butterworth (Ed.), *Language Production, I: Speech and Talk* (pp. 337–372). London: Academic Press.

Perkell, J. (1986). Coarticulatory strategies: Preliminary implications of a detailed analysis of lower lip protrusion gestures. *Speech Communication*, **5**, 47–68.

Pierrehumbert, J. (1980). The phonology and phonetics of English intonation. PhD Thesis, MIT.

Pierrehumbert, J. and Liberman, M. (1982). Modeling the fundamental frequency of the voice (Review of Cooper and Sorenson (1981)). *Contemporary Psychology*, **27**, 690–692.

Pike, K. (1945). *The Intonation of American English*. Ann Arbor, MI: University of Michigan Press.

Rakerd, B., Sennett, W. and Fowler, C. (1987). Domain-final lengthening and foot-level shortening in spoken English. *Phonetica*, **44**, 147–155.

Raphael, L. (1975). The physiological control of durational control between vowels preceding voiced and voiceless consonants in English. *Journal of Phonetics*, **3**, 25–35.

Reason, J. T. (1979). Actions not as planned. In G. Underwood and R. Stevens (Eds), *Aspects of Consciousness* (vol. 1, 67–90). London: Academic Press.

Recasens, D. (1984). Vowel-to-vowel coarticulation in Catalan VCV sequences. *Journal of the Acoustical Society of America*, **76**, 1624–1635.

Repp, B. (1981). On levels of description in speech research. *Journal of the Acoustical Society of America*, **69**, 1462–1464.

Rosenbaum, D. (1985). Motor programming: A review and scheduling theory. In H. Heuer, U. Kleinbeck and K.-H. Schmidt (Eds), *Motor Behavior: Programming, Control and Acquisition* (pp. 1–33). Berlin: Springer.

Rosenbaum, D., Kenny, S. and Derr, M. (1983). Hierarchical and nonhierarchical control of rapid movement sequences. *Journal of Experimental Psychology: Human Perception and Performance*, **9**, 86–102.

Ryle, G. (1949). *The Concept of Mind*. New York: Barnes and Noble.

Sagey, E. (1986). The representation of features and relations in non-linear phonology. PhD Thesis, MIT.

Saltzman, E. (1986). Task-dynamic coordination of the speech articulators: A preliminary model. In H. Heuer and C. Fromm (Eds), *Experimental Brain Research Series*, vol. 15: *Generation and Modulation of Action Patterns* (pp. 129–144). New York: Springer.

Saltzman, E. and Kelso, J. A. S. (1987). Skilled actions: A task-dynamic approach. *Psychological Review*, **94**, 84–106.

Saltzman, E. and Munhall, K. (1989). A dynamical approach to gestural patterning in speech production. *Ecological Psychology*, **1**, 333–382.

Selkirk, E. (1980a). The role of prosodic categories in English word stress. *Linguistic Inquiry*, **11**, 563–605.

Selkirk, E. (1980b). *On Prosodic Structure and its Relation to Syntactic Structure*. Bloomington, IN: Indiana University Linguistics Club.

Selkirk, E. (1984). *Phonology and Syntax: The Relation Between Sound and Structure*. Cambridge, MA: MIT Press.

Shaiman, S. and Abbs, J. (1987). Phonetic task-specific utilization of sensorimotor activity. Paper presented to the American Speech and Hearing Association.

Shattuck-Hufnagel, S. (1979). Speech errors as evidence for a serial-ordering mechanism in sentence production. In W. Cooper and E. Walker (Eds), *Sentence Processing* (pp. 295–342). Hillsdale, NJ: Erlbaum.

Shattuck-Hufnagel, S. (1983). Sublexical units and suprasegmental structure in speech production planning. In P. MacNeilage (Ed.), *The Production of Speech* (pp. 109–136). New York: Springer.

Shattuck-Hufnagel, S. (1986). The representation of phonologial information during speech production planning: Evidence from vowel errors in spontaneous speech. *Phonology Yearbook*, **3**, 117–149.

Shattuck-Hufnagel, S. (1987). The role of word-onset consonants in speech production planning: New evidence from speech errors. In E. Keller and M. Gopnik (Eds), *Motor and Sensory Processing of Language* (pp. 17–52). Hillsdale, NJ: Erlbaum.

Shattuck-Hufnagel, S. and Klatt, D. (1979). Minimal use of features and markedness in speech production. *Journal of Verbal Learning and Verbal Behavior*, **18**, 41–55.

Shields, J., McHugh, A. and Martin, J. (1974). Reaction time to phonemic targets as a function of rhythmic cues in continuous speech. *Journal of Experimental Psychology*, **102**, 250–255.

Simon, H. (1980). How to win at twenty questions with nature. In R. Cole (Ed.), *Perception and Production of Fluent Speech* (pp. 535–548). Hillsdale, NJ: Erlbaum.

Stemberger, J. (1983). *Speech Errors and Theoretical Phonology: A Review*. Bloomington, IN: Indiana University Linguistics Club.

Stemberger, J. (1985). An interactive activation model of language production. In A. Ellis (Ed.), *Progress in the Psychology of Language*, vol. 1 (pp. 143–186). London: Erlbaum.

Stemberger, J. and MacWhinney, B. (1986). Frequency and the lexical storage of regularly inflected words. *Memory and Cognition*, **14**, 17–26.

Sternberg, S., Monsell, S., Knoll, R. and Wright, C. (1978). The latency and duration of rapid movement sequences: Comparison of speech and typing. In G. Stelmach (Ed.), *Information Processing in Motor Control and Learning* (pp. 117–152). New York: Academic Press.

Sternberg, S., Wright, C., Monsell, S. and Knoll, R. (1980). Motor programs in rapid speech: Additional evidence. In R. Cole (Ed.), *Perception and Production of Fluent Speech* (pp. 507–534). Hillsdale, NJ: Erlbaum.

Summers, W. V. (1987). Effects of stress and final-consonant voicing on vowel production. *Journal of the Acoustical Society of America*, **82**, 847–863.

Sussman, H., MacNeilage, P. and Hanson, R. (1973). Labial and mandibular dynamics during the production of bilabial consonants: Preliminary observations. *Journal of Speech and Hearing Research*, **16**, 385–396.

Sussman, H. and Westbury, J. (1981). The effects of antagonist gestures in temporal and amplitude parameters of anticipatory labial coarticulation. *Journal of the Acoustical Society of America*, **46**, 16–24.

Terzuolo, C. and Viviani, P. (1979). The central representation of learned motor patterns. In R. Talbott and D. Humphrey (Eds), *Posture and Movement* (pp. 113–121). New York: Raven Press.

Treiman, R. (1983). The structure of spoken syllables: Evidence from novel word games. *Cognition*, **15**, 49–74.

Treiman, R. (1984). On the status of final consonant clusters in English. *Journal of Verbal Learning and Verbal Behavior*, **23**, 343–356.

Treiman, R. (1986). On the status of final consonant clusters in English. *Journal of Memory and Language*, **25**, 476–491.

Tuller, B., Kelso, J. A. S. and Harris, K. (1982). Interarticulator phasing as an index of temporal regularity in speech. *Journal of Experimental Psychology: Human Perception and Performance*, **8**, 460–472.

Umeda, N. (1982). 'F_0 declination' is situation dependent. *Journal of Phonetics*, **10**, 279–290.

van der Hulst, H. and Smith, N. (1982). An overview of autosegmental and metrical phonologies. In H. van der Hulst and N. Smith (Eds), *The Structure of Phonological Representations*, Part I (pp. 1–46). Dordrecht, The Netherlands: Foris Publications.

Vayra, M., Avesani, C. and Fowler, C. (1984). Patterns of temporal compression in spoken Italian. In M. P. R. van den Broecke and A. Cohen (Eds), *Proceedings of the Tenth International Congress of Phonetic Sciences* (pp. 541–546). Dordrecht, The Netherlands: Foris Publications.

Weismer, G. (1985). Speech breathing: Contemporary views and findings. In R. Daniloff (Ed.), *Speech Science* (pp. 47–72). San Diego, CA: College-Hill Press.

Weiss, P. (1941). Self-differentiation of the basic pattern of coordination. *Comparative Psychology Monographs*, **17**, 21–96.

Chapter 10

Handwriting Movement Control

Hans-Leo Teulings

Motor Control Laboratory, Arizona State University, USA

1 INTRODUCTION

Among the many motor activities – displacement of the body, maintaining posture, grasping and manipulating objects – handwriting distinguishes itself in that it is a learned and generally practiced human skill. For that reason, the motor control aspects of handwriting are both interesting and important. Being a learned skill, handwriting is related to typewriting, speech, sign language and Morse coding. This chapter focuses on psychological, neurological, biomechanical and computational theories of handwriting production and intends to draw parallels with these related skills, and especially with typewriting. Handwriting may have many features in common with these related motor skills so that a unified theory of these skills seems feasible. However, a unified cognitive theory of all motor skills, including grasping, posture, gait, jumping or navigation is still lacking. This chapter intends to present the skill of handwriting in the context of other motor skills and general motor concepts. However, handwriting skill includes only a limited domain of the basic motor skills. This may limit generalization of the knowledge of the handwriting motor system to other motor skills, but at the same time this limited domain allows simpler theories. The domain of handwriting skill is limited by the following basic features:

(1) The aim is to translate a two-dimensional graphical structure into a fixed sequence of movements. Performance is concerned mainly with the spatial structure rather than with the temporal structure.
(2) Although seemingly continuous, the handwriting movement can be considered as a sequence of discrete actions, similar to the typewriting strokes. Namely, the handwriting movement forms a discrete sequence of ballistic movement segments, or handwriting strokes, which are executed at a near-maximum rate of about 10 strokes per second, just like typewriting strokes.
(3) Handwriting requires only small movement amplitudes (e.g. 0.5 cm), small flexions and extensions, and small force levels so that biomechanical constraints are minimal.

Handbook of Perception and Action, Volume 2
ISBN 0-12-516162-X

(4) The movement patterns are the result of an abstract motor program, which can be executed largely independent of visual feedback, proprioceptive feedback, friction, gravity, inertia, instructed speed, writing size, and muscles and limbs involved.

Cursive script can be recorded using a commercial digitizing tablet connected to a computer. As the position of the pen tip on the tablet is digitized at a fixed, high frequency, all kinds of time functions such as positions, velocities, accelerations in horizontal and vertical directions can be estimated (Teulings and Maarse, 1984; Teulings and Thomassen, 1979) (Figure 10.1). When recording the movement of the pen tip during fluent writing the tangential (or absolute) velocity time function will show a sequence of unimodal peaks: the ballistic 'strokes'. A closer look reveals that the time moments of the valleys between the velocity peaks mostly correspond with time moments of high curvature (i.e. the reverse of the curve radius, or the radius of the hitting circle). It appears that after each ballistic stroke the movement direction is changing sharply to another target in the writing plane.

1.1 Recent Overviews

The motor aspects of handwriting have gained attention in an international and multidisciplinary context resulting in various edited volumes (Barbe, Lucas and Wasylyk, 1984; Kao, van Galen and Hoosain, 1986; Plamondon and Leedham, 1990; Plamondon, Suen and Simner, 1989; Thomassen, van Galen and de Klerk, 1985 – in Dutch and geared towards educationalists; van Galen, Thomassen and Wing, 1991; Wann, Wing and Søvik, 1991; Wing, 1979). Also several monographs have been devoted to specific ares of handwriting such as biomechanical and computational modeling of trajectory formation (Dooijes, 1984; Maarse, 1987; MacDonald, 1966; Raibert, 1977; Schomaker, 1991), top-down handwriting movement control model (Teulings, 1988), and educational and developmental aspects (Blöte, 1988; Meulenbroek, 1989; Mojet, 1989; Sassoon, 1988; Søvik, 1975; Wann, 1988). Recently, several overviews have appeared on drawing and handwriting: an integrated handwriting model of mainly the higher levels of control (van Galen, 1991), several intriguing topics of handwriting motor control (Rosenbaum, 1991), neurophysiological aspects for the purpose of forensic expertise (Baier and Bullinger-Baier, 1989) and signature verification (Lorette and Plamondon, 1990). The overviews that overlap perhaps the most with the present one are by Thomassen and van Galen (1992), who included a brief history of the art of writing, and by Thomassen and Teulings (1993), who described the handwriting movement in less technical terms. Finally, Wing (1978) deserves attention because of the overview of less known, early work on programming and biomechanical aspects of handwriting.

Experimental handwriting research as a multidisciplinary approach toward understanding of human motor control, also known as 'graphonomics', is concerned with the dynamical measurement of handwriting. Handwriting research is often brought into connection with graphology, which attempts to study how to draw conclusions about personality from pages of (static) handwriting trajectories. However, the complex discipline of graphology is still remote from its empirical foundation (Tripp, Fluckiger and Weinberg, 1957; Wing and Watts, 1989).

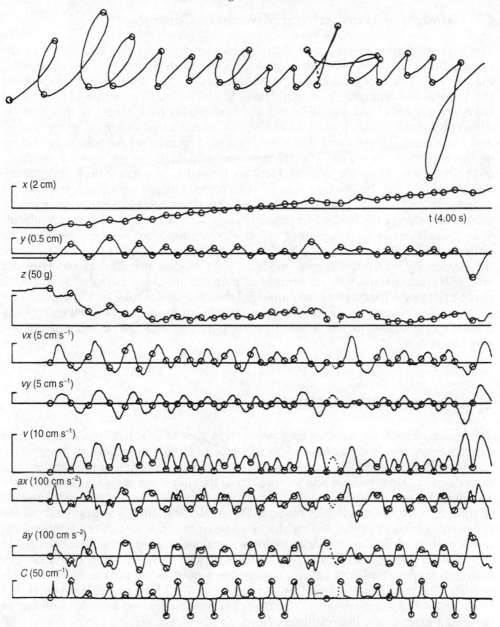

Figure 10.1. *A recorded handwriting pattern with the time functions: x, horizontal coordinate; y, vertical coordinate; z, axial pen pressure; vx, horizontal velocity; vy, vertical velocity; v, absolute velocity; ax, horizontal acceleration; ay, vertical acceleration; C, curvature, i.e. the inverse of curve radius, in calibrated scales. Circles indicate the segmentation points between ballistic strokes on the basis of relative minima of v. Dotted traces refer to movements above the paper.*

1.2 Models of Handwriting Movement Control

The present chapter attempts to organize for the first time the knowledge of the handwriting motor system from global to detailed models in three sections: macroscopic, microscopic and computational models. Within each of these sections the models are arranged from high level to low level. The macroscopic models have several serial and parallel working modules. A new aspect is that entirely different paradigms, such as slips of the pen, effects of neurological disturbances, and movement latencies and durations, provide a consistent picture of the nature of these discrete modules. The microscopic models focus on specific modules of the handwriting motor system. Here all limited-scope, qualitative and quantitative models can be found. Finally, the computational models focus on the generation and simulation of handwriting movements (i.e. dynamic pen movements). Because of the limited frequency bandwidth of the handwriting apparatus, four parameters per stroke are theoretically required to describe handwriting patterns with sufficient accuracy. In this chapter a first attempt is made to compare the parsimony of computational models. Most models use four parameters per stroke; if more parameters are employed then the model is performing almost a curve fit; if fewer parameters are employed then the model may be intelligent. This is interesting if a computational model intends to mimic certain aspects of the biomedical structure of the handwriting apparatus or of the architecture of the nervous system.

2 MACROSCOPIC MODELS

The motor process of handwriting production can be divided into a number of subprocesses, which are supposed to take place in separate modules. The macroscopic models are modular models, and describe a large portion of the handwriting motor system. First the case will be considered that the subprocesses operate strictly sequentially, and subsequently the strategy that subprocesses operate in a time-sharing or a (partially) parallel fashion. The modular models subsume part of the typewriting motor system, which shares some of the modules of the handwriting motor system while some other modules are analogous. Under the assumption that modules possess general principles of the motor system, research based on key pressing, tapping and typewriting is sometimes used to support models of handwriting. The modules discerned are central modules. More peripheral effects due to nerve transmission, peripheral feedback and muscle-force generation will not be discussed extensively. Interesting, but also not discussed, are macroscopic effects of reduction of physiological stress during calligraphy and handwriting (Kao and Robinson, 1987).

Segmenting behavior into serial modules has been one of the main aims of traditional motor research (Sanders, 1980). Evidence for separate modules has also been found in handwriting production. Higher-level modules have been hypothesized on the basis of slips of the pen (Ellis, 1982; van Nes, 1971, 1985), neurological disturbances (Caramazza, Miceli and Villa, 1986; Margolin, 1984), while lower-level modules have been hypothesized on the basis of data on movement dynamics such as delays in movement initiation or movement execution (van Galen, 1991; van Galen and Teulings, 1983).

2.1 Neurological Evidence for Functional Modules

Modularity is not just a way to capture a complex system but is also based upon neurological data. Modularity may explain the great flexibility of human behavior. For example, the sequence of motor commands can be fed to any set of muscles such that writing at different sizes or with different limbs still produces similar writing patterns (Bernstein, 1967). Correlations of psychomotor features across subjects suggest single modules responsible for certain features: for example, timing speed (Keele and Hawkins, 1982), timing accuracy and force-amplitude accuracy (Keele, Ivry and Pokorny, 1987) seem to correlate between finger and arm. On the other hand, timing accuracy and force-amplitude accuracy do not seem to be correlated. This suggests that different modules are responsible for timing and for force control (Keele, Ivry and Pokorny, 1987). Moreover, neurological evidence suggests that timing computations depend on the cerebellum while force regulation depends on the basal ganglia (Keele and Ivry, 1991).

The more or less specific disturbances caused by anatomically localized lesions in neurological patients are also in favor of functional modules. For example, both oral and handwritten spelling showed similar frequencies of disruptions, suggesting that a hypothetical common module such as a graphemic buffer is impaired (Caramazza, Miceli and Villa, 1986). Analogously, Boyle and Canter (1987) observed in a patient with a left-hemispheric infarct that letter sequence errors were similar in the patient's handwriting, typewriting and speech. This confirms that a single, common, high-level module exists which underlies the errors. Furthermore, neocortical lesions may lead to more specific letter formation errors whereas basal ganglia disruptions (e.g. Parkinson's disease) rather lead to improper neuromuscular activity to execute adequate letter sizes (Margolin and Wing, 1983). In agreement with this, Teulings and Stelmach (1991, 1992) found evidence that Parkinsonian handwriting shows more impairment in terms of force amplitudes than durations. Dal Bianco (1944) (quoted by Denier van der Gon and Thuring, 1965) states that particular cerebellar injuries may cause movement disturbances which are more related to the horizontal, left–right movement than to the vertical, up–down movement. In summary, these observations suggest that specific component skills are disrupted in patients with anatomically localized impairments.

Interesting observations were made by Patterson and Wing (1989), which suggest that even storage of handwriting patterns may be modular. This conclusion was based upon a patient suffering from a left parietal stroke who showed disruption of the lower-case cursive-script allographs but relatively little disruption of the upper-case handprint allographs. The cursive-script allographs also took much more time to prepare than to execute, which indicates that it may be a retrieval problem. Furthermore, sometimes a similar cursive-script allograph was produced instead of the correct one (e.g. 'a' instead of 'g'). Remarkably, there were no problems in the patient's signature. There was also no problem in spelling. This suggests that well-defined parts of the motor-pattern store or of motor-pattern retrieval were disrupted.

2.2 Overview of Handwriting and Typewriting Modules

Figure 10.2 provides an overview of the modules discerned in the handwriting or typewriting motor system and probably also in the motor systems describing

The letters to be written are in the
Graphemic Buffer
(containing the graphemic code, i.e. the orthographic information of a word)
↓
The buffer's contents are sent to the
Allographic Store
(containing the allographic code, i.e. the letter shapes in the context of a syllable)
↓
The retrieved code is stored into the
Allographic Buffer
↓
and sent to the
Graphic Motor-Pattern Store
(containing the graphic motor-pattern code, i.e. the stroke sequence of an allograph)
↓
The retrieved code is stored into the
Graphic Motor-Pattern Buffer
↓
At movement initiation the buffer's code is updated by the
Parameter Setting Process
(set nonmuscle specific parameters, e.g. stroke size)
↓
and the
Motor Initiation Process
(set muscle specific parameters, e.g. stroke orientation, force)
↓
Nerve transmission, activation of synapses and internal feedback yield
Muscle Contractions
↓
so that the pen tip moves, which can be analyzed after
Recording and Processing

Figure 10.2. *An overview of the handwriting modules, their contents and the operations taking place between and inside them. The graphemic buffer is common for handwriting and typewriting. The lower-level modules may be analogous for typewriting.*

related skills. The modules are primarily based upon Ellis (1982). His model comprises two parallel input paths to a central, cognitive system to perceive spoken and written information, and two parallel output paths to produce speech and handwriting. Certain modules concern retrieval from a long-term memory, the storage into a short-term buffer, the ordered retrieval from a short-term buffer, or merely updating the contents of a buffer by the substitution of specific parameters.

Margolin (1984) introduced a typing branch analogous to the above handwriting branch. He suggested that the graphemic code is transformed into the allographic code, both in typing and in writing. Then, analogous to the graphic motor-pattern code, a 'typing motor-pattern code' is generated, specifying the sequence of key strokes. To complete the analogy with the handwriting motor system, first the nonmuscle-specific and then the muscle-specific parameters are substituted. In this section, findings on handwriting and typewriting are fitted into a single framework.

2.3 Higher-Level Modules Reflected by Slips of the Pen

Errors in speech, typewriting and handwriting (Ellis, 1982), or 'slips of the tongue', 'slips of the finger' or 'slips of the pen', respectively, provide interesting possibilities to hypothesize the existence of a specific sequence of modules. The highest-level module that we wish to consider here is the *graphemic buffer* (Figure 10.3). This buffer contains the graphemic code needed to spell the to-be-produced word correctly. A grapheme is a letter without details as to whether it is a capital or lower case, handprint or any specific shape of cursive-script letter (Figure 10.4). Therefore, the graphemic code does not yet specify the shape. In the graphemic buffer there can be confusion between identical graphemes but different *allographs* (e.g. 'to English' ⇒ 'to eng...'). Furthermore, anticipations and perseverations (e.g. 'Cognitive' ⇒ 'Go...') may occur at this graphemic level where identical graphemes, e.g. 'g' and 'G', interact. It may be noted that the writer discovers the slip of the pen soon after it was made and stops writing so that it is unknown how the writing pattern would have been completed. Similarly, in typewriting, the interkey period immediately after an erroneous key press is prolonged, although the typing sequence is mostly not interrupted (Salthouse, 1984).

The contents of the graphemic buffer are sent to an allographic store in order to retrieve the *allographic code* which specifies the shape of each grapheme (but not the strokes' sequence). Different shapes of a grapheme are called *allographs*. At this level, confusion between identical allographs may occur. The mutually affecting allographs may be separated by several letter positions in a word, for example omissions of one of the two identical allographs occurring in a word (i.e. letter masking) (e.g. 'satisfactory' ⇒ 'satifa...'; 'listening' ⇒ 'listeing') and haplographies (e.g. 'dependence' ⇒ 'depence'). These errors rarely occur between different allographs of the same grapheme (e.g. 'Multimeter' ⇒ 'Multie...') (Ellis, 1982; van Nes, 1985), which confirms the assumption that letter masking occurs at the allographic level rather than at the graphemic level.

The retrieved allographic code is temporarily stored in the *allographic buffer*. Ellis concluded that the allographic code describes the strokes of a grapheme but not their sequence or execution directions so that reversals (e.g. 'p' versus 'g' in 'pagoda' ⇒ 'padoga') and substitutions (e.g. 'b' versus 'p' in 'Ambiguous' ⇒ 'Amp...') involving similar allographs may occur. Similar allographs have similar shapes but the strokes may be performed in different orders. That these errors occur at a lower level than the previous errors may be derived from the observations that there is no context allograph facilitating letter substitution, and that the affected allographs are only a few letter positions apart.

The proper stroke sequence is retrieved by sending the allographic code to the *graphic motor-pattern store*, yielding the graphic motor-pattern code. Extending the

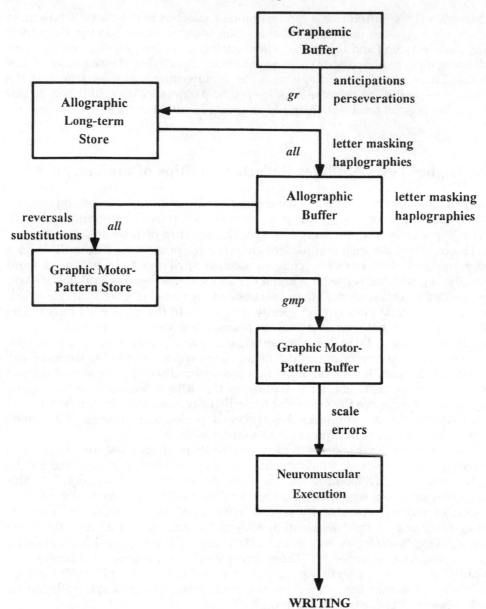

WRITING

Figure 10.3. *The various slips of the pen occurring at or between different modules. The neuromuscular execution still consists of two modules: the muscle-independent parameter setting and the muscle-dependent motor initiation. gr, Graphemic code; all, allographic code; gmp, graphic motor-pattern code. [From Ellis, 1982.]*

ideas of van Galen (1980), Ellis assumes that the graphic motor-pattern code prescribes the sequence of strokes and also the relative sizes required to perform the allograph but not the absolute size. Subsequently, the graphic motor-pattern code is stored in a graphic motor-pattern buffer, awaiting movement initiation. However, the buffered movement code still has to be completed with the current

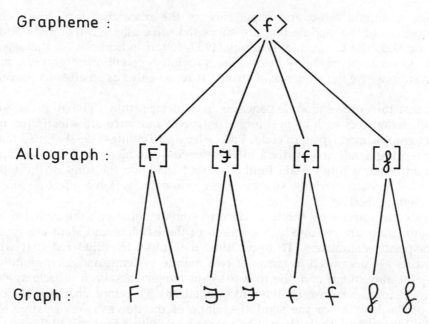

Figure 10.4. *The abstract grapheme 'f' may be represented according to various allographs. Each realization of an allograph is called a graph and shows only variations due to motor noise. [FromEllis, 1982.]*

scale factors like absolute sizes and starting positions. Thus, pattern errors can no longer occur at this level, only scale errors; for example, the size reduction needed to superscript a character may be omitted, but it is rare for the wrong character to be superscripted. Finally, muscle-specific parameters have to be specified, as will be explained next.

2.4 Lower-Level Modules Reflected by Handwriting Movement Dynamics

A different type of paradigm is required to find evidence for distinct modules in the lower level of the motor system. The classic way of distinguishing modules is based on Sternberg's (1969) additive factor method (e.g. Sanders, 1980). This method was successful in the 1980s for discovering serial modules in reaction time paradigms. The method assumes that each module requires some hypothetical processing time, and that the reaction time period is exactly the sum of the processing times of all modules. Then, the mean reaction time equals the sum of the mean processing times. Therefore, if two experimental variables significantly affect the component times of different (sets of) modules, the reaction time data should be additive and not show any interaction between these variables. Even stronger predictions are possible if the component times are statistically independent. Then, not only the means but also the variances are additive. Reversing this logical conclusion yields the speculation that, if two experimental variables show significant main effects and a nonsignificant interaction, they might affect different modules. Common sense and experience of the researcher is used to choose the sequences of the module that are supposed to be affected. Using the additive factor method, van Galen and Teulings (1983) found indications for the existence of two lower-level modules below the previously mentioned graphic motor-pattern store where the sequence of strokes is represented as an abstract movement code.

The first lower-level module concerns 'parameter setting': global, muscle-independent parameters such as position, size, speed and force are substituted in the abstract graphic motor-pattern code. Van Galen and Teulings (1983) argued that the size of writing is not necessarily a muscle-specific parameter because writing size can be adjusted, within certain limits, without changing the roles of the muscles involved. Therefore, writing size is an experimental variable affecting the parameter-setting module.

The second lower-level module concerns 'motor initiation': the actual muscles and motor units are recruited. Orientation of the baseline and slant are typically muscle-specific parameters. To argue this, the autors hypothesized that writing movements are organized in terms of two muscle systems: one corresponding to finger-joint movements and one to wrist-joint movements. Each muscle system is responsible for movements in different orientations. Therefore, changing the orientation of the baseline or the slant (i.e. slope of the downstrokes relative to the baseline; Maarse and Thomassen, 1983) would imply that the roles of these muscle systems change. So orientation of the writing patterns is an experimental variable affecting the latter module.

The data in van Galen and Teulings (1983: Fig. 3) show significant main effects of reaction time as a function of size and orientation but a nonsignificant interaction. For example, reaction time – defined as the latency between imperative stimulus and writing initiation – for the normal orientation and the small letter width (i.e. 0.33 cm) was 651 ms and for the large letter width (i.e. 1 cm) 667 ms (yielding a difference of 16 ms); in the vertical-downward orientation condition it was 710 and 728 ms, respectively (yielding a similar difference of 14 ms, thus rejecting any interaction). These data support a conclusion that two experimental variables exist which may affect different lower-level modules: size probably affects the parameter-setting module, and orientation probably affects the motor-initiation module.

What could be the sense of so many modules after generating the graphic motor-pattern buffer? Van Galen (1980) suggested that the last-minute substitution of global and muscle-specific parameters is more efficient than storing and retrieving them, as many of the lower-level parameters are frequently changing between instances of handwriting production. For example, while writing a line on a page from left to right, the orientation of the hand changes gradually. However, the effectors involved seem to compensate for the varying arm orientations, so that the orientation and slant of the writing pattern vary remarkably little across the line (Maarse, Schomaker and Thomassen, 1986). Therefore, it would not be efficient to store orientation or slant parameters in the graphic motor pattern. Indeed, subjects can easily change the orientation and slant of their writing, either voluntarily or induced by distorted feedback (Pick and Teulings, 1983). Furthermore, this principle of substitution of muscle-specific parameters provides an explanation of the 'motor equivalence' phenomenon: the shape of a movement pattern is only marginally dependent upon the muscles that execute the final movement

(Bernstein, 1967). There is tradeoff between completely stored movements, allowing quick movement preparation, and abstract movement patterns with several processing modules, allowing great flexibility.

2.5 Higher-Level Modules Reflected by Typewriting Errors

In typewriting, higher-level and lower-level modules can be discerned on the basis of typing errors. Rumelhart and Norman (1982) list categories of typewriting errors. Perhaps the highest-level error is the capture error, i.e. the pattern is captured by another but similar word ('efficiency' ⇒ 'efficient'), which typically occurs at the abstract representation of the typing patterns in the graphemic buffer. As the graphemic buffer is providing output to both the typewriting and the handwriting motor system, one may expect these errors also in handwriting (Margolin, 1984). Another high-level error is the alternation reversal ('these' ⇒ 'thses'), where the wrong, but maybe related, movement is selected. One could hypothesize that these errors occur in the typewriting analogy of the allographic buffer.

The next lower-level typing errors concern the proper sequence of the keys. One could hypothesize that these errors occur in the typewriting analogy of the graphic motor-pattern buffer, i.e. the 'typing motor-pattern buffer': transposition ('because' ⇒ 'becuase'), and doubling ('Screen' ⇒ 'Scrren'). Shaffer (1976) reports that transposition errors often occur when both hands alternate keys in an out-of-phase manner (e.g. 'went down' ⇒ 'wne todnw'), so the transposition errors are probably rarely found in handwriting. Rumelhart and Norman's (1982) model of the timing and sequencing of keystrokes simulates exactly these types of error. Their typing model will be explained at the end of this section.

2.6 Lower-Level Modules Reflected by Typewriting Movement Dynamics

After generating the typing motor-pattern code, various categories of 'mis-strokes' or 'substitutions' may occur. The nature of these errors suggests that they could be produced in the module analogous to the parameter-setting module in handwriting. Grudin (1983) investigated video recordings of instances of these mis-strokes and suggests that they are not just aiming errors but actually have been planned as a clear movement to the wrong key. The typing errors of experts and novices consist mostly of 'horizontal mis-strokes', i.e. hitting the wrong key in the same row as the correct one. Often the wrong finger was selected to hit its usual key. Less frequent are 'vertical mis-strokes', where the appropriate finger moves in the wrong direction to the higher or the lower row of keys. Even less frequent but still interesting are 'homologous errors', where the corresponding finger of the opposite hand is activated. These errors indicate that wrist, hand, finger and their movement directions do not need to be specified in a fixed sequence, but are independently substituted into a 'matrix'. Interestingly, the keystroke after a mis-stroke is delayed (Salthouse, 1984), which suggests that individual keystrokes are monitored instead of producing whole groups of keystrokes as 'ballistic typing chunks'.

The lowest-level typing error may be the intrusion or insertion error, resulting from a movement-aiming error, such that the finger lands at a position between two keys. Here, movement amplitudes in horizontal or vertical directions were not properly selected. This seems a typical error occurring in a module analogous to the parameter-setting module in the handwriting model. Of course, there are still many unclassified 'mis-strokes' and omissions in typewriting. However, the ones mentioned here seem to suggest at least close parallels between multimodule models of typewriting and handwriting.

2.7 Feedback in Handwriting

A serial-module model is appropriate to the extent that feedback loops between modules are not essential. This may indeed be the case in fast, single-phasic reaching movements. However, in continuous handwriting, not all parts of the writing pattern need to be prepared before movement can start, but rather subsequent parts of the movement may be prepared during production of the first part, while gradually correcting on the basis of earlier feedback. In his multimodule model, Ellis (1982) included feedback loops but he stated that they play a marginal role in fast, overlearned handwriting movements under stable execution conditions. The main reason is that handwriting is performed as fast as 100 ms per stroke, so that any central processing will be too slow to monitor stroke formation. For example, a sudden increase or decrease of pen-to-paper friction results in an immediate effect upon stroke size. It takes several strokes to restore stroke size (Denier van der Gon and Thuring, 1965) (Figure 10.5). Even the electromyogram

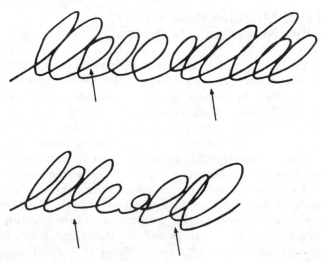

Figure 10.5. *The influence of a sudden increase of the pen-to-paper friction (left arrows) and the restoration of the original pen-to-paper friction (right arrows). Several strokes of at least 100 ms are required to recover from the distortion, which was not internally anticipated. [From Denier van der Gon and Thuring, 1965.]*

(EMG) in fast movements seems at least during the first 100 ms to be independent of proprioceptive feedback, as shown in conditions where the movement was blocked unexpectedly (Wadman *et al.*, 1979).

Furthermore, the speed of writing seems little affected by the absence of visual feedback (Smyth and Silvers, 1987); however, global parameters, such as instructed size changes, are performed more accurately with than without vision (Burton *et al.*, 1990). Also, distortion of visual feedback using rotation and shear transformations show some global effects, although the subjects did not realize the type of distortion. Distorted orientation and slant show a gradual and partial correction toward the writer's usual orientation and slant (Pick and Teulings, 1983).

Although visual feedback is not used for monitoring the current strokes, it still appears that specific slips of the pen occur in the absence of visual feedback. When suppressing visual feedback, subjects appear to have a poor control of the number of stroke repetitions or letter repetitions (Lebrun and Rubio, 1972). Interestingly, patients with lesions in the right hemisphere seem to show similar disruptions, e.g. 'comptable' ⇒ 'comnptabble', suggesting that the visual representation is used to monitor the writing process.

2.8 Serial-and-Parallel Model of Handwriting

Previously, the motor system was considered as a sequence of serial modules, where each module represents a specific process. In strictly serial modules, a module needs to deliver its results before the subsequent module can start processing. However, this seems unlikely in continuous motor tasks such as cursive script: during writing a sentence, the later parts of the sentence may still need to be prepared. Therefore, all modules are active simultaneously, i.e. in parallel.

Perhaps the earliest evidence for online programming was reported by Klapp and Wyatt (1976). They investigated a Morse task consisting of sequences of two key presses, in a 'choice reaction time' paradigm. It appeared that reaction time was lengthened in the more complex Morse patterns (i.e. short–long, or long–short) as compared with simpler patterns (i.e. short–short, or long–long). However, with practice the reaction time was less and less affected by the second key press. This indicates that much of the programming of the second key press is done during the first key press. Accordingly, both duration of the first key press and the interval between first and second key presses were longer when the second key press was the more complex long one, as compared with the more simple shorter key press.

The phenomenon of slowed movement execution during loads due to preparation of later parts of the movement is also observed in 'simple reaction time' conditions, where the movement pattern has already been prepared to some extent and the subject is merely waiting for the 'go signal' to start the execution. Sternberg *et al.* (1978) investigated speech and typewriting sequences in simple reaction time conditions. By postulating a speech unit as a single stress group and a typewriting unit as a single keystroke, it appeared that both movement latency of the first unit and the execution time per unit increased about equally for each unit in the total sequence. The increase was approximately 10 ms per unit, although the effect reduces with exercise. Apparently the total number of units but not the complexity per unit is relevant for the movement latency. For example, the 10 ms increase in reaction time is independent of the number of syllables or connecting words per stress group (i.e. word complexity). Sternberg *et al.* suggested an exhaustive unit-retrieval process from an unsorted, nonreducing buffer was followed by a separate unit-unpacking module. The buffer could be the analogy of the midlevel graphic motor-pattern retrieval in handwriting. The retrieval effects depend upon the number of major movement units and become manifest as delays before and during movement execution. The unit-unpacking module could be the analogy of the lower-level modules of parameter setting and motor initiation in handwriting. The unpacking effects depend upon the complexity of each unit separately so that movement latency is affected by the unpacking of the first unit only.

Interestingly, the increases of reaction time and movement time with the number of units is also observed if all (speech) units are identical: they seem even to be retrieved and executed at a significantly lower rate than if they were different units (Sternberg *et al.*, 1978). The same was observed in handwriting for sequences of identical allographs (Teulings, Thomassen and van Galen, 1983) and, surprisingly, also for sequences of identical syllables (van Galen, 1990). Of course, in choice reaction conditions, sequences of identical units are still initiated faster, probably because only one unit needs to be retrieved from the higher-level graphemic buffer (Teulings, Thomassen and van Galen, 1983).

Initially, the Sternbergian increase of both movement latency and movement duration as a function of the number of units in the string could not be replicated in handwriting (Hulstijn and van Galen, 1983; Teulings, Mullins and Stelmach, 1986). It has been hypothesized that under time pressure, which is the case in these simple reaction time experiments, subjects tend to preprogram largely the whole sequence rather than only the beginning. Van Galen, Meulenbroek and Hylkema (1986) eliminated time pressure by letting the subjects initiate and perform the writing pattern at their own pace after a 'go' signal. Under these conditions, the Sternbergian movement latency and duration effects as a function of sequence length in handwriting became manifest. A speculation as to why especially identical units cause an extra slowing down of movement execution is that these sequences give rise to specific errors, e.g. Lebrun and Rubio (1972) reported counting errors (under reduced visual feedback) in patterns containing repetitions. Furthermore, Rumelhart and Norman's (1982) typewriting model provides special provisions for adjacent and for nonadjacent occurrences of identical keystrokes (see end of this section).

A serial-and-parallel model has been proposed by van Galen (1991) in order to explain the specific effects of parallel multimodule processing in handwriting. *Serial* stands for the notion that several sequential modules are discerned, ranging from the highly abstract intention of formulating a message to performing the appropriate muscle contractions. *Parallel* stands for the notion that all modules are active during movement production. In the multimodule model the output of the higher-level module is transmitted to the next lower-level module, so that the higher-level module is available to process subsequent parts of the writing movement. At the same time, the unit programming at the high-level module may be large, whereas it is hierarchically divided into smaller low-level units (Povel and Collard, 1982; Rosenbaum, Kenny and Derr, 1983; Sternberg, Knoll and Turock, 1990). This suggests that in the higher-level module more wide-ranging errors may occur than in the lower-level modules, and that it is reasonable to suppose that the reverse holds. Furthermore, the more abstract movement information is processed at the higher-level module, which needs to be done with greater anticipation with respect to its execution. In the opposite case, the more concrete movement information may be processed at the lowest level of the motor system, which can probably be done immediately prior to executing the corresponding movement.

The model to explain the differential effects due to the processing demands at higher and lower levels may be completed in two ways. According to one model, a higher-level module may take more processing time for a particular complication and consequently delivers results to the next lower module slightly later. This would imply that the corresponding part of the writing movement arrives at the lowest level with some delay. Thus, the execution of a complicating part of the writing pattern is delayed. Although reasonable, this is not what is observed. The observations rather support a second model, which says that the processing that takes place in a module consumes central processing resources. This implies that execution of the current movement is slowed down at the very moment that higher-level processing is done, analogously to a timesharing computer system. The unique consequence of the latter model is that the higher the level of the module that produces the processing load, the greater the delay prior to outputting the corresponding part of the written pattern. This becomes manifest as movement delays at a specific time prior to producing the complex part. Therefore, the opposite of the rationale seems reasonable: the greater the delay prior to the outputting of a complex part, the higher the level of the processing module involved.

Van Galen, Meulenbroek and Hylkema (1986) tested the consistency of this hypothesis by proposing three complexity levels: the syllable, the allograph and the stroke structure, which are supposed to cause programming complexities at the levels of the graphemic, allographic and graphic motor-pattern buffers, respectively. Their subjects wrote pseudowords at their own pace after a 'go' signal. Complexity at the syllable level was varied by adding letters after the third (target) letter (e.g. 'feb' versus 'febel'). This caused mainly a longer movement latency (286 versus 298 ms). The complexity at letter level was manipulated by increasing the complexity of the third letter itself ('l' versus 'b', e.g. 'fel', 'felel' and 'feleb' versus 'feb', 'febeb' and 'febel'). This caused a longer duration of the letter immediately prior to the manipulated letter (270 versus 273 ms, which would be a small difference for reaction times, but is significant for movement times). The movement latency and the durations of the other letters were hardly affected. The complexity at the stroke level was manipulated by varying the connecting stroke between the second and the third allographs. Its complexity depends upon whether the connecting stroke has a constant sense of rotation (e.g. 'ega') or a change of sense

Table 10.1. *Programming unit, variable affecting complexity and the scope of the resulting delays, in various modules or buffers*

Module/buffer	Programming unit	Complexity variable	Delays
Graphemic	Word or stress group	Syllable structure	Word latency
Allographic	Syllable	Allograph structure	Previous allograph
Graphic motor-pattern	Allograph	Stroke complexity	Previous strokes

of rotation (e.g. 'egu'). This caused a longer duration of the strokes of the allograph prior to the connecting stroke (397 versus 405 ms). In summary, these data support the notion that the higher-level modules consume processing demands in parallel to the lower-level modules, while the lower the level, the narrower scale the influence and the smaller the unit of programming (Table 10.1). Furthermore, repetition of a unit of programming causes slowing down of the execution.

2.9   Serial-and-Parallel Model of Typewriting

The parallel preparation of successive key presses in typewriting has been suggested by many researchers as an explanation of the observed high typing rates of about 10 key presses per second. There is ample evidence that this high speed of typewriting is only possible if several keystrokes are prepared in parallel. If only a preview of a single letter is given, typewriting slows down dramatically (Salthouse, 1984). Gentner, Grudin and Conway (1980) and Larochelle (1982) showed that finger movements are not initiated according to the sequence in which they are going to press the keys, but start moving a variable time ahead, so that each finger arrives just in time at the right key. Indeed, Gentner (1983) states that, with practice, the sequential strategy of typewriting is converted into a more and more parallel strategy, while the cognitive constraints are solved and more hard motor constraints remain. With practice, several fingers are observed to be moving simultaneously, each towards its respective target key.

The parallel preparation of key presses has been captured in a model suggested by Rumelhart and Norman (1982). Although it is both microscopic model and a computational model it is included in this section because it covers several of the modules discussed before, and because it illustrates the parallel processing introduced previously. The model generates interkeystroke duration patterns which are so natural that they cannot be discriminated from the timing patterns generated by human typists. This is remarkable as the simulation was based on an isochronous timer with delays based on those required for hand and finger movements. Furthermore, several types of human typewriting errors could be simulated. In this 'activation triggered schema' (ATS) model a schema is understood as a motor program which, in turn, may be called subschemata, or child schemata, or subprograms, thereby passing specific parameters analogously to a computer subroutine. These subschemata may also employ local processing of feedback from 'extension detectors' of the finger relative to the target key. The master schema contains the letters to type a word and is analogous to the graphemic buffer in handwriting. This schema calls the subschemata to type the individual letters, which are analogous to the allographic buffer in handwriting. These subschemata, in turn, call lower-level subschemata controlling the finger, hand and arm muscles until internal position feedback indicates that the appropriate finger has reached the planned key. The latter subschemata are analogous to the graphic motor-pattern buffer, parameter setting and movement initiation in handwriting.

When starting to type a word, the subschemata of the constituent letters are activated according to their order in the words to follow. The model does not allow two identical letters to be activated simultaneously. If two identical letters are adjacent, a 'double schema' is generated with an activation just above the activation

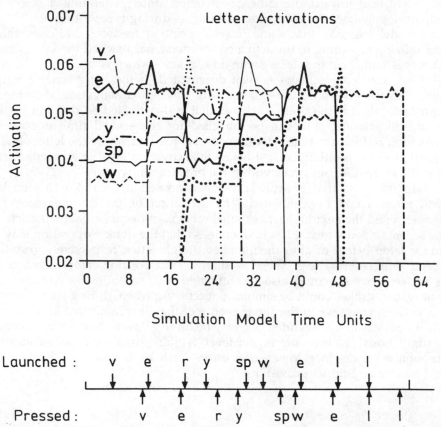

Figure 10.6. *Patterns of activation of the key press schemata, required to set up the string 'very ⟨space⟩ w...'. As soon as the finger reaches the target key, the key press command is launched. After pressing the first 'e', the schema for the second key press of letter 'e', the double schema D, and the schema for the key press of letter 'l' are set up in order to complete the second word 'well'. [Adapted from Rumelhart and Norman, 1982.]*

of the letter to be doubled. On the other hand, if two identical letters occur nonadjacently in the words to be typed, then the second occurrence and all following letters will be blocked until the first occurrence of that particular letter has been executed and deactivated. Furthermore, in order to simulate motor noise some random variations are superimposed upon the activation levels (Figure 10.6).

How do the fingers move toward the appropriate keys? Each letter schema obtains parameters describing the hand and finger that has to press the key. Furthermore, each finger has its own, specified movement limits toward upper and lower rows and inner and outer columns of keys. Therefore, hand and arm movements also need to be involved to reach some keys. The model hypothesizes that the hand is pushed and pulled toward the target positions of all the activated letter schemata in proportion to their activation. So the fingers and the hand are pulled toward the most activated schema, which represents the first key to be pressed. However, the other activated schemata pull the fingers and their hand to some extent also toward the subsequent letters, thus generating a smooth and anticipatory movement of the hands and fingers during typewriting.

The model suggests that some internal position feedback indicates that the finger, moving according to the activated schemata, has reached the key. A ballistic key press is launched and, after some time, a key – which is hopefully the correct one – is hit. The letter schema is then deactivated. If the letter schema with the highest activation has a double schema with still higher activation, then the letter is launched, but it is the double schema that is deactivated so that the particular letter is still activated and can be launched for the second time in succession. Deactivation is done until the activation level is reached where the letter obtains its appropriate serial position, i.e. just below the activation level of its predecessor, or zero if the letter does not occur within the preparation window.

Due to the noise that is artificially superimposed upon the activation levels, several errors could be simulated. The activation of the double schema may increase beyond the next highest activated schema or decrease below the activation of the schema upon which it has to operate, so that the double operation may work upon the letter before or after the intended double letter, respectively, resulting in the usual double errors (e.g. 'sheer' ⇒ 'sherr'). Transposition errors – even multiple ones between hands – could also be simulated (e.g. 'vitamins' ⇒ 'ivtmaisn'). Furthermore, mis-strokes could be simulated, occurring when, during launching a key, hands and fingers move under the influence of the other, activated schemata. As a result, a key near to the intended one may be hit (e.g. 'awareness' ⇒ 'awareneww'). The simulations produce no higher-level typing errors such as captures and alternation reversals, nor lower-level errors such as homologies, because these would require additional provisions.

2.10   Empirical Evidence of Movement Units in Handwriting

The previous sections intended to establish several abstract processing modules. Each of these modules operates with larger or smaller units of programming of handwriting, typewriting or speech. The elementary, mechanically based handwriting movement unit may still be the ballistic stroke, i.e. the trajectory between successive minima of the absolute velocity. However, there is little evidence that strokes form a higher-level organizational unit (Hulstijn and van Galen, 1988; Teulings, Mullins and Stelmach, 1986; Wing, 1978). Hulstijn and van Galen found that the unit of programming depends on the amount of practice. Unfamiliar and unpracticed patterns are considered as a sequence of stroke units, whereas highly practiced stroke sequences may form a single unit at the higher level. Van Galen (1991) suggests a gradual reduction of the units of programming when going from the higher-level modules to the lower-level modules: word, syllable, allograph and stroke, respectively.

Teulings, Thomassen and van Galen (1983) investigated whether a complete allograph or a single stroke forms a movement unit. Their subjects performed all pairs of the allographs 'e', 'u', 'n' and 'j' in a reaction time paradigm with various kinds of advance information: both allographs, only the first allograph, only the second alograph, or no allograph. Usually, the allographs 'e' and 'u' are produced by counterclockwise strokes and 'n' and 'j' by clockwise strokes. It was hypothesized that, if strokes form movement units, then pairs like 'eu' (called similar pairs) consist of a sequence of similar strokes and should show the same reaction times and movement times as identical pairs (e.g. 'ee'). On the other hand, if allographs form movement units, then similar pairs should show the same data as nonsimilar pairs (e.g. 'en'). Only the latter hypothesis appeared to hold. Pairs of identical allographs yield short choice reaction times whereas both pairs of similar and nonsimilar allographs yield long choice reaction times. Furthermore, identical pairs were executed at a lower rate in all choice reaction and simple reaction conditions. These data are compatible with the model that complete allographs form units.

There are more observations to support the idea that each single allograph forms a unit. Meulenbroek and van Galen (1989) found that the strokes belonging to an allograph are systematically different from the connecting strokes between allographs: the latter tend to be longer in time and size, and more noisy. Noise was expressed by the number, frequency and density of dysfluencies and by relatively more high-frequency components. Also between-allograph widths are more variable than the widths of the allographs themselves (Burton *et al.*, 1990). Even if connecting stroke and allograph stroke are virtually identical, differences have been found: Meulenbroek and van Galen (1989) conducted a controlled experiment where adult subjects wrote several times a six-letter word containing 'uu'. Here, the (within-allograph) upstroke of the 'u' is virtually indistinguishable from the upstroke connecting both 'u's. Again, the connecting stroke was more variable. Another example is that with experience and age (from 8-year-olds to adults) each writer acquires a handwriting style which is more and more individual and deviant from the original instruction method. Between each pair of allographs a different connecting stroke may exist, so that connecting strokes may be formed more freely than within-allograph strokes. Therefore, connecting strokes appear to become more easily individual (e.g. Sassoon, Nimmo-Smith and Wing, 1989). Finally, because of their higher number of degrees of freedom, connecting strokes are more sensitive to withdrawal of visual feedback: between-subject differences of connecting strokes increase more than those of strokes within an allograph (Meulenbroek and van Galen, 1989).

In this context it is interesting to mention results by Maarse and Thomassen (1983), who showed that the directions of the upstrokes, which form mostly connecting strokes, are less stable both within and between conditions. The conditions were formed by instructing the subjects to write normally, at increased width or at decreased width. In summary, most empirical evidence supports the allographs as a higher-level unit of handwriting, but apparently this does not reject the hypotheses of larger or smaller units at higher or lower levels, or under certain conditions of practice, respectively.

2.11 Empirical Evidence of Movement Units in Typewriting

It seems reasonable to consider a keystroke as a unit in typewriting, because it is so discrete as compared to the fluent and continuous handwriting movement. Indeed, Sternberg *et al.* (1978) found similar effects in keystrokes as in stress groups, which seemed to fit the properties of a movement unit best. Typewriting strokes are produced at about the same rate as handwriting strokes. However, several handwriting strokes form higher-level allograph units, so that one may wonder whether there are higher-level movement units of several typewriting strokes. Logan (1982) found that when subjects received a 'stop' signal during their typewriting they could inhibit the very last letter of a word very well. This indicates that the unit in typewriting is smaller than a word, and that a keystroke is still a useful unit in typewriting.

3   MICROSCOPIC MODELS

In the previous section the complex handwriting motor system was segmented into various serial-and-parallel modules. An attempt was made also to integrate the typewriting motor system. In the present section, specific modules and processes will be discussed on a more detailed, microscopic scale. The highest-level module concerns the graphemic module, which outputs to the lower-level modules of the handwriting, typewriting and speech motor systems (Ellis, 1982; Margolin, 1984). The graphemic code is translated into the allographic code, which is unique for each of these modalities. The allographic code prescribes the shapes of the graphemes in terms of the strokes required but not the sequence or execution directions of the strokes. This information is retrieved from the graphic motor-pattern store when translating the allographic code into the graphic motor-pattern code. The sequence and directions of the strokes are mostly chosen according to some rules, summarized in the *grammar of action*. The translation between these buffers will be discussed first. The module to be discussed next concerns the graphic motor-pattern store. Not only movement sequences and directions are stored here, but also other motor information to the extent that it is not substituted by the lower-level modules of the nonmuscle-specific parameter setting or the muscle-specific motor initiation. The fixed motor information could be understood as a motor program. The third module to be discussed concerns the lowest-level motor initiation module, where the motor system is dealing with muscle- (or limb-)dependent parameters. Strokes in different directions require different sets of muscle–limb systems, with different features, resulting in main axes of movement in handwriting. Finally, an overview is presented of all conditions and modules that contribute to the time required to produce specific movement times. The large number of factors affecting movement time seems to be an indication that durations are not stored in the graphic motor-pattern but are generated by various modules.

3.1   Grammar of Action

As explained in the previous section on macroscopic models, the allographic code is retrieved from the allographic store and temporarily stored in the allographic buffer. Confusion between allographs with similar shapes but different stroke sequences made Ellis (1982) hypothesize a module where the movement code specifies only the shape of the pattern but not its stroke sequence. The sequence of strokes is established after retrieving the graphic motor-pattern code. If familiar writing patterns are produced, the sequence of strokes is fixed and well learned.

However, if new patterns have to be produced, an efficient sequence will be chosen on the spot, which appears to satisfy a limited set of rules. This set of rules is known as a *grammar of action*, originally proposed by Goodnow and Levine (1973), and extended for handwriting by Thomassen, Tibosch and Maarse (1989), van Sommers (1984) and others.

A graphic pattern may in principle be produced according to numerous sequences and directions of the constituting strokes. Thomassen, Tibosch and Maarse (1989) indicated that the number of different stroke sequences required to copy a geometric pattern increases explosively with the number of segments n as $n!\, 2^n$. However, reading habits, writing instructions, biomechanical effector properties, opportunity for visual guidance and efficiency lead to a reduction in the number of sequences to a few usual sequences, which are chosen by most subjects. The grammar of action specifying preferences to perform the segments may also be the compound result of maturation of the motor system and handwriting skill as several developmental trends and transitions have been observed (Goodnow and Levine, 1973; Nihei, 1983; Thomassen and Teulings, 1979, 1983b; Thomassen, Tibosch and Maarse, 1989; van Sommers, 1984).

The order of stroke production in simple geometric patterns composed of straight horizontal and vertical segments was investigated systematically by Thomassen, Meulenbroek and Tibosch (1991). They observed that five weighted rules could predict nearly 88% of the observed production sequences correctly. These rules are in decreasing order of their weight:

(1) Threading (i.e. continuing without pen lift).
(2) Starting at the extreme left.
(3) Anchoring (i.e. lifting the pen and repositioning it at a segment drawn earlier).
(4) Starting with verticals.
(5) Starting at the top.

Some patterns require conflicting rules to be traded off: e.g. rule 3 is traded off with rule 1; rule 5 is traded off with rule 2. The stroke sequence of patterns where all rules were satisfied simultaneously were less variable, and both reaction and movement times were shorter than in patterns requiring choices to be made between conflicting rules. In patterns requiring tradeoff between various rules, the latencies were longer while the movement times were not longer but even shorter. Therefore, these very high-level decision processes consume central resources long before actually producing the pattern (Thomassen, Meulenbroek and Tibosch, 1991). After extended practice the sequence of strokes of a pattern becomes established as a time-ordered structure in the graphic motor-pattern store.

3.2 Motor Program

Various definitions of a motor program exist. It is generally accepted that a motor program consists of an abstract memory structure containing codes capable of being transformed into movement patterns (Schmidt *et al.*, 1979). A motor program is a controlled sequence, produced by hierarchical units (Keele, Cohen and Ivry, 1990), which is somehow stored in a person's long-term motor memory. As the sequence of strokes is represented in the motor program, the motor program seems most compatible with the graphic motor-pattern code.

Handwriting, typewriting, speech, gesture and gait patterns are indeed highly personal (Cutting and Kozlowski, 1977; Schmidt *et al.*, 1979). Handwriting and signatures, in particular, are considered as personal, motoric fingerprints (Rosenbaum, 1991; Stockholm, 1979). The idiosyncrasy of handwriting is not due to each person's specific handwriting instruction, as children who receive the same writing instruction soon develop their personal handwriting. The sources of personal handwriting features are rather the individual storage of handwriting movements in the graphic motor-pattern store (invariant storage hypothesis) or the individual training of the lower-level movement processing modules (invariant process hypothesis). The individual training could result in individual movement features caused by the muscle-independent parameter setting or the muscle-dependent motor initiation (Soechting, Lacquaniti and Terzuolo, 1986; van Emmerik and Newell, 1989). Some global handwriting features, generated by those lower-level modules, appear so individual that they can be used to identify a writer by analyzing an arbitrary sentence of handwriting. A discriminative set is formed by some global, dynamic features: mean axial pen pressure (i.e. axial pen-to-paper pressure), mean absolute pen velocity in downstrokes, sum of the pen-down durations divided by the total writing time; and by some global, static features: handwriting slant and horizontal extent of the strokes (Maarse, Schomaker and Teulings, 1988).

Nevertheless, there is strong evidence for the invariant storage hypothesis. For example, handwriting storage seems to be hierarchically organized (Patterson and Wing, 1989). Hierarchical storage may also explain why related allographs in adult handwriting show similarities, e.g. between the descenders in 'g' and 'y' or the ascenders in 'l' and 'b'. These complex stroke similarities seem unlikely to be caused by the lower-level processes. The invariant storage hypothesis can also explain the 'motor equivalence' phenomenon (Bernstein, 1967), that the shape of handwriting patterns is rather independent of the limbs and muscles involved. There is a striking shape resemblance between a person's handwriting pattern of normal size and the same pattern performed much larger, or when using other limbs, such that different muscles are involved (Bernstein, 1967; Denier van der Gon and Thuring, 1965; Katz, 1951; Keele, Cohen and Ivry, 1990; Lacquaniti, 1989; Marsden, 1982; Merton, 1972; Raibert, 1977; Stelmach and Teulings, 1983; Teulings, Thomassen and van Galen, 1983; Wing, 1990; Wright, 1990; and others). In terms of the multimodule model, this can be understood by pointing out that writing patterns are stored independently of muscles and limbs, whereas the muscle-specific aspects are substituted in the lowest-level motor-initiation module.

If a motor program is repeated several times, the invariant storage hypothesis predicts many invariant movement features across the resulting replications. By reversing this rationale, which is reasonable, invariant features might stem from those movement parameters that are stored in the motor program, i.e. the graphic motor-pattern code. Additional consistency of invariant features may help to provide further evidence that certain movement parameters are stored in the motor program. Additional consistency can be provided by showing that a supposedly invariant feature does not change when irrelevant execution conditions are changed.

The identification of invariant features is the key to estimating the underlying motor parameters of the motor program. Therefore, invariances have to be expressed on a common scale so that they can be compared. The invariance of a certain feature can be expressed by its signal-to-noise ratio (SNR), defined here as the ratio of the standard deviation of the mean stroke pattern sd(signal') to the mean standard deviation of the differences between the individual stroke patterns and the mean stroke patterns sd(noise). Actually, an unbiased estimator for the noise standard deviation is:

$$sd(signal)^2 = sd(signal')^2 - sd(noise)^2/n$$

where n equals the number of replications used to estimate the mean, although this may yield negative estimates (Teulings and Schomaker, 1993). Any overall variations cause overestimation of sd(noise) so that these small overall variations need to be normalized by a factor, although a rate parameter for time, for example, does not seem statistically reliable in typewriting (Gentner, 1987). However, these normalizations affect the data only little, so that the effect of an unreliable rate parameter is minor. The SNR of a feature presents a dimensionless measure of the invariance of a feature. Furthermore, $1/SNR^2$ represents the relative noise variance of a feature, and is additive for products of independent features – just as absolute variances of sums or differences of independent features are additive. Therefore, it is possible not only to give absolute measures of invariance but also to show how invariances of various features relate to each other.

If it is known how certain features are related, more conclusions can be drawn. A feature could be invariant solely because this feature is related to another and possibly more invariant feature. The comparison of several related invariant features can be illustrated by considering the simplest one-dimensional mechanical equation, which expresses stroke size s as a function of the net force level, which may be assumed to be proportional to the acceleration a in the frictionless case, and stroke duration t:

$$s = eat^2$$

where e stands for the efficiency of the force–time curves. The efficiency is proportional to the distance traveled – given a certain peak force and duration – and is highest for a block-shaped acceleration–time function, and less for half-cosine or triangular-shaped acceleration–time functions, namely 0.25, $2/\pi^2 \approx 0.20$, and $1/6 \approx 0.17$, respectively. The small dynamical range of the efficiency e as a function of acceleration shape indicates that it is not a powerful parameter to control movements.

It is often observed that timing patterns of stokes are remarkably invariant across replications (Denier van der Gon and Thuring, 1965; Viviani and Terzuolo, 1980). However, stroke duration and peak force per stroke are negatively correlated so that it can be understood that the resulting stroke size s is more invariant than either of its factors a and t (Teulings, Thomassen and van Galen, 1986). If the a and t features were generated independently by the motor program, their relative noise variances would add to the relative noise variance of the s feature. However, the s feature shows smaller relative noise variances than the a or t features. This is compatible with a negative correlation between the a and t features. Furthermore, if global writing time or if writing size are deliberately varied by the subject, the s feature appears to change in a more predictable way according to a linear transformation than the a and t features. These two findings suggest that the s feature is more closely related to an underlying movement parameter of the motor program whereas the a and t features are rather related to movement parameters derived at lower levels. In other words, the spatial structure in terms of the relative stroke sizes are more likely to be represented in the graphic motor-pattern code than stroke durations or force levels. This is indeed what one would expect in motor tasks such as handwriting, where the task is specified in the spatial domain and not in the temporal domain.

A person's signature is generally accepted as a motoric fingerprint. The problem of signature verification or identification is interesting to the extent that it requires searching of those parameters that are probably stored in the graphic motor-pattern code and that may be both difficult to suppress or to imitate (Lorette and Plamondon, 1990). For that reason, not only the (static) spatial structure, which may be stored in the graphic motor-pattern code, but also the pen pressure as a function of time seems an interesting dynamical feature for automatic signature verification (Crane and Ostrem, 1983). Apart from the uniform, systematic increase of pen pressure toward the end of a word (Kao, 1983), Schomaker and Plamondon (1991) state that axial pen pressure seems to be a centrally stored pattern, as the pen–force pattern is relatively invariant and not related to the allograph shapes or any biomechanical effects. However, because of its unclear relationship with allograph shapes, pen pressure is of little use for automatic, online handwriting recognition.

Newell and van Emmerik (1989) recorded the vertical component of the pen-tip position and simultaneously the vertical movement components of the hand, wrist, elbow and shoulder joints. They studied right-handers, who wrote with their dominant and with their nondominant hands, and analogously left-handers. The two subject groups employed different coordination patterns in terms of the correlations between joint angles, when writing with their dominant hands. These coordination patterns are again different for loops, circles (i.e. loops without left-to-right movement) and signatures (Lacquaniti et al., 1987; Soechting, Lacquaniti and Terzuolo, 1986; van Emmerik and Newell, 1989). An interesting phenomenon is that both groups of subjects could transfer their invariant coordination patterns to the nondominant side. This means that left- and right-handers using their nondominant limb still do not resemble right- or left-handers, respectively. Importantly, the multijoint coordination patterns seem to be acquired strategies, which have been stored in some lower-level central module, and they are not due to the neurobiomechanical hardware. This seems to support the invariant processing hypothesis.

Van Emmerik and Newell (1989, 1990) realized that the left-to-right writing habit may be responsible for the very different coordination patterns observed in left- and right-handers. Indeed, when performing tasks without left-to-right translation (e.g. circles) the coordination patterns between left- and right-handers become more similar. Writing habits apparently influence the way handwriting movements are produced. This was also found by Thomassen and Teulings (1979), who observed counterclockwise preferences for both left and right hands in schoolchildren and adults when performing drawing patterns (e.g. circles, triangles). These preferences may come from the handwriting habit to form cursive-script letters counterclockwise. Accordingly, children of the age of 5 years, who were not yet exposed to handwriting, showed anatomically based preferences (e.g. mirror symmetry for both hands). However, in fast, uncontrolled scribbling movements, as well as continuous circles of maximum speed, anatomical preferences of the writing apparatus play a predominant role in all age categories. Although handwriting patterns are the result of abstract motor programs stored in the graphic motor-pattern buffer in a muscle- and limb-independent way (e.g. Klapp, 1977), whereas the latter parameters are substituted at the lower-level modules, this does not mean that there are no anatomical factors involved. Muscle- and limb-specific effects play a minor role or are corrected for in the motor program. In fact, the latter examples show that anatomical factors and habits may become manifest under certain conditions.

3.3 Main Axes in Handwriting

Muscle- and limb-specific parameters are substituted in the lowest-level module: the motor-initiation module. This module has to deal with the asymmetric properties of the handwriting apparatus. As the handwriting apparatus has no rotational symmetry, its properties are likely to depend upon movement direction. Indeed, back-and-forth movements generated by flexing and extending the finger joints take about 1.3 times longer than those by the wrist joint (McAllister, 1900; Teulings, Thomassen and Maarse, 1989). Wrist-joint movements and finger-joint movements correspond to nearly orthogonal directions or main axes, each with characteristic properties: wrist-joint movements are fast and finger-joint movements are slow, whereas movements in intermediate directions have intermediate stroke durations. The idea of main axes is not new. Denier van der Gon and Thuring (1965) referred to Dal Bianco (1944), who found that movements along the more horizontal axis were disturbed in patients with cerebellar injury, whereas movements along the perpendicular axis were not. The latter author concluded that movements can well be organized in body-oriented orthogonal axes.

Some authors (for example, Dooijes, 1983; Maarse, Schomaker and Thomassen, 1986; Plamondon and Lamarche, 1986) define *subjective main axes* by asking the subjects to produce voluntary wrist-joint movements and finger movements without wrist movements. These main axes are often oblique. Dooijes (1983) called them *principal directions* and supposed that they moved at constant speed from left to right during writing. He found that the subjects were able to reproduce their voluntary main axes accurately, even after 1 year. Maarse, Schomaker and Thomassen (1986) and Plamondon and Lamarche (1986) estimated main axes ('principal axes' or 'natural axes') in a similar way. The directions varied relatively little as a function of arm rotation, e.g. when writing from left to right across a line, which suggests that these preferred directions are not purely biomechanically determined.

In order to understand the direction-dependent characteristics of the handwriting apparatus, its biomechanical structure is analyzed in terms of degrees of freedom. Each joint of the handwriting apparatus is either a hinge-like or a universal joint. A hinge-like joint requires specification of only one angle (one degree of freedom), whereas a universal joint requires specification of two angles (two degrees of freedom). Neglecting the two universal joints of elbow and shoulder, which are actively involved in handwriting (van Emmerik and Newell, 1989, 1990), the hand–finger system has in total at least 10 degrees of freedom. Namely, the wrist joint possesses two degrees of freedom (dorsal/palmar flexion and ulnar/radial abduction). The thumb and the index finger each possess four degrees of freedom: one for each of the two peripheral finger joints (flexion/ extension), and two for the proximal one (flexion/extension and adduction/abduction). The other fingers do not move independently from the index finger and therefore do not contribute to the degrees of freedom of the handwriting apparatus. However, not all passive or theoretical degrees of freedom are used in handwriting. In order to assure the necessary pen grip, the thumb and fingers are kept opposed. Furthermore, the pen is not supposed to rotate around its axial axis. Finally, the pen tip remains in touch with the paper during cursive writing. Thus the wrist joint has only one effective degree of freedom, formed by a fixed combination of palmar flexion and radial abduction/dorsal flexion and ulnar abduction, depending upon supination/pronation of the forearm. The thumb–fingers system has two, or maybe more, effective degrees of freedom. One component represents the back-and-forth movements to and from the hand palm by flexion/extension of both thumb joints and finger joints, and the other component represents the back-and-forth movements parallel to the hand by simultaneous flexion/extension of thumb joints and the extension/flexion of finger joints. Therefore strokes in intermediate directions use three degrees of freedom.

This analysis in terms of degrees of freedom gives rise to an interesting prediction about the accuracy of movements in various directions. Wrist movements have one degree of freedom and allow the near-perfect production of large circle segments (e.g. with radius 15 cm), which can be well approximated by straight segments in normal stroke lengths of 0.5 cm (Dooijes, 1983). Therefore trajectory inaccuracy can be expressed by the average distance of each stroke from its minimum-squares fitted line. However, finger movements have two degrees of freedom and therefore require coordination between the two (or more) synergistic muscle systems. For example, it is only possible to draw a straight line if the two synergistic muscle systems are initiated simultaneously, despite unequal nerve transmission delays. Uneven initiation causes loops or blunt curves at stroke endings (Schomaker, Thomassen and Teulings, 1989). Furthermore, the force-versus-time patterns need to be proportional; if not, a curved stroke results. Therefore movements with two or more effective degrees of freedom produce less accurate pen trajectories. Finally, intermediate movement directions have three degrees of freedom and produce even less accurate trajectories than the pure finger movements. Hence, the wrist and the finger movement directions can be identified by their capability to produce relatively straight back-and-forth movements. These special movement directions, which have relatively high spatial accuracies, appear to coincide with the directions of extreme stroke durations and also with those of extreme stroke lengths (Teulings, Thomassen and Maarse, 1989). Table 10.2 summarizes the directional properties of the writing apparatus. Opposite to the accuracy of the straightness is the accuracy of the movement amplitude: wrist movements are less accurate than finger movements, as established in Fitts' speed–accuracy tradeoff tasks (Langolf, Chaffin and Foulke, 1976) (see Section 4 for

Table 10.2. *Various features and properties, which may differ for wrist and finger movements, and which may either have an intermediate or cumulative effect for movements of the wrist and fingers combined*

	Joints involved		
Feature	Wrist	Wrist and finger	Finger
Direction (degrees)*	+45	Intermediate	−45
Preferred duration (ms)	120	Intermediate	160
Preferred size (mm)	9	Intermediate	6
Degrees of freedom	1	3	2
Accuracy of straightness (mm)	0.04	>0.07	0.07
Fitts' speed–accuracy (ms per bit)	43	?	26

*Relative to baseline (0 degrees); slant is +70 degrees; most frequent upward movement is +45 degrees.

a discussion on Fitts' law). The net difference seems small in typical handwriting movements with durations of about 140 ms, but increases for precision movements requiring more than about 200 ms.

An interesting finding is that both movement axes are orthogonal and have average directions of +45 and −45 degrees with respect to the baseline of handwriting. The average slant of handwriting was 70 degrees relative to the baseline, and did not coincide or correlate with any of the main axes. This is in agreement with the observation that slant as well as the directions of the subjective main axes appeared highly independent of arm orientation, which changes when writing across the line (Maarse, Schomaker and Thomassen, 1986). Slant was estimated by the most frequent (opposite) direction of downstrokes. Although visual slant was actually a few degrees steeper, this estimator was robust with respect to instructed stretching of writing (Maarse and Thomassen, 1983). Only the most frequent upward stroke direction, representing the connecting strokes between allographs, coincides more or less with the direction of the wrist-joint extensions (Teulings, Thomassen and Maarse, 1989).

3.4 Factors Influencing Movement Duration

The preferred frequency of the handwriting apparatus appears to be close to 5 Hz (Maarse, Schomaker and Thomassen, 1986; Teulings and Maarse, 1984; Teulings, Thomassen and Maarse, 1989). The speed of handwriting in terms of strokes per second varies with the maximum speeds of several different motor tasks involving other muscles, such as tapping with the finger, thumb, hand, arm or foot (for an overview, see Keele and Hawkins, 1982). The latter authors suggest that a central timekeeper with unpredictable transmission delays could form the limiting factor for these speeds. On the other hand, Morasso, Mussa Ivaldi and Ruggiero (1983) and van Galen and Schomaker (1992) suggest rather that the inertia and the peripheral nerve–muscle system may act as a biomechanical low-pass filter of the higher-frequency nerve signals. At least there seems to be a physiologically determined maximum speed of repetitive movements. Previously, various conditions have been discussed, causing processing loads at the higher-level modules of the handwriting motor system, which become manifest as small delays:

(1) Online preparation of complex syllable structures and syllable repetition.
(2) Allograph selection, allograph complexity and allograph repetition.
(3) Stroke sequence selection within an allograph.
(4) Online preparation of complex connecting strokes.
(5) Direction of a stroke.

These factors cause only marginal movement duration effects; the major effects on movement duration are due to the relative sizes and shapes of the strokes. The traditional view (Denier van der Gon and Thuring, 1965) is that the average duration of handwriting strokes does not depend upon their average size ('isochrony'). The principle of isochrony can be extended to the substroke level ('isogony'). Isogony says that trajectories of equal change of direction are performed in equal amounts of time (Viviani and Terzuolo, 1980, 1982). This, in turn, implies at the microscopic scale that angular velocity ω of the handwriting trajectory is constant, or that pen speed v is directly proportional to the radius of curvature r: $v = \omega/r$.

However, more refined predictions are possible. In general, the above approximations do not hold in extreme writing sizes, e.g. on a blackboard (Thomassen and Teulings, 1983b), in more complex patterns consisting of strokes of different sizes (Teulings, Thomassen and van Galen, 1986) or in curvilinear strokes (Lacquaniti, Terzuolo and Viviani, 1983). In order to make these different and conflicting relationships consistent, three contextual levels have been discerned by Thomassen and Teulings (1985). In each context, specific time versus size relationships appear to exist. The compound effect is the product of three factors because these three contextual levels form concentric shells:

(1) Macro context (i.e. a word in the context of other words of different overall sizes).
(2) Meso context (i.e. a single stroke in the context of other strokes of different sizes).
(3) Micro context (i.e. the local curve radius in the context of the curvilinear trace of a single stroke).

In macro context complete writing patterns are considered in isolation. As mentioned earlier, in the frictionless case, stroke size s is proportional to the peak muscle force (or peak acceleration a) and the stroke duration t squared: $s = eat^2$, where e is an efficiency factor, characterizing the effect of a particular shape of the force-time curve. The efficiency e plays a minor role in controlling stroke sizes in handwriting (Teulings, Thomassen and van Galen, 1986). The shapes of the force–time curves are indeed quite constant (Plamondon and Maarse, 1989).

It appears that the time to produce a writing pattern is virtually independent of its size, provided that the average stroke sizes are not too big, i.e. between 0.25 and 1 cm (Denier van der Gon and Thuring, 1965; Michel, 1971; Thomassen and Teulings, 1984; although not in agreement with Wing, 1980). The duration is apparently limited by the frequency bandwidth of the handwriting apparatus so that size increase is entirely produced by force increase. Consequently, duration t is constant in the range of normal writing sizes so that peak force a is proportional to stroke size s. On the other hand, in large writing sizes, i.e. much larger than 1 cm, as when writing on the blackboard, force levels may become very high and may reach a ceiling. Thomassen and Teulings (1984) found that the height of this ceiling depends on the instructed pace or time pressure. Therefore, when producing large writing sizes or arm movements, it is the force that seems constant, whereas size variations are programmed entirely by variation of duration (Wadman *et al.* 1979). Thus, in macro context, a power relationship between t and s can be proposed:

$$t = ks^b \qquad (b = 0 \text{ if } s < 1\,\text{cm})$$

$$(b = 1/2 \text{ if } s \gg 1\,\text{cm})$$

where k is constant per context and instruction.

Apart from the force level approaching a ceiling, there may still be another mechanism that causes larger writing patterns to be produced more slowly, as suggested by Keele (1982): namely, relative accuracy is not necessarily kept under control when instructed to write larger. The most natural assumption would be that the subjects keep a constant relative accuracy so that writing patterns of various sizes appear very similar. For a large range of movement amplitudes, Fitts' law reliably predicts that aiming movement time depends only upon the relative accuracies (see Section 4 for a discussion of Fitts' law). This would suggest that movement time does not depend upon movement size. However, when writing size increases, the arm becomes more involved and the fingers less so (Meulenbroek *et al.*, 1993). The critical observation is that arm movements require more time for a specific relative accuracy than do hand or finger movements, namely 106 ms per bit, versus 43 or 26 ms per bit, respectively (Langolf, Chaffin and Foulke, 1976). This holds for stroke durations longer than about 200 ms, which may occur in precision movements. In order to maintain the required relative accuracy in larger writing sizes, where mainly arm movements are involved, the motor system may deliberately choose a lower rate. This hypothesis seems to be supported to some extent by data presented by Wright (1991). He showed that writing with the arm was indeed slower than writing with the fingers within a small ascender-to-descender size range of 1.5–2.5 cm, although the reliable difference was as small as 5 ms per stroke. However, there are some small inconsistencies in this hypothesis. For example, writing time as a function of size of the two affector systems did not seem to interact (Wright, 1991), whereas the speed–accuracy relationships clearly do (Langolf, Chaffin and Foulke, 1976). Furthermore, finger movements, which show the highest accuracy, are not the fastest movements (see Table 10.2). Another difficulty to disentangle finger and wrist movements versus arm movements is the 'hysteresis' observed, i.e. when increasing or decreasing writing sizes, the effector systems already involved tend to continue their contribution. Therefore, the relative contribution of these effector systems may depend upon the movements performed immediately beforehand.

Meso context refers to the adjacency of strokes of different sizes (such as in the cursive-script word 'pellet'). The specific problem for the motor system is the abrupt adjustment of peak force or stroke duration, leading to a size increase from the 'e' to 'l'. Denier van der Gon and Thuring (1965) suggested a pure time increase with no increase of peak force level, as in large movement sizes in macro context, but most observations are compatible with an increase of both time and force. This seems likely because a pure increase of peak force, without slowing the movement, may take several strokes (Denier van der Gon and Thuring, 1965; Stelmach and Teulings, 1983). Thomassen and Teulings (1985) suggested the following power function to describe the relationship between duration t and size s in meso context:

$$t = ks^b \quad (b = \pm 0.33)$$

The data of 'el' or 'le' pairs by Greer and Green (1983), Hollerbach (1981), Thomassen and Schomaker (1986), Thomassen and Teulings (1985) and Wing (1980) yield values for $b = 0.22, 0.34, 0.34, 0.38$ and 0.41, respectively. Indeed, there is only marginal consistency, which may mean that b depends upon the subject and upon various unknown conditions. At least, b seems clearly within the range of the extreme values of 0.0 and 0.5, which occur in macro context.

Finally, micro context describes the time needed per infinitesimal part of the writing trajectory, which is equivalent to the local pen speed v. An estimator of 'local size' is the curve radius r of the circle, which fits the curve at that point. An estimator of 'local duration' is the inverse angular velocity, i.e. $r/v = 1/\omega$. Lacquaniti, Terzuolo and Viviani (1983) observed that, in a large variety of drawing tasks, a more complex relationship holds than the one suggested by the isogony principle, namely:

$$1/\omega = r/v = kr^b \quad (b = 2/3) \quad \text{(two-thirds power law)}$$

where k is a constant gain factor which depends upon meso and macro context. This relationship can be derived for perfectly sinusoidal movements, i.e. two equal-frequency movement components without left-to-right translation, which produces only arbitrary ellipses. The relationship holds to some extent for a narrow-frequency bandwidth movement, consisting of two independent movement components (e.g. horizontal and vertical) which are piecewise sinusoids–as in large, fluent scribbling movements. However, the two-thirds power law does not hold for normal handwriting. Thomassen and Teulings (1985) studied the behavior of the value b and the correlation between $\log(r/v)$ and $\log(r)$ for various writing patterns and simulated patterns. A normal handwriting pattern yields virtually the same values as a random walk pattern: $b = 0.41$ (instead of 2/3) and correlation 0.83 (instead of 1.0, ideally). Also alternating small and big loops (e.g. 'elel') yield values close to those of a random walk. Only continuous ellipses and 'llll' patterns yield values that are closer to the ideal value than to those of a random walk: $b = 0.59$ and correlations as high as 0.95. That the two-thirds power law does not seem to hold for handwriting in general is probably due to the wide frequency bandwidth of handwriting (Teulings and Maarse, 1984) and the left-to-right trend, although this trend is probably only taking place during the upstrokes (Maarse and Thomassen, 1983; Thomassen and Teulings, 1983a). Wann, Nimmo-Smith and Wing (1988) also observed significant deviations from the two-thirds power law in large, repetitive ellipses produced at lower than maximal rates. The velocity patterns become skewed, due to faster accelerations than decelerations. Therefore, they suggested a 'wobbling-mass model', which will be discussed in the next section on computational models. In summary, the two-thirds power law does not seem to describe the instantaneous speed of handwriting strokes accurately enough.

The observation that so many parameters affect movement durations provides additional evidence that durations are not stored in the graphic motor-pattern code (Teulings, Thomassen and van Galen, 1986). Instead, the pattern of durations is the result of various time-consuming actions (Lacquaniti, Terzuolo and Viviani, 1983), which mainly take place at the lower-level modules of parameter setting and motor initiation. A similar line of evidence exists for typewriting. There appears to be no global typing-rate parameter (Gentner, 1987). The interkey intervals are rather the result of fixed actions required to move to each subsequent key, as Rumelhart and Norman (1982) have demonstrated in their typewriting simulation model. The more complex handwriting motor system has not yet been captured by an extended model. There is a class of computational models of the writing movement which employ only a limited set of features of the writing pattern itself in order to reconstruct an existing writing pattern. However, the symbolic computational models may allow more than simply reproducing existing writing patterns by substituting parts of the writing patterns by symbolic units, so that new writing patterns can also be generated. None of the computational models is so detailed that these central and peripheral effects can also be generated.

4 COMPUTATIONAL MODELS

Computational models focus on the quantitative simulation of the pen movements in handwriting. The aim is to generate handwriting movements with limited sets of parameters, which may relate to certain neurophysiological variables of the motor program or the biomechanical architecture of the handwriting apparatus. These models may at least suggest the validity of certain models, although it is impossible to draw firm conclusions. Furthermore, the models may indicate the complexity of the handwriting motor system.

4.1 Theoretical Minimum Number of Parameters

According to the sampling theorem (Jerri, 1977), the minimum number of (isochronous) samples required to reconstruct a time function of duration T and limited frequency bandwidth W, equals $2WT$. This requires sampling of the handwriting movement at the Nyquist frequency, which is equal to $2W$. Handwriting consists actually of two time functions: one for the horizontal and one for the vertical component. Under the worst-case assumption that both components are independent, $4WT$ parameters are required to describe exactly a handwriting segment of duration T. The frequency spectrum of handwriting shows a predominant frequency of 5 Hz and a gradual descent to noise level at about $W = 10$ Hz (Teulings and Maarse, 1984). The durations of the fastest ballistic strokes, which are easiest to simulate, are about 0.1 s. Therefore, four parameters per ballistic stroke allow the exact description of the handwriting movement in space and time. A more realistic estimate of the 'equivalent bandwidth' of the nonhomogeneous frequency spectrum is slightly smaller than the maximum bandwidth, typically $W = 7$ Hz. This explains why low-pass filtering of frequencies lower than 7 Hz deteriorates the shape of a handwriting pattern (Teulings and Thomassen, 1979). The average duration of ballistic strokes is slightly longer than the minimum duration, typically $T = 0.14$ s. Again, on average four parameters per stroke are required to reconstruct the writing signal completely.

Perhaps the most unintelligent computational model to describe the handwriting movement adequately would sample isochronously and simultaneously (and infinitely accurately) x and y coordinates at the Nyquist frequency $f = 2W = 2/0.14$ s $= 14$ Hz. Of course, when sampling handwriting with discrete, finite-accuracy digitizers (e.g. 0.002 cm resolution, 0.004 cm accuracy) (Meeks and Kuklinski, 1990), higher sampling frequencies (e.g. 100 Hz) are required, especially if time derivatives have to be estimated (Teulings and Maarse, 1984). It will appear that many more intelligent computational models also employ four parameters per stroke and seem no more parsimonious than this unintelligent computational model. Some models even use more than four parameters – which is not parsimonious – and seem to perform a curve fit. The migration of the computational models runs from the original models, generating horizontal and vertical force components, via orientation-free models, mass-spring models, to symbolic and biomechanical models.

The average number of parameter updates per ballistic stroke provides a measure for the parsimony of a model. The initial parameter settings are not counted if they hold for all handwriting patterns. Two properties of a model may yield a further reduction of the 'effective number of parameters', although this has not been applied to the models for reasons of comparability. The first property is the implementation of symbolic or hierarchical representations of movement units, e.g. allographs, or parts of them. For example, if the set of parameters that generates an allograph can be reused for each replication in all contexts, then the total number of parameters of a pattern equals the number of 'allograph identifiers'. The number of parameters for the actual allograph is merely a constant initial condition.

The second property yielding a reduction in the information contents of the set of parameters is the quantization of a parameter into a few discrete levels. Normally, parameters are scalars, with a finite number of 'effective quantization' levels due to the limited accuracy of the handwriting motor system. The ratio of parameter quantization and effective quantization yields the reduction factor of the number of effective parameters of a model. The number of effective quantization levels in normal handwriting strokes can be derived from the speed–accuracy tradeoff according to Fitts' law. Fitts' law says that the duration of reciprocal aiming movements of amplitude A toward a target of width W increases linearly with the information measure $\log_2(2A/W)$ in 'bits'. The factor of 2 expresses that A is actually the radius of the circle of diameter $2A$ within which all possible aiming movements of amplitude A are found. The duration increases with instructed accuracy according to 26 and 43 ms per bit for the finger and wrist movements, respectively, in a wide range of amplitudes and accuracies (Langolf, Chaffin and Foulke, 1976). This suggests that during a typical handwriting stroke of 140 ms the finger and wrist movements produce 5.4 and 3.2 bits, corresponding to the number of effective quantization levels $2A/W$ of 40 and 10, respectively. It may be speculated that, if both finger and wrist movements are controlled independently, each stroke contains 8.6 bits, corresponding to 400 discrete strokes, which incidentally equals the empirical finding that a self-organizing net of strokes of at least 400 cells provides an adequate description of the handwriting strokes for automatic recognition (Schomaker and Teulings, 1990).

When also taking the different offsets into account, the speed–accuracy tradeoff relationships for finger, wrist and arm movements yield similar values of the relative accuracy, namely, 2.6 bits for stroke durations of 140–200 ms, corresponding to six effective quantization levels. The signal-to-noise ratio (SNR) yields similar values of the effective number of quantization levels in a more adequate task than the Fitts task, namely in a real handwriting task, where stroke durations are about 140 ms. The SNR is the ratio of the standard deviations of the movement amplitude sd(signal) and of the movement noise sd(noise) (see Section 3). The relationship between the strict sizes A and W and the standard deviations is exactly $A = 2\text{sd(signal)}$ and approximately $W = 4\text{sd(noise)}$: namely, a Gauss-shaped probability distribution between $+$ and -2sd(noise) corresponds to 95% hits within target W. Therefore, the number of effective quantization levels per component in a real handwriting task is $2A/W = \text{SNR}$. The observed SNRs of about 6 in patterns of the vertical stroke sizes (Teulings, Thomassen and van Galen, 1986) suggest a lower number of effective quantization levels per component, which seems understandable as handwriting is more complex than reciprocal movements.

4.2 X and Y Force Models

One of the earliest characterizations of handwriting movements was presented by Denier van der Gon and Thuring (1965). Their statements are interesting in that they provided a simple representation of the pen-point movement in handwriting. They suggested that the ratios of the stroke lengths are programmed by the duration ratios of the accelerative force bursts whereas overall size is programmed by force amplitude. The pen-to-paper and internal frictional forces were supposed to be negligible relative to inertial or accelerating forces. Finally, they suggested that movements are programmed in terms of separate horizontal and vertical components. This model has inspired many computational models of handwriting. Denier van der Gon, Thuring and Strackee (1962) used analog force generators with fixed force rises up to a fixed amplitude. Vredenbregt and Koster (1971) have successfully regenerated handwriting. They used electromotors for horizontal and vertical movement components and manually adjusted the start and stop moments of fixed amplitude currents (or forces or accelerations). They found that changes in the vertical component distorted the generated writing trajectory about twice as much as large changes in the horizontal component. Under the condition of fixed force amplitudes for each of the two sets of agonists and antagonists involved, each stroke requires four parameters: the stop moment of the agonist force causing the acceleration, and the start moment of the antagonistic force causing the decelerating force, respectively, for horizontal and vertical components independently. The agonist force has already started in the previous stroke and the antagonist force will stop in the next stroke, so that these parameters are not reckoned to the current stroke. If the force amplitude per component were a parameter also, this would require two more parameters per stroke and the model would no longer be parsimonious.

Dooijes (1983) presented an equally parsimonious computational model of handwriting by assuming that the accelerating and decelerating force amplitudes vary per stroke, but that the stop moment of the accelerating and the start moment of the decelerating forces coincide. A 'bang-bang' force pattern results. Furthermore, instead of orthogonal axes, oblique axes are used, derived separately from the subject's preferred hand and finger movements. The axes are moving at constant speed from left to right. The question arises as to whether more realistic generation models exist than this bang-bang force pattern, and which are still parsimonious.

MacDonald (1966) examined the shape of the acceleration bursts during handwriting. The finger movements produced rectangular acceleration functions, while the wrist movements produced rather trapezoid acceleration functions, and the lower arm movements rather triangular acceleration functions. These force patterns occurred only in the 'stroke-controlled' or ballistic movements (i.e. strokes taking less than 250 ms, with a single acceleration and a single deceleration phase). However, 'continuously controlled' movements (i.e. slower strokes) are produced at such a low rate that they show multiple acceleration phases per velocity phase (Maarse *et al.*, 1987). Finally, extra force bursts occur when the pen tip suddenly 'sticks' to the paper ('static friction' or 'Coulomb friction'), which occurs where movement direction reverses such as in cursive allographs 'c' or 'u'. This frictional force was hard to describe, but Denier van der Gon and Thuring (1965) suggested that friction may be neglected with respect to the accelerating or inertial force. Viscous force, which increases with velocity, also appeared to be negligible with respect to the inertial force: $k = \pi m / T < 0.1$, where T is the stroke duration, and m the effective mass of the hand.

Plamondon and Maarse (1989) compared the accuracy of reconstruction of the writing trajectories generated by several of these models and their variants. They showed that many of the models can be represented by second-order or third-order transmission systems. The order of a system is the highest time derivative needed to relate the input and the output signal. The zeroth, first or second time derivatives of the input represent the input signal itself, the rate of change of the input signal and the acceleration of the input signal, respectively. To estimate the order, the nerve–muscle interface and a muscle–pen (or hand–paper) interface were described separately.

The nerve–muscle interface can be derived from Hill's relationship (Dijkstra *et al.*, 1973) and expresses the muscle-force output $F(t)$ as a function time, the relative nerve activation level $g(t)$ (ranging from 0 to 1), the muscle's maximal isometric force F_{max}, its shortening speed $v(t)$, and its maximum shortening speed v_{max}:

$$F(t) = \{[(F_{max} + a)\,v_{max}]/[v(t) + v_{max}] - a\}\,g(t)$$

where a is the muscle constant. For the forefinger muscles, v_{max} corresponds to pen speeds of 20 cm/s, whereas the highest pen speeds in normal size handwriting are nearer 10 cm/s, so that $v(t) \ll v_{max}$. Furthermore, the minimum activation and deactivation times of the system are about 20 ms, whereas normal handwriting strokes have durations of at least 100 ms. Therefore, handwriting movements are well within the range of the physiological muscle specifications, so that $F(t) \approx F_{max}g(t)$ (Plamondon and Maarse, 1989). This forms a zeroth-order transmission system. Furthermore, the nerve activation level $g(t)$ is assumed to depend only upon the first and the zeroth time derivatives of the nerve firing rate so that the nerve–muscle interface is probably a first-order response system to the neural firing rate.

The muscle–pen interface can be described by a damped spring-mass system:

$$F(t) = m \cdot a(t) + fv \cdot v(t) + k \cdot r(t) + f \cdot Fz \cdot |v(t)|$$

where $r(t)$ is the off-equilibrium distance and $v(t)$ and $a(t)$ are its first and second time derivatives, or velocity and acceleration, respectively, and $|v(t)|$ is the speed irrespective of direction. Fz is the pen-to-paper pressure and m, fv, k and f are the equivalent mass, the viscous friction constant, the muscle stiffness and the pen-to-paper friction, respectively (see also Wing, 1978; Dooijes, 1983). As the second time derivative (i.e. the acceleration $a(t)$) is the highest time derivative of position, this is a second-order transmission system. The order of the total transmission system is therefore 3. However, if the nervous system is anticipating the first-order internal transformation, the order of the total system may be as low as 2. The system order of the models defined in the acceleration domain therefore requires two integrations and is at least 2, and that defined in the velocity domain requires only one integration so that the system order is at least 1. The order had to be augmented by 1 if the shape of the pattern was a symmetrical trapezoid, a symmetrical triangle or an exponential function (containing one adjustable parameter), or by 2 if it was Gaussian or sinusoid (containing two parameters). Examples of second-order systems are to be found in Denier van der Gon *et al.* (1962, 1965), Dooijes (1983), Eden (1962), Hollerbach (1981) and Mermelstein and Eden (1964). They consist of component movements along two axes, without friction or elasticity, and two or three acceleration levels: positive, zero and negative. Examples of third-order systems are put forward by MacDonald (1966) using trapezoid acceleration patterns and by Yasuhara (1975) incorporating exponential acceleration patterns and some internal friction.

These and several other models were compared in terms of the spatial error between original and regenerated handwriting patterns, defined as the average distance relative to the stroke length. More precisely, the spatial error was calculated by the average of the surfaces between the recorded and the regenerated strokes, divided by their squared lengths. To regenerate a handwriting pattern, the effective accelerations and durations of the positive and negative phases were estimated for the horizontal and the vertical acceleration components separately. These phases represent force bursts in horizontal and vertical directions, respectively. Analogously, the phases of the velocity components were estimated on behalf of the velocity domain models. These phases represent 'ballistic component strokes' as the components were analyzed separately. The shapes of the positive and negative phases could be approximated by rectangular, symmetrical trapezoid, symmetrical triangular, half-sinusoid, Gaussian or exponential rise-and-decay time functions (Figure 10.7). The numbers of phases per component equals approximately the number of ballistic strokes. Therefore, four parameters per ballistic stroke are required: the durations and the effective accelerations or velocities for the horizontal and vertical components.

It appeared that most models accurately reproduced the handwriting patterns. The models defined in the acceleration domain were slightly worse than those defined in the velocity domain. Small spatial errors were achieved

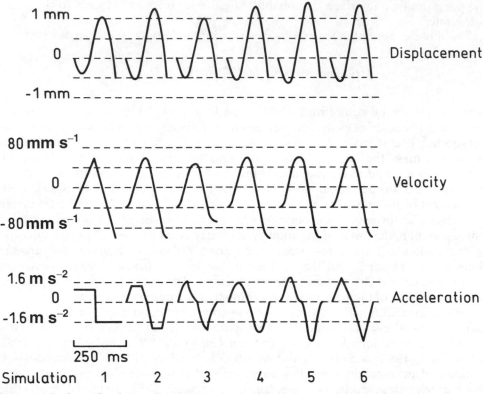

Figure 10.7. *Some fitted time functions per stroke in acceleration domain with: 1, rectangular; 2, symmetrical trapezoid; 3, exponential rise and decay; 4, half-sinusoid; 5, Gaussian; and 6, symmetrical triangular shape, and their shapes in velocity and displacement domains. [From Plamondon and Maarse, 1989.]*

by approximating the acceleration components by rectangular or trapezoid functions, or by approximating the velocity components by several reasonable patterns, such as sinusoidal, Gaussian or triangular time functions. There was no difference in accuracy between models of different system orders.

4.3   Orientation-Free Force Models

There is a class of models which do not assume any specific x or y axes, nor axes related to biomechanical joints. Morasso and Mussa Ivaldi (1982) and Morasso, Mussa Ivaldi and Ruggiero (1983) state that movement patterns are unlikely to be described in terms of joint angles but rather in some spatial reference frame, which does not need to be the body-oriented horizontal coordinates. They assumed that discrete 'circular strokes' are generated in a discontinuous process while the inertia of the finger–hand–arm system smooths the movement by acting as a low-pass filter (van Galen and Schomaker, 1992) (Figure 10.8). Circular strokes are defined

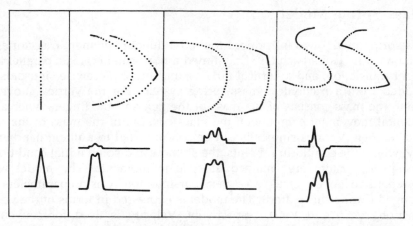

Figure 10.8. *Examples of the performance of the circular-stroke composition model for four movement patterns in the four frames. Dots are equally spaced in time. Each frame shows the simulated movement pattern (top left), the underlying circular strokes with Gaussian velocity time functions (top right), and the curvature and absolute velocity time functions (bottom). [From Morasso, Mussa Ivaldi and Ruggiero, 1983.]*

as: (1) a circle segment of specific curve radius, arc length and orientation, such that it is tangential to the trace at the point of peak velocity or inflection; (2) having a half-phase of a Gaussian velocity function during the interval from the previous absolute velocity peak to the current peak and the other half-phase from the current peak to the next peak; (3) each half overlapping in time with the previous and the following circular strokes, respectively. Overlapping circular strokes are averaged sample by sample. Therefore, six parameters per ballistic stroke are needed: its curve radius, arc length, orientation, peak velocity, duration between previous and following velocity peak, and the asymmetric position of the peak velocity between the previous and following ones. The accuracy of this model does not seem as high as that of the simpler models, which were based on component movements per axis (Plamondon and Maarse, 1989).

In another paper Plamondon (1989) provides a model which allows a more accurate reconstruction of writing patterns. As in the previous model, absolute velocity is approximated by a piecewise Gaussian function but, instead of the previous constant radius approximation and the concept of overlap, the angular velocity is also approximated by a piecewise Gaussian function. Thus, again, two parallel motor signals are required but they do not refer to Cartesian axes. The piecewise Gaussian functions are generated by a hypothetical velocity nerve signal, consisting of a sequence of rectangular time functions (Plamondon, 1989). The height of each block represents the gain of the muscular speed generator. In order to simulate sharp movement reversals, discontinuities had to be inserted in the angular velocity. The cursive-script word 'bug', containing about 12 ballistic strokes, could be reconstructed very accurately, using 60 parameters for the tangential velocity and 52 parameters for the angular velocity. Therefore, as many as nine parameters per ballistic stroke were used, which is much more than the minimum of four parameters per stroke.

4.4   Mass-Spring Model

The mass-spring model was introduced to model fluent movement trajectories in a parsimonious way. Hollerbach (1981) assumed a horizontal (x) axis, parallel to the left-to-right translation, and a vertical (y) axis, and fitted piecewise sinusoids as if they resulted from a frictionless mass-spring system. For the vertical movement component, the mass consists of the mass of the pen and the fingers whereas, for the horizontal movement component, the mass consists of the mass of the whole hand and the pen. Various sinusoids can be concatenated to a fluent handwriting trajectory, where the equilibrium points, the stiffness and some initial conditions of the mass-spring system are changed at specific moments. The model would generate repetitive loops such as 'eeee' very parsimoniously as no parameters need to be changed during this pattern. The model is expressed in terms of the velocity time functions $Vx(t)$ and $Vy(t)$, respectively. Velocity is used for convenience instead of position or acceleration, which would also be sinusoids:

$$Vx(t) = Vx\_\text{peak} \cdot \sin(\omega x \cdot t + \varphi x) + c$$

$$Vy(t) = Vy\_\text{peak} \cdot \sin(\omega y \cdot t + \varphi y)$$

where $Vx\_$peak and $Vy\_$peak are the velocity amplitudes, ωx and ωy are angular frequencies or frequencies multiplied by 2π, and φx and φy are the initial phases, respectively. The constant velocity, horizontal left-to-right movement c is added to the horizontal component.

Some simplifications can be made. Clearly, only $\varphi x - \varphi y = \varphi$ is relevant as the initial phase can be set in the initial condition. Furthermore, the basic setting of the peak velocities in both horizontal and vertical directions can be chosen to be equal to twice the horizontal left-to-right velocity, i.e. $Vx\_$peak $= Vy\_$peak $= 2c$. So repetitive loops are generated by circular movements, while the center of the circle moves with half the circling speed. Finally, the horizontal and vertical frequencies may be chosen to be equal, i.e. $\omega x = \omega y = \omega$. Unequal frequencies would only be needed in patterns like '8'. Various basic patterns can be generated by modulating φ: upright loops ($\varphi = 90$ degrees), slanted loops ($\varphi = 60$ degrees), guirlands ($\varphi = 30$ degrees), waves ($\varphi = 0$ degrees) and arcades ($\varphi = -30$ degrees). Another important parameter to influence stroke shape is the horizontal velocity Vx at the moments where Vy changes from upward to downward (i.e. at the top of a stroke): $Vx = c - Vx\_$peak $\cdot \sin(\varphi)$. Hence, if a sharp movement reversal has to be programmed such as at the top of allograph 'c', requiring Vx to change sign, the parameters φ, $Vx\_$peak or c may be adjusted simultaneously.

Ascenders and descenders can be generated by increasing $Vy\_$peak and by decreasing ω, similar to the observed change of both force and duration in meso context. In order to maintain a stable baseline, $Vy\_$peak should only be changed at the segmentation points where the upward movement turns into a downward movement or vice versa, i.e. $Vy = 0$. These upper and lower segmentation points correspond with the boundaries of ballistic strokes, i.e. points of minimum absolute velocities. An ascender can be generated at a lower segmentation point and a descender can be generated at an upper segmentation point. However, if only $Vy\_$peak is adjusted, between 'e' and 'l', then the slant would change as well, so that at least two parameters have to be adjusted simultaneously. The second parameter to be changed follows from the expression of the slant, which was defined here by the complementary angle needed to shear the writing trace so that slanted loops obtain vertical mirror symmetry. This measure appeared to fit well the slant perceived by subjects (see also Maarse and Thomassen, 1983). The slant β in terms of model parameters is: $\beta = \arctan\ [Vy\_\mathrm{peak}/(Vx\_\mathrm{peak}\cdot\cos(\varphi))]$, which again depends upon one or more parameters. When generating an ascender, Vy_peak was to be increased, so that either φ or Vx_peak has to be changed as well, in order to maintain slant.

Another way to vary stroke length in meso context is to decrease only angular frequency ω, which does not affect slant and may seem more suitable. However, observations of size variation in meso context show that both duration and force are varied (see Section 3). This suggests adjustment of both ω and Vy_peak, respectively. As several model parameters have to be changed simultaneously, it is not easy to suppose that these parameters form a realistic representation in the graphic motor-pattern code. Other functions could have been used instead of sinusoid velocity functions, e.g. triangular functions, which correspond with rectangular functions in the acceleration domain (Plamondon and Maarse, 1989), yielding: $\beta = \arctan\ (Vy\_\mathrm{peak}/Vx\_\mathrm{peak})$, which contains only an amplitude ratio and which would involve fewer parameters. If trapezoid functions had been used in the acceleration domain, the latter would still hold but for a limited range of phase φ.

An example of a simulation of the letter sequence 'elye', counting 11 ballistic strokes, requires 30 parameter changes and time moments and 10 initial parameter settings, which may be pattern dependent. This yields only 3.6 parameters per

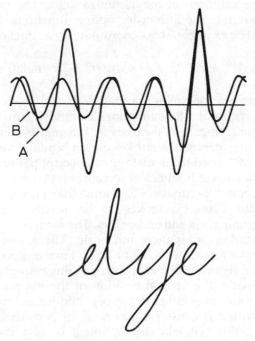

Figure 10.9. *Vertical (A) and horizontal (B) velocity components generated by the mass-spring model and the resultant writing trajectory. [From Hollerbach, 1981.]*

stroke, which is parsimonious indeed, as it is less than 4 (Figure 10.9). Although the model would generate repetitive loops parsimoniously, it appeared difficult to generate more complex repetitive patterns like 'ellellell...'. Furthermore, normal handwriting does not have a predominant sinusoidal movement (Teulings and Maarse, 1984), nor a constant left-to-right trend (Thomassen and Teulings, 1983a), because in that case there would not have been any problem to satisfy the two-thirds power law in micro context (see Section 3).

4.5 Symbolic and Biomechanical Models

There is yet another motor principle apart from the principle of a mass-spring system: minimizing the mean squared rate of force change. In the frictionless case (and when reducing the writing apparatus to a single-joint stick-and-point-mass system) the rate of force change can be approximated by the third time derivative of the horizontal and vertical position time functions, which is known as jerk. This appears to generate realistic, smooth aiming movement patterns (Edelman and Flash, 1987; Flash and Hogan, 1985; Nelson, 1983). For example, in straight movements the minimum jerk model generates Gaussian-shaped lines with Gaussian velocity functions that have peak velocities $V\_\max = 1.875s/T$, where s equals the stroke size and T the stroke duration. Edelman and Flash (1987) suppose in their 'minimum jerk model' that cursive script consists of a sequence of curved segments. For curved segments the minimum jerk model needed to be extended by adding a 'via point' near the point of maximum curvature (Flash and Hogan, 1985). Such a curved segment will be called here a 'via stroke'. A via stroke corresponds to a pair of 'ballistic strokes'. The solutions of the minimization of the mean squared jerk with a via point constraint are fifth-order spline functions for the x and y coordinates separately. For example, the x coordinate as a function of time t is:

$$x(t) = ax0 + ax1 \cdot t + ax2 \cdot t^2 + \cdots + ax5 \cdot t^5 + px \cdot \max(0, t - t1)^5$$

where $ax0 \ldots ax5$ and px are the spline parmeters and $t1$ is the optimized time parameter to reach the via point. The minimum jerk model shows that reconstruction of the handwriting movements on the basis of 'kinematics from shape' matches experimental data well, e.g. curved via strokes obtain bimodal velocity patterns.

Edelman and Flash (1987) tried to simulate cursive-script patterns and found that a limited set of basic via strokes is sufficient to represent cursive script: hook (like cursive 'i' without dot), cup (like cursive 'v'), gamma (like cursive 'l') and oval (like cursive 'o') (Figure 10.10). These via strokes can be classified on the basis of the configuration of the beginning, via and end-points. The form of the basic via strokes are invariant under rotation, translation and scale. There were a few discrete parameters: each via stroke was either small or large. Furthermore, vertical velocity may or may not change direction at the via point, yielding retrograde or regular via strokes, respectively. Finally, the vertical position of the via point relative to the baseline and letter-body size may either be: upper, middle or lower. Variability of fast and sloppy handwriting is considered as random perturbation of the movement parameters. Using this symbolic description it is, in principle, possible to generate novel letter sequences in a particular handwriting, or to automatically recognize online handwriting (Edelman, Flash and Ullman, 1990).

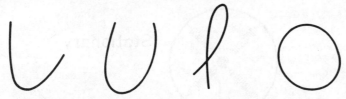

Figure 10.10. *The four basic via strokes: hook, cup, gamma and oval, respectively. All cursive characters can be represented as combinations of rotated, translated and scaled versions of these via strokes. [From Edelman and Flash, 1987.]*

However, the minimum jerk model with only via point constraints does only allow simulation of the hook. While trying to generate the other three basic via strokes it appeared that additional via points did not provide a solution as it is unclear which other via point to select apart than the natural one near the point of maximum curvature. Instead, other constraints should be added, which should satisfy the kinematics-from-shape principle: the direction (i.e. dy/dx) at the beginning and end-points of the via stroke. Because of the border condition of zero velocities and accelerations, the direction is undefined, so that, according to a mathematical rule, the direction of the lowest nonzero derivatives has to be used, which turns out to be jerk. But when jerk needs to be constrained, it does not make sense to minimize mean squared jerk. Instead, the mean squared fourth time derivative (i.e. snap) should be minimized. This yields a seventh-order spline function, analogous to the fifth-order spline function above. The 'minimum snap model' still requires a via point because without this the accuracy turns out to be poor.

The minimum snap model employs 18 parameters per via stroke: $ax0, \ldots ax7$, px, $ay0, \ldots, t1$). However, most parameters, and even duration $t1$ until the via point, are fixed by the boundary conditions. The boundary conditions are that the beginning and end of the via strokes should have a continuous and smooth connection to the adjacent via strokes, i.e. equal horizontal and vertical positions, velocities, accelerations and jerks. Furthermore, two boundary conditions from the via point yield eight fixed parameters per via stroke. The two minimization equations for $x(t)$ and $y(t)$ per via stroke fix two more parameters. Therefore, six parameters per via stroke, i.e. only three parameters per ballistic stroke, are required: x and y positions of beginning and via points, direction and amplitude of the jerk at the beginning point, and the mean absolute jerk.

Wann, Nimmo-Smith and Wing (1988) showed that the minimum jerk model generates movements which satisfy the two-thirds power law (Lacquaniti, Terzuolo and Viviani, 1983; see also Section 3). However, both models generate symmetric velocity functions, which are not observed in movements that are slower than maximally fast. In slower movements, velocity patterns are more skewed with peak velocity occurring earlier than halfway. Wann *et al.* wondered how the motor system, which can sense only joint angle, stretch and the rate of stretch, is able to minimize jerk at all. They suggested extending the minimum jerk model by a psychological model, without claiming its biomechanical validity, where an inertial mass is suspended with springs that have a certain stiffness inside the viscoelastic limb (Figure 10.11). The extent of off-balance and its rate of change allow detection of acceleration and its rate of change (i.e. jerk), respectively. Furthermore, if it is

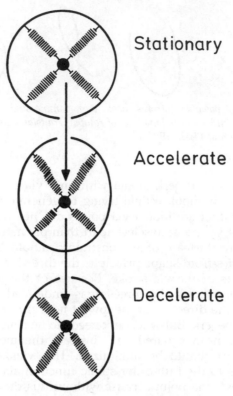

Stationary

Accelerate

Decelerate

Figure 10.11. *Representation of a viscoelastic model which attempts to extend the minimum jerk model. The mass inside the body (e.g. the arm) is suspended by surrounding tissues, represented by damped springs. As the body accelerates, the distortions of the surrounding tissues provide information about direction and extent of the acceleration and its rate of change, i.e. jerk. In this model, the mean squared jerk of the mass is minimized, instead of that of the outside of the body. [From Wann, Nimmo-Smith and Wing, 1988.]*

assumed that instead of the limb the suspended mass is moving according to the minimum jerk model, then the sum of the jerk of the limb plus the jerk of the mass relative to the limb has to be minimized. Simulations at low speeds, where stiffness is low, confirm that this extended minimum jerk model generates the skewed velocity patterns that are in accordance with empiric data. Recently, Plamondon (1991) provided another explanation for the skewed velocity profiles by assuming a set of independent (parallel) subsystems, each producing an arbitrary probability density of a velocity command. The net result is a probability density which is the product of all these component probability densities. Therefore, its logarithm is the sum of a number of arbitrary probability densities, which iterates to a log-normal probability density for the velocity signal of an aiming movement. This generates also an asymmetric velocity pattern.

A fully symbolic model to simulate handwriting has been presented by Schomaker, Thomassen and Teulings (1989). Input to the model is an arbitrary text in terms of a sequence of allographs, analogous to the allographic buffer. The output is cursive-script movement of the writer's own style of handwriting.

Interesting features of this model are the implementation of visual feedback, and the writer-specific motor memory, analogous to the graphic motor-pattern store (symbolic letter descriptions). Visual feedback monitors only the baseline and lineation levels. It is implemented by an exponentially decaying lineation memory, which adjusts vertical sizes of subsequent strokes after an inappropriate stroke size causes a departure from the imaginary baseline and lineation levels.

The symbolic letter descriptions of the allographs were trained on the basis of a corpus of a writer's handwriting. Thus, each allograph is represented by a sequence of strokes, where each stroke is represented by four stroke parameters: dX (horizontal displacement per stroke), dY (vertical displacement per stroke), T (compound stroke duration) and C (stroke-shape factor). Pen status may form a fifth feature but in cursive script it is more parsimonious to insert (penup) and (pendown) commands at appropriate times. In the previous models pen status was not included. These parameters have been based upon the average of several manually selected replications of the same allograph in various contexts. Averaging is allowed as context effects are only marginal, especially for spatial features (Schomaker and Thomassen, 1986; Thomassen and Schomaker, 1986). The strokes of an allograph appear indeed to be retrieved as complete units (Teulings, Thomassen and van Galen, 1983).

At the symbolic module the spatial features have been quantized; dX/dY could be: close, normal or far; dY could be: descender, base, body or ascender. However, in natural handwriting, quantization of the vertical positions of the beginning and end of a stroke may be more fine-grained than four levels. Therefore each level was split up into two or three sublevels (e.g. body-plus, body, body-minus, etc. but ascender-plus and descender-minus were omitted), yielding a total of 10 lineation levels for vertical position.

Although there is no evidence that relative durations are represented in motor memory (Teulings, Thomassen and van Galen, 1986), the 'compound stroke duration' T is used as a parameter conveniently to interpret the required 'stroke-shape factor' C: namely, the interval between successive zero crossings in the X velocity component (i.e. $t1$ ($vx = 0$) and $t2$ ($vx = 0$), respectively) can be defined as the X stroke duration, and similarly for the Y stroke duration. The compound stroke duration is defined as the average of the X and the Y stroke durations:

$$T = \{[t2\,(vx = 0) - t1\,(vx = 0)] + [t2\,(vy = 0) - t1\,(vy = 0)]\}\,/2$$

so that T ranges between 50 and 150 ms. The stroke-shape factor C is defined as the time interval between two nearby zero crossings of X and Y velocities, relative to the compound stroke duration T:

$$C = [t1\,(vx = 0) - t1\,(vy = 0)]\,/\,T$$

The shape factor is a generalized phase difference between X and Y velocity time functions. If the X velocity component is ahead of the Y component, then the stroke shape will form (part of) a counterclockwise loop (i.e. $-1.5 < C < 0$). In the opposite case, the stroke shape will form (part of) a clockwise loop (i.e. $0 < C < 1.5$). In the special case that the X and Y zero crossings occur simultaneously ($C = 0$), there will be a sharp stroke ending, followed by a movement reversal (Figure 10.12).

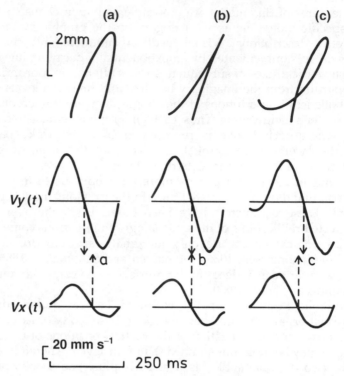

Figure 10.12. *Basic stroke shapes and their relative timing in the velocity domain. (a) Blunt, clockwise stroke transition, where the zero crossing of the horizontal velocity occurs after that of the vertical velocity, yielding shape factor C > 0. (b) Sharp stroke ending, where both zero crossings occur simultaneously, yielding shape factor C = 0. (c) Counterclockwise looping stroke transition, where the zero crossing of the horizontal velocity occurs before that of the vertical velocity, yielding shape factor C < 0. [From Schomaker, Thomassen and Teulings, 1989.]*

The procedure to translate the allographic code input into the required movement patterns is as follows. In the symbolic module, specific connecting strokes have to be inserted between pairs of allographs and punctuation signs. The connecting stroke depends upon the final stroke of the preceding allograph and the initial stroke of the subsequent allograph. The parameters of the connecting stroke have been estimated by the average of the replications in similar contexts in the corpus of handwriting. For example, the connecting stroke in 'me' is assumed to be similar to that in 'ne'. The 'cursive connections grammar' contains the generic rules that prescribe the connecting strokes to be inserted. For example, the input 'an ad...' is expanded to: '(pendown) (a) (base to midline, clockwise, close progression) (n) (base to base-plus, sharp ending, close progression) (penup) (space) (pendown) (a) (base to midline, sharp ending, normal progression) (d)'.

Subsequently, at the quantitative level, the strokes per allograph are selected from a sort of graphic motor-pattern store. The 'quantitative letter descriptors' describe the strokes in terms of dX, dY, T and C. The compound stroke duration T and the shape factor C allow the approximation of the moments in time where X and Y velocities change sign. In order to generate the kinematics of a handwriting trajectory, a general form of the velocity pattern is selected. For convenience, a sinusoid velocity time function is selected to fit between successive zero crossings of X and Y velocities, which appeared to approximate handwriting movement patterns relatively well (Plamondon and Maarse, 1989).

Although only four parameters per stroke are used to generate handwriting patterns, the effective number of parameters is less; namely, certain stroke sequences, representing allographs, can be retrieved by just one parameter: the allograph identifier. Furthermore, dY is quantized. Interestingly, the generated handwriting patterns do not form a curve fit of a particular pattern, but appear as noisy as individual replication of the same pattern, while showing the personal traits of the original writer. Also, in reality, a writer cannot reproduce a writing pattern exactly (Teulings, Thomassen and van Galen, 1986). Analogously to assessing the typewriting model in Rumelhart and Norman (1982), a quality measure is needed, which tells to what extent the generated pattern is within the natural variations of the writer. The correlations of the horizontal and vertical stroke sizes and durations between the original patterns appeared to be of the same order as those between the simulated pattern and the original ones. Therefore, the simulated pattern fits well within the set of the original patterns of handwriting so that the present simulation model is sufficiently accurate.

4.6 Summary

Many other computational models for specific purposes such as automatic online handwriting recognition and signature verification exist. Appropriate models attempt to describe the handwriting pattern in a parsimonious set of parameters, which may suggest that these parameters are less sensitive to motor noise and primarily express the underlying movement information. However, in online handwriting recognition systems, a redundant set of higher- and lower-level features may have advantages, as the self-learning expert system may be able to select the statistically relevant features itself. It appears that many models require the theoretical minimum of about four parameters per stroke. Models with more emphasis on curve fitting may require more parameters. However, the accurate regeneration of writing patterns does not need to be the final target, since the motor system does not allow the accurate reproduction of a movement pattern either. Therefore, the symbolic models seem attractive as they may show the same kind of noise when reproducing a handwriting pattern as if a writer were reproducing the pattern.

5 CONCLUSION

This chapter has presented several theories on handwriting production, ranging from motor-pattern representation and retrieval to trajectory formation. It was intended to describe the theories in common terms, in order to proceed in the direction of the unification of motor theories, and particularly of handwriting motor theories, and related skills such as typewriting, sign language and speech. Eventually, this may lead to application of this motor knowledge in more remote domains of motor skills, such as grasping, posture, gait, jumping and navigation. Various theories of different scope support the notion of modularity of the motor system. Understanding the motor system of handwriting may lead to a well-founded top-down approach for various important questions in handwriting research. They include the following:

(1) How can the body of motor knowledge presented here be integrated into the world of motor control?
(2) What developmental paths are followed in the various modules as a function of maturation, exercise, ageing or nerve diseases?
(3) Can changes in the generation model – be it theoretical, procedural, empirically based or neurally inspired – simulate the above changes in motor behavior?
(4) What automatically estimated motor characteristics can serve as measures of 'neurological fitness' in child development, or as a precursor for a nerve disease?
(5) What do children learn during handwriting instruction, and can immediate feedback via computer-assisted instruction help?
(6) Which features of the allograph shapes are appropriate for automatic handwriting recognition, and for reconstruction of the intended motor programs?
(7) Which features of the motor programs and the translation processes are subject-specific so that they may serve for writer identification and verification in handwriting expertise?

ACKNOWLEDGEMENTS

The writing of this paper was supported by Esprit Project 5204 'Papyrus': 'Pen And Paper Input Recognition Using Script' and Aim Project 11520 'Camarc II: Computer Aided Movement Analysis in Rehabilitation Context II'. I wish to thank Gerard van Galen and Arnold Thomassen for supportive comments on the earlier versions of this manuscript, Steven Keele and Herbert Heuer for their critical remarks on later versions, and Eric Helsper, Don Gentner and Tamar Flash for useful comments on the previous version.

REFERENCES

Baier, P. E. and Bullinger-Baier, M. (1989). Dynamik der Handschrift und neurophysiologische Grundlagen des Schreibens. In W. Conrad and B. Stier (Eds), *Grundlagen, Methoden, und Ergebnisse der forensischen Schriftundersuchung: Festschrift für Lothar Michel* (pp. 189–211). Lübeck: Schmidt-Römhild.

Barbe, W. B., Lucas, V. H. and Wasylyk, T. M. (Eds) (1984). *Handwriting: Basic Skills for Effective Communication*. Columbus, OH: Zaner-Bloser.

Bernstein, N. (1967). *The Coordination and Regulation of Movements*. Oxford: Pergamon.

Blöte, A. W. (1988). The development of writing behavior. PhD Thesis, University of Leiden.

Boyle, M. and Canter, G. J. (1987). Neuropsychological analysis of a typewriting disturbance following cerebral damage. *Brain and Language*, **30**, 147–164.

Burton, A. W., Pick, H. L., Holmes, C. and Teulings, H. L. (1990). The independence of horizontal and vertical dimensions in handwriting with and without vision. *Acta Psychologica*, **75**, 201–212.

Caramazza, A., Miceli, G. and Villa, G. (1986). The role of the (output) phonological buffer in reading, writing, and repetition. *Cognitive Neuropsychology*, **3**, 37–76.

Crane, H. C. and Ostrem, J. S. (1983). Automatic signature verification using a three-axis force-sensitive pen. *IEEE Transactions on Systems, Man, and Cybernetics*, **13**, 329–337.

Cutting, J. E. and Kozlowski, L. T. (1977). Recognizing friends by their walk: Gait perception without familiarity cues. *Bulletin of the Psychonomic Society*, **9**, 353–356.

Dal Bianco, P. (1944). Zur Koordination schwunghafter Bewegungen und ihrer Störungen bei Kleinhirnschädigungen. *Deutscher Zeitschrift für Nervenheilkunde*, **136**, 184–211.

Denier van der Gon, J. J. and Thuring, J. Ph. (1965). The guiding of human writing movements. *Biological Cybernetics*, **2**, 145–148.

Denier van der Gon, J. J., Thuring, J. Ph. and Strackee, J. (1962). A handwriting simulator. *Physics in Medical Biology*, **6**, 407–414.

Dijkstra, Sj., Denier van der Gon, J. J., Blangé, T., Karemaker, J. M. and Kramer, A. E. J. L. (1973). A simplified sliding-filament muscle model for simulation purposes. *Biological Cybernetics*, **12**, 94–101.

Dooijes, E. H. (1983). Analysis of handwriting movements. *Acta Psychologica*, **54**, 99–114.

Dooijes, E. H. (1984). Analysis of handwriting movements. PhD Thesis, University of Amsterdam.

Edelman, S. and Flash, T. (1987). A model of handwriting. *Biological Cybernetics*, **57**, 25–36.

Edelman, S., Flash, T. and Ullman, S. (1990). Reading cursive handwriting by alignment of letter prototypes. *International Journal of Computer Vision*, **5**, 303–331.

Eden, M. (1962). Handwriting and pattern recognition. *IRE Transactions on Information Theory*, **8**, 160–166.

Ellis, A. W. (1979). Slips of the pen. *Visible Language*, **13**, 265–282.

Ellis, A. W. (1982). Spelling and writing (and reading and speaking). In A. W. Ellis (Ed.), *Normality and Pathology in Cognitive Functions* (pp. 113–146). London: Academic Press.

Flash, T. and Hogan, N. (1985). The coordination of arm movements: An experimentally confirmed mathematical model. *Journal of Neuroscience*, **5**, 1688–1703.

Gentner, D. R. (1983). The acquisition of typewriting skill. *Acta Psychologica*, **54**, 233–248.

Gentner, D. R. (1987). Timing of skilled motor performance: Tests of the proportional duration model. *Psychological Review*, **94**, 255–276.

Gentner, D. R., Grudin, J. T. and Conway, E. (1980). Finger movements in transcription typing. Technical Report No. 8001. La Jolla. University of California, San Diego, Center for Human Information Processing.

Goodnow, J. J. and Levine, R. A. (1973). The grammar of action: Sequence and syntax in children's copying. *Cognitive Psychology*, **4**, 82–98.

Greer, K. L. and Green, D. W. (1983). Context and motor control in handwriting. *Acta Psychologica*, **54**, 205–215.

Grudin, J. (1983). Non-hierarchic specification of components in transcription typewriting. *Acta Psychologica*, **54**, 249–262.

Hollerbach, J. M. (1981). An oscillation theory of handwriting. *Biological Cybernetics*, **39**, 139–156.

Hulstijn, W. and van Galen, G. P. (1983). Programming in handwriting: Reaction time and movement time as a function of sequence length. *Acta Psychologica*, **54**, 23–49.

Hulstijn, W. and van Galen, G. P. (1988). Levels of motor programming in writing familiar and unfamiliar symbols. In A. M. Colley and J. R. Beech (Eds), *Cognition and Action in Skilled Behavior* (pp. 65–85). Amsterdam: North-Holland.

Jerri, A. J. (1977). The Shannon sampling theorem–its various extensions and applications: A tutorial review. *Proceedings of the IEEE*, **65**, 1565–1596.

Kao, H. S. R. (1983). Progressive motion variability in handwriting. *Acta Psychologica*, **54**, 149–163.

Kao, H. S. R. and Robinson, L. (1987). Heartrate deceleration in graphonomic acts: Drawing, calligraphy and handwriting. In R. Plamondon, C. Y. Suen, J. G. Deschenes and G. Poulin (Eds), *Proceedings of the Third International Symposium on Handwriting and Computer Applications* (pp. 123–125). Montreal: Ecole Polytechnique.

Kao, H. S. R., van Galen, G. P. and Hoosain, R. (Eds) (1986). *Graphonomics: Contemporary Research in Handwriting*. Amsterdam: North-Holland.

Katz, D. (1951). *Gestalt Psychology: Its Nature and Significance*. London: Methuen.

Keele, S. W. (1982). Component analysis and concepts of skill. In J. A. Scott Kelso (Ed.), *Human Motor Behavior: An Introduction* (pp. 143–159). Hillsdale, NJ: Erlbaum.

Keele, S. W., Cohen, A. and Ivry, R. (1990). Motor programs: Concepts and issues. In: M. Jeannerod (Ed.), *Attention and Performance*, vol. XIII: *Motor Representation and Control* (pp. 77–111). Hillsdale, NJ: Erlbaum.

Keele, S. W. and Hawkins, H. L. (1982). Explorations of individual differences relevant to high level skill. *Journal of Motor Behavior*, **14**, 3–23.

Keele, S. W. and Ivry, R. I. (1991). Does the cerebellum provide a common computation for diverse tasks: A timing hypothesis. In A. Diamond (Ed.), The development and neural bases of higher cognitive functions. *Annals of the New York Academy of Sciences*, **608**, 179–211.

Keele, S. W., Ivry, R. I. and Pokorny, R. A. (1987). Force control and its relation to timing. *Journal of Motor Behavior*, **19**, 96–114.

Klapp, S. T. (1977). Response programming, as assessed by reaction time, does not establish commands to particular muscles. *Journal of Motor Behavior*, **9**, 301–312.

Klapp, S. T. and Wyatt, E. P. (1976). Motor programming within a sequence of responses. *Journal of Motor Behavior*, **8**, 19–26.

Lacquaniti, F. (1989). Central representations of human limb movement as revealed by studies of drawing and handwriting. *Trends in Neuroscience*, **12**, 287–291.

Lacquaniti, F., Ferrigo, G., Pedotti, A., Soechting, J. F. and Terzuolo, C. (1987). Changes in spatial scale in drawing and handwriting: Kinematic contributions by proximal and distal joints. *Journal of Neuroscience*, **7**, 819–828.

Lacquaniti, F., Terzuolo, C. and Viviani, P. (1983). The law relating the kinematic and figural aspects of drawing movements. *Acta Psychologica*, **54**, 115–130.

Langolf, G. D., Chaffin, D. B. and Foulke, J. A. (1976). An investigation of Fitts' law using a wide range of movement amplitudes. *Journal of Motor Behavior*, **8**, 113–128.

Larochelle, S. (1982). The initiation and duration of movements in skilled typewriting. *IPO Annual Progress Report*, **17**, 116–122.

Lebrun, Y. and Rubio, S. (1972). Réduplications et omissions graphiques chez des patients atteints d'une lésion hémisphérique droite. *Neuropsychologia*, **10**, 249–251.

Logan, G. D. (1982). On the ability to inhibit complex movements: A stop-signal study in typewriting. *Journal of Experimental Psychology and Human Performance*, **8**, 778–792.

Lorette, G. and Plamondon, R. (1990). Dynamic approaches to handwritten signature verification. In R. Plamondon and G. Leedham (Eds), *Computer Processing of Handwriting* (pp. 21–47). Singapore: World Scientific.

Maarse, F. J. (1987). The study of handwriting movement: Peripheral models and signal processing techniques. PhD Thesis. Lisse, The Netherlands: Swets and Zeitlinger.

Maarse, F. J., Meulenbroek, R. G. J., Teulings, H. L. and Thomassen A. J. W. M. (1987). Computational measures for ballistic handwriting. In R. Plamondon, C. Y. Suen, J. G. Deschenes and G. Poulin (Eds), *Proceedings of the Third International Symposium on Handwriting and Computer Applications* (pp. 16–18). Montreal: Ecole Polytechnique.

Maarse, F. J., Schomaker, L. R. B. and Teulings, H. L. (1988). Automatic identification of writers. In G. Mulder and G. van der Veer (Eds), *Human–Computer Interaction: Psychonomic Aspects* (pp. 353–360). Berlin: Springer.

Maarse, F. J., Schomaker, L. R. B. and Thomassen, A. J. W. M. (1986). The influence of changes in the effector coordinate systems on handwriting movements. In H. S. R. Kao, G. P. van Galen and R. Hoosain (Eds), *Graphonomics: Contemporary Research in Handwriting* (pp. 33–46). Amsterdam: North-Holland.

Maarse, F. J. and Thomassen, A. J. W. M. (1983). Produced and perceived writing slant: Difference between up and down strokes. *Acta Psychologica*, **54**, 131–147.

MacDonald, J. S. (1966). Experimental studies of handwriting signals. Massachusetts Institute of Technology; Research Laboratory Electronics: Technical Report No. 433, March.

Margolin, D. I. (1984). The neuropsychology of writing and spelling: Semantic, phonological, motor and perceptual processes. *Quarterly Journal of Experimental Psychology: Human Experimental Psychology*, **36A**, 459–489.

Margolin, D. I. and Wing, A. M. (1983). Agraphia and micrographia: Clinical manifestations of motor programming and performance disorders. *Acta Psychologica*, **54**, 263–283.

Marsden, C. D. (1982). The mysterious function of the basal ganglia: The Robert Wartenburg Lecture. *Neurology*, **32**, 514–539.

McAllister, C. N. (1900). Researches on movements used in handwriting. *Studies from the Yale Psychological Laboratory*, **8**, 21–63.

Meeks, M. L. and Kuklinski, T. T. (1990). Measurement of dynamic digitizer performance. In R. Plamondon and G. Leedham (Eds), *Computer Processing of Handwriting* (pp. 89–110). Singapore: World Scientific.

Mermelstein, P. and Eden, M. (1964). Experiments on computer recognition of connected handwritten words. *Information Control*, **7**, 255–270.

Merton, P. A. (1972). How we control the contraction of our muscles. *Scientific American*, **226**, 30–37.

Meulenbroek, R. G. L. (1989). A study of handwriting production: Educational and developmental aspects. PhD Thesis, University of Nijmegen.

Meulenbroek, R. G. J., Rosenbaum, D. A. Thomassen, A. J. W. M. and Schomaker, L. R. B. (1993). Limb-segment selection in drawing behavior. *Quarterly Journal of Experimental Psychology*, **46**, 273–299.

Meulenbroek, R. G. J. and van Galen, G. P. (1989). The production of connecting strokes in cursive writing: Developing co-articulation in 8 to 12 year-old children. In R. Plamondon, C. Y. Suen and M. Simner (Eds), *Computer Recognition and Human Production of Handwriting* (pp. 273–286). Singapore: World Scientific.

Michel, F. (1971). Etude expérimentale de la vitesse du geste graphique. *Neuropsychologia*, **9**, 1–13.

Mojet, J. W. (1989). Kenmerken van schrijfvaardigheid: Procesaspecten van het schrijven bij zes- tot twaalfjarigen. PhD Thesis, University of Leiden. De Lier: ABC.

Morasso, P. and Mussa Ivaldi, F. A. (1982). Trajectory formation and handwriting: A computational model. *Biological Cybernetics*, **45**, 131–142.

Morasso, P. and Mussa Ivaldi, F. A. (1987). Computational models for handwriting. In R. Plamondon, C. Y. Suen, J. G. Deschenes and G. Poulin (Eds), *Proceedings of the Third International Symposium on Handwriting and Computer Applications* (pp. 11–13). Montreal: Ecole Polytechnique.

Morasso, P., Mussa Ivaldi, F. A. and Ruggiero, C. (1983). How a discontinuous mechanism can produce continuous patterns in trajectory formation and handwriting. *Acta Psychologica*, **54**, 83–98.

Nelson, W. L. (1983). Physical principles for economies of skilled movement. *Biological Cybernetics*, **46**, 135–147.

Newell, K. M. and van Emmerik, K. M. (1989). The acquisition of coordination: Preliminary analysis of learning to write. *Human Movement Science*, **8**, 17–32.

Nihei, Y. (1983). Development change in covert principles for the organization of strokes in drawing and handwriting. *Acta Psychologica*, **54**, 221–232.

Patterson, K. E. and Wing, A. M. (1989). Processes in handwriting: A case for case. *Cognitive Neuropsychology*, **6**, 1–23.

Pick, H. L., Jr and Teulings, H. L. (1983). Geometric transformations of handwriting as a function of instruction and feedback. *Acta Psychologica*, **54**, 327–340.

Plamondon, R. (1989). Handwriting control: A functional model. In R. M. J. Cotterill (Ed.), *Models of Brain Function* (pp. 563–574). London: Cambridge University Press.

Plamondon, R. (1991). On the origin of asymmetric bell-shaped velocity profiles in rapid-aiming movements. In J. Requin and G. E. Stelmach (Eds), *Tutorials in Motor Neuroscience* (pp. 283–295). NATO ASI Series. Dordrecht, The Netherlands: Kluwer.

Plamondon, R. and Lamarche, F. (1986). Modelization of handwriting: A system approach. In H. S. R. Kao, G. P. van Galen and R. Hoosain (Eds), *Graphonomics: Contemporary Research in Handwriting* (pp. 169–183). Amsterdam: North-Holland.

Plamondon, R. and Leedham, G. (Eds) (1990). *Computer Processing of Handwriting*. Singapore: World Scientific.

Plamondon, R. and Maarse, F. J. (1989). An evaluation of motor models of handwriting. *IEEE Transactions on Systems, Man, and Cybernetics*, **19**, 1060–1072.

Plamondon, R., Suen, C. Y. and Simner, M. (Eds) (1989). *Computer Recognition and Human Production of Handwriting*. Singapore: World Scientific.

Povel, D. J. and Collard, R. (1982). Structural factors in patterned finger tapping. *Acta Psychologica*, **52**, 107–123.

Raibert, M. H. (1977). Motor control and learning by the state–space model. Technical Report, Artificial Intelligence Laboratory, MIT AI-TR-439.

Rosenbaum, D. A. (1991). *Human Motor Control*. New York: Academic Press.

Rosenbaum, D. A., Inhof, A. W. and Gordon, A. M. (1984). Choosing between movement sequences: A hierarchical editor model. *Journal of Experimental Psychology*, **113**, 373–393.

Rosenbaum, D. A., Kenny, S. B. and Derr, M. A. (1983). Hierarchical control of rapid movement sequences. *Journal of Experimental Psychology: Human Perception and Performance*, **9**, 86–102.

Rumelhart, D. E. and Norman, D. A. (1982). Simulating skilled typists: A study of skilled cognitive-motor performance. *Cognitive Science*, **6**, 1–36.

Salthouse, T. A. (1984). Effects of age and skill in typing. *Journal of Experimental Psychology: General*, **113**, 345–371.

Sanders, A. F. (1980). Stage analysis of reaction processes. In G. E. Stelmach and J. Requin (Eds), *Tutorials in Motor Behavior* (pp. 331–354). Amsterdam: North-Holland.

Sassoon, R. S. (1988). Joins in children's handwriting: The effects of different models and teaching methods. PhD Thesis, University of Reading.

Sassoon, R. S., Nimmo-Smith, I. and Wing, A. M. (1989). Developing efficiency in cursive handwriting: An analysis of 't' crossing behavior in children. In R. Plamondon, C. Y. Suen and M. Simner (Eds), *Computer Recognition and Human Production of Handwriting* (pp. 287–297). Singapore: World Scientific.

Schmidt, R. A. (1975). A schema theory of discrete motor skill learning. *Psychological Review*, **82**, 225–260.

Schmidt, R. A., Zelaznik, H., Hawkins, B., Frank, J. S. and Quinn, J. T. (1979). Motor-output variability: A theory for the accuracy of rapid motor acts. *Psychological Review*, **86**, 415–451.

Schomaker, L. R. B. (1991). Simulation and recognition of handwriting movements: A vertical approach to modeling human motor behavior. PhD Thesis, University of Nijmegen.

Schomaker, L. R. B. and Plamondon, R. (1991). The relation between pen force and pen point kinematics in handwriting. *Biological Cybernetics*, **63**, 277–289.

Schomaker, L. R. B. and Teulings, H. L. (1990). A handwriting recognition system based on properties of the human motor system. In C. Y. Suen (Ed.) *Frontiers in handwriting recognition* (pp. 195–209). Montreal: CENPARMI.

Schomaker, L. R. B. and Thomassen, A. J. W. M. (1986). On the use of and limitations of averaging handwriting signals; programming in handwriting. In H. S. R. Kao, G. P. Van Galen and R. Hoosain (Eds). *Graphonomics: Contemporary research in handwriting* (pp. 225–252). Amsterdam: North-Holland.

Schomaker, L. R. B. Thomassen, A. J. W. M. and Teulings, H. L. (1989). A computational model of cursive handwriting. In R. Plamondon, C. Y. Suen and M. Simner (Eds), *Computer Recognition and Human Production of Handwriting* (pp. 153–177). Singapore: World Scientific.

Shaffer, L. H. (1976). Intention and performance. *Psychological Review, 83*, 375–393.

Smyth, M. M. and Silvers, G. (1987). Functions of vision in the control of handwriting. *Acta Psychologica, 65*, 47–64.

Soechting, J. F., Lacquaniti, F. and Terzuolo, C. (1986). Coordination of arm movements in three-dimensional space: Sensorimotor mapping during drawing movements. *Neuroscience, 17*, 295–311.

Søvik, N. (1975). *Developmental Cybernetics of Handwriting and Graphic Behavior*. Oslo: Universitets Forlaget.

Stelmach, G. E. and Teulings, H. L. (1983). Response characteristics of prepared and restructured handwriting. *Acta Psychologica, 54*, 51–67.

Sternberg, S. (1969). The discovery of processing stages: Extension of Donders' method. *Acta Psychologica, 30*, 276–315.

Sternberg, S., Knoll, R. L. and Turock, D. L. (1990). Hierarchical control in the execution of action sequences: Tests of two invariance properties. In M. Jeannerod (Ed.), *Attention and Performance*, vol. XIII: *Motor Representation and Control* (pp. 3–55). Hillsdale, NJ: Erlbaum.

Sternberg, S., Monsell, S., Knoll, R. L. and Wright, C. E. (1978). The latency and duration of rapid movement sequences: Comparisons of speech and typewriting. In G. E. Stelmach (Ed.), *Information Processing in Motor Control and Learning* (pp. 117–152). New York: Academic Press.

Stockholm, E. (1979). Recognition of a writer as a function of his method of writing. *Perceptual and Motor Skills, 49*, 483–488.

Teulings, H. L. (1988). Handwriting-movement control: Research into different levels of the motor system. PhD Thesis, University of Nijmegen.

Teulings, H. L. and Maarse, F. J. (1984). Digital recording and processing of handwriting movements. *Human Movement Science, 3*, 193–217.

Teulings, H. L., Mullins, P. A. and Stelmach, G. E. (1986). The elementary units of programming in handwriting. In H. S. R. Kao, G. P. van Galen and R. Hoosain (Eds), *Graphonomics: Contemporary Research in Handwriting* (pp. 21–32). Amsterdam: North-Holland.

Teulings, H. L. and Schomaker, L. R. B. (1993). Invariant properties between stroke features in handwriting. *Acta Psychologica, 82*, 69–88.

Teulings, H. L. and Stelmach, G. E. (1991). Control of stroke size, peak acceleration, and stroke duration in Parkinsonian handwriting. *Human Movement Science, 10*, 315–333.

Teulings, H. L. and Stelmach, G. E. (1992). Simulation of impairment of force amplitude and force timing in Parkinsonian handwriting. In G. E. Stelmach and J. Requin (Eds), *Tutorials in Motor Behavior*, vol. III (pp. 425–442). Amsterdam: North-Holland.

Teulings, H. L. and Thomassen, A. J. W. M. (1979). Computer-aided analysis of handwriting movements. *Visible Language, 13*, 218–231.

Teulings, H. L., Thomassen, A. J. W. M. and Maarse, F. J. (1989). A description of handwriting in terms of main axes. In R. Plamondon, C. Y. Suen and M. Simner (Eds), *Computer Recognition and Human Production of Handwriting* (pp. 193–211). Singapore: World Scientific.

Teulings, H. L., Thomassen, A. J. W. M. and van Galen, G. P. (1983). Preparation of partly precued handwriting movements: The size of movement units in writing. *Acta Psychologica, 54*, 165–177.

Teulings, H. L., Thomassen, A. J. W. M. and van Galen, G. P. (1986). Invariants in handwriting: The information contained in a motor program. In H. S. R. Kao, G. P. van Galen and R. Hoosain (Eds), *Graphonomics: Contemporary Research in Handwriting* (pp. 305–315). Amsterdam: North-Holland.

Thomassen, A. J. W. M., Keuss, P. J. G. and van Galen, G. P. (Eds) (1984). *Motor Aspects of Handwriting: Approaches to Movement in Graphic Behavior*. Amsterdam: North-Holland.

Thomassen, A. J. W. M., Meulenbroek, R. G. J. and Tibosch, H. J. C. M. (1991). Latencies and kinematics reflect graphic production rules. *Human Movement Science,* **10,** 271–289.

Thomassen, A. J. W. M. and Schomaker, L. R. B. (1986). Between-letter context effects in handwriting trajectories. In H. S. R. Kao, G. P. van Galen and R. Hoosain (Eds), *Graphonomics: Contemporary Research in Handwriting* (pp. 253–272). Amsterdam: North-Holland.

Thomassen, A. J. W. M. and Teulings, H. L. (1979). The development of directional preference in writing movements. *Visible Language,* **13,** 299–313.

Thomassen, A. J. W. M. and Teulings, H. L. (1983a). Constancy in stationary and progressive handwriting. *Acta Psychologica,* **54,** 179–196.

Thomassen, A. J. W. M. and Teulings, H. L. (1983b). The development of handwriting. In M. Martlew (Ed.), *The Psychology of Written Language: Developmental and Educational Perspectives* (pp. 179–213). New York: John Wiley.

Thomassen, A. J. W. M. and Teulings, H. L. (1984). The development of directional preference in writing movements. In W. B. Barbe, V. H. Lucas and T. M. Wasylyk (Eds), *Handwriting: Basic Skills for Effective Communication* (pp. 367–376). Columbus, OH: Zaner-Bloser.

Thomassen, A. J. W. M. and Teulings, H. L. (1985). Time, size, and shape in handwriting: Exploring spatio-temporal relationships at different levels. In J. A. Michon and J. B. Jackson (Eds), *Time, Mind, and Behavior* (pp. 253–263). Heidelberg: Springer.

Thomassen, A. J. W. M., Teulings, H. L. and Schomaker, L. R. B. (1988). Real-time processing of cursive writing and sketched graphics. In G. Mulder and G. van der Veer (Eds), *Human–Computer Interaction: Psychonomic Aspects* (pp. 334–352). Berlin: Springer.

Thomassen, A. J. W. M., Tibosch, H. J. C. M. and Maarse, F. J. (1989). The effect of context on stroke direction and stroke order in handwriting. In R. Plamondon, C. Y. Suen and M. Simner (Eds), *Computer Recognition and Human Production of Handwriting* (pp. 213–230). Singapore: World Scientific.

Thomassen, A. J. W. M. and van Galen, G. P. (1992). Handwriting as a motor task: Experimentation, modeling and simulation. In J. J. Summers (Ed.), *Approaches to the Study of Motor Control and Learning* (pp. 113–144). Amsterdam: North-Holland.

Thomassen, A. J. W. M., van Galen, G. P. and de Klerk, L. F. W. (Eds) (1985). *Studies over de Schrijfmotoriek: Theorie en Toepassing in het Onderwijs.* Lisse, The Netherlands: Swets and Zeitlinger.

Tripp, C. A., Fluckiger, F. A. and Weinberg, G. H. (1957). Measurement of handwriting variables. *Perceptual and Motor Skills,* **7,** 279–294.

van Emmerik, R. E. A. and Newell, K. M. (1989). The relationship between pen-point and joint kinematics in handwriting and drawing. In R. Plamondon, C. Y. Suen and M. Simner (Eds), *Computer Recognition and Human Production of Handwriting* (pp. 231–248). Singapore: World Scientific.

van Emmerik, R. E. A. and Newell, K. M. (1990). The influence of task and organismic constraints on intralimb and pen-point kinematics in a drawing task. *Acta Psychologica,* **73,** 171–190.

van Galen, G. P. (1980). Storage and retrieval of handwriting patterns: A two stage model of complex behavior. In G. E. Stelmach and J. Requin (Eds), *Tutorials in Motor Behavior* (pp. 567–578). Amsterdam: North-Holland.

van Galen, G. P. (1990). Phonological and motoric demands in handwriting: Evidence for discrete transmission of information. *Acta Psychologica,* **74,** 259–275.

van Galen, G. P. (1991). Handwriting: Issues for a psychomotor theory. *Human Movement Science,* **10,** 165–191.

van Galen, G. P., Meulenbroek, R. G. J. and Hylkema, H. (1986). On the simultaneous processing of words, letters and strokes in handwriting: Evidence for a mixed linear and parallel model. In H. S. R. Kao, G. P. van Galen and R. Hoosain (Eds), *Graphonomics: Contemporary Research in Handwriting* (pp. 5–20). Amsterdam: North-Holland.

van Galen, G. P. and Schomaker, L. R. B. (1992). Fitts' law as a low-pass filter effect on muscle stiffness. *Human Movement Science*, **11**, 11–21.

van Galen, G. P. and Teulings, H. L. (1983). The independent monitoring of form and scale parameters in handwriting. *Acta Psychologica*, **54**, 9–22.

van Galen, G. P., Thomassen, M. J. W. M. and Wing, A. M. (Eds) (1991). Handwriting. *Human Movement Science*, **10**, 2–3.

van Nes, F. L. (1971). Errors in the motor programme for handwriting. *IPO Annual Progress Report*, **6**, 61–63.

van Nes, F. L. (1985). Verschrijvingen als informatiebron bij de studie van schrijfprocessen. In A. J. W. M. Thomassen, G. P. van Galen and L. F. W. de Klerk (Eds), *Studies over de Schrijfmotoriek: Theorie en Toepassing in het Onderwijs* (pp. 87–110). Lisse, The Netherlands: Swets and Zeitlinger.

van Sommers, P. (1984). *Drawing and Cognition: Descriptive and Experimental Studies of Graphic Production Processes*. Cambridge: Cambridge University Press.

Viviani, P. and Terzuolo, C. (1980). Space–time invariance in learned motor skills. In G. E. Stelmach and J. Requin (Eds), *Tutorials in Motor Behavior* (pp. 525–533). Amsterdam: North-Holland.

Viviani, P. and Terzuolo, C. (1982). Trajectory determines movement dynamics. *Neuroscience*, **7**, 431–437.

Vredenbregt, J. and Koster, W. G. (1971). Analysis and synthesis of handwriting. *Philips Technical Review*, **32**, 73–78.

Vredenbregt, J., Koster, W. G. and Kirchhof, J. W. (1968). On the tolerances in the timing programme of synthesized letters. *IPO Annual Progress Report*, **3**, 95–97.

Wadman, W. J., Denier van der Gon, J. J., Geuze, R. H. and Mol, C. R. (1979). Control of fast goal-directed arm movements. *Journal of Human Movement Studies*, **5**, 3–17.

Wann, J. P. (1988). The control of fine-motor trajectories. Unpublished PhD Thesis, University of Cambridge.

Wann, J. P., Nimmo-Smith, I. and Wing, A. M. (1988). Relation between velocity and curvature in movement: Equivalence and divergence between power law and minimum-jerk model. *Journal of Experimental Psychology: Human Perception and Performance*, **14**, 622–637.

Wann, J. P., Wing, A. M. and Søvik, N. (Eds) (1991). *The Development of Graphic Skills: Research Perspectives and Educational Implications*. London: Academic Press.

Wing, A. M. (1978). Response timing in handwriting. In G. E. Stelmach (Ed.), *Information Processing in Motor Control and Learning* (pp. 153–172). New York: Academic Press.

Wing, A. M. (Ed.) (1979). *Visible Language*, **13**.

Wing, A. M. (1980). The height of handwriting. *Acta Psychologica*, **46**, 141–152.

Wing, A. M. (1990). Etude de la variabilité dans la forme spatiale de l'écriture cursive. In C. Sirat, J. Irigoin and E. Poulle (Eds), *L'écriture: Le Cerveau, l'Oeil et la Main Bibliologia* (pp. 127–137). Turnhout: Brepols.

Wing, A. M. and Watts, F. (1989). Developmental dynamics of handwriting: A new approach to appraising the relation between handwriting and personality. *Proceedings of the Fourth IGS Conference: Development of Graphic Skills*. Trondheim: University Press.

Wright, C. E. (1990). Generalized motor programs: reexamining claims of effector independence in writing. In M. Jeannerod (Ed.), *Attention and Performance*, vol. XIII (pp. 294–320). Hillsdale, NJ: Erlbaum.

Wright, C. E. (1991). Temporal invariance in handwriting. *5th Handwriting Conference of the IGS: Motor Control of Handwriting* (pp. 86–89). Tempe, AZ.

Yasuhara, M. (1975). Experimental studies of handwriting process. Rep. Univ. Electro-Comm. 25-2 (Sci. and Tech. Sect.), 233–254.

Index

*For core concepts and keywords, please refer to the
Table of Contents as well.*